New Insights in the Genetics and Genomics of Adrenocortical Tumors and Pheochromocytomas

New Insights in the Genetics and Genomics of Adrenocortical Tumors and Pheochromocytomas

Editor

Peter Igaz

MDPI • Basel • Beijing • Wuhan • Barcelona • Belgrade • Manchester • Tokyo • Cluj • Tianjin

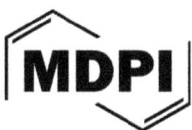

Editor
Peter Igaz
Department of Endocrinology
Semmelweis University
Budapest
Hungary

Editorial Office
MDPI
St. Alban-Anlage 66
4052 Basel, Switzerland

This is a reprint of articles from the Special Issue published online in the open access journal *Cancers* (ISSN 2072-6694) (available at: www.mdpi.com/journal/cancers/special_issues/adrenocortical_pheochromocytomas).

For citation purposes, cite each article independently as indicated on the article page online and as indicated below:

LastName, A.A.; LastName, B.B.; LastName, C.C. Article Title. *Journal Name* **Year**, *Volume Number*, Page Range.

ISBN 978-3-0365-3358-2 (Hbk)
ISBN 978-3-0365-3357-5 (PDF)

© 2022 by the authors. Articles in this book are Open Access and distributed under the Creative Commons Attribution (CC BY) license, which allows users to download, copy and build upon published articles, as long as the author and publisher are properly credited, which ensures maximum dissemination and a wider impact of our publications.

The book as a whole is distributed by MDPI under the terms and conditions of the Creative Commons license CC BY-NC-ND.

Contents

About the Editor vii

Preface to "New Insights in the Genetics and Genomics of Adrenocortical Tumors and Pheochromocytomas" ix

Peter Igaz
New Insights in the Genetics and Genomics of Adrenocortical Tumors and Pheochromocytomas
Reprinted from: *Cancers* **2022**, *14*, 1094, doi:10.3390/cancers14041094 1

Yi-Yao Chang, Chien-Ting Pan, Zheng-Wei Chen, Cheng-Hsuan Tsai, Shih-Yuan Peng and Chin-Chen Chang et al.
KCNJ5 Somatic Mutations in Aldosterone-Producing Adenoma Are Associated with a Greater Recovery of Arterial Stiffness
Reprinted from: *Cancers* **2021**, *13*, 4313, doi:10.3390/cancers13174313 5

Hung-Wei Liao, Kang-Yung Peng, Vin-Cent Wu, Yen-Hung Lin, Shuei-Liong Lin and Wei-Chou Lin et al.
Characteristics of a Novel $ATP2B3$ $K416_F418delinsN$ Mutation in a Classical Aldosterone-Producing Adenoma
Reprinted from: *Cancers* **2021**, *13*, 4729, doi:10.3390/cancers13184729 19

Siyuan Gong, Martina Tetti, Martin Reincke and Tracy Ann Williams
Primary Aldosteronism: Metabolic Reprogramming and the Pathogenesis of Aldosterone-Producing Adenomas
Reprinted from: *Cancers* **2021**, *13*, 3716, doi:10.3390/cancers13153716 31

Ariadni Spyroglou, George P. Piaditis, Gregory Kaltsas and Krystallenia I. Alexandraki
Transcriptomics, Epigenetics, and Metabolomics of Primary Aldosteronism
Reprinted from: *Cancers* **2021**, *13*, 5582, doi:10.3390/cancers13215582 51

Scott M. MacKenzie, Hannah Saunders, Josie C. van Kralingen, Stacy Robertson, Alexandra Riddell and Maria-Christina Zennaro et al.
Circulating microRNAs as Diagnostic Markers in Primary Aldosteronism
Reprinted from: *Cancers* **2021**, *13*, 5312, doi:10.3390/cancers13215312 71

André Marquardt, Laura-Sophie Landwehr, Cristina L. Ronchi, Guido di Dalmazi, Anna Riester and Philip Kollmannsberger et al.
Identifying New Potential Biomarkers in Adrenocortical Tumors Based on mRNA Expression Data Using Machine Learning
Reprinted from: *Cancers* **2021**, *13*, 4671, doi:10.3390/cancers13184671 87

Péter István Turai, Zoltán Herold, Gábor Nyirő, Katalin Borka, Tamás Micsik and Judit Tőke et al.
Tissue miRNA Combinations for the Differential Diagnosis of Adrenocortical Carcinoma and Adenoma Established by Artificial Intelligence
Reprinted from: *Cancers* **2022**, *14*, 895, doi:10.3390/cancers14040895 101

Karina C. F. Tosin, Edith F. Legal, Mara A. D. Pianovski, Humberto C. Ibañez, Gislaine Custódio and Denise S. Carvalho et al.
Newborn Screening for the Detection of the *TP53* R337H Variant and Surveillance for Early Diagnosis of Pediatric Adrenocortical Tumors: Lessons Learned and Way Forward
Reprinted from: *Cancers* **2021**, *13*, 6111, doi:10.3390/cancers13236111 115

Marco Lo Iacono, Soraya Puglisi, Paola Perotti, Laura Saba, Jessica Petiti and Claudia Giachino et al.
Molecular Mechanisms of Mitotane Action in Adrenocortical Cancer Based on In Vitro Studies
Reprinted from: *Cancers* **2021**, *13*, 5255, doi:10.3390/cancers13215255 131

Sakshi Jhawar, Yasuhiro Arakawa, Suresh Kumar, Diana Varghese, Yoo Sun Kim and Nitin Roper et al.
New Insights on the Genetics of Pheochromocytoma and Paraganglioma and Its Clinical Implications
Reprinted from: *Cancers* **2022**, *14*, 594, doi:10.3390/cancers14030594 143

Shahida K. Flores, Cynthia M. Estrada-Zuniga, Keerthi Thallapureddy, Gustavo Armaiz-Peña and Patricia L. M. Dahia
Insights into Mechanisms of Pheochromocytomas and Paragangliomas Driven by Known or New Genetic Drivers
Reprinted from: *Cancers* **2021**, *13*, 4602, doi:10.3390/cancers13184602 159

Balazs Sarkadi, Istvan Liko, Gabor Nyiro, Peter Igaz, Henriett Butz and Attila Patocs
Analytical Performance of NGS-Based Molecular Genetic Tests Used in the Diagnostic Workflow of Pheochromocytoma/Paraganglioma
Reprinted from: *Cancers* **2021**, *13*, 4219, doi:10.3390/cancers13164219 173

María Monteagudo, Paula Martínez, Luis J. Leandro-García, Ángel M. Martínez-Montes, Bruna Calsina and Marta Pulgarín-Alfaro et al.
Analysis of Telomere Maintenance Related Genes Reveals *NOP10* as a New Metastatic-Risk Marker in Pheochromocytoma/Paraganglioma
Reprinted from: *Cancers* **2021**, *13*, 4758, doi:10.3390/cancers13194758 195

Peter Istvan Turai, Gábor Nyírő, Henriett Butz, Attila Patócs and Peter Igaz
MicroRNAs, Long Non-Coding RNAs, and Circular RNAs: Potential Biomarkers and Therapeutic Targets in Pheochromocytoma/Paraganglioma
Reprinted from: *Cancers* **2021**, *13*, 1522, doi:10.3390/cancers13071522 217

Letizia Canu, Soraya Puglisi, Paola Berchialla, Giuseppina De Filpo, Francesca Brignardello and Francesca Schiavi et al.
A Multicenter Epidemiological Study on Second Malignancy in Non-Syndromic Pheochromocytoma/Paraganglioma Patients in Italy
Reprinted from: *Cancers* **2021**, *13*, 5831, doi:10.3390/cancers13225831 233

Margo Dona, Maaike Lamers, Svenja Rohde, Marnix Gorissen and Henri J. L. M. Timmers
Targeting the Redox Balance Pathway Using Ascorbic Acid in *sdhb* Zebrafish Mutant Larvae
Reprinted from: *Cancers* **2021**, *13*, 5124, doi:10.3390/cancers13205124 249

About the Editor

Peter Igaz

Dr. Peter Igaz is full professor of internal medicine and endocrinology. He is currently the head of the Department of Endocrinology at the Department of Internal Medicine and Oncology, Semmelweis University. Between July 2016 and May 2020, he served as the director of the 2nd Department of Internal Medicine, Semmelweis University, which under his leadership was awarded the Center of Excellence Title of the European Neuroendocrine Tumor Society in 2019. He is Co-Head of this ENETS Center of Excellence. In 2020, his research group was awarded the title of Research Center of Excellence by the European Network for the Study of Adrenal Tumors (ENSAT). He has boarding exams in internal medicine, endocrinology and clinical genetics. Beside his medical degree (MD), Dr. Igaz has degrees in biology (MSc, molecular biology) and laws (JD). He was awarded the PhD in 1999 and the Doctor of Sciences (DSc) by the Hungarian Academy of Sciences in 2013. His research focus includes the study of microRNAs, bioinformatics, adrenal tumors, hereditary endocrine neoplasia syndromes. Dr. Igaz has authored over 150 scientific papers and edited three books (Igaz P (Ed.): Circulating microRNAs in disease diagnostics and their potential biological relevance, Springer, 2015 and Igaz P-Patócs A (Eds): Genetics of Endocrine Diseases and Syndromes, Springer, 2019, Igaz P (Ed.): Practical Clinical Endocrinology, Springer, 2021).

Preface to "New Insights in the Genetics and Genomics of Adrenocortical Tumors and Pheochromocytomas"

This Special Issue/Article Collection of papers published in *Cancers* under the title "New Insights in the Genetics and Genomics of adrenocortical tumors and pheochromocytomas"presents recent advancements in the fascinating field of adrenal endocrine oncology.

Adrenal tumors are common, and their prevalence increases with age. Most are indolent hormonally inactive tumors that are discovered incidentally during imaging aimed at diseases of other organs (adrenal incidentaloma). On the other hand, hormone production in both adrenocortical and adrenomedullary tumors (pheochromocytoma) is associated with significant morbidity and mortality. Primary aldosteronism is mostly caused by unilateral adenomas or bilateral hyperplasia and it is the most common cause of secondary endocrine hypertension. Both malignant adrenocortical and adrenomedullary tumors are rare but with a poor prognosis. There are several issues warranting ongoing molecular and clinical investigations in these tumors such as questions of their pathogenesis and difficulties in diagnosis and treatment.

Molecular genetics and genomics studies have uncovered several novel aspects of these tumors in recent years including novel pathogenic pathways, molecular classifications and biomarkers, moreover, novel treatment options are envisaged.

This Special Issue book includes an editorial and 16 papers presenting contemporary issues in the research of this field. An editorial, 10 research papers and six reviews are presented discussing three main topics: i. primary aldosteronism, ii. adrenocortical cancer, and iii. pheochromocytoma, which is the human tumor with the highest heritability. The papers cover a wide spectrum of different features such as molecular genetics, epigenetics and even metabolomics.

I hope that the readers of this Special Issue book will gain a useful overview of this research field.

Peter Igaz
Editor

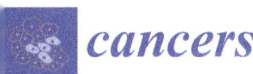

Editorial

New Insights in the Genetics and Genomics of Adrenocortical Tumors and Pheochromocytomas

Peter Igaz [1,2,3]

1 Department of Endocrinology, ENS@T Research Center of Excellence, Faculty of Medicine, Semmelweis University, H-1083 Budapest, Hungary; igaz.peter@med.semmelweis-univ.hu; Tel.: +36-1-266-0816
2 Department of Internal Medicine and Oncology, Faculty of Medicine, Semmelweis University, H-1083 Budapest, Hungary
3 MTA-SE Molecular Medicine Research Group, Eötvös Loránd Research Network, H-1083 Budapest, Hungary

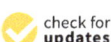

Citation: Igaz, P. New Insights in the Genetics and Genomics of Adrenocortical Tumors and Pheochromocytomas. *Cancers* **2022**, *14*, 1094. https://doi.org/10.3390/cancers14041094

Received: 13 February 2022
Accepted: 17 February 2022
Published: 21 February 2022

Publisher's Note: MDPI stays neutral with regard to jurisdictional claims in published maps and institutional affiliations.

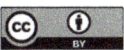

Copyright: © 2022 by the author. Licensee MDPI, Basel, Switzerland. This article is an open access article distributed under the terms and conditions of the Creative Commons Attribution (CC BY) license (https://creativecommons.org/licenses/by/4.0/).

This article collection includes 16 scientific papers that present the current state of the art of genetics and genomics research in the fascinating field of adrenal tumors. In recent years, significant advancements in genetics, epigenetics and genomics have been made, and in our Special Issue, several of these issues are presented by international leaders of the field.

Adrenal tumors include adrenocortical and adrenomedullary tumors. Among adrenocortical tumors, hormonally inactive, benign adenomas are the most common, but hormone secretion is associated with significant morbidity and mortality. Primary aldosteronism represents the most frequent hormonally active adrenocortical tumor syndrome that is a common cause of secondary hypertension, being responsible for 5–10% of all cases. Primary aldosteronism is almost invariably caused by a benign, unilateral adenoma or bilateral hyperplasia. Malignant adrenocortical cancer (ACC) is rare and has a poor prognosis; moreover, its management is difficult due to difficulties in diagnosis and treatment. Adrenomedullary tumors, pheochromocytomas (and their extra-adrenal counterparts, i.e., paragangliomas) are also associated with significant morbidity and mortality due to severe hypertension, cardiovascular complications and, in some cases, metastatic disease.

The manuscripts in this Special Issue discuss the genetic–epigenetic–genomic issues of three major adrenal-tumor-related diseases: primary aldosteronism, adrenocortical cancer and pheochromocytoma/paraganglioma.

Recent studies have shown that a significant proportion of aldosterone-producing adrenocortical adenomas harbor somatic mutations in a subset of genes mostly coding ion channels. The disease phenotype might be associated with some genetic variants, as the article by Chang et al. shows greater recovery from arterial stiffness in adenomas harboring *KCNJ5* somatic mutations [1]. The molecular features of a novel mutation in the *ATP2B3* gene are presented in detail in the article by Liao et al. [2]. By using advanced bioinformatics approaches, Gong et al. characterized the metabolome and tissue microenvironment in aldosterone-producing adenomas and showed metabolic reprogramming toward fatty acid β-oxidation and glycolysis; moreover, an immunosuppressive tissue microenvironment was also found [3]. In a systematic review, Spyroglou et al. present recent developments in the transcriptomics, epigenetics and metabolomics of primary aldosteronism [4]. MicroRNAs belonging to the group of non-coding RNA molecules are also investigated as circulating markers in primary aldosteronism [5].

The diagnosis of adrenocortical cancer is challenging. There is no available preoperative, bloodborne marker of malignancy, but even the histological diagnosis of malignancy is often difficult. Moreover, prognostic markers are warranted to aid in the clinical management of patients. Artificial-intelligence-based approaches can be used to uncover novel markers, as presented in two studies of this Special Issue. Marquardt et al. revealed novel transcriptomic markers with prognostic relevance [6], whereas in the study by our research group (Turai et al.) microRNA combination markers for adrenocortical malignancy with high diagnostic performance are presented [7]. A peculiar feature of adrenocortical cancer is represented by the high incidence of pediatric ACC in southern Brazil due to a founder mutation in the *TP53* gene. Prognostic factors, newborn screening, surveillance and treatment costs are discussed in the article by Tosin et al. [8]. The treatment of adrenocortical cancer is also problematic, as mitotane is the only available adrenal-specific drug with several side effects and a narrow therapeutic range. Moreover, its mechanism of action is only partially elucidated. In their review article, Lo Iacono present in vitro data of mitotane action highlighting controversial issues [9].

Pheochromocytoma/paraganglioma (PPGL) is associated with the highest heritability among human tumors, as about 40% of tumors are associated with germ-line mutations of susceptibility genes. Recent advancements in the genetics of PPGL are presented by Jhawar et al. [10], and the relevance of genetic findings in the clinical management of PPGL patients is detailed in the review by Flores et al. [11]. The molecular methods and their analytical performance for genetic diagnosis are crucial, as presented by Sarkadi et al. [12].

The diagnosis of PPGL malignancy is challenging, as there is no reliable histological or blood-borne marker for metastatic disease. A new metastasis risk gene, NOP10, which is related to telomere maintenance, has been reported by Monteagudo et al. [13], and the potential for non-coding RNA markers is presented in our review [14].

In an interesting original study by Canu et al. on a large Italian cohort, the increased incidence of various secondary malignancies in non-syndromic PPGL patients is documented [15]. This observation is relevant regarding the surveillance and follow-up strategy for PPGL patients.

Alterations in the mitochondrial respiratory chain and redox balance are major pathogenic factors in a subgroup of PPGL. The article by Dona et al. presents a novel zebrafish model that could be efficiently used for the study of PPGL [16].

I do hope that the articles included in this Special Issue will be helpful for the readers to gain an insight into this rapidly involving and dynamic field of endocrine oncology.

Funding: P.I. received funding from the Hungarian National Research, Development and Innovation Office (NKFIH) grant K134215 and from the National Research, Development and Innovation Fund by the Ministry of Innovation and Technology of Hungary (Project no. TKP2021-EGA-24) financed under the [TKP2021-EGA] funding scheme.

Conflicts of Interest: The author declares no conflict of interest.

References

1. Chang, Y.Y.; Pan, C.T.; Chen, Z.W.; Tsai, C.H.; Peng, S.Y.; Chang, C.C.; Lee, B.C.; Liao, C.W.; Peng, K.Y.; Chiu, Y.W.; et al. KCNJ5 Somatic Mutations in Aldosterone-Producing Adenoma Are Associated with a Greater Recovery of Arterial Stiffness. *Cancers* **2021**, *13*, 4313. [CrossRef] [PubMed]
2. Liao, H.W.; Peng, K.Y.; Wu, V.C.; Lin, Y.H.; Lin, S.L.; Lin, W.C.; Chueh, J.S.; On Behalf Of Taipai Study Group. Characteristics of a Novel ATP2B3 K416_F418delinsN Mutation in a Classical Aldosterone-Producing Adenoma. *Cancers* **2021**, *13*, 4729. [CrossRef] [PubMed]
3. Gong, S.; Tetti, M.; Reincke, M.; Williams, T.A. Primary Aldosteronism: Metabolic Reprogramming and the Pathogenesis of Aldosterone-Producing Adenomas. *Cancers* **2021**, *13*, 3716. [CrossRef] [PubMed]
4. Spyroglou, A.; Piaditis, G.P.; Kaltsas, G.; Alexandraki, K.I. Transcriptomics, Epigenetics, and Metabolomics of Primary Aldosteronism. *Cancers* **2021**, *13*, 5582. [CrossRef] [PubMed]
5. MacKenzie, S.M.; Saunders, H.; van Kralingen, J.C.; Robertson, S.; Riddell, A.; Zennaro, M.C.; Davies, E. Circulating microRNAs as Diagnostic Markers in Primary Aldosteronism. *Cancers* **2021**, *13*, 5312. [CrossRef] [PubMed]
6. Marquardt, A.; Landwehr, L.S.; Ronchi, C.L.; di Dalmazi, G.; Riester, A.; Kollmannsberger, P.; Altieri, B.; Fassnacht, M.; Sbiera, S. Identifying New Potential Biomarkers in Adrenocortical Tumors Based on mRNA Expression Data Using Machine Learning. *Cancers* **2021**, *13*, 4671. [CrossRef] [PubMed]
7. Turai, P.I.; Herold, Z.; Nyirő, G.; Borka, K.; Micsik, T.; Tőke, J.; Szücs, N.; Tóth, M.; Patócs, A.; Igaz, P. Tissue miRNA Combinations for the Differential Diagnosis of Adrenocortical Carcinoma and Adenoma Established by Artificial Intelligence. *Cancers* **2022**, *14*, 895. [CrossRef]

8. Tosin, K.C.F.; Legal, E.F.; Pianovski, M.A.D.; Ibañez, H.C.; Custódio, G.; Carvalho, D.S.; Figueiredo, M.M.O.; Hoffmann Filho, A.; Fiori, C.; Rodrigues, A.L.M.; et al. Newborn Screening for the Detection of the TP53 R337H Variant and Surveillance for Early Diagnosis of Pediatric Adrenocortical Tumors: Lessons Learned and Way Forward. *Cancers* **2021**, *13*, 6111. [CrossRef] [PubMed]
9. Lo Iacono, M.; Puglisi, S.; Perotti, P.; Saba, L.; Petiti, J.; Giachino, C.; Reimondo, G.; Terzolo, M. Molecular Mechanisms of Mitotane Action in Adrenocortical Cancer Based on In Vitro Studies. *Cancers* **2021**, *13*, 5255. [CrossRef] [PubMed]
10. Jhawar, S.; Arakawa, Y.; Kumar, S.; Varghese, D.; Kim, Y.S.; Roper, N.; Elloumi, F.; Pommier, Y.; Pacak, K.; Del Rivero, J. New Insights on the Genetics of Pheochromocytoma and Paraganglioma and Its Clinical Implications. *Cancers* **2022**, *14*, 594. [CrossRef] [PubMed]
11. Flores, S.K.; Estrada-Zuniga, C.M.; Thallapureddy, K.; Armaiz-Peña, G.; Dahia, P.L.M. Insights into Mechanisms of Pheochromocytomas and Paragangliomas Driven by Known or New Genetic Drivers. *Cancers* **2021**, *13*, 4602. [CrossRef] [PubMed]
12. Sarkadi, B.; Liko, I.; Nyiro, G.; Igaz, P.; Butz, H.; Patocs, A. Analytical Performance of NGS-Based Molecular Genetic Tests Used in the Diagnostic Workflow of Pheochromocytoma/Paraganglioma. *Cancers* **2021**, *13*, 4219. [CrossRef] [PubMed]
13. Monteagudo, M.; Martínez, P.; Leandro-García, L.J.; Martínez-Montes, Á.M.; Calsina, B.; Pulgarín-Alfaro, M.; Díaz-Talavera, A.; Mellid, S.; Letón, R.; Gil, E.; et al. Analysis of Telomere Maintenance Related Genes Reveals NOP10 as a New Metastatic-Risk Marker in Pheochromocytoma/Paraganglioma. *Cancers* **2021**, *13*, 4758. [CrossRef] [PubMed]
14. Turai, P.I.; Nyírő, G.; Butz, H.; Patócs, A.; Igaz, P. MicroRNAs, Long Non-Coding RNAs, and Circular RNAs: Potential Biomarkers and Therapeutic Targets in Pheochromocytoma/Paraganglioma. *Cancers* **2021**, *13*, 1522. [CrossRef] [PubMed]
15. Canu, L.; Puglisi, S.; Berchialla, P.; De Filpo, G.; Brignardello, F.; Schiavi, F.; Ferrara, A.M.; Zovato, S.; Luconi, M.; Pia, A.; et al. A Multicenter Epidemiological Study on Second Malignancy in Non-Syndromic Pheochromocytoma/Paraganglioma Patients in Italy. *Cancers* **2021**, *13*, 5831. [CrossRef] [PubMed]
16. Dona, M.; Lamers, M.; Rohde, S.; Gorissen, M.; Timmers, H. Targeting the Redox Balance Pathway Using Ascorbic Acid in sdhb Zebrafish Mutant Larvae. *Cancers* **2021**, *13*, 5124. [CrossRef] [PubMed]

Article

KCNJ5 Somatic Mutations in Aldosterone-Producing Adenoma Are Associated with a Greater Recovery of Arterial Stiffness

Yi-Yao Chang [1,2,3,4], Chien-Ting Pan [5], Zheng-Wei Chen [5], Cheng-Hsuan Tsai [3,6], Shih-Yuan Peng [3], Chin-Chen Chang [7], Bo-Ching Lee [7], Che-Wei Liao [8], Kang-Yung Peng [3], Yu-Wei Chiu [2,9], Chia-Hung Chou [10], Vin-Cent Wu [11], Li-Yu Daisy Liu [12], Chi-Sheng Hung [3,13,*] and Yen-Hung Lin [3,13,*]

1. National Taiwan University College of Medicine Graduate Institute of Clinical Medicine, Taipei 100, Taiwan; rollerpapa@mail.chihlee.edu.tw
2. Cardiology Division of Cardiovascular Medical Center, Far Eastern Memorial Hospital, New Taipei City 220, Taiwan; dtmed005@saturn.yzu.edu.tw
3. Division of Cardiology, Department of Internal Medicine, National Taiwan University Hospital and National Taiwan University College of Medicine, Taipei 100, Taiwan; d09421005@ntu.edu.tw (C.-H.T.); sypeng@ntu.edu.tw (S.-Y.P.); kangyung@ntu.edu.tw (K.-Y.P.)
4. Center of General Education, Chihlee University of Technology, New Taipei City 220, Taiwan
5. Department of Internal Medicine, National Taiwan University Hospital Yun-Lin Branch, Yun-Lin 640, Taiwan; y04444@ms1.ylh.gov.tw (C.-T.P.); librajohn7@hotmail.com (Z.-W.C.)
6. Department of Internal Medicine, National Taiwan University Hospital Jin-Shan Branch, New Taipei City 220, Taiwan
7. Department of Medical Imaging, National Taiwan University Hospital and National Taiwan University College of Medicine, Taipei 100, Taiwan; ccchang@ntuh.gov.tw (C.-C.C.); bclee@ntuh.gov.tw (B.-C.L.)
8. Department of Medicine, National Taiwan University Cancer Center, Taipei 106, Taiwan; A01217@ntucc.gov.tw
9. Department of Computer Science and Engineering, Yuan Ze University, Taoyuan City 320, Taiwan
10. Department of Obstetrics and Gynecology, National Taiwan University Hospital and National Taiwan University College of Medicine, Taipei 100, Taiwan; d03421008@ntu.edu.tw
11. Division of Nephrology, Department of Internal Medicine, National Taiwan University Hospital and National Taiwan University College of Medicine, Taipei 100, Taiwan; q91421028@ntu.edu.tw
12. Department of Agronomy, Biometry Division, National Taiwan University, Taipei 106, Taiwan; lyliu@ntu.edu.tw
13. Cardiovascular Center, National Taiwan University Hospital, Taipei 100, Taiwan
* Correspondence: 009578@ntuh.gov.tw (C.-S.H.); yenhunglin@ntuh.gov.tw (Y.-H.L.); Tel.: +88-62-2312-3456 (C.-S.H.); +88-62-2312-3456 (Y.-H.L.)

Simple Summary: Primary aldosteronism (PA) is the most common form of secondary hypertension and induces various cardiovascular injuries. Aldosterone-producing adenoma (APA) is one of the major forms of PA. The occurrence of APA is closely correlated with somatic mutations, including *KCNJ5*. We described here the impact of *KCNJ5* somatic mutations on arterial stiffness excluding the influence of age, sex, and blood pressure status. We found *KCNJ5* mutation carriers had similar arterial stiffness before surgery, but greater improvement of arterial stiffness after adrenalectomy compared with non-carriers. Hence, APA patients with *KCNJ5* mutations had a greater improvement in arterial stiffness after adrenalectomy than those without mutations.

Abstract: Primary aldosteronism is the most common form of secondary hypertension and induces various cardiovascular injuries. In aldosterone-producing adenoma (APA), the impact of *KCNJ5* somatic mutations on arterial stiffness excluding the influence of confounding factors is uncertain. We enrolled 213 APA patients who were scheduled to undergo adrenalectomy. *KCNJ5* gene sequencing of APA was performed. After propensity score matching (PSM) for age, sex, body mass index, blood pressure, number of hypertensive medications, and hypertension duration, there were 66 patients in each group with and without *KCNJ5* mutations. The mutation carriers had a higher aldosterone level and lower log transformed brachial–ankle pulse wave velocity (baPWV) than the non-carriers before PSM, but no difference in log baPWV after PSM. One year after adrenalectomy, the mutation carriers had greater decreases in log plasma aldosterone concentration, log aldosterone–renin activity ratio, and log baPWV than the non-carriers after PSM. Only the mutation carriers had a significant decrease in log baPWV after surgery both before and after PSM. *KCNJ5* mutations were not correlated with baseline baPWV after PSM but were significantly correlated with ΔbaPWV after surgery both before and after PSM. Conclusively, APA patients with *KCNJ5* mutations had a greater regression in arterial stiffness after adrenalectomy than those without mutations.

Keywords: *KCNJ5* somatic mutation; pulse wave velocity; aldosterone-producing adenoma; adrenalectomy; propensity score matching; arterial stiffness

1. Introduction

Primary aldosteronism (PA) is the most common form of secondary endocrine hypertension, which accounts for 5–15% of all cases of hypertension [1–3]. Excessive aldosterone results in various vascular structure injuries. Previous animal studies have shown that aldosterone infusion in uninephrectomized rats accompanied with a high sodium diet could cause increased arterial stiffness associated with fibronectin accumulation [4]. In addition, this effect was independent of wall stress as shown by normotensive controls and reversal of vascular damage by treatment with an aldosterone antagonist [4]. In clinical studies, increased carotid–femoral pulse wave velocity (PWV), which represents increased arterial stiffness, has been noted in patients with PA compared to patients with essential hypertension (EH) after adjusting for all clinical variables including 24 h blood pressure [5]. These effects on arteries have been shown to be reversed after adrenalectomy [6,7].

Aldosterone-producing adenoma (APA) is one of the major subtypes of PA, and it can be cured by adrenalectomy [8,9]. Channelopathies resulting from somatic mutations have been identified as the main pathogenesis of APA in recent years [10–14]. Mutations of the *KCNJ5* gene (coding for G protein-activated inward rectifier potassium channels [10]) are the most common, with a prevalence rate of around 40% in Western countries [15–17] but 55–75% in Asian countries [18–21]. Some common clinical phenotypes in both Western and Asian APA patients with *KCNJ5* mutations have been observed, including younger age, higher aldosterone level, lower potassium level, and higher hypertension cure rate [15–17,22]. However, differences in sex and tumor size have not been found in most Asian studies [20,23,24].

Previous studies have reported associations between *KCNJ5* somatic mutations and worse left ventricular remodeling but better recovery after adrenalectomy [22,25]. However, only a few studies have investigated the impact of *KCNJ5* somatic mutations on arterial stiffness. Previous studies have reported a lower PWV in APA patients with *KCNJ5* mutations compared to those without mutations [23,24]. However, a younger age in patients with mutations would cause a lower PWV, which would then interfere with the interpretation of the effect of *KCNJ5* mutations. In contrast, an earlier study from our group showed that APA patients with *KCNJ5* mutations had comparable PWV to patients without *KCNJ5* mutations both before and after matching for age, sex, and body mass index [26]. In addition, the influence of *KCNJ5* mutations on the change in PWV after adrenalectomy is still unclear.

This study was designed to investigate the role of *KCNJ5* mutations on arterial stiffness and its reversal after adrenalectomy. We used propensity score matching (PSM) analysis to attenuate possible confounding factors.

2. Materials and Methods

2.1. Patients

In this prospective study, we enrolled 213 APA patients who were scheduled to undergo adrenalectomy from January 2007 to May 2019 at National Taiwan University Hospital. The medical histories, including demographic data, severity of blood pressure, and medications of all patients were reviewed carefully. Serum biochemical and brachial–ankle pulse wave velocity (baPWV) data were acquired at the initial evaluation of the patients, and again 1 year after adrenalectomy. Cure was defined as patients who had normalized blood pressure (systolic blood pressure (SBP) < 140 mmHg and diastolic blood pressure (DBP) < 90 mmHg) independently of any antihypertensive drugs after adrenalectomy, which is the same as the definition of "completely clinically cured" proposed by the Primary Aldosteronism Surgical Outcomes (PASO) group [27]. Informed consent was obtained from all patients prior to inclusion in the study, and the study was approved by the Ethics Committee of National Taiwan University Hospital (approval number: 200611031R).

2.2. Laboratory Measurements

Plasma aldosterone concentration (PAC) was measured using a commercial radioimmune assay kit (Aldosterone Maia Kit; Adaltis Italia, Bologna, Italy). Plasma renin activity (PRA) was measured according to the generation of angiotensin-I in vitro using a commercial radioimmune assay kit (DiaSorin, Stillwater, MN, USA). The aldosterone-to-renin ratio (ARR) was calculated as the PAC divided by the PRA.

2.3. Diagnostic Criteria for Aldosterone-Producing Adenomas

The diagnosis of APA was confirmed according to the consensus of the Taiwan Society of Aldosteronism [28] and "modified four corner criteria" after adrenalectomy [29,30] as follows: (1) excess aldosterone production in accordance with an ARR > 35, TAIPAI score > 60% [31], and seated post-saline loading PAC > 16 ng/dL or urine aldosterone > 12 μg/24 h [32]; (2) adenoma on a CT scan; (3) lateralization of excessive aldosterone secretion according to adrenal venous sampling or dexamethasone suppression NP-59 single-photon emission computed tomography (SPECT/CT) [33]; (4) adenoma in histopathological analysis after adrenalectomy, and subsequently either a biochemical cure pattern with improvement of hypertension or clinical cure pattern of hypertension without antihypertensive drugs.

2.4. Arterial Stiffness Evaluation

We measured the baPWV of the patients in a supine position with an autonomic waveform analyzer (Colin VP-2000, Omron Inc., Kyoto, Japan) after a rest of at least 15 min. The analyzer recorded bilateral brachial and tibial arterial pressure waveforms, phonocardiogram, and electrocardiogram. The time difference from brachial to ankle arterial pressure wave was determined according to the wave front velocity theory [34]. The distance between arm and ankle was expressed as a linear equation of height. The baPWV was calculated as the distance divided by the time difference. Finally, the average of right and left baPWV values in each patient was used for further analysis.

2.5. Adrenalectomy

All of the APA patients underwent laparoscopic adrenalectomy via a lateral transperitoneal approach by experienced laparoscopic surgeons.

2.6. Histopathologic Studies

Adrenal specimens were blindly assessed by an experienced pathologist. Nodules comprised of adrenal cortical cells and clearly demarcated by a pseudo-capsule were defined as adenomas [35]. Adenomas were differentiated from nodular hyperplasia if they were isolated and well-circumscribed [36].

2.7. Genomic DNA Extraction and Sequencing of the KCNJ5 Gene

Adrenal specimens were stored at −80 °C after adrenalectomy. Genomic DNA was extracted using a QIAamp DNA mini kit (Qiagen, Hilden, Germany) from 213 peritumoral adrenal cortices.

We analyzed the coding regions of the genomic DNA via exome sequencing. The entire coding sequence (exons 2–3) and flanking regions of the *KCNJ5* gene were amplified and sequenced using four sets of gene-specific primers as reported previously [37] (listed in Table S1). GoTaq® Master Mix (Promega Corporation, Madison, WI, USA) was used for the PCR reactions with an annealing temperature of 58 °C. GenepHlow™ Gel/PCR Kits (Geneaid, Taipei, Taiwan ROC) were used to extract DNA fragments from PCR. Sanger sequencing of PCR products was carried out using a 3730 DNA Analyzer (Applied Biosystems, Foster City, CA, USA).

2.8. Statistical Analysis

SPSS for Windows version 25.0 (SPSS Inc., Chicago, IL, USA) with the R-3.3 plugin extension was used for the propensity score matching (PSM) analysis. A 1:1 matching ratio was adopted. Propensity scores were assessed using a non-parsimonious multiple logistic regression model including the following probable confounding variables in patients with and without *KCNJ5* somatic mutations: age, sex, body mass index (BMI), SBP, DBP, number of hypertensive medications, and duration of hypertension. The balance of the selected covariates for matching between the matched groups was subsequently examined.

All continuous variables were presented as mean ± SD. Non-normally distributed variables were presented as median and interquartile range, including PAC, PRA, and ARR. The equality of two proportions was evaluated using the Pearson chi-square test. Comparisons of continuous data between two groups were conducted using the Student's t test for normally distributed variables or the Wilcoxon rank-sum test for non-normally distributed variables. Comparisons of continuous data before and after adrenalectomy were performed using paired t tests. PAC, PRA, and ARR data were log-transformed due to non-normal distribution as determined by the Kolmogorov–Smirnov test for further regression analysis. Correlations of *KCNJ5* mutations with baseline log baPWV and the change in log baPWV after adrenalectomy before and after PSM were analyzed using linear regression analysis with different adjustment models.

3. Results

3.1. Clinical and Biochemical Data of All APA Patients before and after Matching

Of the 213 APA patients who received adrenalectomy, 126 (59.2%) had *KCNJ5* somatic mutations. Of these 126 mutation carriers, sequencing of adenoma specimens demonstrated that 75 patients had p.Gly151Arg (c.451G > A or c.451G > C), 45 had p.Leu168Arg (c.503T > G), 3 had p.Thr158Ala (c.472A > G), and 3 had p.Glu145Gln (c.433G > C) mutations in the heterozygous state.

The *KCNJ5* mutation carriers were younger ($p < 0.001$), had a shorter duration of hypertension ($p = 0.018$), higher DBP ($p = 0.003$), higher aldosterone level ($p < 0.001$), higher ARR ($p = 0.003$), and lower potassium level ($p < 0.001$) (Table 1).

After 1:1 PSM for age, sex, BMI, SBP, DBP, duration of hypertension, and number of hypertensive medications, there were 66 patients in each group (*KCNJ5* mutation carrier group and non-carrier group). The matched APA patients with *KCNJ5* mutations had a lower rate of angiotensin-converting enzyme inhibitor (ACEI) or angiotensin II blocker (ARB) use ($p = 0.037$), higher aldosterone level ($p = 0.012$), higher ARR ($p = 0.017$), and lower potassium level ($p < 0.001$) than the non-carriers (Table 1).

3.2. baPWV of All APA Patients before and after Matching

Before PSM, the patients with *KCNJ5* mutations had a lower log baPWV ($p = 0.046$) compared to the non-carriers (Table 1). After PSM, there was no significant difference in log baPWV between the two groups (Table 1).

3.3. The Change in Clinical Data after Adrenalectomy before and after Matching

One year after adrenalectomy, the APA patients with *KCNJ5* mutations had a significantly higher cure rate (79% vs. 61%, $p = 0.004$) before PSM, and borderline higher cure rate (79% vs. 64%, $p = 0.055$) after PSM.

Before PSM, the APA patients with *KCNJ5* mutations had a greater decrease in SBP ($p = 0.002$), DBP ($p = 0.003$), number of hypertensive drugs ($p = 0.001$), log PAC ($p < 0.001$), log PRA ($p = 0.034$), and log ARR ($p = 0.001$), and greater increase in creatinine ($p = 0.009$)

and potassium ($p < 0.001$) compared to the patients without *KCNJ5* mutations (Table 2). After PSM, the decrease in log PAC ($p = 0.033$) and log ARR ($p = 0.015$) and increase in potassium ($p < 0.001$) were still significantly higher in the matched APA patients with *KCNJ5* mutations than in those without *KCNJ5* mutations (Table 2).

Table 1. Baseline clinical data of APA patients with and without *KCNJ5* mutations before and after PSM.

Variables	Before Propensity Score Matching			After Propensity Score Matching *		
Patient Characteristics	*KCNJ5* (+) (n = 126)	*KCNJ5* (−) (n = 87)	p	*KCNJ5* (+) (n = 66)	*KCNJ5* (−) (n = 66)	p
Age, years	47.3 ± 10.3	55.3 ± 10.5	<0.001	50.3 ± 9.6	52.5 ± 10.1	0.190
Sex, male	53(42%)	36(36%)	0.921	27(41%)	27(41%)	1.000
Height, cm	164 ± 8	163 ± 9	0.213	163 ± 8	163 ± 9	0.763
Weight, kg	66 ± 13	67 ± 14	0.774	67 ± 12	66 ± 14	0.930
Body mass index, kg/m^2	24.5 ± 3.5	25.1 ± 3.8	0.248	24.9 ± 3.7	24.8 ± 3.7	0.914
Duration of hypertension, years	6.5 ± 6.0	9.0 ± 8.6	0.018	7.0 ± 6.1	8.4 ± 8.5	0.281
SBP, mm Hg	156 ± 22	151 ± 21	0.114	153 ± 22	152 ± 21	0.930
DBP, mm Hg	94 ± 15	89 ± 13	0.003	90 ± 14	90 ± 13	0.923
Diabetes mellitus	10(8%)	12(14%)	0.189	8(12%)	7(11%)	0.786
Dyslipidemia	21(17%)	20(23%)	0.321	15(23%)	15(23%)	1.000
Number of anti-hypertensive drugs	2.1 ± 1.1	1.9 ± 1.1	0.251	1.9 ± 1.0	2.0 ± 1.0	0.670
Hypertension medication type						
ACEI/ARB	50(40%)	44(50%)	0.172	26(39%)	38(58%)	0.037
α -Blocker	34(27%)	15(17%)	0.097	15(23%)	13(20%)	0.673
β -Blocker	44(35%)	30(34%)	0.858	20(30%)	22(33%)	0.711
CCB	93(74%)	57(65%)	0.183	45(68%)	44(67%)	0.854
Diuretics except aldosterone antagonist	8(6%)	9(10%)	0.210	3(5%)	8(12%)	0.118
Aldosterone antagonist	37(29%)	18(21%)	0.203	19(29%)	12(18%)	0.153
Vasodilator	9(7%)	6(7%)	0.963	3(5%)	4(6%)	0.700
Laboratory parameters						
Creatinine, mg/dL	0.87 ± 0.34	0.89 ± 0.29	0.694	0.89 ± 0.42	0.92 ± 0.31	0.718
Potassium, mmol/L	3.3 ± 0.6	3.8 ± 0.4	<0.001	3.3 ± 0.6	3.8 ± 0.5	<0.001
PAC [†], ng/dL	51(45)	34(23)	<0.001	46(42)	34(22)	0.012
PRA [†], ng/mL/h	0.17(0.52)	0.28(0.70)	0.171	0.17(0.45)	0.36(0.78)	0.090
ARR [†], ng/dL per ng/mL/h	271(737)	134(429)	0.003	254(619)	118(361)	0.017
Log PAC	1.69 ± 0.28	1.53 ± 0.27	<0.001	1.66 ± 0.29	1.55 ± 0.27	0.026
Log PRA	−0.74 ± 0.73	−0.60 ± 0.82	0.167	−0.75 ± 0.71	0.54 ± 0.89	0.133
Log ARR	2.44 ± 0.78	2.12 ± 0.80	0.005	2.41 ± 0.73	2.08 ± 0.86	0.022
baPWV [†], cm/s	1554(428)	1661(445)	0.088	1559(414)	1571(422)	0.831
log baPWV	3.20 ± 0.07	3.22 ± 0.08	0.046	3.21 ± 0.07	3.21 ± 0.08	0.530

Values are expressed as mean SD, median (interquartile range), or number (percentage). SBP, systolic blood pressure; DBP, diastolic blood pressure; ACEI, angiotensin-converting enzyme inhibitor; ARB, angiotensin II blocker; ARR, aldosterone–renin ratio; CCB, calcium channel blocker; PAC, plasma aldosterone concentration; PRA, plasma renin activity; ARR, aldosterone–renin activity ratio. * 1:1 matched for age, sex, BMI, SBP, DBP, duration of hypertension, and number of anti-hypertension drugs between the *KCNJ5*(+) and *KCNJ5*(−) groups. [†] Expressed as median and interquartile range.

For the change in log baPWV, the APA patients with *KCNJ5* mutations had a significantly greater decrease than the patients without *KCNJ5* mutations both before ($p = 0.014$) and after ($p = 0.040$) PSM (Figure 1A,D).

3.4. Paired Comparisons of Clinical Data in All Patients before PSM before and after Adrenalectomy, and Comparisons of Parameters 1 Year after Surgery between the APA Patients with and without Mutations

Before PSM, both the APA patients with and without *KCNJ5* mutations had significant decreases in SBP, DBP, number of hypertensive drugs, and log ARR, and both groups had significant increases in creatinine, potassium, and log PRA after adrenalectomy (Table 3).

However, only the APA patients with KCNJ5 mutations had a significant decrease in log PAC ($p < 0.001$) and log baPWV ($p < 0.001$) after adrenalectomy, which was not found in the patients without KCNJ5 mutations (Figure 1B,C).

Table 2. Changes of clinical data of APA patients with and without KCNJ5 mutation after adrenalectomy before and after PSM.

Variables	Before Propensity Score Matching			After Propensity Score Matching *		
Patient Characteristics	KCNJ5 (+) (n = 106)	KCNJ5 (−) (n = 74)	p	KCNJ5 (+) (n = 58)	KCNJ5 (−) (n = 58)	p
ΔSBP, mmHg	−26 ± 22	−16 ± 22	0.002	−24 ± 23	−16 ± 23	0.085
ΔDBP, mmHg	−13 ± 16	−7 ± 13	0.003	−10 ± 14	−7 ± 14	0.142
ΔNumber of hypertensive drugs	−1.7 ± 1.1	−1.2 ± 1.1	0.001	−1.6 ± 1.1	−1.3 ± 1.1	0.052
ΔCreatinine, mg/dL	0.19 ± 0.36	0.07 ± 0.22	0.009	0.18 ± 0.38	0.06 ± 0.23	0.427
ΔPotassium, mmol/L	1.1 ± 0.7	0.4 ± 0.6	<0.001	1.1 ± 0.8	0.5 ± 0.6	<0.001
Δlog PAC	−0.24 ± 0.35	−0.05 ± 0.35	<0.001	−0.19 ± 0.36	−0.04 ± 0.35	0.033
Δlog PRA	0.99 ± 0.95	0.68 ± 0.99	0.034	0.99 ± 0.93	0.67 ± 1.03	0.082
Δlog ARR	−1.23 ± 1.04	−0.72 ± 1.00	0.001	−1.18 ± 1.02	−0.71 ± 1.00	0.015

Values are expressed as mean SD, median (interquartile range). SBP, systolic blood pressure; DBP, diastolic blood pressure; PAC, plasma aldosterone concentration; PRA, plasma renin activity; ARR, aldosterone–renin activity ratio. * 1:1 matched for age, sex, BMI, SBP, DBP, duration of hypertension, and number of anti-hypertension drugs between the KCNJ5(+) and KCNJ5(−) groups.

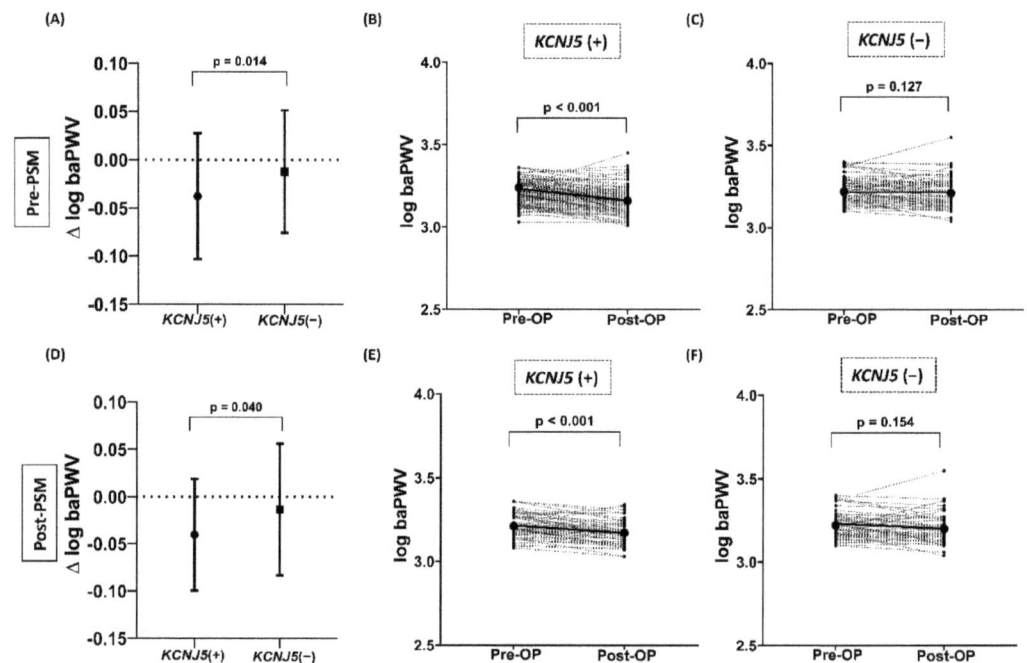

Figure 1. The changes in log baPWV after adrenalectomy between the APA patients with and without KCNJ5 mutations before and after PSM. (A) Before PSM, the decrease in log baPWV after adrenalectomy was significantly greater in the patients with KCNJ5 mutations than in those without mutations. (D) Even after PSM, the decrease in log baPWV after adrenalectomy was still significantly greater in the patients with KCNJ5 mutations than in those without mutations. (B,C) Before PSM, only the patients with KCNJ5 mutations had a significant decrease in log baPWV, and this was not seen in the patients without KCNJ5 mutations. (E,F) After PSM, still only the patients with KCNJ5 mutations had a significant decrease in log baPWV, and again this was not seen in the patients without KCNJ5 mutations. APA, aldosterone-producing adenoma; baPWV, brachial–ankle pulse wave velocity.

Table 3. Paired comparisons of clinical data and pulse wave velocity data of all patients before and after adrenalectomy according to the status of *KCNJ5* mutations and the comparisons of parameters after operations between APA patients with and without mutations.

Variables	KCNJ5 (+)			KCNJ5 (−)			
Patient Characteristics	Baseline (n = 106)	Post-OP 1Y (n = 106)	p	Baseline (n = 74)	Post-OP 1Y (n = 74)	p	p §
SBP, mm Hg	157 ± 22	130 ± 16	<0.001	152 ± 21	136 ± 19	<0.001	0.044
DBP, mm Hg	95 ± 15	82 ± 11	<0.001	89 ± 12	82 ± 11	<0.001	0.862
Number of hypertensive drugs	2.1 ± 1.1	0.4 ± 0.8	<0.001	1.9 ± 1.1	0.7 ± 1.0	<0.001	0.010
Creatinine, mg/dL	0.88 ± 0.36	1.07 ± 0.61	0.001	0.90 ± 0.31	0.96 ± 0.33	0.014	0.171
Potassium, mmol/L	3.3 ± 0.7	4.4 ± 0.4	<0.001	3.8 ± 0.5	4.2 ± 0.4	<0.001	0.081
Log PAC	1.71 ± 0.26	1.47 ± 0.23	<0.001	1.53 ± 0.27	1.49 ± 0.26	0.262	0.589
Log PRA	−0.74 ± 0.78	0.99 ± 0.95	<0.001	−0.55 ± 0.84	0.68 ± 0.99	<0.001	0.248
Log ARR	2.45 ± 0.82	1.21 ± 0.65	<0.001	2.08 ± 0.81	1.36 ± 0.73	<0.001	0.182
Log baPWV *	3.20 ± 0.07	3.16 ± 0.08	<0.001	3.22 ± 0.08	3.21 ± 0.09	0.127	<0.001

Values are expressed as mean SD, median (interquartile range). SBP, systolic blood pressure; DBP, diastolic blood pressure; PAC, plasma aldosterone concentration; PRA, plasma renin activity; ARR, aldosterone–renin activity ratio; baPWV, brachial–ankle pulse wave velocity.
* There were 103 patients and 65 patients with and without *KCNJ5* mutations, respectively, that took a PWV exam one year after operation.
§ p value comparing the parameters after operations between APA patients with and without *KCNJ5* mutations.

In addition, the patients with *KCNJ5* mutations had a significantly lower SBP ($p = 0.044$), number of hypertensive drugs ($p = 0.010$), and log baPWV ($p < 0.001$) 1 year after adrenalectomy compared to those without mutations.

3.5. Paired Comparisons of Clinical Data in Matched Patients before and after Adrenalectomy

After PSM, both the APA patients with and without *KCNJ5* mutations had significant decreases in SBP, DBP, number of hypertensive drugs, and log ARR, and both groups had significant increases in potassium and log PRA after adrenalectomy (Table 4). However, only the APA patients with *KCNJ5* mutations had a significant increase in creatinine ($p = 0.001$) and decrease in log PAC ($p < 0.001$) and log baPWV ($p < 0.001$) after adrenalectomy, which was not found in the patients without *KCNJ5* mutations (Figure 1E,F).

Table 4. Paired comparison of clinical data and pulse wave velocity data of matched * patients before and after adrenalectomy according to the status of *KCNJ5* mutations.

Variables	KCNJ5 (+)			KCNJ5 (−)			
Patient Characteristics	Baseline (n = 58)	Post-OP 1Y (n = 58)	p	Baseline (n = 58)	Post-OP 1Y (n = 58)	p	p §
SBP, mm Hg	154 ± 23	131 ± 15	<0.001	152 ± 20	136 ± 19	<0.001	0.092
DBP, mm Hg	92 ± 14	81 ± 10	<0.001	90 ± 12	84 ± 11	0.001	0.194
Number of hypertensive drugs	2.0 ± 1.0	0.4 ± 0.8	<0.001	2.0 ± 1.0	0.7 ± 1.0	<0.001	0.013
Creatinine, mg/dL	0.91 ± 0.45	1.09 ± 0.75	0.001	0.94 ± 0.32	1.01 ± 0.35	0.083	0.469
Potassium, mmol/L	3.3 ± 0.7	4.3 ± 0.4	<0.001	3.8 ± 0.5	4.3 ± 0.4	<0.001	0.472
Log PAC	1.68 ± 0.30	1.49 ± 0.22	<0.001	1.55 ± 0.27	1.50 ± 0.26	0.339	0.836
Log PRA	−0.75 ± 0.77	0.24 ± 0.62	<0.001	−0.52 ± 0.91	0.15 ± 0.75	<0.001	0.462
Log ARR	2.42 ± 0.79	1.24 ± 0.64	<0.001	2.07 ± 0.86	1.35 ± 0.72	<0.001	0.390
log baPWV †	3.21 ± 0.06	3.17 ± 0.07	<0.001	3.22 ± 0.08	3.20 ± 0.09	0.154	0.045

Values are expressed as mean SD, median (interquartile range). SBP, systolic blood pressure; DBP, diastolic blood pressure; PAC, plasma aldosterone concentration; PRA, plasma renin activity; ARR, aldosterone–renin activity ratio; baPWV, brachial–ankle pulse wave velocity.
* 1:1 matched for age, sex, BMI, SBP, DBP, duration of hypertension, and number of anti-hypertension drugs between the *KCNJ5* (+) and *KCNJ5* (−) groups. † After PSM, there were 55 patients and 52 patients with and without *KCNJ5* mutations, respectively, that took a PWV exam one year after operation. § p value comparing the parameters after operations between APA patients with and without *KCNJ5* mutations.

In addition, the matched patients with *KCNJ5* mutations had a significantly higher number of hypertensive drugs ($p = 0.013$), and log baPWV ($p = 0.045$) 1 year after adrenalectomy compared to those without mutations.

3.6. Correlation of KCNJ5 Mutations with Baseline log baPWV and the Change in log baPWV before and after PSM

Before PSM, the patients with *KCNJ5* mutations were correlated with baseline log PWV in Model 1 analysis ($p = 0.046$, without adjustments) (Table 5). However, after adjusting for age and sex (Model 2 analysis), the correlation between *KCNJ5* mutations and baseline log PWV was no longer significant. This was also found in subsequent analysis models. In contrast, the patients with *KCNJ5* mutations were correlated with the change in log PWV in all of the analysis models, including unadjusted (Model 1, $p = 0.014$), adjusted for age and sex (Model 2, $p = 0.017$), adjusted for age, sex, SBP, and DBP (Model 3, $p = 0.043$), and adjusted for age, sex, SBP, DBP, hypertensive drugs, and hypertension duration (Model 4, $p = 0.039$).

Table 5. Correlation of *KCNJ5* mutations with baseline log baPWV and the change of log baPWV after adrenalectomy of APA patients before and after PSM.

Model	Pre-PSM		Post-PSM	
	Pre-OP log baPWV	Δ log baPWV	Pre-OP log baPWV	Δ log baPWV
Model 1	β = −0.137, $p = 0.046$ (−0.043, 0.000)	β = −0.190, $p = 0.014$ (−0.046, −0.005)	β = −0.055, $p = 0.530$ (−0.036, 0.019)	β = −0.199, $p = 0.040$ (−0.051, −0.001)
Model 2	β = 0.065, $p = 0.293$ (−0.009, 0.029)	β = −0.194, $p = 0.017$ (−0.047, −0.005)	β = 0.004, $p = 0.959$ (−0.023, 0.024)	β = −0.191, $p = 0.049$ (−0.050, 0.000)
Model 3	β = 0.025, $p = 0.644$ (−0.013, 0.021)	β = −0.161, $p = 0.043$ (−0.043, −0.001)	β = −0.002, $p = 0.980$ (−0.021, 0.020)	β = −0.194, $p = 0.036$ (−0.049, −0.002)
Model 4	β = 0.020, $p = 0.721$ (−0.014, 0.020)	β = −0.166, $p = 0.039$ (−0.043, −0.001)	β = −0.001, $p = 0.982$ (−0.021, 0.021)	β = −0.187, $p = 0.043$ (−0.048, −0.001)

Model 1 unadjusted. Model 2 adjusted for age, sex. Model 3 adjusted for age, sex, SBP, DBP. Model 4 adjusted for age, sex, SBP, DBP, number of hypertensive drugs, hypertension duration.

After PSM, the patients with *KCNJ5* mutations were not correlated with baseline log PWV in any of the analysis models (Table 5). In contrast, the patients with *KCNJ5* mutations were correlated with the change in log PWV in all of the analysis models, including unadjusted (Model 1, $p = 0.040$), adjusted for age and sex (Model 2, $p = 0.049$), adjusted for age, sex, SBP, and DBP (Model 3, $p = 0.036$), and adjusted for age, sex, SBP, DBP, hypertensive drugs, and hypertension duration (Model 4, $p = 0.043$).

4. Discussion

The major findings of this study were as follows. First, the APA patients with *KCNJ5* mutations had lower baseline baPWV compared to those without mutations; however, there was no difference after matching for age, sex, and blood pressure. Second, after adrenalectomy, the patients with *KCNJ5* mutations had a greater decrease in baPWV compared to those without mutations both before and after matching. Third, only the patients with *KCNJ5* mutations had a significant improvement in baPWV after adrenalectomy, and this was not seen in those without mutations either before or after matching. Finally, *KCNJ5* mutations were correlated with the change in baPWV even after adjusting for age, sex, and baseline blood pressure status both before and after matching.

Arterial stiffness can be caused by various etiologies, including age, hypertension, and hyperglycemia. PWV is a global cardiovascular indicator of arterial stiffness [38]. A pulse wave is produced from the ejection of blood from the heart. PWV is the speed of a pulse wave propagating to the periphery and is calculated as the distance of a pulse wave travelled divided by the time difference [39]. baPWV was developed around 20 years ago, and it is widely used to measure PWV due to its simplicity, convenience, and reliable reproducibility, especially in Japan and Asian countries [40,41]. Recent studies have shown that baPWV is a good predictor of cardiovascular events [42–45]. In a meta-analysis including 18 studies [43], Vlachopoulos et al. reported that an increase in baPWV of 1 m/s was correlated with increases of 12%, 13%, and 6% in total cardiovascular events, cardiovascular mortality, and all-cause mortality, respectively.

In a vascular smooth muscle cell study, aldosterone was shown to increase collagen synthesis [46]. In an animal study, aldosterone infusion accompanied with a high sodium diet in rats was shown to cause increased arterial stiffness as evidenced by fibronectin accumulation. Moreover, this effect was independent of wall stress as shown by normotensive controls and reversal of vascular damage by treatment with an aldosterone antagonist [4]. In clinical studies, patients with PA have also been shown to have a higher PWV compared to patients with EH [5], even after adjusting for blood pressure [5,47], and this effect was reversed after adrenalectomy [6,7]. In addition, the severity of PWV has been correlated with serum aldosterone level [48]. Taken together, these studies all imply that excessive aldosterone increases arterial stiffness.

The *KCNJ5* gene is the most common site of somatic mutations in APA patients, especially in Asian countries [18–21]. *KCNJ5* mutations have been reported to increase intracellular calcium concentrations and induce activation of calcium signaling, leading to the overexpression of CYP11B2 and increase in aldosterone production [10]. APA patients with *KCNJ5* mutations have been reported to be younger, have a higher aldosterone level, lower potassium level, and higher hypertension cure rate compared to those without mutations in previous studies [15–17,22]. However, age, blood pressure and aldosterone level may influence the PWV in APA patients, and this may account for the diverse results reported in previous studies about the effect of *KCNJ5* mutations on PWV [23,24,26].

Our previous study revealed that APA patients with *KCNJ5* mutations had a higher left ventricular mass, and subsequently a greater regression in mass after adrenalectomy than those without mutations [25]. However, the impact of *KCNJ5* mutations on the change in PWV after adrenalectomy is still uncertain. In a study from Japan, Kitamoto et al. [23] reported a lower baseline baPWV in patients with *KCNJ5* mutations compared to those without mutations, and only patients with mutations had a significant decrease in baPWV. However, their study only enrolled a relatively small number of cases with follow-up baPWV data after adrenalectomy (33 with mutations and 5 without mutations), and subsequent data of comparisons in changes between the two groups were not available. In addition, the baseline age was younger in the patients with mutations, which may have interfered with the interpretation of lower baseline baPWV and greater change in baPWV in the patients with mutations, since younger patients generally have a lower baPWV after excluding other confounding factors. In contrast, an earlier study from our group showed that APA patients with *KCNJ5* mutations had a comparable PWV to patients without mutations both before and after matching for age, sex, and body mass index [26]. In addition, the post-operative decrease in PWV was numerically higher in the APA patients with *KCNJ5* mutations, although the difference did not reach significance ($p = 0.106$). This may have been due to the small number of enrolled patients [26].

In the present study, before PSM, the APA patients with *KCNJ5* mutations had a lower baPWV compared to those without mutations, however there was no difference after matching for age, sex, and blood pressure status. Before PSM, the patients with mutations were younger and had a shorter duration of hypertension, which may have contributed to the lower baPWV compared to those without mutations. However, after matching for age and blood pressure status, including the duration of hypertension, the difference in baPWV between the two groups diminished. This implies that a younger age and shorter hypertension duration may have accounted for the lower baPWV in the patients with *KCNJ5* mutations before PSM.

In the current study, we also found that the patients with *KCNJ5* mutations had a larger decrease in baPWV after adrenalectomy both before and after PSM compared to those without mutations. This finding was not shown in a previous study in Japan [23]. Our previous study showed a numerically higher baPWV post-operatively but without significance in APA patients with *KCNJ5* mutations comparable to those without mutations [26], and the current study confirms this finding both before and after PSM. Comparing the current study with our previous study, we enrolled more patients in the current study, which may be why the difference in baPWV reached statistical significance. The possible causes of a greater decrease in baPWV after surgery in patients with *KCNJ5* mutations include the following. First, the decreases in serum PAC level and ARR were greater in the patients with *KCNJ5* mutations than in those without mutations both before and after PSM. One previous study showed a correlation between serum aldosterone level and the severity of PWV [48]. Therefore, a greater decrease in aldosterone level after adrenalectomy may contribute to greater reversal of baPWV. Second, the rate of residual hypertension was lower in the patients with *KCNJ5* mutations after adrenalectomy. In addition, SBP (before PSM) and the number of hypertensive drugs (before and after PSM) were lower in the patients without *KCNJ5* mutations. Taken together, these findings imply better blood pressure status in the patients with *KCNJ5* mutations compared to those without mutations. The association between hypertension and arterial stiffness has been well established [49]. Therefore, this may account for the smaller reversal in baPWV after surgery in the patients without mutations. Third, in another recent study by our group, we found that the presence of *KCNJ5* mutations was associated with a lower incidence of subclinical hypercortisolism [50]. APA patients with subclinical hypercortisolism have been reported to have a higher incidence of comorbidities, including heart disease, cardiovascular events history, diabetes, and metabolic syndrome [51]. The higher incidence of subclinical hypercortisolism and subsequent comorbidity in APA patients without *KCNJ5* mutations compared to those with *KCNJ5* mutations may therefore also contribute to a smaller reversal in baPWV after surgery.

Limitations

There are several limitations to this study. First, even though we used PSM to decrease discrepancies in age, sex, BMI, blood pressure, duration of hypertension, and number of hypertensive medications between the patients with and without *KCNJ5* mutations, unknown bias is still possible, and this may have caused an imbalance in baPWV between the two study groups. Second, we did not check somatic mutations other than *KCNJ5*, such as *ATP1A1*, *ATP2B3* [52], *CACNA1D* [53], and *CTNNB1* [54], hence we had no idea about the effects of these genes on baPWV. Third, the usage rates of ACEIs/ARBs in the APA patients with *KCNJ5* mutations were lower compared to those without mutation after matching. However, in previous studies, ACEIs or ARBs have been shown to improve arterial stiffness in patients with hypertension [55–57]. Therefore, the lower usage rates of ACEIs/ARBs in the patients with mutations may have caused the smaller decrease in baPWV, but this did not affect the final result of greater reversal of baPWV in patients with mutations. Fourth, since *KCNJ5* gene mutations present heterogeneity between Asian and Western populations, the results of this study may not be completely applicable to Western populations. Fifth, the use of aldosterone antagonists may influence the study results. However, the number of patients who use aldosterone antagonists was small, and it was not adequate for subgroup analysis. Sixth, we did not have the long-term follow-up data of baPWV of these patients. Whether the discrepancy of the changes of baPWV between the two groups persists or not is uncertain.

5. Conclusions

Compared to the APA patients without *KCNJ5* mutations, those with *KCNJ5* mutations had comparable baseline arterial stiffness but a greater regression in arterial stiffness after adrenalectomy independently of age or blood pressure.

Supplementary Materials: The following are available online at https://www.mdpi.com/article/10.3390/cancers13174313/s1, Table S1: Primer sequences of *KCNJ5*.

Author Contributions: Conceptualization, Y.-Y.C. and Y.-H.L.; methodology, Y.-H.L.; software, Y.-Y.C.; validation, Z.-W.C., C.-H.T. and S.-Y.P.; formal analysis, Y.-Y.C., C.-C.C., B.-C.L., C.-H.C. and K.-Y.P.; investigation, C.-W.L. and C.-T.P.; resources, Y.-W.C., V.-C.W., C.-S.H. and Y.-H.L.; data curation, L.-Y.D.L.; writing—original draft preparation, Y.-Y.C.; writing—review and editing, L.-Y.D.L., C.-S.H. and Y.-H.L.; visualization, Y.-Y.C.; supervision, L.-Y.D.L. and Y.-H.L.; project administration, Y.-H.L.; funding acquisition, Y.-H.L. All authors have read and agreed to the published version of the manuscript.

Funding: This study was supported by Ministry of Science and Technology (MOST 106-2314-B-002-169-MY3, 107-2314-B-002-264-MY3), National Taiwan University Hospital (NTUH 107-A141, 108-A141, 109-A141, 108-N01, 109-S4673, VN109-21, UN109-054), Far Eastern Memorial Hospital and National Taiwan University Hospital Joint Research Program (110-FTN23), Excellent Translational Medicine Research Projects of National Taiwan University College of Medicine, and National Taiwan University Hospital (109C 101-43). The funders had no role in study design, data collection and analysis, decision to publish, or preparation of the manuscript.

Institutional Review Board Statement: The study was conducted according to the guidelines of the Declaration of Helsinki and approved by the Ethics Committee of National Taiwan University Hospital.

Informed Consent Statement: Informed consent was obtained from all subjects involved in the study.

Data Availability Statement: The data presented in this study are available on request from the corresponding author.

Acknowledgments: The authors thank the staff of the Second Core Lab of the Department of Medical Research at National Taiwan University Hospital for technical assistance and all of the staff of Taiwan Primary Aldosteronism Study Group (TAIPAI study group). Membership of the Taiwan Primary Aldosteronism Investigation (TAIPAI) Study Group: Che-Hsiung Wu (Chi-Taz Hospital, PI of Committee); Vin-Cent Wu (NTUH, PI of Committee); Yen-Hung Lin (NTUH, PI of Committee); Hung-Wei Chang (Far Eastern Clinics, PI of Committee); Lian-Yu Lin (NTUH, PI of Committee); Fu-Chang Hu (Harvard Statistics, Site Investigator); Kao-Lang Liu (NTUH, PI of Committee); Shuo-Meng Wang (NTUH, PI of Committee); Kuo-How Huang (NTUH, PI of Committee); Yung-Ming Chen (NTUH, PI of Committee); Chin-Chen Chang (NTUH, PI of Committee); Shih-Cheng Liao (NTUH, PI of Committee); Ruoh-Fang Yen (NTUH, PI of Committee); and Kwan-Dun Wu (NTUH, Director of Coordinating Center).

Conflicts of Interest: The authors declare no conflict of interest. The funders had no role in the design of the study; in the collection, analyses, or interpretation of data; in the writing of the manuscript, or in the decision to publish the results.

References

1. Funder, J.W.; Carey, R.M.; Mantero, F.; Murad, M.H.; Reincke, M.; Shibata, H.; Stowasser, M.; Young, W.F., Jr. The management of primary aldosteronism: Case detection, diagnosis, and treatment: An endocrine society clinical practice guideline. *J. Clin. Endocrinol. Metab.* **2016**, *101*, 1889–1916.
2. Käyser, S.C.; Dekkers, T.; Groenewoud, H.J.; van der Wilt, G.J.; Carel Bakx, J.; van der Wel, M.C.; Hermus, A.R.; Lenders, J.W.; Deinum, J. Study heterogeneity and estimation of prevalence of primary aldosteronism: A systematic review and meta-regression analysis. *J. Clin. Endocrinol. Metab.* **2016**, *101*, 2826–2835.
3. Buffolo, F.; Monticone, S.; Burrello, J.; Tetti, M.; Veglio, F.; Williams, T.A.; Mulatero, P. Is primary aldosteronism still largely unrecognized? *Horm. Metab. Res.* **2017**, *49*, 908–914.
4. Lacolley, P.; Labat, C.; Pujol, A.; Delcayre, C.; Benetos, A.; Safar, M. Increased carotid wall elastic modulus and fibronectin in aldosterone-salt-treated rats: Effects of eplerenone. *Circulation* **2002**, *106*, 2848–2853.
5. Strauch, B.; Petrák, O.; Wichterle, D.; Zelinka, T.; Holaj, R.; Widimský, J., Jr. Increased arterial wall stiffness in primary aldosteronism in comparison with essential hypertension. *Am. J. Hypertens.* **2006**, *19*, 909–914.
6. Strauch, B.; Petrák, O.; Zelinka, T.; Wichterle, D.; Holaj, R.; Kasalický, M.; Safařík, L.; Rosa, J.; Widimský, J., Jr. Adrenalectomy improves arterial stiffness in primary aldosteronism. *Am. J. Hypertens.* **2008**, *21*, 1086–1092.
7. Lin, Y.H.; Lin, L.Y.; Chen, A.; Wu, X.M.; Lee, J.K.; Su, T.C.; Wu, V.C.; Chueh, S.C.; Lin, W.C.; Lo, M.T.; et al. Adrenalectomy improves increased carotid intima-media thickness and arterial stiffness in patients with aldosterone producing adenoma. *Atherosclerosis* **2012**, *221*, 154–159.

8. Amar, L.; Plouin, P.F.; Steichen, O. Aldosterone-producing adenoma and other surgically correctable forms of primary aldosteronism. *Orphanet J. Rare Dis.* 2010, 5, 9.
9. Rossi, G.P.; Di Bello, V.; Ganzaroli, C.; Sacchetto, A.; Cesari, M.; Bertini, A.; Giorgi, D.; Scognamiglio, R.; Mariani, M.; Pessina, A.C. Excess ldosterone is associated with alterations of myocardial texture in primary aldosteronism. *Hypertension* 2002, 40, 23–27.
10. Choi, M.; Scholl, U.I.; Yue, P.; Bjorklund, P.; Zhao, B.; Nelson-Williams, C.; Ji, W.; Cho, Y.; Patel, A.; Men, C.J.; et al. K+ channel mutations in adrenal aldosterone-producing adenomas and hereditary hypertension. *Science* 2011, 331, 768–772.
11. El Zein, R.M.; Boulkroun, S.; Fernandes-Rosa, F.L.; Zennaro, M.C. Molecular genetics of conn adenomas in the era of exome analysis. *Presse Med.* 2018, 47, e151–e158.
12. De Sousa, K.; Boulkroun, S.; Baron, S.; Nanba, K.; Wack, M.; Rainey, W.E.; Rocha, A.; Giscos-Douriez, I.; Meatchi, T.; Amar, L.; et al. Genetic, cellular, and molecular heterogeneity in adrenals with aldosterone-producing adenoma. *Hypertension* 2020, 75, 1034–1044.
13. Nanba, K.; Omata, K.; Gomez-Sanchez, C.E.; Stratakis, C.A.; Demidowich, A.P.; Suzuki, M.; Thompson, L.D.R.; Cohen, D.L.; Luther, J.M.; Gellert, L.; et al. Genetic characteristics of aldosterone-producing adenomas in blacks. *Hypertension* 2019, 73, 885–892.
14. Nanba, K.; Omata, K.; Else, T.; Beck, P.C.C.; Nanba, A.T.; Turcu, A.F.; Miller, B.S.; Giordano, T.J.; Tomlins, S.A.; Rainey, W.E. Targeted molecular characterization of aldosterone-producing adenomas in white americans. *J. Clin. Endocrinol. Metab.* 2018, 103, 3869–3876.
15. Fernandes-Rosa, F.L.; Williams, T.A.; Riester, A.; Steichen, O.; Beuschlein, F.; Boulkroun, S.; Strom, T.M.; Monticone, S.; Amar, L.; Meatchi, T.; et al. Genetic spectrum and clinical correlates of somatic mutations in aldosterone-producing adenoma. *Hypertension* 2014, 64, 354–361.
16. Boulkroun, S.; Beuschlein, F.; Rossi, G.P.; Golib-Dzib, J.F.; Fischer, E.; Amar, L.; Mulatero, P.; Samson-Couterie, B.; Hahner, S.; Quinkler, M.; et al. Prevalence, clinical, and molecular correlates of kcnj5 mutations in primary aldosteronism. *Hypertension* 2012, 59, 592–598.
17. Lenzini, L.; Rossitto, G.; Maiolino, G.; Letizia, C.; Funder, J.W.; Rossi, G.P. A meta-analysis of somatic kcnj5 k(+) channel mutations in 1636 patients with an aldosterone-producing adenoma. *J. Clin. Endocrinol. Metab.* 2015, 100, E1089–E1095.
18. Wu, V.C.; Wang, S.M.; Chueh, S.J.; Yang, S.Y.; Huang, K.H.; Lin, Y.H.; Wang, J.J.; Connolly, R.; Hu, Y.H.; Gomez-Sanchez, C.E.; et al. The prevalence of ctnnb1 mutations in primary aldosteronism and consequences for clinical outcomes. *Sci. Rep.* 2017, 7, 39121.
19. Taguchi, R.; Yamada, M.; Nakajima, Y.; Satoh, T.; Hashimoto, K.; Shibusawa, N.; Ozawa, A.; Okada, S.; Rokutanda, N.; Takata, D.; et al. Expression and mutations of kcnj5 mrna in japanese patients with aldosterone-producing adenomas. *J. Clin. Endocrinol. Metab.* 2012, 97, 1311–1319.
20. Zheng, F.-F.; Zhu, L.-M.; Nie, A.-F.; Li, X.-Y.; Lin, J.-R.; Zhang, K.; Chen, J.; Zhou, W.-L.; Shen, Z.-J.; Zhu, Y.-C.; et al. Clinical characteristics of somatic mutations in the chinese patients with aldosterone-producing adenoma. *Hypertension* 2015, 65, 622–628.
21. Hong, A.R.; Kim, J.H.; Song, Y.S.; Lee, K.E.; Seo, S.H.; Seong, M.-W.; Shin, C.S.; Kim, S.W.; Kim, S.Y. Genetics of aldosterone-producing adenoma in korean patients. *PLoS ONE* 2016, 11, e0147590.
22. Rossi, G.P.; Cesari, M.; Letizia, C.; Seccia, T.M.; Cicala, M.V.; Zinnamosca, L.; Kuppusamy, M.; Mareso, S.; Sciomer, S.; Iacobone, M.; et al. Kcnj5 gene somatic mutations affect cardiac remodelling but do not preclude cure of high blood pressure and regression of left ventricular hypertrophy in primary aldosteronism. *J. Hypertens.* 2014, 32, 1514–1521, discussion 1522.
23. Kitamoto, T.; Suematsu, S.; Matsuzawa, Y.; Saito, J.; Omura, M.; Nishikawa, T. Comparison of cardiovascular complications in patients with and without kcnj5 gene mutations harboring aldosterone-producing adenomas. *J. Atheroscler. Thromb.* 2015, 22, 191–200.
24. Wu, V.C.; Huang, K.H.; Peng, K.Y.; Tsai, Y.C.; Wu, C.H.; Wang, S.M.; Yang, S.Y.; Lin, L.Y.; Chang, C.C.; Lin, Y.H.; et al. Prevalence and clinical correlates of somatic mutation in aldosterone producing adenoma-taiwanese population. *Sci. Rep.* 2015, 5, 11396.
25. Chang, Y.Y.; Tsai, C.H.; Peng, S.Y.; Chen, Z.W.; Chang, C.C.; Lee, B.C.; Liao, C.W.; Pan, C.T.; Chen, Y.L.; Lin, L.C.; et al. Kcnj5 somatic mutations in aldosterone-producing adenoma are associated with a worse baseline status and better recovery of left ventricular remodeling and diastolic function. *Hypertension* 2021, 77, 114–125.
26. Chang, C.H.; Hu, Y.H.; Tsai, Y.C.; Wu, C.H.; Wang, S.M.; Lin, L.Y.; Lin, Y.H.; Satoh, F.; Wu, K.D.; Wu, V.C. Arterial stiffness and blood pressure improvement in aldosterone-producing adenoma harboring kcnj5 mutations after adrenalectomy. *Oncotarget* 2017, 8, 29984–29995.
27. Williams, T.A.; Lenders, J.W.M.; Mulatero, P.; Burrello, J.; Rottenkolber, M.; Adolf, C.; Satoh, F.; Amar, L.; Quinkler, M.; Deinum, J.; et al. Outcomes after adrenalectomy for unilateral primary aldosteronism: An international consensus on outcome measures and analysis of remission rates in an international cohort. *Lancet Diabetes Endocrinol.* 2017, 5, 689–699.
28. Wu, V.C.; Hu, Y.H.; Er, L.K.; Yen, R.F.; Chang, C.H.; Chang, Y.L.; Lu, C.C.; Chang, C.C.; Lin, J.H.; Lin, Y.H.; et al. Case detection and diagnosis of primary aldosteronism—the consensus of taiwan society of aldosteronism. *J. Formos. Med. Assoc.* 2017, 116, 993–1005.
29. Rossi, G.P.; Belfiore, A.; Bernini, G.; Desideri, G.; Fabris, B.; Ferri, C.; Giacchetti, G.; Letizia, C.; Maccario, M.; Mallamaci, F.; et al. Comparison of the captopril and the saline infusion test for excluding aldosterone-producing adenoma. *Hypertension* 2007, 50, 424–431.
30. Wu, V.C.; Chang, H.W.; Liu, K.L.; Lin, Y.H.; Chueh, S.C.; Lin, W.C.; Ho, Y.L.; Huang, J.W.; Chiang, C.K.; Yang, S.Y.; et al. Primary aldosteronism: Diagnostic accuracy of the losartan and captopril tests. *Am. J. Hypertens.* 2009, 22, 821–827.
31. Wu, V.C.; Yang, S.Y.; Lin, J.W.; Cheng, B.W.; Kuo, C.C.; Tsai, C.T.; Chu, T.S.; Huang, K.H.; Wang, S.M.; Lin, Y.H.; et al. Kidney impairment in primary aldosteronism. *Clin. Chim. Acta* 2011, 412, 1319–1325.

32. Schwartz, G.L.; Turner, S.T. Screening for primary aldosteronism in essential hypertension: Diagnostic accuracy of the ratio of plasma aldosterone concentration to plasma renin activity. *Clin. Chem.* **2005**, *51*, 386–394.
33. Chao, C.T.; Wu, V.C.; Kuo, C.C.; Lin, Y.H.; Chang, C.C.; Chueh, S.J.; Wu, K.D.; Pimenta, E.; Stowasser, M. Diagnosis and management of primary aldosteronism: An updated review. *Ann. Med.* **2013**, *45*, 375–383.
34. McDonald, D.A. Regional pulse-wave velocity in the arterial tree. *J. Appl. Physiol.* **1968**, *24*, 73–78.
35. Nomura, K.; Toraya, S.; Horiba, N.; Ujihara, M.; Aiba, M.; Demura, H. Plasma aldosterone response to upright posture and angiotensin ii infusion in aldosterone-producing adenoma. *J. Clin. Endocrinol. Metab.* **1992**, *75*, 323–327.
36. Novitsky, Y.W.; Kercher, K.W.; Rosen, M.J.; Cobb, W.S.; Jyothinagaram, S.; Heniford, B.T. Clinical outcomes of laparoscopic adrenalectomy for lateralizing nodular hyperplasia. *Surgery* **2005**, *138*, 1009–1017.
37. Azizan, E.A.B.; Murthy, M.; Stowasser, M.; Gordon, R.; Kowalski, B.; Xu, S.; Brown, M.J.; O'Shaughnessy, K.M. Somatic mutations affecting the selectivity filter of kcnj5 are frequent in 2 large unselected collections of adrenal aldosteronomas. *Hypertension* **2012**, *59*, 587–591.
38. Laurent, S.; Boutouyrie, P.; Asmar, R.; Gautier, I.; Laloux, B.; Guize, L.; Ducimetiere, P.; Benetos, A. Aortic stiffness is an independent predictor of all-cause and cardiovascular mortality in hypertensive patients. *Hypertension* **2001**, *37*, 1236–1241.
39. Munakata, M. Brachial-ankle pulse wave velocity in the measurement of arterial stiffness: Recent evidence and clinical applications. *Curr. Hypertens. Rev.* **2014**, *10*, 49–57.
40. Cortez-Cooper, M.Y.; Supak, J.A.; Tanaka, H. A new device for automatic measurements of arterial stiffness and ankle-brachial index. *Am. J. Cardiol.* **2003**, *91*, 1519–1522.
41. Wang, J.W.; Zhou, Z.Q.; Hu, D.Y. Prevalence of arterial stiffness in north china, and associations with risk factors of cardiovascular disease: A community-based study. *BMC Cardiovasc. Disord.* **2012**, *12*, 119.
42. Ninomiya, T.; Kojima, I.; Doi, Y.; Fukuhara, M.; Hirakawa, Y.; Hata, J.; Kitazono, T.; Kiyohara, Y. Brachial-ankle pulse wave velocity predicts the development of cardiovascular disease in a general japanese population: The hisayama study. *J. Hypertens.* **2013**, *31*, 477–483, discussion 483.
43. Vlachopoulos, C.; Aznaouridis, K.; Terentes-Printzios, D.; Ioakeimidis, N.; Stefanadis, C. Prediction of cardiovascular events and all-cause mortality with brachial-ankle elasticity index: A systematic review and meta-analysis. *Hypertension* **2012**, *60*, 556–562.
44. Sheng, C.S.; Li, Y.; Li, L.H.; Huang, Q.F.; Zeng, W.F.; Kang, Y.Y.; Zhang, L.; Liu, M.; Wei, F.F.; Li, G.L.; et al. Brachial-ankle pulse wave velocity as a predictor of mortality in elderly chinese. *Hypertension* **2014**, *64*, 1124–1130.
45. Snijder, M.B.; Stronks, K.; Agyemang, C.; Busschers, W.B.; Peters, R.J.; van den Born, B.J. Ethnic differences in arterial stiffness the helius study. *Int. J. Cardiol.* **2015**, *191*, 28–33.
46. Callera, G.E.; Touyz, R.M.; Tostes, R.C.; Yogi, A.; He, Y.; Malkinson, S.; Schiffrin, E.L. Aldosterone activates vascular p38map kinase and nadph oxidase via c-src. *Hypertension* **2005**, *45*, 773–779.
47. Ambrosino, P.; Lupoli, R.; Tortora, A.; Cacciapuoti, M.; Lupoli, G.A.; Tarantino, P.; Nasto, A.; Di Minno, M.N. Cardiovascular risk markers in patients with primary aldosteronism: A systematic review and meta-analysis of literature studies. *Int. J. Cardiol.* **2016**, *208*, 46–55.
48. Park, S.; Kim, J.B.; Shim, C.Y.; Ko, Y.G.; Choi, D.; Jang, Y.; Chung, N. The influence of serum aldosterone and the aldosterone-renin ratio on pulse wave velocity in hypertensive patients. *J. Hypertens.* **2007**, *25*, 1279–1283.
49. Cecelja, M.; Chowienczyk, P. Dissociation of aortic pulse wave velocity with risk factors for cardiovascular disease other than hypertension: A systematic review. *Hypertension* **2009**, *54*, 1328–1336.
50. Peng, K.Y.; Liao, H.W.; Chan, C.K.; Lin, W.C.; Yang, S.Y.; Tsai, Y.C.; Huang, K.H.; Lin, Y.H.; Chueh, J.S.; Wu, V.C. Presence of subclinical hypercortisolism in clinical aldosterone-producing adenomas predicts lower clinical success. *Hypertension* **2020**, *76*, 1537–1544.
51. Tang, L.; Li, X.; Wang, B.; Ma, X.; Li, H.; Gao, Y.; Gu, L.; Nie, W.; Zhang, X. Clinical characteristics of aldosterone- and cortisol-coproducing adrenal adenoma in primary aldosteronism. *Int. J. Endocrinol.* **2018**, *2018*, 4920841.
52. Beuschlein, F.; Boulkroun, S.; Osswald, A.; Wieland, T.; Nielsen, H.N.; Lichtenauer, U.D.; Penton, D.; Schack, V.R.; Amar, L.; Fischer, E.; et al. Somatic mutations in atp1a1 and atp2b3 lead to aldosterone-producing adenomas and secondary hypertension. *Nat. Genet.* **2013**, *45*, 440–444.
53. Scholl, U.I.; Goh, G.; Stolting, G.; de Oliveira, R.C.; Choi, M.; Overton, J.D.; Fonseca, A.L.; Korah, R.; Starker, L.F.; Kunstman, J.W.; et al. Somatic and germline cacna1d calcium channel mutations in aldosterone-producing adenomas and primary aldosteronism. *Nat. Genet.* **2013**, *45*, 1050–1054.
54. Scholl, U.I.; Healy, J.M.; Thiel, A.; Fonseca, A.L.; Brown, T.C.; Kunstman, J.W.; Horne, M.J.; Dietrich, D.; Riemer, J.; Kücükköylü, S.; et al. Novel somatic mutations in primary hyperaldosteronism are related to the clinical, radiological and pathological phenotype. *Clin. Endocrinol.* **2015**, *83*, 779–789.
55. Shahin, Y.; Khan, J.A.; Chetter, I. Angiotensin converting enzyme inhibitors effect on arterial stiffness and wave reflections: A meta-analysis and meta-regression of randomised controlled trials. *Atherosclerosis* **2012**, *221*, 18–33.
56. Frimodt-Møller, M.; Kamper, A.L.; Strandgaard, S.; Kreiner, S.; Nielsen, A.H. Beneficial effects on arterial stiffness and pulse-wave reflection of combined enalapril and candesartan in chronic kidney disease—A randomized trial. *PLoS ONE* **2012**, *7*, e41757.
57. Anan, F.; Takahashi, N.; Ooie, T.; Yufu, K.; Hara, M.; Nakagawa, M.; Yonemochi, H.; Saikawa, T.; Yoshimatsu, H. Effects of valsartan and perindopril combination therapy on left ventricular hypertrophy and aortic arterial stiffness in patients with essential hypertension. *Eur. J. Clin. Pharmacol.* **2005**, *61*, 353–359.

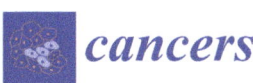

Article

Characteristics of a Novel *ATP2B3* K416_F418delinsN Mutation in a Classical Aldosterone-Producing Adenoma

Hung-Wei Liao [1],[†], Kang-Yung Peng [2],[†], Vin-Cent Wu [2], Yen-Hung Lin [2], Shuei-Liong Lin [2], Wei-Chou Lin [3], Jeff S. Chueh [4],* and on behalf of (TAIPAI) Study Group[‡]

1. Chinru Clinic, Taipei 116, Taiwan; lhw898@gmail.com
2. Department of Internal Medicine, National Taiwan University Hospital, Taipei 110, Taiwan; kangyung@ntu.edu.tw (K.-Y.P.); q91421028@ntu.edu.tw (V.-C.W.); yenhunglin@ntuh.gov.tw (Y.-H.L.); linsl@ntu.edu.tw (S.-L.L.)
3. Department of Pathology, National Taiwan University Hospital, National Taiwan University College of Medicine, Taipei 100, Taiwan; weichou8@ntuh.gov.tw
4. Department of Urology, College of Medicine, National Taiwan University, National Taiwan University Hospital, Taipei 110, Taiwan
* Correspondence: scchueh@ntu.edu.tw; Tel.: +886-2-23123456 (ext. 63098)
† These authors contributed equally to this work.
‡ Membership of the (TAIPAI) Study Group is provided in the Acknowledgments.

Simple Summary: The *ATP2B3* channel mutation is a rare cause of primary aldosteronism (PA). *ATP2B3* gene mutation leads to the dysfunction of calcium channel that pumps calcium ion out of the cell and accumulates intracellular calcium signal to stimulate aldosterone synthesis. In the present study, we found a novel somatic *ATP2B3* K416_F418delinsN mutation in a PA patient, and proved its functionality by demonstrating aldosterone hyper-function in the mutant-transfected adrenal cell-line. The *ATP2B3* K416_F418delinsN mutation resulted from the deletion from nucleotides 1248 to 1253. The translated amino acid sequence from 416 to 418 as lysine-phenylalanine-phenylalanine was deleted and an asparagine was inserted due to the merging of residual nucleotide sequences.

Abstract: In patients with primary aldosteronism (PA), the prevalence of *ATP2B3* mutation is rare. The aim of this study is to report a novel *ATP2B3* mutation in a PA patient. Based on our tissue bank of aldosterone-producing adenomas (APA), we identified a novel somatic *ATP2B3* K416_F418delinsN mutation. The affected individual was a 53 year-old man with a 4 year history of hypertension. Computed tomography (CT) showed bilateral adrenal masses of 1.6 (left) and 0.5 cm (right) in size. An adrenal venous sampling (AVS) showed a lateralization index (LI) of 2.2 and a contralateral suppression index (CLS) of 0.12; indicating left functional predominance. After a left unilateral adrenalectomy, he achieved partial biochemical and hypertension–remission. This classical adenoma harbored a novel *ATP2B3* K416_F418delinsN somatic mutation, which is a deletion from nucleotides 1248 to 1253. The translated amino acid sequence from 416 to 418, reading as lysine-phenylalanine-phenylalanine, was deleted; however, an asparagine was inserted due to merging of residual nucleotide sequences. The CYP11B2 immunohistochemistry staining demonstrated strong immunoreactivity in this classical adenoma. The *ATP2B3* K416_F418delinsN mutation is a functional mutation in APA, since HAC15 cells, a human adrenal cell line, transfected with the mutant gene showed increased CYP11B2 expression and aldosterone production.

Keywords: aldosterone producing adenoma; ATP2B3; K416-F418delinsN mutation; primary aldosteronism

1. Introduction

Primary aldosteronism (PA) is originally classified into unilateral hyperaldosteronism and bilateral hyperaldosteronism (BHA) [1]. BHA is mainly related to bilateral idiopathic hyperplasia, which could not be detected by computed tomography (CT) [1–3]. Bilateral aldosterone producing adenoma (APA) [4] could be detected as bilateral detectable mass by CT but is a rare finding [1]. The pathogenesis of patients affected by bilateral PA, thought related to BHA, could not be confirmed, because few patients with bilateral PA underwent adrenalectomy, and no such adrenal tissues could be obtained for further investigation. Many somatic mutant genes have been identified that enhance aldosterone secretion; in particular, mutations in *KCNJ5* [5], *CACNA1D* [6], *CACNA1H* [7], *CLCN2* [8], *ATP1A1* [9], and *ATP2B3* [9] genes have been identified. These mutant genes are often related to changes in the function or permeability of ion channels or ion pumps across cell membranes [10].

The aldosterone synthase (CYP11B2) transcription and aldosterone production rely on increased intracellular calcium signaling [10]. After stimulation, zona glomerulosa cells are depolarized and voltage-gated calcium (Ca^{2+}) channels on cellular membrane are activated. Subsequently, an influx of extracellular calcium occurs and increases intracellular calcium concentrations and downstream signaling. The ion channel ATP2B3, a Ca^{2+} ATPase type 3, is a protein pump over cellular membrane that exports intracellular calcium out of cells [11]. The mutated *ATP2B3* in aldosterone-producing cells may reduce efflux of calcium ions from cytoplasm, accumulate intracellular calcium, and stimulate aldosterone production [12].

The prevalence of *ATP2B3* mutation in PA is quite low [9]; ranging 1.6% [9]~0.9% [13] from European cohorts. In our previous report, the prevalence of mutated *ATP2B3* gene among our PA patients in Taiwan was 0.5% [14]. In this research, we described a novel mutation of *ATP2B3* K416_F418delinsN in an APA patient who underwent ipsilateral adrenalectomy, and illustrated his clinical characteristics.

2. Materials and Methods

2.1. Ethics Statement

Ethics approval (approval number 200611031R) was approved by the Institutional Review Committee of National Taiwan University Hospital. Before participating in the study, we obtained a written informed consent form from all participants to collect and study clinical data.

2.2. Diagnosis of PA

Based on the Taiwan standard TAIPAI protocol and the consensus on hyperaldosteronism, the referral of patients with hypertension was screened, confirmed and subtyped for PA patients [15,16]. Prior to the PA screening and confirmation test, all original antihypertensive drugs were discontinued for at least 21 days. We prescribed doxazosin and/or diltiazem during the evaluation phase as needed to control markedly hypertension. The diagnosis of PA in patients with hypertension was according to the abnormal hypersecretion of aldosterone and met the criteria [16–26].

2.3. Genomic DNA Extraction

Tumoral and adjacent adrenal tissue's genomic DNA was extracted by using QIAamp DNA mini kit (Qiagen, Hilden, Germany); genomic DNA from peripheral whole blood was extracted by using Blood DNA Isolation Kit (Geneaid Biotech; New Taipei City, Taiwan) according to the manufacturer's instructions.

2.4. ATP2B3 Gene Sequencing

The coding regions containing well- characterized mutations of *ATP2B3* gene were amplified and sequenced by using gene-specific primers and the BigDye® Terminator v3.1 Cycle Sequencing Kit (Applied Biosystems Inc., Foster City, CA, USA) on the 3730 DNA Analyzer (Applied Biosystems, Foster City, CA, USA). The primers of polymerase chain reaction (PCR) used to amplify fragments for *ATP2B3* direct sequencing followed that from a previous report [21] (forward CCTGGGCTGTTTATCCTGAA, reverse CCCCAGTTTCCGAGTCTGTA). The sequences analysis was performed by using the DNAStar Lasergene SeqMan Pro 7.1.0 software (DNAStar Inc., Madison, WI, USA).

2.5. Immunohistochemistry of Resected Tissues

The CYP11B2 and 17α-hydroxylase (CYP17A1) mouse monoclonal antibody, CYP11B1 rat monoclonal antibody (generous gifts from Professor Celso Gomez-Sanchez [27]), and HSD3B mouse monoclonal antibody (Abnova, Taipei, Taiwan) were used for immunohistochemistry (IHC) [28]. The polymerized horseradish peroxidase (HRP)-anti-mouse conjugate method (Novolink; Novocastra Laboratories Ltd., Newcastle Upon Tyne, UK) was used to stain sections of paraffin-embedded adrenal tumors and surrounding tissues according to the manufacturer's instructions [14]. The images were captured by Olympus BX51 fluorescence microscope combined with Olympus DP72 camera and cell Sens Standard 1.14 software (Olympus, Hamburg, Germany) was used for image analysis.

2.6. Culture of Cell Line

We used HAC15 cell, a human adrenocortical cell line, which express aldosterone synthase, CYP11B2, and secrete aldosterone for aldosterone production study. The HAC 15 cell line was obtained from generous Dr. Silvia Monticone [29]. HAC15 cells were cultured in HAC15 complete media containing DMEM:F12 (1:1) supplemented with 10% cosmic calf serum, 1× ITS, 1% penicillin–streptomycin and 100 μg/mL primocin at 37 °C. We used humidified incubator with 5% CO_2 to incubate the cultured cells, as previously reported [17].

2.7. Plasmid and Transfection

We used PCR-assisted, site-directed mutagenesis for the plasmids, expressing the wild-type and mutant *ATP2B3* genes and cloning into the pIRES-GFP-puro vector. PCR-based direct sequencing confirmed that the mutation was successfully cloned into the vector. Moreover, 3×10^6 cells HAC15 cells were transiently transfected with 3 μg pIRES-GFP empty vector, pIRES-GFP-wild-type *ATP2B3* or pIRES-GFP *ATP2B3* K416_F418delinsN using the Amaxa Cell Line Nucleofector Kit R (Lonza, Cologne, Germany) and the Nucleofector I (program X-005), according to the instructions of the manufacturer. After transfection, we seeded the HAC15 cells with a density of 1×10^6 cells/well into a 6-well plate. Furthermore, 72 h after the transfection, the cells and culture supernatants were harvested for Western blot analysis and aldosterone measurement.

2.8. Western Blot Analysis

Using RIPA buffer (50 mM Tris base pH 8, 150 mM NaCl, 1% NP40, 0.10% SDS) containing a protease inhibitor (Roche Diagnostics, Indianapolis, IN, USA), proteins were isolated from whole cell extracts. After we centrifuged the cell lysates, the supernatants were mixed with 3× sample buffer (30% glycerol, 15% 2-mercaptoethanol and 1% bromophenol blue). The proteins were separated through 12% SDS-PAGE gels and electrophoretic transferred to PVDF membranes. The membranes were then blocked by incubating in the BlockPRO™ blocking buffer (Visual Protein Biotechnology, Taipei, Taiwan) for 1 h blocking buffer containing anti-CYP11B2 mouse monoclonal antibody (a kind gift from Professor Celso Gomez-Sanchez) and anti-GAPDH antibody were incubated overnight at 4 °C. Extensive washing was conducted by Tris-buffered saline containing 0.1% Tween-20 (TBST) buffer. We further incubated the transfer membranes in blocking buffer that contained HRP-conjugated secondary antibodies for 1.5 h. Subsequently, the membranes were washed with TBST three times. Enhanced chemiluminescent reagent (Thermo Scientific, Rockford, IL, USA) was applied at a ratio of 1:1. Reagents for Chemiluminescence detection (Millipore, Billerica, MA, USA) were used to detect protein levels, and UVP Biospectrum 810 imaging system (Ultra Violet Products Ltd., Cambridge, UK) was used for visualization. We quantified protein expression in each sample by using UVP software (Ultra Violet Products Ltd., Cambridge, UK). A densitometry analysis of each protein band was normalized to GAPDH levels and expressed as a relative fold change when compared with the non-transfected control.

2.9. Analysis of Aldosterone

The culture supernatants were collected 72 h after cells transfected with *ATP2B3* K416_F418delinsN mutant or wild type plasmids to measure aldosterone concentration (ALDO-RIACT RIA kit, Cisbio Bioassays, Codolet, France) [28].

2.10. Statistical Analysis

The experimental differences between the transfected gene groups were analyzed by one-way ANOVA with post hoc least significant difference test (LSD) tests. A two-sided p value < 0.05 was defined as statistically significant. All of the statistical analyses were performed using IBM SPSS statistics version 19 (IBM Corp, Armonk, NY, USA) software.

3. Results

3.1. Identifying the ATP2B3 K416_F418delinsN Gene and Demographics of the Specific Patient

In DNA samples extracted from APA tumor tissues, we identified the mutant *ATP2B3* gene in a left adrenal adenoma. The affected individual was a 53 year-old man. He had a history of hypertension for more than 4 years and presented with uncontrollable hypertension and hypokalemia (2.8 mEq/L) for further survey. After the standardized screening and confirmation tests, his PA was diagnosed. A computer tomography scan showed a left 1.6 cm and a right 0.5 cm adrenal masses. An adrenal venous sampling (AVS) showed functionally predominant aldosterone hypersecretion over his left adrenal gland (Table 1). The lateralization index (LI) was 2.2 and the contralateral suppression index (CLS) was 0.12. The result of the iodine-131 6-beta-iodomethyl-19-norcholesterol adrenal scintigraphy (NP-59 scan) was also compatible with a functional left adrenal adenoma. After a left adrenalectomy, his hypertension achieved clinical partial remission, with reduced doses of anti-hypertensive medications (Table 1). In the postoperative biochemical tests, hypokalemia was resolved; however, the aldosterone to renin ratio (ARR) remained high. Therefore, biochemical outcome reached only partial success [30].

This novel *ATP2B3* K416_F418delinsN somatic mutation was identified only in the resected adrenal tissue, but not in peripheral blood cells and adjacent adrenal tissue. The *ATP2B3* K416_F418delinsN somatic mutation resulted from the deletion at nucleotide 1248 to 1253 as GTTCTT (Figure 1). The resulting amino acid sequence showed the deletion of 416 lysine (Lys, K), 417 phenylalanine (Phe, F) and 418 phenylalanine (Phe, F) due to the deletion of the nucleotide from 1248 to 1253 (Figure 1). However, a new amino acid, asparagine, was found due to merged nucleotides from 1246, 1247 and 1254. Therefore, the original amino acid sequence as lysine-phenylalanine- phenylalanine was not encoded, but instead a new amino acid, asparagine, was inserted.

3.2. The Immunochemistry Staining of CYP11B2 on Excised Adrenal Tissue

The gross slide section showed a well-demarcated and easily identified classical APA in the excised adrenal gland. The steroid 18-hydroxylase (CYP11B2; aldosterone synthase) IHC staining showed intense density within that compact zona glomerulosa (ZG)-like adenoma (Figure 2). No CYP11B2 IHC staining was found in the adjacent adrenal cortical tissues. For other steroidogenesis related enzymes, such as 3β-Hydroxysteroid dehydrogenase (HSD3B), 17α-hydroxylase (CYP17A1), and 11β-hydroxylase (CYP11B1), their IHC staining was not enhanced in the adenoma, but was observed in the adjacent adrenal gland tissues.

Table 1. The basal characteristics of the uPA patient with adenoma harboring ATP2B3 K416-F418delinsN deletion patient.

Variables	ATP2B3 K416_F418delinsN Mutation
Age (years old)	53
Sex	male
Body weight (kg)	75
BMI (kg/m^2)	25.95
CT mass size (cm)	Left: 1.6; Right: 0.5
AVS (aldosterone, ng/dL)/cortisol (μg/dL)	
CLS	0.12
LI	2.2
NP-59	Bilateral adrenal gland hyperfunction with left side predominance
Hypertension duration (years)	4
SBP (mm Hg)	197
SBP 12 mon	158
DBP (mm Hg)	92
DBP 12 mon	88
Aldosterone level (ng/dL) [†]	59.3
PRA (ng/mL/hr) [†]	0.55
ARR(ng/dL per ng/mL/h)	107.82
K (mEq/L) [†]	2.8
At 12 months after adrenalectomy	
Aldosterone level	30.5
PRA	0.09
K (mEq/L) [†]	4.0
ARR (ng/dL per ng/mL/h)	338.33
Clinical success	partial success [§]
Biochemical success	partial success

Abbreviations: ARR, aldosterone renin ratio; BMI, body mass index; CLS: contralateral suppression index; DBP, diastolic blood pressure; K, potassium; LI, lateralization index; NP-59, The iodine-131 6-beta-iodomethyl-19-norcholesterol adrenal scintigraphy; PA, primary aldosteronism; PRA, plasma renin activity; SBP, systolic blood pressure. [§] Partial success represents that the same blood pressure as before surgery but with less antihypertensive medication or decreased BP by the same or less antihypertensive medication. [†] Obtained after withholding drugs that interfere with the renin-angiotensin system.

3.3. The Aldosterone Synthase of ATP2B3 K416-F418delinsN Mutation

We transfected the mutant ATP2B3 K416_F418delinsN gene to HAC15 cells and investigated the physiological effects of this novel mutation. The expression of CYP11B2 in mutant-gene transfected cells was increased compared to that of control cells transfected with empty vector or wild type ATP2B3 (Figure 3). The aldosterone levels in the supernatant of the culture medium were higher in mutant-gene transfected cells compared to that from control vector or the wild type cells. Thus, the deletion of amino acid expression of lysine, and two phenylalanine residues from 416 to 418, along with an insertion of asparagine, showed a gain-of-function mutation at ATP2B3 channel for aldosterone over-production.

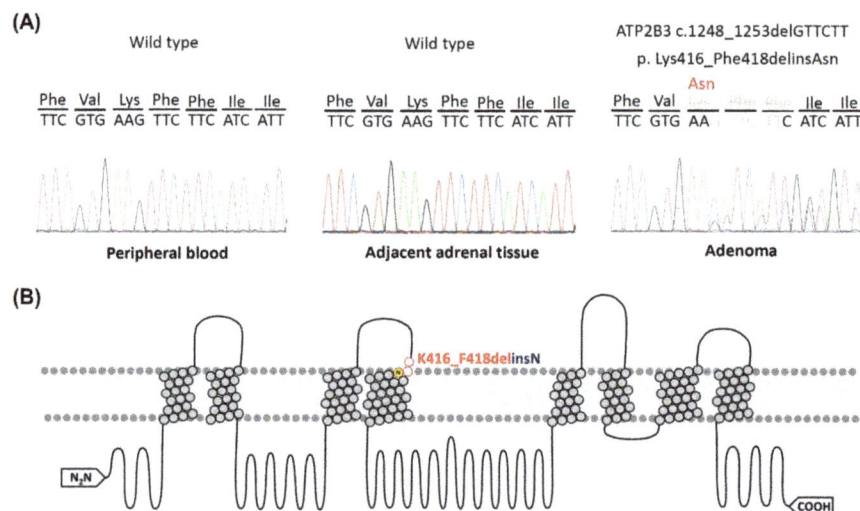

Figure 1. A novel *ATP2B3* K416-F418delinsN mutation in classical APA. (**A**) The deletion at nucleotide 1248 to 1253 as GTTCTT in the *ATP2B3* K416-F418delinsN gene was identified in a patient with APA in the resected adrenal adenoma. The amino acid residue 416 to 418 of ATP2B3 protein was substituted from lysine (Lys) and 2 phenylalanine (Phe) to asparagine (Asn) insertion. The letters for nucleotide bases represented as following: C, cytosine; G, guanine; T, thymine; (**B**) the protein secondary structure of mutant ATP2B3 channel was demonstrated. The yellow circle N represented insertion of amino acid, asparagine. The model was based on Protter software application [31] (http://wlab.ethz.ch/protter/start/ (accessed on 22 July 2021) [32]).

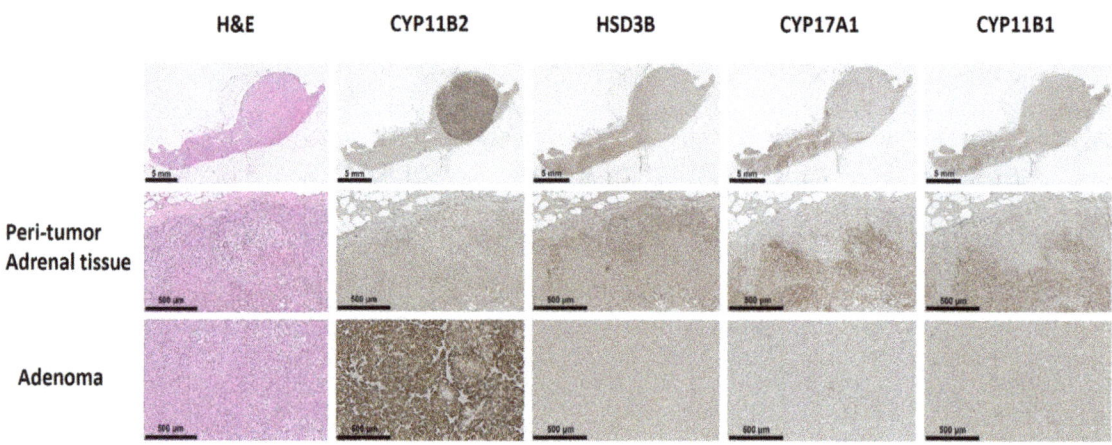

Figure 2. The immunohistochemistry staining in unilateral PA patients with the *ATP2B3* K416-F418delinsN mutations. The CYP11B2 and other steroidogenesis related enzyme IHC staining was conducted. The CYP11B2 immunoactivity was stained intensely within the adenoma, but did not stain in the adjacent adrenal gland tissue. Of note, HSD3B, CYP17A1 and CYP11B1 did not observed with adenoma but scattered in the residual adrenal gland tissue. Scale bar represented 500 μm.

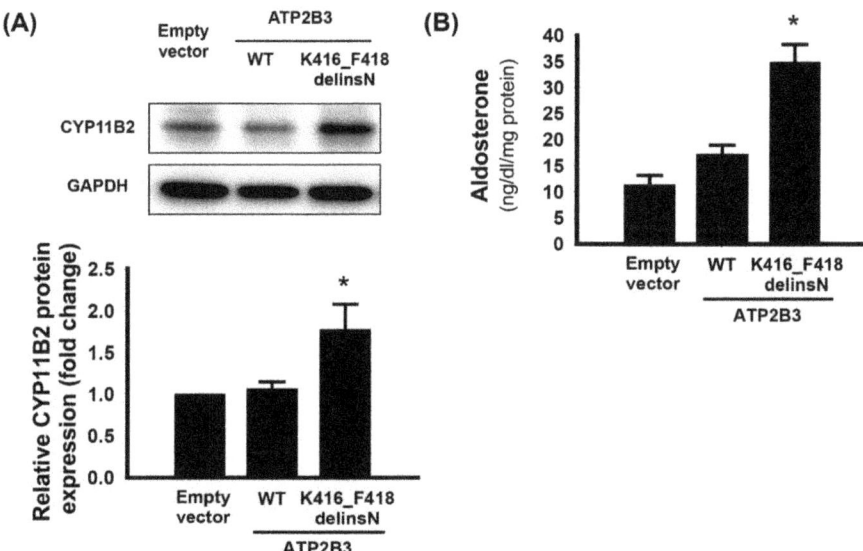

Figure 3. The CYP11B2 synthase and aldosterone production in the HAC 15 cells with transfected *ATP2B3* K416_F418delinsN. The aldosterone synthase, CYP1B2, expression and supernatant aldosterone levels were analyzed at 72 h after plasmid transfection. (**A**) The cells transfected with *ATP2B3* K416_F418delinsN had increased CYP11B2 protein expression in compared with the cells transfected with wild type cells; (**B**) The aldosterone levels of supernatant in the culture cells also increased in transfected group compared with the wild type cells. The data are presented as the means ± SD of three independent experiments in the transfected wild type and mutant cells. * $p < 0.05$ represented significant difference. The uncropped Western Blot image can be found in Figure S2.

4. Discussion

In this study, we found a novel functional somatic *ATP2B3* K416_F418delinsN mutant gene from our APA tissue bank. The histopathological examination showed a well-defined compact, ZG-like classical adenoma and intense immunoreactivity to CYP11B2 staining. The cells transfected with the indicated mutant gene demonstrated increased CYP11B2 expression and elevated aldosterone levels in the culture supernatant when compared with that of the wild-type cells. Moreover, we have used Sanger sequencing to confirm that there were no other conventional and well-characterized aldosterone-driving gene mutations, including *KCNJ5*, *ATP1A1*, *CACNA1D*, and *CTNNB1*, in the adenoma harboring with *ATP2B3* K416_F418delinsN mutation (Figure S1).

4.1. Calcium Channel and Somatic Mutations in APA

The transcription of *CYP11B2* could be activated by intracellular calcium signaling [33]. Consistently increased cytoplasmic calcium concentration or stimulation may lead to the excessive production of aldosterone [34], which is the main mechanism of PA. Mutant KCNJ5, and CLCN2 ion channels are involved in cellular membrane depolarization and subsequently activate voltage-gated Ca^{2+} channels to increase Ca^{2+} influx [34,35] into cytoplasm. However, ion channels of CACNA1D and CACNA1H control the entry of extracellular calcium, and enhance the Ca^{2+} permeability with their mutant voltage-gated Ca^{2+} channels. Unlike other channels that increase intracellular calcium by affecting Ca^{2+} entry, the mutated ATP2B3 ion channel reduces Ca^{2+} export from cytoplasm. Thus, there are two possible ways to increase stimulating signaling in ATP2B3 ion channel [11]: (1) reduce clearance of intracellular calcium and directly stimulating *CYP11B2* transcription, and (2) accumulation of cation leads to Na^+ influx and subsequently depolarizes the cellular membrane and activates a downstream reaction [11].

4.2. Mutant ATP2B3 and APA

ATP2B3 ion channel belongs to plasma membrane Ca^{2+} ATPase (PMCA) transporter. The *ATP2B3* mutant APAs have higher serum aldosterone levels and lower potassium levels compared to other mutant genes related to APA [36].

Our index patient with *ATP2B3* K416_F418delinsN had uncontrollable hypertension and hypokalemia at presentation. In accordance with our finding, most identified *ATP2B3* mutation in APA were expressed mainly in ZG-like cells [37]. The IHC showed condensed CYP11B2 staining in the adenoma, but not in the peri-tumoral region. Therefore, the source of excess aldosterone could arise from the classical adenoma, in concordance with the location of the mutant gene. We have also confirmed that the adrenal tissue adjacent to the adenoma, besides that from white blood cells, carried wild-type *ATP2B3* gene by using Sanger sequencing (showed in the Figure 1A and Table S1).

4.3. Bilateral Asymmetric Manifestations of the APA

This patient had bilateral adrenal masses, and CT showed a larger mass on the left side. The LI of AVS was 2.2 (>2.0) [38], indicating a left functional predominance. The CLS was 0.12 (<1.0) [39,40], indicating the suppression of the right adrenal gland. The preoperative diagnosis was unilateral PA over the left adrenal gland. However, 1 year after left unilateral adrenalectomy, blood pressure control only achieved partial success. The serum potassium level was normalized from 2.8 to 4.0 mEq/L. However, the ARR after unilateral adrenalectomy remained high. According to the PASO consensus, the biochemical outcome achieved only partial success [30]. Thus, from the functional and clinical responses, this patient with *ATP2B3* K416_F418delinsN mutation may have abnormal contralateral adrenal gland and bilateral asymmetric aldosterone secretion. However, before the left total adrenalectomy, the aldosterone secretion from the right adrenal gland was suppressed by the left functional adenoma initially; once the patient underwent left adrenalectomy, the suppression from the left adrenal was gone, and the aldosterone secretion from the right adrenal gland, probably in the form of multiple aldosterone-producing micronodules (mAPM) or APA, may take over and contribute to the bilateral asymmetric disease, and led to his incomplete blood pressure and biochemical recovery.

4.4. Clinical Implication and Study Limitations

Different mutant genes of PA have specific pathophysiological, clinical and biochemical manifestations [36]. Identifying functional genes in PA would help physicians determine the course of the disease and make decision on treatment and follow-up. Patients with *ATP2B3* mutant APA have obvious aldosterone and potassium abnormalities [36]. Most reported that APA harboring *ATP2B3* mutant was unilateral APA. Our finding of this new mutation will help researchers in this field to incorporate this mutation in their future routine screening of the possible mutation spots, and the actual prevalence of this novel mutation will be further assured. Although left APA was confirmed by the AVS and resected, the pathophysiological characteristics in the contralateral adenoma could not be obtained. Furthermore, we have only one APA patient harboring this novel *ATP2B3* K416_F418delinsN gene and could not conclude a general relationship between the genotype and phenotype.

5. Conclusions

In conclusion, we identified a patient with an APA harboring a novel *ATP2B3* K416_F418delinsN somatic mutation. He became a partial hypertension-remission and biochemical success after unilateral adrenalectomy. HAC15 cells harboring this *ATP2B3* K416_F418delinsN somatic mutation increased CYP11B2 synthesis and aldosterone production. The immunohistochemistry staining showed a compact and well demarcated ZG-like adenoma, with intense CYP11B2 expression. Thus, this novel somatic mutation of *ATP2B3* K416_F418delinsN functionally increased aldosterone secretion, and it also showed a distinct histopathologic pattern, as well as an important clinical signature.

Supplementary Materials: The following are available online at https://www.mdpi.com/article/10.3390/cancers13184729/s1, Figure S1. Sanger sequencing analysis of tumor DNAs for conventional and well-characterized aldosterone-driving gene mutations, including *KCNJ5*, *ATP1A1*, *CACNA1D*, and *CTNNB1*, in the adenoma harboring with *ATP2B3* K416_F418delinsN mutation, Figure S2. Uncropped Western Blot images from Figure 3 in the main text, Table S1. Primers used for Sanger sequencing.

Author Contributions: Conceptualization, K.-Y.P. and V.-C.W.; methodology, K.-Y.P.; software, H.-W.L.; validation, Y.-H.L., S.-L.L. and W.-C.L.; formal analysis, H.-W.L. and K.-Y.P.; investigation, V.-C.W.; resources, V.-C.W.; data curation, K.-Y.P.; writing—original draft preparation, H.-W.L. and K.-Y.P.; writing—review and editing, V.-C.W. and J.S.C.; visualization, K.-Y.P. and V.-C.W.; supervision, J.S.C.; project administration, V.-C.W.; funding acquisition, V.-C.W. All authors have read and agreed to the published version of the manuscript.

Funding: This project was supported by National Health Research Institutes [PH-102-SP-09)], Ministry of Science and Technology, Taiwan, R.O.C. [MOST107-2314-B-002-026-MY3, 108-2314-B-002-058, 109-2314-B-002-174-MY3], National Taiwan University Hospital [109-S4634, PC-1264, PC-1309, VN109-09, UN109-041, UN110-030], Grant MOHW110-TDU-B-212-124005 and Mrs. Hsiu-Chin Lee Kidney Research Fund.

Institutional Review Board Statement: Ethics approval was approved by the Institutional Review Committee of National Taiwan University Hospital (approval number 200611031R; extended approval date: 3 August 2020).

Informed Consent Statement: Before participating in the study, a written informed consent statement for clinical data collection and research was obtained from all participants.

Data Availability Statement: The data are all included in the manuscript or can be acquired from the corresponding author.

Acknowledgments: The authors thank the staff of the Second Core Lab in the Department of Medical Research of National Taiwan University Hospital for technical assistance. Membership of the Taiwan Primary Aldosteronism Investigation (TAIPAI) Study Group: Tai-Shuan Lai; Vin-Cent Wu; Shao-Yu Yang; Kao-Lang Liu; Chin-Chen Chang; Bo-Chiag Lee; Shuo-Meng Wang; Kuo-How Huang; Po-Chih Lin; Yen-Hung Lin; Lian-Yu Lin; Shih-Cheng Liao; Ruoh-Fang Yen; Ching-Chu Lu; Shih-Chieh Jeff Chueh (National Taiwan University Hospital ,Taipei, Taiwan); Chieh-Kai Chan (NTUH Hsin-Chu branch); Leay-Kiaw Er; Ya-Hui Hu; Chia-Hui Chang; Che-Hsiung Wu; Yao-Chou Tsai (Taipei Tzu Chi Hospital, Buddhist Tzu Chi Medical Foundation, Taipei, Taiwan); Chen-Hsun Ho (Taipei Medical University-Shuang Ho Hospital, Ministry of Health and Welfare); Wei-Chieh Huang(Taipei Veterans General Hospital); Ying-Ying Chen (MacKay Memorial Hospital); Kwan-Dun Wu (National Taiwan University Hospital ,Taipei, Taiwan NTUH, Director of Coordinating Center).

Conflicts of Interest: No conflict of interest is declared. No financial conflict of interest exists.

References

1. Omata, K.; Satoh, F.; Morimoto, R.; Ito, S.; Yamazaki, Y.; Nakamura, Y.; Anand, S.K.; Guo, Z.; Stowasser, M.; Sasano, H.; et al. Cellular and Genetic Causes of Idiopathic Hyperaldosteronism. *Hypertension* **2018**, *72*, 874–880. [CrossRef]
2. Young, W.F. Diagnosis and treatment of primary aldosteronism: Practical clinical perspectives. *J. Intern. Med.* **2019**, *285*, 126–148. [CrossRef]
3. Kuo, C.-C.; Wu, V.-C.; Huang, K.-H.; Wang, S.-M.; Chang, C.-C.; Lu, C.-C.; Yang, W.-S.; Tsai, C.-W.; Lai, C.-F.; Lee, T.-Y.; et al. Verification and evaluation of aldosteronism demographics in the Taiwan Primary Aldosteronism Investigation Group (TAIPAI Group). *J. Renin-Angiotensin-Aldosterone Syst.* **2011**, *12*, 348–357. [CrossRef] [PubMed]
4. Wu, V.-C.; Chueh, S.; Chang, H.; Lin, W.-C.; Liu, K.-L.; Li, H.; Lin, Y.-H.; Wu, K.-D.; Hsieh, B. Bilateral aldosterone-producing adenomas: Differentiation from bilateral adrenal hyperplasia. *Qjm* **2007**, *101*, 13–22. [CrossRef]
5. Choi, M.; Scholl, U.I.; Yue, P.; Björklund, P.; Zhao, B.; Nelson-Williams, C.; Ji, W.; Cho, Y.; Patel, A.; Men, C.J.; et al. K+ Channel Mutations in Adrenal Aldosterone-Producing Adenomas and Hereditary Hypertension. *Science* **2011**, *331*, 768–772. [CrossRef] [PubMed]
6. Scholl, U.I.; Goh, G.; Stölting, G.; De Oliveira, R.C.; Choi, M.; Overton, J.D.; Fonseca, A.L.; Korah, R.; Starker, L.F.; Kunstman, J.; et al. Somatic and germline CACNA1D calcium channel mutations in aldosterone-producing adenomas and primary aldosteronism. *Nat. Genet.* **2013**, *45*, 1050–1054. [CrossRef] [PubMed]

7. Daniil, G.; Fernandes-Rosa, F.L.; Chemin, J.; Blesneac, I.; Beltrand, J.; Polak, M.; Jeunemaitre, X.; Boulkroun, S.; Amar, L.; Strom, T.M.; et al. CACNA1H Mutations Are Associated with Different Forms of Primary Aldosteronism. *EBioMedicine* **2016**, *13*, 225–236. [CrossRef] [PubMed]
8. Fernandes-Rosa, F.L.; Daniil, G.; Orozco, I.J.; Göppner, C.; El Zein, R.; Jain, V.; Boulkroun, S.; Jeunemaitre, X.; Amar, L.; Lefebvre, H.; et al. A gain-of-function mutation in the CLCN2 chloride channel gene causes primary aldosteronism. *Nat. Genet.* **2018**, *50*, 355–361. [CrossRef]
9. Beuschlein, F.; Boulkroun, S.; Osswald, A.; Wieland, T.; Nielsen, H.N.; Lichtenauer, U.D.; Penton, D.; Schack, V.R.; Amar, L.; Fischer, E.; et al. Somatic mutations in ATP1A1 and ATP2B3 lead to aldosterone-producing adenomas and secondary hypertension. *Nat. Genet.* **2013**, *45*, 441–442. [CrossRef]
10. Seccia, T.M.; Caroccia, B.; Gomez-Sanchez, E.P.; Gomez-Sanchez, C.E.; Rossi, G.P. The Biology of Normal Zona Glomerulosa And Aldosterone-Producing Adenoma: Pathological Implications. *Endocr. Rev.* **2018**, *39*, 1029–1056. [CrossRef]
11. Tauber, P.; Aichinger, B.; Christ, C.; Stindl, J.; Rhayem, Y.; Beuschlein, F.; Warth, R.; Bandulik, S. Cellular Pathophysiology of an Adrenal Adenoma-Associated Mutant of the Plasma Membrane Ca2+-ATPase ATP2B3. *Endocrinology* **2016**, *157*, 2489–2499. [CrossRef] [PubMed]
12. Fernandes-Rosa, F.L.; Boulkroun, S.; Zennaro, M.-C. Genetic and Genomic Mechanisms of Primary Aldosteronism. *Trends Mol. Med.* **2020**, *26*, 819–832. [CrossRef] [PubMed]
13. Williams, T.A.; Monticone, S.; Schack, V.R.; Stindl, J.; Burrello, J.; Buffolo, F.; Annaratone, L.; Castellano, I.; Beuschlein, F.; Reincke, M.; et al. Somatic ATP1A1, ATP2B3, and KCNJ5 Mutations in Aldosterone-Producing Adenomas. *Hypertension* **2014**, *63*, 188–195. [CrossRef]
14. Wu, V.-C.; Wang, S.-M.; Chueh, S.-C.J.; Yang, S.-Y.; Huang, K.-H.; Lin, Y.-H.; Wang, J.-J.; Connolly, R.; Hu, Y.-H.; Gomez-Sanchez, C.E.; et al. The prevalence of CTNNB1 mutations in primary aldosteronism and consequences for clinical outcomes. *Sci. Rep.* **2017**, *7*, 39121. [CrossRef] [PubMed]
15. Chao, C.-T.; Wu, V.-C.; Kuo, C.-C.; Lin, Y.-H.; Chang, C.-C.; Chueh, S.J.; Wu, K.-D.; Pimenta, E.; Stowasser, M. Diagnosis and management of primary aldosteronism: An updated review. *Ann. Med.* **2013**, *45*, 375–383. [CrossRef] [PubMed]
16. Wu, V.-C.; Hu, Y.-H.; Er, L.K.; Yen, R.-F.; Chang, C.-H.; Chang, Y.-L.; Lu, C.-C.; Chang, C.-C.; Lin, J.-H.; Lin, Y.-H.; et al. Case detection and diagnosis of primary aldosteronism—The consensus of Taiwan Society of Aldosteronism. *J. Formos. Med. Assoc.* **2017**, *116*, 993–1005. [CrossRef] [PubMed]
17. Peng, K.-Y.; Chang, H.-M.; Lin, Y.-F.; Chan, C.-K.; Chang, C.-H.; Chueh, S.-C.J.; Yang, S.-Y.; Huang, K.-H.; Lin, Y.-H.; Wu, V.-C.; et al. miRNA-203 Modulates Aldosterone Levels and Cell Proliferation by Targeting Wnt5a in Aldosterone-Producing Adenomas. *J. Clin. Endocrinol. Metab.* **2018**, *103*, 3737–3747. [CrossRef] [PubMed]
18. Peng, K.-Y.; Liao, H.-W.; Chan, C.-K.; Lin, W.-C.; Yang, S.-Y.; Tsai, Y.-C.; Huang, K.-H.; Lin, Y.-H.; Chueh, J.S.; Wu, V.-C. Presence of Subclinical Hypercortisolism in Clinical Aldosterone-Producing Adenomas Predicts Lower Clinical Success. *Hypertension* **2020**, *76*, 1537–1544. [CrossRef] [PubMed]
19. Wu, V.-C.; Kuo, C.-C.; Wang, S.-M.; Liu, K.-L.; Huang, K.-H.; Lin, Y.-H.; Chu, T.-S.; Chang, H.-W.; Lin, C.-Y.; Tsai, C.-T.; et al. Primary aldosteronism: Changes in cystatin C-based kidney filtration, proteinuria, and renal duplex indices with treatment. *J. Hypertens.* **2011**, *29*, 1778–1786. [CrossRef]
20. Wu, V.-C.; Lo, S.-C.; Chen, Y.-L.; Huang, P.-H.; Tsai, C.-T.; Liang, C.-J.; Kuo, C.-C.; Kuo, Y.-S.; Lee, B.-C.; Wu, E.-L.; et al. Endothelial Progenitor Cells in Primary Aldosteronism: A Biomarker of Severity for Aldosterone Vasculopathy and Prognosis. *J. Clin. Endocrinol. Metab.* **2011**, *96*, 3175–3183. [CrossRef]
21. Wu, V.-C.; Huang, K.-H.; Peng, K.-Y.; Tsai, Y.-C.; Wu, C.-H.; Wang, S.-M.; Yang, S.-Y.; Lin, L.-Y.; Chang, C.-C.; Lin, Y.-H.; et al. Prevalence and clinical correlates of somatic mutation in aldosterone producing adenoma-Taiwanese population. *Sci. Rep.* **2015**, *5*, 11396. [CrossRef]
22. Wu, V.-C.; Chueh, S.-C.; Chang, H.-W.; Lin, L.-Y.; Liu, K.-L.; Lin, Y.-H.; Ho, Y.-L.; Lin, W.-C.; Wang, S.-M.; Huang, K.-H.; et al. Association of Kidney Function With Residual Hypertension After Treatment of Aldosterone-Producing Adenoma. *Am. J. Kidney Dis.* **2009**, *54*, 665–673. [CrossRef] [PubMed]
23. Wu, V.-C.; Yang, S.-Y.; Lin, J.-W.; Cheng, B.-W.; Kuo, C.-C.; Tsai, C.-T.; Chu, T.-S.; Huang, K.-H.; Wang, S.-M.; Lin, Y.-H.; et al. Kidney impairment in primary aldosteronism. *Clin. Chim. Acta* **2011**, *412*, 1319–1325. [CrossRef] [PubMed]
24. Wu, V.-C.; Chang, H.-W.; Liu, K.-L.; Lin, Y.-H.; Chueh, S.-C.; Lin, W.-C.; Ho, Y.-L.; Huang, J.-W.; Chiang, C.-K.; Yang, S.-Y.; et al. Primary Aldosteronism: Diagnostic Accuracy of the Losartan and Captopril Tests. *Am. J. Hypertens.* **2009**, *22*, 821–827. [CrossRef] [PubMed]
25. Wu, V.-C.; Wang, S.-M.; Chang, C.-H.; Hu, Y.-H.; Lin, L.-Y.; Lin, Y.-H.; Chueh, S.-C.J.; Chen, L.; Wu, K.-D. Long term outcome of Aldosteronism after target treatments. *Sci. Rep.* **2016**, *6*, 32103. [CrossRef] [PubMed]
26. Chan, C.-K.; Yang, W.-S.; Lin, Y.-H.; Huang, K.-H.; Lu, C.-C.; Hu, Y.-H.; Wu, V.-C.; Chueh, J.S.; Chu, T.-S.; Chen, Y.-M. Arterial Stiffness is Associated with Clinical Outcome and Cardiorenal Injury in Lateralized Primary Aldosteronism. *J. Clin. Endocrinol. Metab.* **2020**, *105*. [CrossRef]
27. Gomez-Sanchez, C.E.; Qi, X.; Velarde-Miranda, C.; Plonczynski, M.W.; Parker, C.R.; Rainey, W.; Satoh, F.; Maekawa, T.; Nakamura, Y.; Sasano, H.; et al. Development of monoclonal antibodies against human CYP11B1 and CYP11B2. *Mol. Cell. Endocrinol.* **2014**, *383*, 111–117. [CrossRef]

28. Peng, K.-Y.; Liao, H.-W.; Chueh, J.S.; Pan, C.-Y.; Lin, Y.-H.; Chen, Y.-M.; Chen, P.-Y.; Huang, C.-L.; Wu, V.-C. Pathophysiological and Pharmacological Characteristics of *KCNJ5* 157-159delITE Somatic Mutation in Aldosterone-Producing Adenomas. *Biomedicines* **2021**, *9*, 1026. [CrossRef]
29. Monticone, S.; Hattangady, N.G.; Penton, D.; Isales, C.M.; Edwards, M.A.; Williams, T.A.; Sterner, C.; Warth, R.; Mulatero, P.; Rainey, W.E. a Novel Y152C KCNJ5 mutation responsible for familial hyperaldosteronism type III. *J. Clin. Endocrinol. Metab.* **2013**, *98*, E1861–E1865. [CrossRef]
30. Williams, T.A.; Lenders, J.W.M.; Mulatero, P.; Burrello, J.; Rottenkolber, M.; Adolf, C.; Satoh, F.; Amar, L.; Quinkler, M.; Deinum, J.; et al. Outcomes after adrenalectomy for unilateral primary aldosteronism: An international consensus on outcome measures and analysis of remission rates in an international cohort. *Lancet Diabetes Endocrinol.* **2017**, *5*, 689–699. [CrossRef]
31. Omasits, U.; Ahrens, C.; Müller, S.; Wollscheid, B. Protter: Interactive protein feature visualization and integration with experimental proteomic data. *Bioinformatics* **2014**, *30*, 884–886. [CrossRef] [PubMed]
32. Protter Software Application. Available online: http://wlab.ethz.ch/protter/start/ (accessed on 22 July 2021).
33. Nanba, K.; Chen, A.; Nishimoto, K.; Rainey, W.E. Role of Ca2+/Calmodulin-Dependent Protein Kinase Kinase in Adrenal Aldosterone Production. *Endocrinology* **2015**, *156*, 1750–1756. [CrossRef]
34. Seidel, E.; Schewe, J.; Scholl, U.I. Genetic causes of primary aldosteronism. *Exp. Mol. Med.* **2019**, *51*, 1–12. [CrossRef] [PubMed]
35. Fernandes-Rosa, F.L.; Boulkroun, S.; Zennaro, M.-C. Somatic and inherited mutations in primary aldosteronism. *J. Mol. Endocrinol.* **2017**, *59*, R47–R63. [CrossRef] [PubMed]
36. Fernandes-Rosa, F.L.; Williams, T.A.; Riester, A.; Steichen, O.; Beuschlein, F.; Boulkroun, S.; Strom, T.M.; Monticone, S.; Amar, L.; Meatchi, T.; et al. Genetic Spectrum and Clinical Correlates of Somatic Mutations in Aldosterone-Producing Adenoma. *Hypertension* **2014**, *64*, 354–361. [CrossRef]
37. Itcho, K.; Oki, K.; Ohno, H.; Yoneda, M. Update on Genetics of Primary Aldosteronism. *Biomedicines* **2021**, *9*, 409. [CrossRef] [PubMed]
38. Rossi, G.P.; Auchus, R.J.; Brown, M.; Lenders, J.W.; Naruse, M.; Plouin, P.F.; Satoh, F.; Young, W.F. An Expert Consensus Statement on Use of Adrenal Vein Sampling for the Subtyping of Primary Aldosteronism. *Hypertension* **2014**, *63*, 151–160. [CrossRef]
39. Kline, G.; Chin, A.; So, B.; Harvey, A.; Pasieka, J. Defining contralateral adrenal suppression in primary aldosteronism: Implications for diagnosis and outcome. *Clin. Endocrinol.* **2015**, *83*, 20–27. [CrossRef]
40. Lee, J.; Kang, B.; Ha, J.; Kim, M.-H.; Choi, B.; Hong, T.-H.; Kang, M.I.; Lim, D.-J. Clinical outcomes of primary aldosteronism based on lateralization index and contralateral suppression index after adrenal venous sampling in real-world practice: A retrospective cohort study. *BMC Endocr. Disord.* **2020**, *20*, 114. [CrossRef] [PubMed]

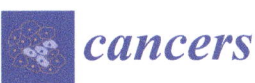

Article

Primary Aldosteronism: Metabolic Reprogramming and the Pathogenesis of Aldosterone-Producing Adenomas

Siyuan Gong [1], Martina Tetti [1,2], Martin Reincke [1] and Tracy Ann Williams [1,2,*]

[1] Medizinische Klinik und Poliklinik IV, Klinikum der Universität München, Ludwig-Maximilians-Universität München, 80336 Munich, Germany; Siyuan.Gong@med.uni-muenchen.de (S.G.); martina.tetti@med.uni-muenchen.de (M.T.); Martin.Reincke@med.uni-muenchen.de (M.R.)
[2] Department of Medical Sciences, Division of Internal Medicine and Hypertension, University of Turin, 10126 Turin, Italy
* Correspondence: tracy.williams@med.uni-muenchen.de; Tel.: +49-089-4400-52137

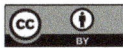

Citation: Gong, S.; Tetti, M.; Reincke, M.; Williams, T.A. Primary Aldosteronism: Metabolic Reprogramming and the Pathogenesis of Aldosterone-Producing Adenomas. *Cancers* **2021**, *13*, 3716. https://doi.org/10.3390/cancers13153716

Academic Editor: Adam E. Frampton

Received: 2 June 2021
Accepted: 21 July 2021
Published: 23 July 2021

Publisher's Note: MDPI stays neutral with regard to jurisdictional claims in published maps and institutional affiliations.

Copyright: © 2021 by the authors. Licensee MDPI, Basel, Switzerland. This article is an open access article distributed under the terms and conditions of the Creative Commons Attribution (CC BY) license (https://creativecommons.org/licenses/by/4.0/).

Simple Summary: Primary aldosteronism is a common form of endocrine hypertension often caused by a hyper-secreting tumor of the adrenal cortex called an aldosterone-producing adenoma. Metabolic reprogramming plays a role in tumor progression and influences the tumor immune microenvironment by limiting immune-cell infiltration and suppressing its anti-tumor function. We hypothesized that the development of aldosterone-producing adenomas involves metabolic adaptations of its component tumor cells and intrinsically influences tumor pathogenesis. Herein, we use state-of-the-art computational tools for the comprehensive analysis of array-based gene expression profiles to demonstrate metabolic reprogramming and remodeling of the immune microenvironment in aldosterone-producing adenomas compared with paired adjacent adrenal cortical tissue. Our findings suggest metabolic alterations may function in the pathogenesis of aldosterone-producing adenomas by conferring survival advantages to their component tumor cells.

Abstract: Aldosterone-producing adenomas (APAs) are characterized by aldosterone hypersecretion and deregulated adrenocortical cell growth. Increased energy consumption required to maintain cellular tumorigenic properties triggers metabolic alterations that shape the tumor microenvironment to acquire necessary nutrients, yet our knowledge of this adaptation in APAs is limited. Here, we investigated adrenocortical cell-intrinsic metabolism and the tumor immune microenvironment of APAs and their potential roles in mediating aldosterone production and growth of adrenocortical cells. Using multiple advanced bioinformatics methods, we analyzed gene expression datasets to generate distinct metabolic and immune cell profiles of APAs versus paired adjacent cortex. APAs displayed activation of lipid metabolism, especially fatty acid β-oxidation regulated by PPARα, and glycolysis. We identified an immunosuppressive microenvironment in APAs, with reduced infiltration of CD45+ immune cells compared with adjacent cortex, validated by CD45 immunohistochemistry (3.45-fold, $p < 0.001$). APAs also displayed an association of lipid metabolism with ferroptosis and upregulation of antioxidant systems. In conclusion, APAs exhibit metabolic reprogramming towards fatty acid β-oxidation and glycolysis. Increased lipid metabolism via PPARα may serve as a key mechanism to modulate lipid peroxidation, a hallmark of regulated cell death by ferroptosis. These findings highlight survival advantages for APA tumor cells with metabolic reprogramming properties.

Keywords: adaptive metabolism; adrenal gland; conn adenoma; fatty acid metabolism; ferroptosis; hyperaldosteronism; metabolic reprogramming; β-oxidation; PPARα; tumor microenvironment

1. Introduction

Primary aldosteronism (PA) is the most frequent secondary cause of hypertension characterized by the overproduction of aldosterone relatively autonomous of the renin-angiotensin system. PA is generally classified into unilateral and bilateral forms, which determine the surgical or pharmacological treatment of the disease [1]. The surgical management of unilateral PA has made available, as a side effect, tissue sample specimens for a wide range of scientific studies. Histopathology shows that the surgically removed adrenals mainly display an aldosterone-producing adenoma (APA) with somatic mutations in a few genes that cause constitutive aldosterone production [2–5]. The variants usually occur in genes that encode ion channels or ATPases and function in the regulation of cellular ion homeostasis [6]. Of these, the KCNJ5 inwardly rectifying potassium channel (also called GIRK4) displays the highest prevalence of variants in most reported populations. Furthermore, in vivo observations and in vitro findings suggest that KCNJ5 mutations are likely to also cause cell proliferation [7–9]. The role of somatic mutations in constitutive aldosterone production is well defined, but many other mechanisms may modulate aldosterone production from APAs [10–15]. Regulated forms of cell death, including apoptosis [16] and ferroptosis [17], have also been implicated in the pathogenesis of APAs.

Metabolic reprogramming has a well-characterized role in cancer progression [18]. Increasing evidence suggests that tumor cells must modify their metabolism in response to their elevated energy requirements [19], and metabolic adaptations have been described in many types of cancers [20–22]. Of note, tumor cells undergo metabolic reprogramming that may modify the tumor microenvironment (TME) to fulfill the demands of biosynthesis and growth [23]. Tumor-infiltrating immune cells also rely on nutrients in the TME, and metabolic competition between tumor cells and infiltrating immune cells hamper or eliminate the anti-tumor immune response [23,24]. Furthermore, the high metabolic activity of tumor cells can generate metabolites (e.g., adenosine, kynurenine, and acidosis) that may accumulate to toxic concentrations, target immune suppressive cells and inhibit their function [25–27]. For instance, increased glycolysis in cancer cells (the Warburg effect) produces lactate that acidifies the TME and interferes with immune-cell effector function [28].

Because APAs are hormone-producing adenomas, an increased metabolic demand compared with adjacent tissue would be expected to sustain aldosterone hypersecretion. In this study, we investigated metabolic differences between APAs and paired adjacent cortical tissue to investigate mechanisms of the TME to support the development and progression of an APA.

2. Materials and Methods

2.1. Data Preprocessing

We analyzed microarray gene expression data from GSE64957 [29] and GSE60042 [30] from the Gene Expression Omnibus (GEO) database (https://www.ncbi.nlm.nih.gov/geo/ access date for GSE64957 and GSE60042: 1 January 2021 and 5 April 2021, respectively). GSE64957 comprised a data set from 13 APAs with corresponding paired zona glomerulosa, and zona fasciculata samples (7 APAs with a *KCNJ5* mutation and 6 APAs with no mutation detected). GSE60042 comprised 7 APAs and paired adjacent adrenal cortex tissue samples. GSE64957 Affymetrix microarray raw data were processed using the robust multichip average (RMA) algorithm with R package oligo for background adjustment, quantile normalization, log-transformation, and Combat function of R package sva (surrogate variable analysis) was used for batch correction. The expression matrix of GSE60042 was extracted from series matrix files downloaded from the GEO database using the GEOquery package, followed by standardization using the normalize Between Arrays function of the limma R package. The gene expression datasets were translated into commonly used gene symbols for further analyses.

The R package "limma" was used to clarify differentially expressed genes among paired groups; differentially expressed genes with adjust $p < 0.05$ and $\log_2$ fold change (FC) ($\log_2$FC) >1 were selected for further functional enrichments.

2.2. Patient Samples

Resected adrenal samples for histology and immunohistochemistry analyses were from patients diagnosed with unilateral primary aldosteronism following European Society of Hypertension guidelines [31,32] at the Medizinische Klinik IV, Klinikum Ludwig-Maximilians-Universität München, Munich, Germany, in accordance with local criteria for adrenal venous sampling [33]. These APAs comprised 6 with a *KCNJ5* mutation and 6 without *KCNJ5* mutations (2 *CACNA1D*, 2 *ATP1A1*, and 2 with no mutation detected). These patients gave written informed consent for use of biomaterial for medical research in accordance with the local ethics committee.

2.3. Functional Enrichments

To identify biological processes and pathway enrichment associated with differentially expressed genes, we used the gene set enrichment analysis (GSEA) method based on Gene Ontology (GO), Kyoto Encyclopedia of Genes and Genomes (KEGG), HALLMARK and Reactome gene sets from MSigDB database with the clusterProfiler package of R. The online tools of Metascape® (https://metascape.org access data: 11 April 2021) [34] and g:profiler (https://biit.cs.ut.ee/gprofiler access data: 21 April 2021) [35] were also used to identify pathway interactions, and protein–protein interaction networks, and to comprehensively understand the biology of differentially expressed genes using different independent knowledge bases (e.g., WikiPathways) to summarize the function of identified genes.

2.4. Determination of Tumor Immune Microenvironment and Immune Cell Infiltration Patterns

To assess tumor immune microenvironments, the "Estimation of Stromal and Immune cells in Malignant Tumors using Expression data" (ESTIMATE) algorithm [36] was used to quantify the infiltrating immune cell level (immune score) and stromal content (stromal score) for each sample, using gene expression signatures.

To further evaluate the immune characteristics of APA and adjacent zona glomerulosa cells, single sample GSEA (ssGSEA) [37] analysis was performed to identify the relative proportions of 28 immune cell types in the TME based on the feature gene panels for each immune cell type [38,39]. In addition, the Microenvironment Cell Populations-counter (MCP-counter) algorithm [40,41] was used to calculate stromal cell abundance, including endothelial cells and cancer-associated fibroblasts.

2.5. Identification of Ferroptosis-Related, Immune-Related, and Reactive Oxygen Species (ROS)-Related Genes

The corresponding ferroptosis-related gene list was downloaded from FerrDb [42]. In total, we identified 259 ferroptosis-related genes, including 108 drivers, 69 suppressors, and 111 markers. The immune-related gene lists were obtained from ImmPort (https://www.immport.org/resources access data: 21 December 2020). The ROS-related gene list was collected from the GeneCards database (https://www.genecards.org/ access data: 4 April 2021) using the term "reactive oxygen species", and only genes with a relevance score >7 were considered. All significantly differentially expressed genes were set at adjust p-value < 0.05 and $|\log_2 FC| > 1$.

2.6. Immunohistochemistry

Formalin fixed paraffin-embedded sections of APA tissue were incubated with anti-CD45 primary antibody (#13917; Cell Signaling Technology, Danvers, MA, USA) at 4 °C overnight. Immunohistochemistry staining was performed using ZytoChem Plus HRP Polymer kit (Zytomed, Berlin, Germany) following the manufacturer's instructions and quantified with QuPath (v.0.2.3, University of Edinburgh, Edinburgh, UK) using the positive cell detection feature with empirical parameters.

2.7. Cell Line and Culture Conditions

Human adrenocortical (HAC15) cells (a kind gift from Professor William E. Rainey, University of Michigan, Ann Arbor, MI, USA) were cultured in Dulbecco's Modified Eagle/F12 medium with L-glutamine containing 10% (*v/v*) cosmic calf serum, 1% antibiotic-antimycotic, 1% insulin-transferrin-selenium, and 50 mg/mL gentamycin at 37 °C and 5% CO_2.

2.8. Cell Viability Assay

HAC15 cells (4×10^4 per well) were seeded on 96-well plates for 24 h and then treated with etomoxir (E1905, Sigma-Aldrich, St.Louis, MO, USA). Cell viability was measured using WST-1 assay according to the manufacturer's instructions (Roche Diagnostics GmbH, Mannheim, Germany). Cells without etomoxir treatment were used as a control.

2.9. Statistics

R software (version 4.0.3, Vienna, Austria) and GraphPad Prism 8.0 (GraphPad Software Inc., San Diego, CA, USA) were employed for figures generation and statistical analyses. Differences between the two groups were analyzed through paired *t*-test or paired Wilcoxon test, whereas Kruskal–Wallis test or One-way ANOVA was performed between groups. The statistically significant level was set as $p < 0.05$.

3. Results

3.1. Transcriptome Defined Metabolic Reprogramming towards Fatty Acid β-Oxidation and Glycolysis in APAs

Transcriptome data from GSE60042 were used to analyze the biology of differentially expressed genes in APAs versus paired adjacent adrenal cortex. The top upregulated gene sets were related to oxidative phosphorylation (Figure 1A) consistent with a proteomic analysis of APAs [43].

Transcriptome data from GSE64957 were used to evaluate potential metabolic differences between APAs and paired adjacent zona glomerulosa. Alterations in transcriptome signatures related to metabolic synthesis were distinguished, with striking gene set enrichments in APAs of oxidative phosphorylation, fatty acid metabolism, and glycolysis (Figure 1A,B). Reactome gene sets demonstrated that the most significantly upregulated signaling pathways in APAs were mitochondrial fatty acid β-oxidation and peroxisome proliferator-activated receptor-α (PPARα) (Figure 1C). These data suggest that APAs may oxidize fatty acids as an energy source for tumor growth and/or steroidogenesis through PPARα signaling. We explored potential crosstalk between these signaling pathways using Metascape analyses with ClueGo, a Cystoscope plug-in. These network analyses highlighted that most signaling pathways involved aspects of lipid biology at the core of the pathogenesis of APAs. Furthermore, we demonstrated a functional link between lipid biology and ferroptosis. This is relevant because adrenocortical cells have previously been shown to be highly sensitive to cell death by ferroptosis due to the inhibition of glutathione biosynthesis (Figure 2A) [17,44,45]. Of note, the ferroptosis suppressor gene coding for glutamate-cysteine ligase catalytic subunit (GCLC) and the gene coding for stearoyl-CoA desaturase (SCD) are highly expressed in APAs compared with adjacent zona glomerulosa (Figure 2C). In addition, protein–protein interaction network analysis of differentially expressed genes revealed an upregulation of hub genes involved in glycolysis/gluconeogenesis using the Molecular Complex Detection algorithm (Figure 2B). Collectively, our evidence indicates that metabolic reprogramming towards fatty acid β-oxidation and glycolysis may confer some metabolic advantage to the APA microenvironment that may sustain tumor cell growth and aldosterone overproduction.

The GSE64957 data set was used to evaluate potential metabolic differences between APAs and paired adjacent zona fasciculata. Fatty acid β-oxidation was observed in adjacent zona fasciculata relative to paired adjacent zona glomerulosa (Figure 1D). We further analyzed the upregulated differentially expressed genes in APAs compared with adjacent zona glomerulosa and in paired zona fasciculata, compared with adjacent zona glomerulosa (Figure 2D). APAs specifically overexpressed genes related to glycolysis/gluconeogenesis, whereas genes that were exclusively upregulated in the paired adjacent zona fasciculata were enriched in pathways related to lipid metabolism.

3.2. KCNJ5 Mutations and Metabolic Reprogramming

APAs with *KCNJ5* mutations show an increased proliferative index compared with other APAs [9]. We investigated if *KCNJ5* mutated APAs display distinct metabolic features. We showed that genes involved in glycolysis and lipid metabolism displayed enhanced transcription in *KCNJ5* mutated APAs relative to Wild type APAs (both normalized to their adjacent zona glomerulosa) (Figure 2D).

3.3. Fatty Acid Oxidation Is Required for the Survival of Human Adrenocortical Cells

To further elaborate the functional role of fatty acid oxidation in human adrenal cells, HAC15 cells were treated with etomoxir in culture, an inhibitor of fatty acid oxidation via carnitine palmitoyltransferase-1 inhibition. Etomoxir significantly decreased cell viability of HAC15 cells in a dose-s and time-dependent manner (Figure 3A,B), indicating that fatty acid oxidation may support adrenocortical cell growth.

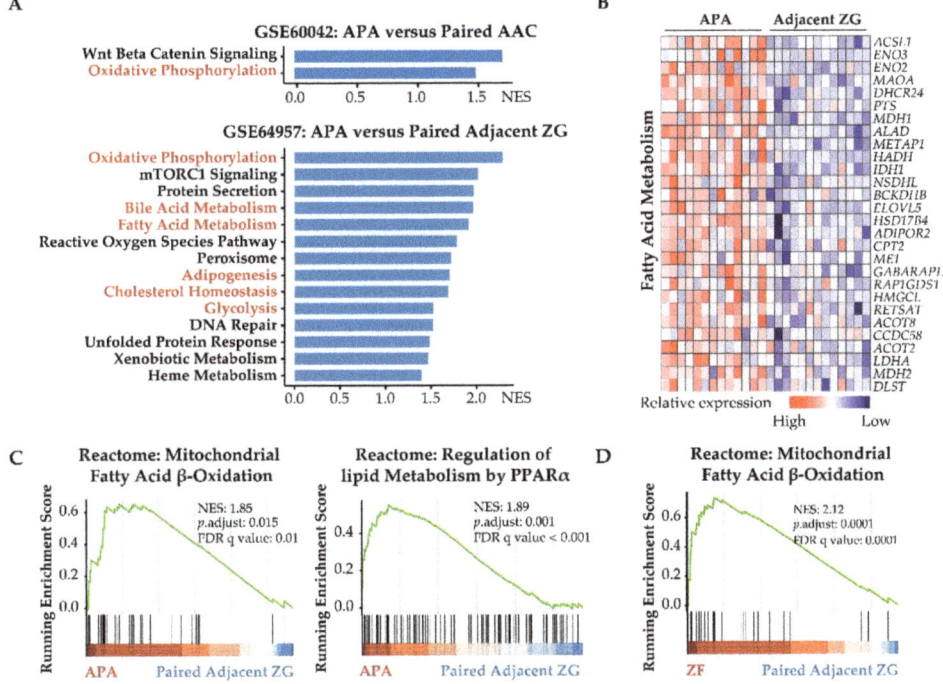

Figure 1. APAs undergo transcriptomic alterations toward increased fatty acid metabolism and glycolysis. (**A**) GSEA showing MSigDB hallmark of upregulated differentially expressed genes in APAs versus AAC (GSE60042) and adjacent ZG (GSE64957). Pathways in red indicate functions related to lipid metabolism and glycolysis. (**B**) Heatmap of the significant upregulated differentially expressed genes with *p* value < 0.05 for fatty acid metabolism in APAs compared with adjacent ZG. (**C**) GSEA plots showing Reactome pathways of lipid biological processes in APAs versus adjacent ZG. (**D**) GSEA plots showing Reactome pathways of mitochondrial fatty acid β-oxidation in ZF versus paired adjacent ZG. APA, aldosterone-producing adenoma; AAC, adjacent adrenal cortex; ZG, zona glomerulosa; ZF, zona fasciculata; NES, normalized enrichment score; FDR, false discovery rate.

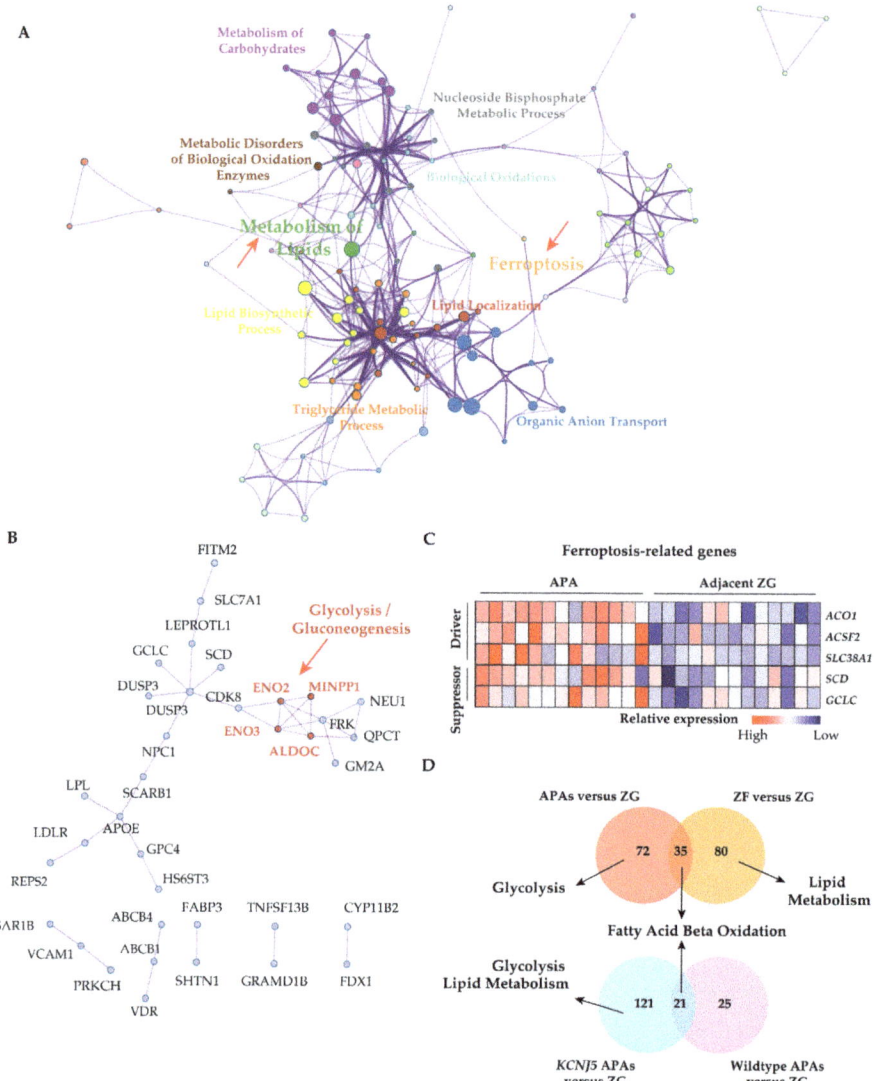

Figure 2. The interaction between lipid metabolism and ferroptosis, and the association of metabolic alterations with adjacent adrenal cortical tissue and APA genotype. (**A**) Metascape functional enrichment analysis of upregulated differentially expressed genes in APAs versus paired adjacent ZG (GSE64957). One node per enriched term, colored by cluster ID. Node size indicates the number of differentially expressed genes involved in the enriched term. (**B**) Protein–protein network using Molecular Complex Detection (MCODE) algorithm. Red fonts represent the core genes of the network involved in the glycolysis/gluconeogenesis pathway. (**C**) Heat map of ferroptosis-related upregulated differentially expressed genes grouped as driver and suppressor in APAs compared paired adjacent ZG. (**D**) Venn diagrams showing the number of unique and overlapping upregulated differentially expressed genes from APAs and adjacent ZF of those APAs to paired adjacent ZG comparisons, and from *KCNJ5* mutated APAs and APAs without mutations (Wild type) to their adjacent ZG comparisons. Top pathways in which the distinct differentially expressed genes from APAs, adjacent ZF, *KCNJ5*-mutated APA, and APA without mutations (Wild type), respectively compared to paired adjacent ZG, using g:profiler online tool. APA, aldosterone-producing adenoma. AAC, adjacent adrenal cortex; ZG, zona glomerulosa; ZF, zona fasciculata; DEGs, differentially expressed genes; NES, normalized enrichment score; FDR, false discovery rate.

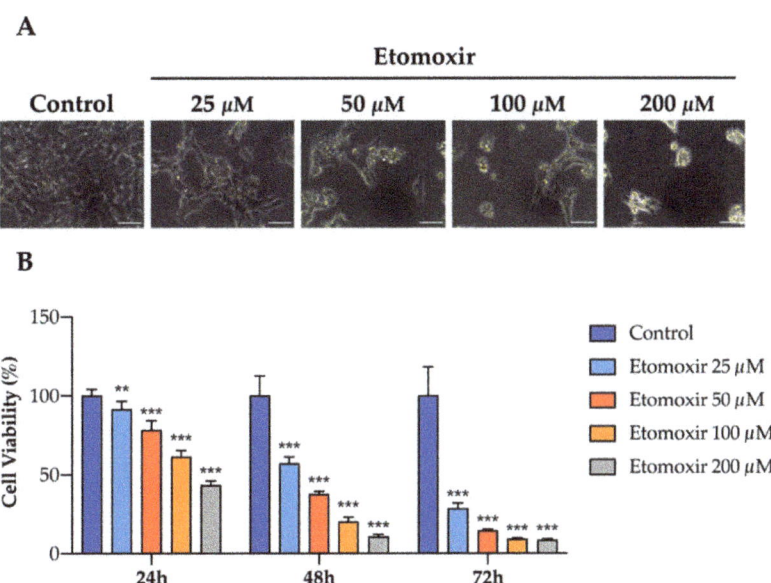

Figure 3. Inhibition of fatty acid oxidation induces cell death in human HAC15 cells. (**A**) Representative images of the effects of etomoxir in HAC15 cells in 6-well plate for 72 h. Scale Bar: 50 μm. (**B**) Cell viability in HAC15 cells treated with increasing concentration of etomoxir (25–200 μM) for 24 h, 48 h, and 72 h. Data are presented as mean ± s.d., One-way ANOVA; ** $p < 0.01$, *** $p < 0.001$.

3.4. Immune Phenotype Alterations in APAs

Dysregulation of tumor cell metabolism is known to contribute to immune evasion within the TME. Therefore, we investigated the effect of metabolic reprogramming of the TME on tumor-infiltrating immune-cell populations in APAs and adjacent adrenal cortical tissue. We used GSEA to screen for downregulated differentially expressed genes in APAs versus paired adjacent adrenal cortex and identified a vast number of immune-related pathways that were relatively increased in adjacent adrenal cortex, including inflammatory response, interferon-gamma response, and IL6 JAK STAT3 signaling (Figure 4A). Further analysis using the ESTIMATE algorithm to predict immune states revealed a statistically significant decrease of the immune and stromal score in APAs compared with paired adjacent adrenal cortex ($p < 0.01$, paired t test, Figure 4C). Collectively, APAs had a higher proportion of tumor cells. To validate these findings, we performed immunohistochemistry analysis of the surface protein CD45, a common marker of immune cells, on 12 formalin-fixed paraffin embedded APA samples with attached adjacent adrenal cortex (Figure 4B). The density and frequency of CD45$^+$ cells per mm^2 were significantly lower in APAs relative to the adjacent adrenal cortex (3.45-fold, $p < 0.001$, paired Wilcoxon test, Figure 4D), which included 6 *KCNJ5*-mutated APAs and 6 APAs without *KCNJ5* mutation. This is consistent with previous studies reporting sparse or no immune-cell infiltration within APAs compared to cortisol-producing adenoma [46]. These findings support the concept of tumor cells within the TME of APAs evading immune surveillance.

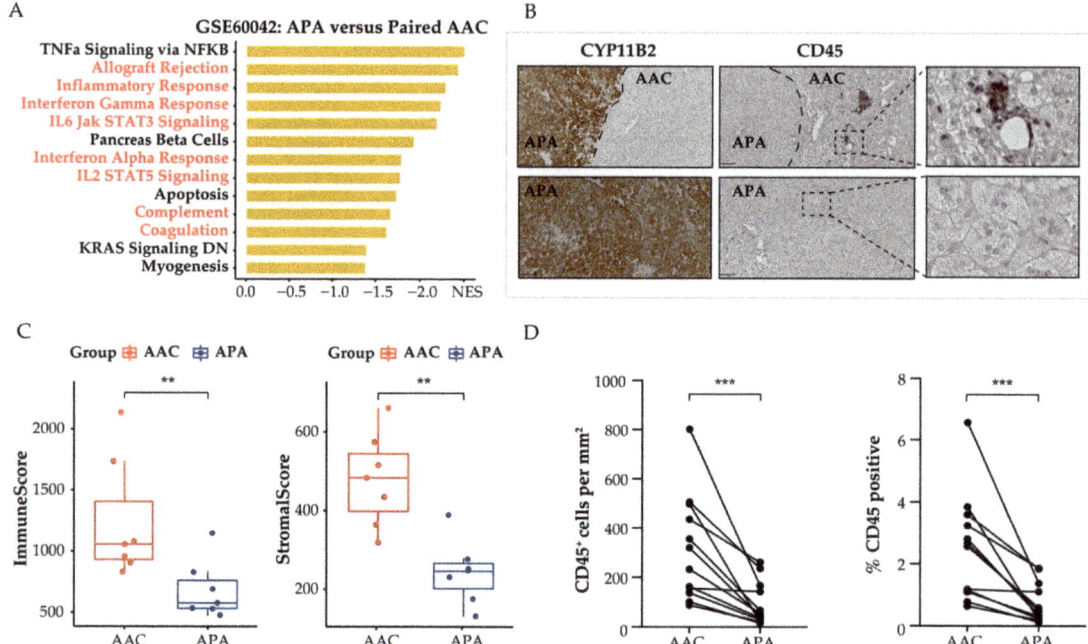

Figure 4. Spatial organization of tumor infiltrating immune cells in APAs versus paired adjacent adrenal cortex (AAC). (**A**) GSEA showing MSigDB hallmark of downregulated differentially expressed genes in APAs versus AAC (GSE60042). Pathways in red indicate functions related to immune response. (**B**) CYP11B2 and CD45 immunohistochemistry staining. The border of APA is defined by the CYP11B2 immunohistochemistry. Scare bar: 100 μm. (**C**) ESTIMATE algorithm showing the distribution of ImmuneScore, StromalScore in APAs versus AAC. ** $p < 0.01$ by paired t test. (**D**) CD45$^+$ immune cell density and positive percentage between APAs and AAC. *** $p < 0.001$ by paired Wilcox test. APA, aldosterone-producing adenoma; AAC, adjacent adrenal cortex; NES, normalized enrichment score.

We used a similar approach to assess tumor-infiltrating immune cells of APAs, paired adjacent zona fasciculata, and adjacent zona glomerulosa (Figure 5A–C). APA had fewer CD45$^+$ immune cells compared with the adjacent zona glomerulosa and adjacent zona fasciculata, suggesting an immunosuppressive microenvironment at the local site of APA. CD45$^+$ immune cells in the adjacent zona fasciculata showed higher levels compared to those in adjacent zona glomerulosa, indicating that fatty acid β-oxidation may not contribute to the immunosuppressive properties of APA.

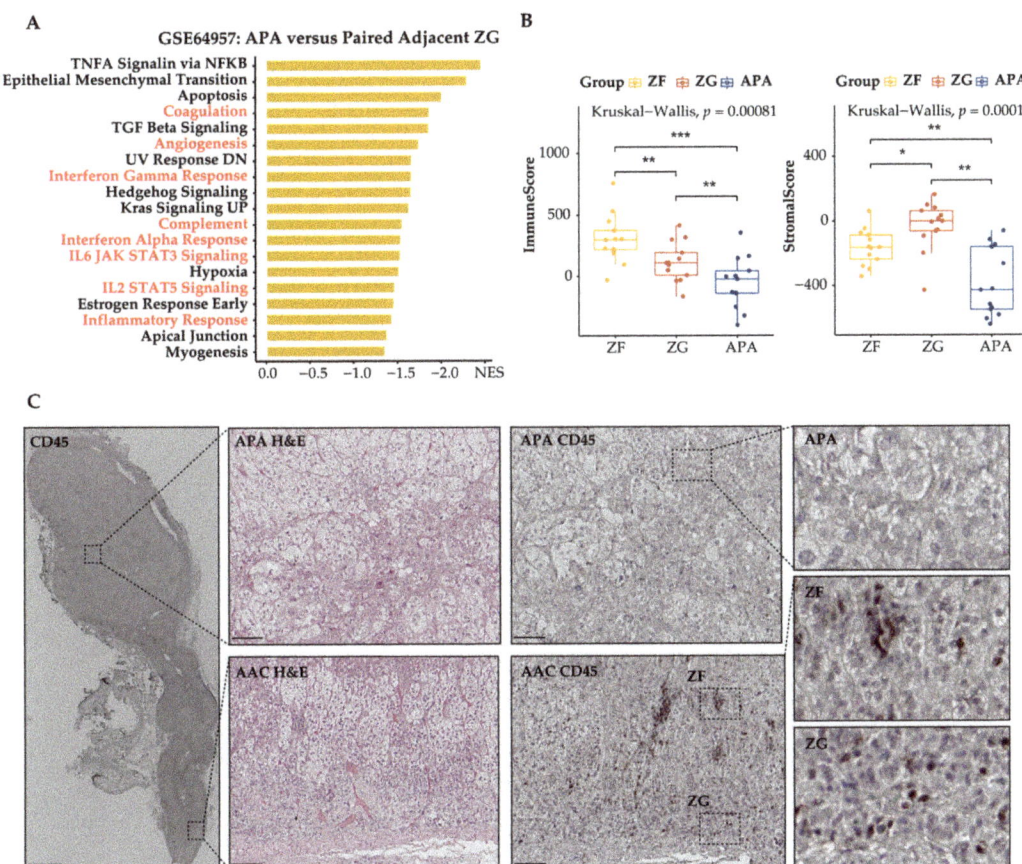

Figure 5. Spatial organization of tumor-infiltrating immune cells in APAs. Tumor-infiltrating immune cells in APAs were determined versus adjacent zona glomerulosa (ZG), and adjacent zona fasciculata (ZF). (**A**) GSEA showing MSigDB hallmark of downregulated differentially expressed genes in APAs versus adjacent ZG (GSE64957). Pathways in red indicate functions related to immune response. (**B**) ESTIMATE algorithm showing the distribution of ImmuneScore, StromalScore among APAs, adjacent ZG, and adjacent ZF. * $p < 0.05$, ** $p < 0.01$, *** $p < 0.001$ by paired Wilcox test. Kruskal–Wallis test was used between groups. (**C**) Immunohistochemistry of H&E and CD45 staining among APA, adjacent ZF, and adjacent ZG. Overview of CD45 image: scale bar 2 mm. Deep zoom images: scare bar 100 μm. APA, aldosterone-producing adenoma; ACC, adjacent adrenal cortex; GSEA, gene set enrichment analysis; NES, normalized enrichment score; ZG, zona glomerulosa; ZF, zona fasciculata.

3.5. Distinct Immune Microenvironment Landscapes in APAs vs. Paired Adjacent Zona Glomerulosa

To further explore differences in the composition of immune cells of APAs and paired adjacent zona glomerulosa, we performed ssGSEA using the MCP-counter algorithm, a method to profile fractions of immune cells by deconvolution of gene expression data, as shown in a heatmap (Figure 6A). Notably, principal component analysis showed two distinct clusters of tumor-infiltrating immune cells of the TME (APAs vs. paired adjacent zona glomerulosa) (Figure 6B). Further, we observed decreased anti-immune cells (e.g., activated and central memory CD4 T cells, effector memory CD8 T cells, and nature killer cells) and increased pro-immune cells (immature dendritic cells) (Figure 6C–F).

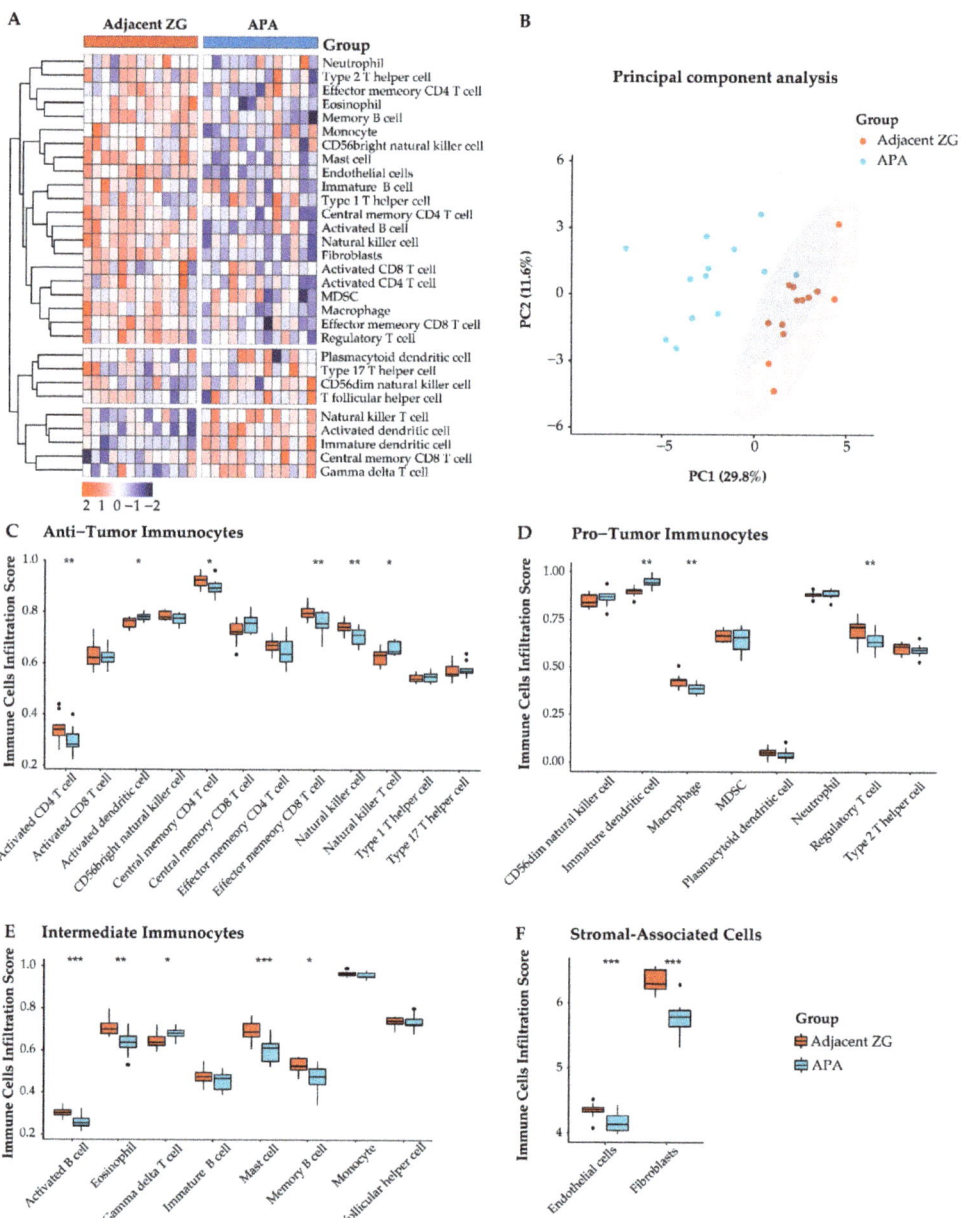

Figure 6. Distinct immune microenvironment landscapes in APA versus paired adjacent zona glomerulosa (ZG). (**A**) Heatmap of 28 tumor infiltration cells between APAs and adjacent ZG (GSE64957). MDSC, myeloid-derived suppressor cells. (**B**) Principal component analysis (PCA) of tumor-infiltrating cells. Two distinct groups were plotted in two-dimensional space: APA and adjacent ZG. PC, principal component. (**C**–**E**) Boxplot of the proportions of tumor microenvironment immune cells in (**A**) using the ssGSEA algorithm. (**F**) Boxplot of the proportions of TME stromal associated cells in (**A**) using MCP-counter algorithm. Box plots: scattered dots, immune score of the two subgroups; middle lines, median value; bottom and top of the boxes, 25th–75th percentiles. ns, not significant; * $p < 0.05$; ** $p < 0.01$; *** $p < 0.001$ by paired Wilcoxon test. APA, aldosterone-producing adenoma; ZG, zona glomerulosa.

3.6. Functional Characterization of Immune-Related Differentially Expressed Genes in APAs

To classify immune-related genes, we intersected the whole dataset of differentially expressed genes with immune-related genes from ImmPort. A total of 31 differentially expressed immune-related genes were identified; 9 of these 31 were upregulated and the remaining 22 genes were downregulated in APAs versus paired adjacent zona glomerulosa (Figure 7A). GO analysis determined downregulated genes related to the immune response were enriched in the pathways related to "cellular response to oxidative stress" (Figure 7B), suggesting that oxidative stress may elicit an inflammatory response in the adjacent zona glomerulosa.

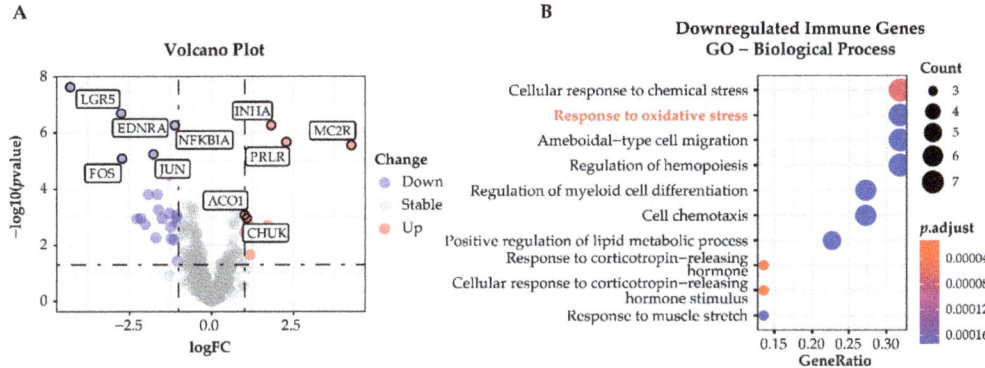

Figure 7. Functional characterization of immune-related differentially expressed genes in APAs versus paired adjacent zona glomerulosa (ZG). (**A**) Volcano Plot showing immune-differentially expressed genes (adjust p-value < 0.05 and $|\log_2 FC| > 1$) in APA versus adjacent ZG (GSE64957). Each point represents a gene. Red and Blue dots represent upregulated and downregulated immune-differentially expressed genes, respectively. (**B**) GO analysis of downregulated immune-differentially expressed genes in (**A**). APA, aldosterone-producing adenoma; ZG, zona glomerulosa.

3.7. Enhanced Anti-Oxidative Response Pathways in APAs

Our analyses indicate that adjacent zona glomerulosa are challenged with increased oxidative stress compared to cells of APAs. To investigate the function of ROS within the context of APA cells, we compared differentially expressed genes functionally related to ROS in APAs vs. paired adjacent zona glomerulosa. We identified 22 upregulated ROS genes and 40 downregulated ROS genes. KEGG analysis of the upregulated ROS genes demonstrated upregulation of several metabolic pathways, including cholesterol metabolism, peroxisome proliferator-activated receptor (PPAR) signaling, aldosterone synthesis, and secretion (Figure 8B), suggesting that ROS may be involved in the regulation of metabolism and/or affected by the intermediates of metabolic alterations. In contrast, the most prominently altered processes of downregulated genes related to ROS were the inflammatory response pathways (Figure 8D). Collectively, the link of ROS with metabolism and the inflammatory response may suggest contributory biological mechanisms to the pathogenesis of APAs.

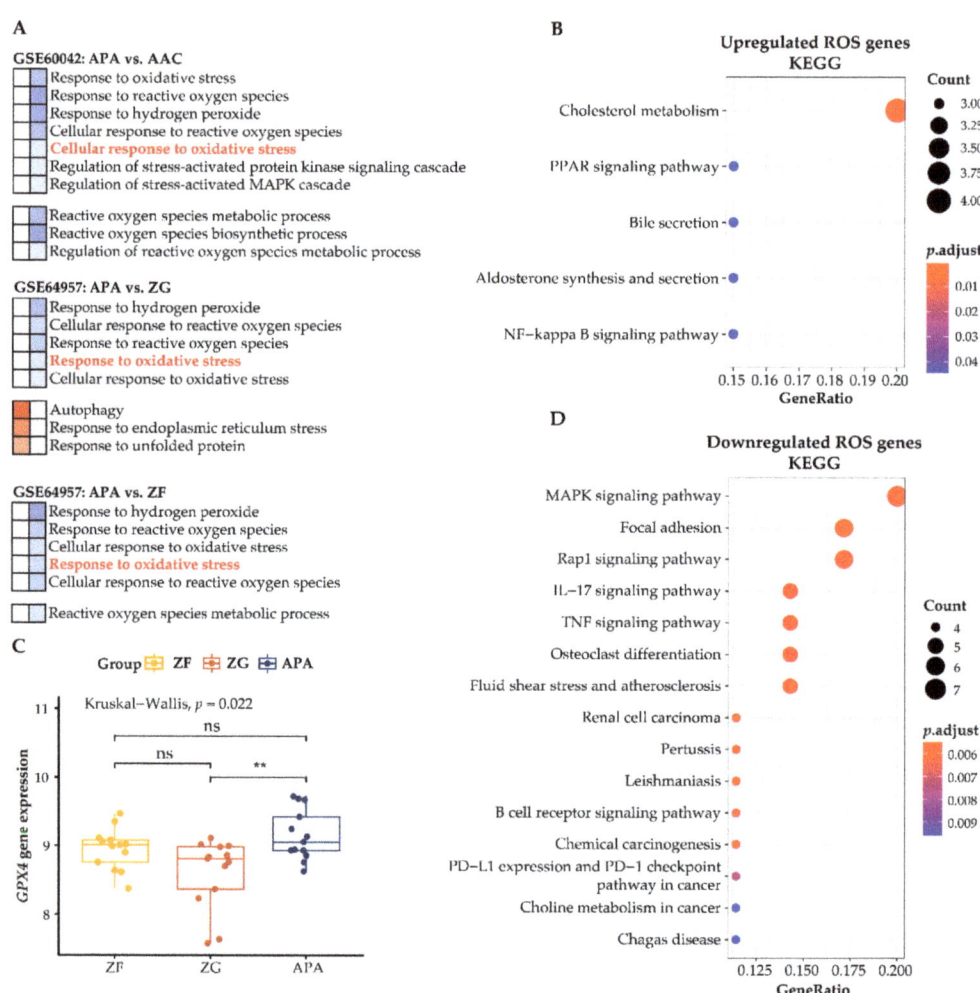

Figure 8. Enhanced antioxidative response pathways in APAs. (**A**) GO analysis of GSEA showing heatmap of ROS-related pathways. Red and blue color indicate upregulated and downregulated pathways ordered by normalized enrichment score in APAs versus AAC, adjacent ZG, and adjacent ZF, respectively. Normalized enrichment score >0 means upregulated pathways (Red), whereas normalized enrichment score <0 means downregulated pathways (Blue). Corresponding pathway enrichments are listed on the side. (**B,D**) indicate KEGG pathways of differentially expressed genes involved in ROS in APA versus adjacent ZG. Overexpressed ROS gene categories associated with metabolism pathways, whereas those downregulated ROS genes are associated with immune-response pathways. (**C**) The *GPX4* gene expression between APAs, adjacent ZG, and adjacent ZF. ** p < 0.01 by paired Wilcoxon test. Kruskal–Wallis test was used between groups. APA, aldosterone-producing adenoma; AAC, adjacent adrenal cortex; ZG, zona glomerulosa; ZF, zona fasciculata; ROS, reactive oxygen species.

To address how APAs accommodate high ROS levels and ameliorate oxidative stress, we summarized ROS-related pathways between APAs versus paired adjacent adrenal cortex, APAs vs. paired adjacent zona glomerulosa, and APAs versus paired adjacent zona fasciculata. In general, all adjacent tissues showed higher enrichment of genes involved in ROS-related pathways such as "cellular response to oxidative stress" (Figure 8A). Therefore, we postulated that adrenocortical tumor cells may increase antioxidant properties to counteract metabolic stress. Accordingly, we determined upregulation of the unfolded protein response pathway in APAs (vs. adjacent zona glomerulosa) [47], which is an adaptive mechanism to relieve endoplasmic reticulum stress and restore cellular metabolic function, thereby promoting the survival of tumor cells. In addition, autophagy, a cellular stress-response mechanism [48] that recycles key metabolites under metabolic stress and promotes cellular adaptation to oxidative stress, was also enhanced in APAs. In addition, glutathione peroxidase 4 (GPX4) mRNA levels, a key enzyme for antioxidant defense, were higher in APAs among groups (Figure 8C). Together, these mechanisms ensure an efficient alleviation of oxidative stress that APA cells encounter during excess aldosterone production and abnormal proliferation.

4. Discussion

In this study we used advanced bioinformatics tools to comprehensively evaluate the TME of APAs. We demonstrated that metabolic reprogramming towards fatty acid β-oxidation and glycolysis is a general feature of APAs that may provide a metabolically favorable environment for tumor growth. Furthermore, we showed an immunosuppressive microenvironment in APA and diverse cellular components of the TME (e.g., immune and stromal cells) between APAs and the adjacent zona glomerulosa.

We showed that lipid metabolism is highly associated with APA tumorigenesis. Metabolism reprogramming enables tumor cells to sustain ATP generation for cell growth, division, and survival. Notably, dysregulation of lipid metabolism has been demonstrated as a prominent metabolic alteration in cancers [49]. In particular, increased β-oxidation of stored lipids provides a source of NAPDH and ATP—approximately six times that of oxidation of carbohydrates—through the oxidation of acetyl-CoA by the tricarboxylic acid (TCA) cycle, thereby facilitating tumor progression [50]. Furthermore, NAPDH is critical for two steps in steroidogenesis pathways in the adrenal gland: (1) the rate-limiting step for the conversion of cholesterol to pregnenolone catalyzed by CYP11A1 and (2) the conversion of deoxycorticosterone to aldosterone catalyzed by CYP11B2 [51,52]. Thus, elevated fatty acid β-oxidation in APAs may stimulate aldosterone synthesis by the high metabolic activity of NAPDH generation in mitochondria. In addition, our bioinformatics studies implied that changes in lipid metabolism in APAs are regulated by PPARα. Previous studies reported that transcriptional activation of PPARα regulates β-oxidation in tissues displaying high energy consumption [53,54]. Consistent with our findings, a previous study demonstrated that fenofibrate, a PPARα agonist, increased angiotensin II-independent *CYP11B2* mRNA expression and aldosterone production in human adrenocortical carcinoma H295R cells, whereas a peroxisome proliferator-activated receptor-γ (PPARγ) agonist either had no effect or reduced aldosterone secretion [55]. These data indicate that high activity of fatty acid β-oxidation induced by PPARα signaling may be crucial for excess aldosterone production.

Further to a role for fatty acid β-oxidation in APA pathogenesis, we reported that glycolysis metabolism may also play a key role, especially in *KCNJ5*-mutated APAs. This latter finding is consistent with a mass spectrometry imaging study that identified the activation of glycolysis pathways in APAs as well as in a subgroup of aldosterone-producing micronodules [56] (previously known as aldosterone-producing cell clusters [57]). In contrast, a high-resolution mass spectrometry imaging map of the normal human adrenal gland reported that glycolysis/gluconeogenesis was found to be significantly increased in the medulla [58]. This finding is consistent with the concept that a metabolic switch to glycolysis confers a selective advantage for tumor growth. However, the underlying mechanism of such metabolic phenotypes is unclear. Of potential interest, lactate infusion alone, or in combination with angiotensin II, results in increased aldosterone secretion from rat zona glomerulosa cells [59]. Therefore, the precise relationship between glycolysis and its metabolites and aldosterone production merits further investigation.

Our study showed the low tumor infiltrating CD45$^+$ lymphocyte density in APAs. Such a scenario is in line with previous reports showing sparse immune cell infiltration using hematoxylin-eosin staining in APAs relative to cortisol-producing adenomas [46].

This alteration in the TME may be accounted for by competition for nutrients in the TME, and glycolysis intermediates forming an acidic microenvironment and thereby suppressing immune activation [27,60]. Another potential mechanism is the promotion of immunosurveillance evasion by activated PPAR signaling [61]. PPARα exerts anti-inflammatory activity, for example, and PPARα agonists mediate a variety of effects on the immune response to reverse acute and chronic liver inflammation [54]. Consistently, PPARα-deficient aged mice show a pro-inflammatory phenotype [62]. In addition, the PPARα agonist fenofibrate caused a reduction in blood pressure, especially in salt-sensitive hypertensive subjects [63], suggesting that PPARα may play a role in regulation of renin–angiotensin–aldosterone system activity, and influence aldosterone secretion. This discrepancy may be explained, however, by its dual influence on systemic and local tumor levels. Furthermore, through expression–signature-based approaches, we observed low effector memory CD8 T cell infiltration in APAs, which is in agreement with a previous study that demonstrated decreased viability of effector T cells in a glucose-restricted medium in vitro [64]. These data suggest that metabolic reprogramming towards glycolysis in APA may impose a hypoglycemic environment, restrict glucose uptake by immune cells and therefore hamper their function. In addition, a previous study showed that the distribution of mast cells is more frequently visualized in the adjacent cortex of APAs [11], consistent with the high mast cell infiltration in adjacent zona glomerulosa relative to APAs in our study.

Active steroidogenesis has been implicated in contributing to high ROS production and oxidative stress, triggering cell death [65]. Our analyses demonstrated that the adjacent cortex is challenged with increased oxidative stress compared to APAs, regions of high steroidogenesis. Our finding of enhanced fatty acid β-oxidation in APAs may explain this apparent paradox because it provides NAPDH, which may counteract ROS toxicity from metabolic stress [66]. Furthermore, fatty acid β-oxidation is increased in zona fasciculata relative to paired zona glomerulosa, likely because glucocorticoid production in normal zona fasciculata produces significantly more cellular ROS than from aldosterone synthesis in normal zona glomerulosa due to 40% of "leaky" electrons in the P450c11β (CYP11B1) system [67]. This would require elevated fatty acid β-oxidation for protection of adrenocortical zona fasciculata cells from ROS. In addition, previous work demonstrated that enhanced glycolysis can combat oxidative stress via increasing glutathione metabolism and maintaining redox balance [68], a potential factor contributing to the larger tumor diameter in APAs with *KCNJ5* mutations. Additionally, our data showed an increased antioxidant response via an enhanced unfolding protein response and autophagy [47,48], suggesting that multiple mechanisms participate in the detoxification of ROS and aid adrenocortical tumor cell survival.

It has been reported that adrenocortical cells are sensitive to ferroptosis-triggering agents, such as RSL3, which can inhibit GPX4 activity [17,45]. Indeed, our data showed elevated *GPX4* expression in APAs compared with adjacent zona glomerulosa. Adrenocortical tumor cells must boost their antioxidant capacity to counteract the lipid peroxidation and oxidative stress induced by steroidogenesis to suppress cell death by ferroptosis. Although studies into the molecular mechanisms underlying the adaptation of APA cells to high ROS generation in the local tumor site to circumvent ferroptosis are not well defined, lipid metabolism likely participates, and in particular fatty acid β-oxidation. This hypothesis is partially supported by Kagan et al., who showed that etomoxir, an inhibitor of mitochondrial fatty acid β-oxidation, enhanced RSL3-induced ferroptosis in mouse embryonic fibroblasts [69]. Further, PPARα activator can reduce lipid peroxidation [70]. Considering the known association of fatty acid β-oxidation with PPARα, PPARα activation may feasibly regulate the susceptibility of adrenocortical cells to lipid peroxidation, a key characteristic of ferroptosis, through β-oxidation. Furthermore, we observed increased *SCD* and *GCLC* mRNA expression in APAs. Two key enzymes catalyze monounsaturated fatty acid synthesis and biosynthesis of glutathione, which protect tumor cells against ferroptosis inducers [71,72]. These exemplify the central hub role of metabolism reprogramming to adapt to metabolic stress.

This study reports a potential role of fatty acid oxidation in supporting adrenocortical cell growth; however, further research is required to delineate the precise mechanisms involved. Our study had several limitations, including the absence of protein-level data corresponding to identified differentially expressed genes related to lipid metabolism with a potential role in APA pathophysiology. In addition, we did not fully characterize the role of oxidative stress (lipid peroxidation) in APA tissues, which warrants further investigation.

5. Conclusions

It is challenging to evaluate the tumorigenic landscape of APAs using experimental methods. As such, it is still unclear how APA tumor adrenocortical cells maintain hypersecretion and cell proliferation despite a nutrient-deprived environment. We address this knowledge gap by shedding light on the energy metabolism and tumor immune microenvironment. Our analyses reveal that metabolic reprogramming involving a switch to fatty acid β-oxidation and glycolysis may stimulate aldosterone production, disturb the TME, mitigate oxidative stress, and support tumor cell survival. Therefore, we highlight metabolic reprogramming as a putative novel mechanism in APA pathophysiology.

Author Contributions: Conceptualization, T.A.W., S.G. and M.R.; data curation, S.G.; formal analysis, S.G. and M.T.; funding acquisition, T.A.W. and M.R.; investigation, S.G.; methodology, T.A.W. and S.G.; project administration, T.A.W.; software, S.G.; supervision, T.A.W.; validation, S.G. and M.T.; writing–original draft, S.G.; writing–review and editing, T.A.W., M.T. and M.R. All authors have read and agreed to the published version of the manuscript.

Funding: This work was financed by the Deutsche Forschungsgemeinschaft (DFG) project number 444776998 to T.A. Williams (WI 5359/2-1) and M. Reincke (RE 752/31-1) and project number 314061271-TRR 205/project B15 to T.A. Williams (within the CRC/Transregio 205/1 "The Adrenal: Central Relay in Health and Disease"). The CRC/Transregio 205/1 also supports the research of M. Reincke. This study was also supported by the European Research Council under the European Union Horizon 2020 research and innovation program (grant agreement No. 694913 to M. Reincke) and the Else Kröner-Fresenius Stiftung in support of the German Conn's Registry-Else-Kröner Hyperaldosteronism Registry (2013_A182, 2015_A171 and 2019_A104 to M. Reincke). Siyuan Gong was supported by the China Scholarship Council (CSC) for supporting her study in LMU Munich.

Institutional Review Board Statement: The study was conducted according to the guidelines of the Declaration of Helsinki, and approved by the Ethics Committee of Ludwig-Maximilians-Universität, München (protocol code 379-10 and 11 January 2012).

Informed Consent Statement: Informed consent was obtained from all subjects involved in the study.

Data Availability Statement: The publicly archived datasets presented in this study can be accessible through GEO series accession number GSE64957 and GSE60042.

Acknowledgments: We thank Isabella-Sabrina Kinker and Petra Rank for their expert technical assistance.

Conflicts of Interest: The authors declare no conflict of interest.

Abbreviation	Definition
PA	Primary aldosteronism
APA	Aldosterone-producing adenoma
AAC	Adjacent adrenal cortex
ZG	Zona glomerulosa
ZF	Zona fasciculata
TME	Tumor microenvironment
ROS	Reactive oxygen species
GO	Gene Ontology
KEGG	Kyoto Encyclopedia of Genes and Genomes
GSEA	Gene set enrichment analysis

MCP-COUNTER	Microenvironment cell populations-counter
ESTIMATE	Estimation of Stromal and Immune cells in Malignant Tumors using Expression data
GCLC	Glutamate-cysteine ligase catalytic subunit
SCD	Stearoyl-CoA desaturase
GPX4	Glutathione peroxidase 4
ATP	Adenosine triphosphate
NADPH	Nicotinamide adenine dinucleotide phosphate
TME	Tumor microenvironment

References

1. Young, W.F. Diagnosis and treatment of primary aldosteronism: Practical clinical perspectives. *J. Intern. Med.* **2019**, *285*, 126–148. [CrossRef] [PubMed]
2. Rege, J.; Nanba, K.; Blinder, A.R.; Plaska, S.; Udager, A.M.; Vats, P.; Kumar-Sinha, C.; Giordano, T.J.; Rainey, W.E.; Else, T. Identification of Somatic Mutations in CLCN2 in Aldosterone-Producing Adenomas. *J. Endocr. Soc.* **2020**, *4*, bvaa123. [CrossRef]
3. Scholl, U.I.; Goh, G.; Stolting, G.; De Oliveira, R.C.; Choi, M.; Overton, J.D.; Fonseca, A.L.; Korah, R.; Starker, L.F.; Kunstman, J.W.; et al. Somatic and germline CACNA1D calcium channel mutations in aldosterone-producing adenomas and primary aldosteronism. *Nat. Genet.* **2013**, *45*, 1050–1054. [CrossRef]
4. Williams, T.A.; Monticone, S.; Schack, V.R.; Stindl, J.; Burrello, J.; Buffolo, F.; Annaratone, L.; Castellano, I.; Beuschlein, F.; Reincke, M.; et al. Somatic ATP1A1, ATP2B3, and KCNJ5 mutations in aldosterone-producing adenomas. *Hypertension* **2014**, *63*, 188–195. [CrossRef]
5. Meyer, L.S.; Handgriff, L.; Lim, J.S.; Udager, A.M.; Kinker, I.S.; Ladurner, R.; Wildgruber, M.; Knosel, T.; Bidlingmaier, M.; Rainey, W.E.; et al. Single-Center Prospective Cohort Study on the Histopathology, Genotype, and Postsurgical Outcomes of Patients With Primary Aldosteronism. *Hypertension* **2021**. [CrossRef] [PubMed]
6. Itcho, K.; Oki, K.; Ohno, H.; Yoneda, M. Update on Genetics of Primary Aldosteronism. *Biomedicines* **2021**, *9*, 409. [CrossRef]
7. Scholl, U.I.; Nelson-Williams, C.; Yue, P.; Grekin, R.; Wyatt, R.J.; Dillon, M.J.; Couch, R.; Hammer, L.K.; Harley, F.L.; Farhi, A.; et al. Hypertension with or without adrenal hyperplasia due to different inherited mutations in the potassium channel KCNJ5. *Proc. Natl. Acad. Sci. USA* **2012**, *109*, 2533–2538. [CrossRef]
8. Tamura, A.; Nishimoto, K.; Seki, T.; Matsuzawa, Y.; Saito, J.; Omura, M.; Gomez-Sanchez, C.E.; Makita, K.; Matsui, S.; Moriya, N.; et al. Somatic KCNJ5 mutation occurring early in adrenal development may cause a novel form of juvenile primary aldosteronism. *Mol. Cell. Endocrinol.* **2017**, *441*, 134–139. [CrossRef] [PubMed]
9. Yang, Y.; Gomez-Sanchez, C.E.; Jaquin, D.; Aristizabal Prada, E.T.; Meyer, L.S.; Knosel, T.; Schneider, H.; Beuschlein, F.; Reincke, M.; Williams, T.A. Primary Aldosteronism: KCNJ5 mutations and Adrenocortical Cell Growth. *Hypertension* **2019**, *74*, 809–816. [CrossRef] [PubMed]
10. Oki, K.; Gomez-Sanchez, C.E. The landscape of molecular mechanism for aldosterone production in aldosterone-producing adenoma. *Endocr. J.* **2020**, *67*, 989–995. [CrossRef]
11. Duparc, C.; Moreau, L.; Dzib, J.F.; Boyer, H.G.; Tetsi Nomigni, M.; Boutelet, I.; Boulkroun, S.; Mukai, K.; Benecke, A.G.; Amar, L.; et al. Mast cell hyperplasia is associated with aldosterone hypersecretion in a subset of aldosterone-producing adenomas. *J. Clin. Endocrinol. Metab.* **2015**, *100*, E550–E560. [CrossRef] [PubMed]
12. Berthon, A.; Drelon, C.; Ragazzon, B.; Boulkroun, S.; Tissier, F.; Amar, L.; Samson-Couterie, B.; Zennaro, M.C.; Plouin, P.F.; Skah, S.; et al. WNT/beta-catenin signalling is activated in aldosterone-producing adenomas and controls aldosterone production. *Hum. Mol. Genet.* **2014**, *23*, 889–905. [CrossRef]
13. Williams, T.A.; Monticone, S.; Morello, F.; Liew, C.C.; Mengozzi, G.; Pilon, C.; Asioli, S.; Sapino, A.; Veglio, F.; Mulatero, P. Teratocarcinoma-derived growth factor-1 is upregulated in aldosterone-producing adenomas and increases aldosterone secretion and inhibits apoptosis in vitro. *Hypertension* **2010**, *55*, 1468–1475. [CrossRef] [PubMed]
14. Decmann, A.; Nyiro, G.; Darvasi, O.; Turai, P.; Bancos, I.; Kaur, R.J.; Pezzani, R.; Iacobone, M.; Kraljevic, I.; Kastelan, D.; et al. Circulating miRNA Expression Profiling in Primary Aldosteronism. *Front. Endocrinol.* **2019**, *10*, 739. [CrossRef]
15. Tombol, Z.; Turai, P.I.; Decmann, A.; Igaz, P. MicroRNAs and Adrenocortical Tumors: Where do we Stand on Primary Aldosteronism? *Horm. Metab. Res.* **2020**, *52*, 394–403. [CrossRef]
16. Williams, T.A.; Monticone, S.; Crudo, V.; Warth, R.; Veglio, F.; Mulatero, P. Visinin-like 1 is upregulated in aldosterone-producing adenomas with KCNJ5 mutations and protects from calcium-induced apoptosis. *Hypertension* **2012**, *59*, 833–839. [CrossRef]
17. Yang, Y.; Tetti, M.; Vohra, T.; Adolf, C.; Seissler, J.; Hristov, M.; Belavgeni, A.; Bidlingmaier, M.; Linkermann, A.; Mulatero, P.; et al. BEX1 Is Differentially Expressed in Aldosterone-Producing Adenomas and Protects Human Adrenocortical Cells From Ferroptosis. *Hypertension* **2021**, *77*, 1647–1658. [CrossRef]
18. Pavlova, N.N.; Thompson, C.B. The Emerging Hallmarks of Cancer Metabolism. *Cell Metab.* **2016**, *23*, 27–47. [CrossRef]
19. Faubert, B.; Solmonson, A.; DeBerardinis, R.J. Metabolic reprogramming and cancer progression. *Science* **2020**, *368*, eaaw5473. [CrossRef]
20. Ligorio, F.; Pellegrini, I.; Castagnoli, L.; Vingiani, A.; Lobefaro, R.; Zattarin, E.; Santamaria, M.; Pupa, S.M.; Pruneri, G.; de Braud, F.; et al. Targeting lipid metabolism is an emerging strategy to enhance the efficacy of anti-HER2 therapies in HER2-positive breast cancer. *Cancer Lett.* **2021**, *511*, 77–87. [CrossRef]

21. Xu, W.; Hu, X.; Anwaier, A.; Wang, J.; Liu, W.; Tian, X.; Zhu, W.; Ma, C.; Wan, F.; Shi, G.; et al. Fatty Acid Synthase Correlates With Prognosis-Related Abdominal Adipose Distribution and Metabolic Disorders of Clear Cell Renal Cell Carcinoma. *Front. Mol. Biosci.* **2020**, *7*, 610229. [CrossRef]
22. Schmidt, D.R.; Patel, R.; Kirsch, D.G.; Lewis, C.A.; Vander Heiden, M.G.; Locasale, J.W. Metabolomics in cancer research and emerging applications in clinical oncology. *CA Cancer J. Clin.* **2021**. [CrossRef]
23. Reina-Campos, M.; Moscat, J.; Diaz-Meco, M. Metabolism shapes the tumor microenvironment. *Curr. Opin. Cell Biol.* **2017**, *48*, 47–53. [CrossRef]
24. Xia, L.; Oyang, L.; Lin, J.; Tan, S.; Han, Y.; Wu, N.; Yi, P.; Tang, L.; Pan, Q.; Rao, S.; et al. The cancer metabolic reprogramming and immune response. *Mol. Cancer* **2021**, *20*, 28. [CrossRef] [PubMed]
25. Ohta, A.; Gorelik, E.; Prasad, S.J.; Ronchese, F.; Lukashev, D.; Wong, M.K.; Huang, X.; Caldwell, S.; Liu, K.; Smith, P.; et al. A2A adenosine receptor protects tumors from antitumor T cells. *Proc. Natl. Acad. Sci. USA* **2006**, *103*, 13132–13137. [CrossRef]
26. Romero-Garcia, S.; Moreno-Altamirano, M.M.; Prado-Garcia, H.; Sanchez-Garcia, F.J. Lactate Contribution to the Tumor Microenvironment: Mechanisms, Effects on Immune Cells and Therapeutic Relevance. *Front. Immunol.* **2016**, *7*, 52. [CrossRef]
27. Leone, R.D.; Powell, J.D. Metabolism of immune cells in cancer. *Nat. Rev. Cancer* **2020**, *20*, 516–531. [CrossRef]
28. Allison, K.E.; Coomber, B.L.; Bridle, B.W. Metabolic reprogramming in the tumour microenvironment: A hallmark shared by cancer cells and T lymphocytes. *Immunology* **2017**, *152*, 175–184. [CrossRef]
29. Zhou, J.; Lam, B.; Neogi, S.G.; Yeo, G.S.; Azizan, E.A.; Brown, M.J. Transcriptome Pathway Analysis of Pathological and Physiological Aldosterone-Producing Human Tissues. *Hypertension* **2016**, *68*, 1424–1431. [CrossRef]
30. Murakami, M.; Yoshimoto, T.; Nakabayashi, K.; Tsuchiya, K.; Minami, I.; Bouchi, R.; Izumiyama, H.; Fujii, Y.; Abe, K.; Tayama, C.; et al. Integration of transcriptome and methylome analysis of aldosterone-producing adenomas. *Eur. J. Endocrinol.* **2015**, *173*, 185–195. [CrossRef]
31. Mulatero, P.; Monticone, S.; Deinum, J.; Amar, L.; Prejbisz, A.; Zennaro, M.C.; Beuschlein, F.; Rossi, G.P.; Nishikawa, T.; Morganti, A.; et al. Genetics, prevalence, screening and confirmation of primary aldosteronism: A position statement and consensus of the Working Group on Endocrine Hypertension of The European Society of Hypertension. *J. Hypertens.* **2020**, *38*, 1919–1928. [CrossRef]
32. Mulatero, P.; Sechi, L.A.; Williams, T.A.; Lenders, J.W.; Reincke, M.; Satoh, F.; Januszewicz, A.; Naruse, M.; Doumas, M.; Veglio, F.; et al. Subtype diagnosis, treatment, complications and outcomes of primary aldosteronism and future direction of research: A position statement and consensus of the Working Group on Endocrine Hypertension of the European Society of Hypertension. *J. Hypertens.* **2020**, *38*, 1929–1936. [CrossRef]
33. Williams, T.A.; Reincke, M. MANAGEMENT OF ENDOCRINE DISEASE: Diagnosis and management of primary aldosteronism: The Endocrine Society guideline 2016 revisited. *Eur. J. Endocrinol.* **2018**, *179*, R19–R29. [CrossRef] [PubMed]
34. Zhou, Y.; Zhou, B.; Pache, L.; Chang, M.; Khodabakhshi, A.H.; Tanaseichuk, O.; Benner, C.; Chanda, S.K. Metascape provides a biologist-oriented resource for the analysis of systems-level datasets. *Nat. Commun.* **2019**, *10*, 1523. [CrossRef] [PubMed]
35. Raudvere, U.; Kolberg, L.; Kuzmin, I.; Arak, T.; Adler, P.; Peterson, H.; Vilo, J. g:Profiler: A web server for functional enrichment analysis and conversions of gene lists (2019 update). *Nucleic Acids Res.* **2019**, *47*, W191–W198. [CrossRef] [PubMed]
36. Yoshihara, K.; Shahmoradgoli, M.; Martinez, E.; Vegesna, R.; Kim, H.; Torres-Garcia, W.; Trevino, V.; Shen, H.; Laird, P.W.; Levine, D.A.; et al. Inferring tumour purity and stromal and immune cell admixture from expression data. *Nat. Commun.* **2013**, *4*, 2612. [CrossRef] [PubMed]
37. Barbie, D.A.; Tamayo, P.; Boehm, J.S.; Kim, S.Y.; Moody, S.E.; Dunn, I.F.; Schinzel, A.C.; Sandy, P.; Meylan, E.; Scholl, C.; et al. Systematic RNA interference reveals that oncogenic KRAS-driven cancers require TBK1. *Nature* **2009**, *462*, 108–112. [CrossRef] [PubMed]
38. Jia, Q.; Wu, W.; Wang, Y.; Alexander, P.B.; Sun, C.; Gong, Z.; Cheng, J.N.; Sun, H.; Guan, Y.; Xia, X.; et al. Local mutational diversity drives intratumoral immune heterogeneity in non-small cell lung cancer. *Nat. Commun.* **2018**, *9*, 5361. [CrossRef]
39. Charoentong, P.; Finotello, F.; Angelova, M.; Mayer, C.; Efremova, M.; Rieder, D.; Hackl, H.; Trajanoski, Z. Pan-cancer Immunogenomic Analyses Reveal Genotype-Immunophenotype Relationships and Predictors of Response to Checkpoint Blockade. *Cell Rep.* **2017**, *18*, 248–262. [CrossRef]
40. Sturm, G.; Finotello, F.; Petitprez, F.; Zhang, J.D.; Baumbach, J.; Fridman, W.H.; List, M.; Aneichyk, T. Comprehensive evaluation of transcriptome-based cell-type quantification methods for immuno-oncology. *Bioinformatics* **2019**, *35*, i436–i445. [CrossRef]
41. Becht, E.; Giraldo, N.A.; Lacroix, L.; Buttard, B.; Elarouci, N.; Petitprez, F.; Selves, J.; Laurent-Puig, P.; Sautes-Fridman, C.; Fridman, W.H.; et al. Estimating the population abundance of tissue-infiltrating immune and stromal cell populations using gene expression. *Genome Biol.* **2016**, *17*, 218. [CrossRef] [PubMed]
42. Zhou, N.; Bao, J. FerrDb: A manually curated resource for regulators and markers of ferroptosis and ferroptosis-disease associations. *Database* **2020**, *2020*. [CrossRef]
43. Swierczynska, M.M.; Betz, M.J.; Colombi, M.; Dazert, E.; Jeno, P.; Moes, S.; Pfaff, C.; Glatz, K.; Reincke, M.; Beuschlein, F.; et al. Proteomic Landscape of Aldosterone-Producing Adenoma. *Hypertension* **2019**, *73*, 469–480. [CrossRef] [PubMed]
44. Belavgeni, A.; Bornstein, S.R.; von Massenhausen, A.; Tonnus, W.; Stumpf, J.; Meyer, C.; Othmar, E.; Latk, M.; Kanczkowski, W.; Kroiss, M.; et al. Exquisite sensitivity of adrenocortical carcinomas to induction of ferroptosis. *Proc. Natl. Acad. Sci. USA* **2019**, *116*, 22269–22274. [CrossRef] [PubMed]

45. Weigand, I.; Schreiner, J.; Rohrig, F.; Sun, N.; Landwehr, L.S.; Urlaub, H.; Kendl, S.; Kiseljak-Vassiliades, K.; Wierman, M.E.; Angeli, J.P.F.; et al. Active steroid hormone synthesis renders adrenocortical cells highly susceptible to type II ferroptosis induction. *Cell Death Dis.* **2020**, *11*, 192. [CrossRef] [PubMed]
46. Kitawaki, Y.; Nakamura, Y.; Kubota-Nakayama, F.; Yamazaki, Y.; Miki, Y.; Hata, S.; Ise, K.; Kikuchi, K.; Morimoto, R.; Satoh, F.; et al. Tumor microenvironment in functional adrenocortical adenomas: Immune cell infiltration in cortisol-producing adrenocortical adenoma. *Hum. Pathol.* **2018**, *77*, 88–97. [CrossRef] [PubMed]
47. Madden, E.; Logue, S.E.; Healy, S.J.; Manie, S.; Samali, A. The role of the unfolded protein response in cancer progression: From oncogenesis to chemoresistance. *Biol. Cell* **2019**, *111*, 1–17. [CrossRef]
48. Peker, N.; Gozuacik, D. Autophagy as a Cellular Stress Response Mechanism in the Nervous System. *J. Mol. Biol.* **2020**, *432*, 2560–2588. [CrossRef] [PubMed]
49. Snaebjornsson, M.T.; Janaki-Raman, S.; Schulze, A. Greasing the Wheels of the Cancer Machine: The Role of Lipid Metabolism in Cancer. *Cell Metab.* **2020**, *31*, 62–76. [CrossRef] [PubMed]
50. Carracedo, A.; Cantley, L.C.; Pandolfi, P.P. Cancer metabolism: Fatty acid oxidation in the limelight. *Nat. Rev. Cancer* **2013**, *13*, 227–232. [CrossRef] [PubMed]
51. Barrett, P.Q.; Guagliardo, N.A.; Klein, P.M.; Hu, C.; Breault, D.T.; Beenhakker, M.P. Role of voltage-gated calcium channels in the regulation of aldosterone production from zona glomerulosa cells of the adrenal cortex. *J. Physiol.* **2016**, *594*, 5851–5860. [CrossRef]
52. Wiederkehr, A.; Szanda, G.; Akhmedov, D.; Mataki, C.; Heizmann, C.W.; Schoonjans, K.; Pozzan, T.; Spat, A.; Wollheim, C.B. Mitochondrial matrix calcium is an activating signal for hormone secretion. *Cell Metab.* **2011**, *13*, 601–611. [CrossRef]
53. Gulick, T.; Cresci, S.; Caira, T.; Moore, D.D.; Kelly, D.P. The peroxisome proliferator-activated receptor regulates mitochondrial fatty acid oxidative enzyme gene expression. *Proc. Natl. Acad. Sci. USA* **1994**, *91*, 11012–11016. [CrossRef]
54. Pawlak, M.; Lefebvre, P.; Staels, B. Molecular mechanism of PPARalpha action and its impact on lipid metabolism, inflammation and fibrosis in non-alcoholic fatty liver disease. *J. Hepatol.* **2015**, *62*, 720–733. [CrossRef]
55. Hardege, I.; Long, L.; Al Maskari, R.; Figg, N.; O'Shaughnessy, K.M. Targeted disruption of the Kcnj5 gene in the female mouse lowers aldosterone levels. *Clin. Sci.* **2018**, *132*, 145–156. [CrossRef]
56. Sun, N.; Meyer, L.S.; Feuchtinger, A.; Kunzke, T.; Knosel, T.; Reincke, M.; Walch, A.; Williams, T.A. Mass Spectrometry Imaging Establishes 2 Distinct Metabolic Phenotypes of Aldosterone-Producing Cell Clusters in Primary Aldosteronism. *Hypertension* **2020**, *75*, 634–644. [CrossRef] [PubMed]
57. Williams, T.A.; Gomez-Sanchez, C.E.; Rainey, W.E.; Giordano, T.J.; Lam, A.K.; Marker, A.; Mete, O.; Yamazaki, Y.; Zerbini, M.C.N.; Beuschlein, F.; et al. International Histopathology Consensus for Unilateral Primary Aldosteronism. *J. Clin. Endocrinol. Metab.* **2021**, *106*, 42–54. [CrossRef] [PubMed]
58. Sun, N.; Wu, Y.; Nanba, K.; Sbiera, S.; Kircher, S.; Kunzke, T.; Aichler, M.; Berezowska, S.; Reibetanz, J.; Rainey, W.E.; et al. High-Resolution Tissue Mass Spectrometry Imaging Reveals a Refined Functional Anatomy of the Human Adult Adrenal Gland. *Endocrinology* **2018**, *159*, 1511–1524. [CrossRef] [PubMed]
59. Lieu, F.K.; Lin, C.Y.; Wang, P.S.; Jian, C.Y.; Yeh, Y.H.; Chen, Y.A.; Wang, K.L.; Lin, Y.C.; Chang, L.L.; Wang, G.J.; et al. Effect of swimming on the production of aldosterone in rats. *PLoS ONE* **2014**, *9*, e87080. [CrossRef] [PubMed]
60. Chang, C.H.; Qiu, J.; O'Sullivan, D.; Buck, M.D.; Noguchi, T.; Curtis, J.D.; Chen, Q.; Gindin, M.; Gubin, M.M.; van der Windt, G.J.; et al. Metabolic Competition in the Tumor Microenvironment Is a Driver of Cancer Progression. *Cell* **2015**, *162*, 1229–1241. [CrossRef]
61. Korpal, M.; Puyang, X.; Jeremy Wu, Z.; Seiler, R.; Furman, C.; Oo, H.Z.; Seiler, M.; Irwin, S.; Subramanian, V.; Julie Joshi, J.; et al. Evasion of immunosurveillance by genomic alterations of PPARgamma/RXRalpha in bladder cancer. *Nat. Commun.* **2017**, *8*, 103. [CrossRef]
62. Poynter, M.E.; Daynes, R.A. Peroxisome proliferator-activated receptor alpha activation modulates cellular redox status, represses nuclear factor-kappaB signaling, and reduces inflammatory cytokine production in aging. *J. Biol. Chem.* **1998**, *273*, 32833–32841. [CrossRef]
63. Gilbert, K.; Nian, H.; Yu, C.; Luther, J.M.; Brown, N.J. Fenofibrate lowers blood pressure in salt-sensitive but not salt-resistant hypertension. *J. Hypertens.* **2013**, *31*, 820–829. [CrossRef]
64. Zhao, E.; Maj, T.; Kryczek, I.; Li, W.; Wu, K.; Zhao, L.; Wei, S.; Crespo, J.; Wan, S.; Vatan, L.; et al. Cancer mediates effector T cell dysfunction by targeting microRNAs and EZH2 via glycolysis restriction. *Nat. Immunol.* **2016**, *17*, 95–103. [CrossRef] [PubMed]
65. Prasad, R.; Kowalczyk, J.C.; Meimaridou, E.; Storr, H.L.; Metherell, L.A. Oxidative stress and adrenocortical insufficiency. *J. Endocrinol.* **2014**, *221*, R63–R73. [CrossRef]
66. Wu, K.C.; Cui, J.Y.; Klaassen, C.D. Beneficial role of Nrf2 in regulating NADPH generation and consumption. *Toxicol. Sci.* **2011**, *123*, 590–600. [CrossRef] [PubMed]
67. Rapoport, R.; Sklan, D.; Hanukoglu, I. Electron leakage from the adrenal cortex mitochondrial P450scc and P450c11 systems: NADPH and steroid dependence. *Arch. Biochem. Biophys.* **1995**, *317*, 412–416. [CrossRef] [PubMed]
68. Choi, J.E.; Sebastian, C.; Ferrer, C.M.; Lewis, C.A.; Sade-Feldman, M.; LaSalle, T.; Gonye, A.; Lopez, B.G.C.; Abdelmoula, W.M.; Regan, M.S.; et al. A unique subset of glycolytic tumour-propagating cells drives squamous cell carcinoma. *Nat. Metab.* **2021**, *3*, 182–195. [CrossRef]

69. Kagan, V.E.; Mao, G.; Qu, F.; Angeli, J.P.; Doll, S.; Croix, C.S.; Dar, H.H.; Liu, B.; Tyurin, V.A.; Ritov, V.B.; et al. Oxidized arachidonic and adrenic PEs navigate cells to ferroptosis. *Nat. Chem. Biol.* **2017**, *13*, 81–90. [CrossRef]
70. Martinez, N.; White, V.; Kurtz, M.; Higa, R.; Capobianco, E.; Jawerbaum, A. Activation of the nuclear receptor PPARalpha regulates lipid metabolism in foetal liver from diabetic rats: Implications in diabetes-induced foetal overgrowth. *Diabetes Metab. Res. Rev.* **2011**, *27*, 35–46. [CrossRef] [PubMed]
71. Tesfay, L.; Paul, B.T.; Konstorum, A.; Deng, Z.; Cox, A.O.; Lee, J.; Furdui, C.M.; Hegde, P.; Torti, F.M.; Torti, S.V. Stearoyl-CoA Desaturase 1 Protects Ovarian Cancer Cells from Ferroptotic Cell Death. *Cancer Res.* **2019**, *79*, 5355–5366. [CrossRef] [PubMed]
72. Gao, M.; Monian, P.; Quadri, N.; Ramasamy, R.; Jiang, X. Glutaminolysis and Transferrin Regulate Ferroptosis. *Mol. Cell* **2015**, *59*, 298–308. [CrossRef] [PubMed]

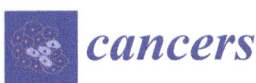

Systematic Review

Transcriptomics, Epigenetics, and Metabolomics of Primary Aldosteronism

Ariadni Spyroglou [1,2], George P. Piaditis [3], Gregory Kaltsas [4,†] and Krystallenia I. Alexandraki [1,*,†]

1. 2nd Department of Surgery, Aretaieio Hospital Athens, Medical School, National and Kapodistrian University of Athens, 11528 Athens, Greece; aspyroglou@gmail.com or ariadni.spyroglou@usz.ch
2. Clinic for Endocrinology, Diabetology and Clinical Nutrition, University Hospital Zurich, CH-8091 Zurich, Switzerland
3. Department of Endocrinology and Diabetes Center, G. Gennimatas General Hospital, 11527 Athens, Greece; edk-pgna@otenet.gr
4. Endocrine Unit, First Department of Propaedeutic Medicine, Laiko University Hospital, Medical School, National and Kapodistrian University of Athens, 11527 Athens, Greece; gregory.kaltsas@gmail.com
* Correspondence: alexandrakik@gmail.com
† Equally contributing senior authors.

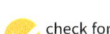

Simple Summary: Improvement in the understanding of the development of primary aldosteronism, the most common cause of endocrine hypertension and mainly caused by aldosterone producing adenomas or hyperplasia, has been continuously accomplished over the past several years. Herein, we summarize the major milestones in the field, including utilization of the newest available molecular techniques to not only shed light on the mechanisms involved in disease development but also to assist in the identification of disease subtypes with distinct laboratory and molecular findings, enabling the personalized treatment of the patients.

Citation: Spyroglou, A.; Piaditis, G.P.; Kaltsas, G.; Alexandraki, K.I. Transcriptomics, Epigenetics, and Metabolomics of Primary Aldosteronism. *Cancers* **2021**, *13*, 5582. https://doi.org/10.3390/cancers13215582

Academic Editor: Peter Igaz

Received: 23 August 2021
Accepted: 5 November 2021
Published: 8 November 2021

Publisher's Note: MDPI stays neutral with regard to jurisdictional claims in published maps and institutional affiliations.

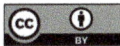

Copyright: © 2021 by the authors. Licensee MDPI, Basel, Switzerland. This article is an open access article distributed under the terms and conditions of the Creative Commons Attribution (CC BY) license (https://creativecommons.org/licenses/by/4.0/).

Abstract: Introduction: Primary aldosteronism (PA) is the most common cause of endocrine hypertension, mainly caused by aldosterone-producing adenomas or hyperplasia; understanding its pathophysiological background is important in order to provide ameliorative treatment strategies. Over the past several years, significant progress has been documented in this field, in particular in the clarification of the genetic and molecular mechanisms responsible for the pathogenesis of aldosterone-producing adenomas (APAs). Methods: Systematic searches of the PubMed and Cochrane databases were performed for all human studies applying transcriptomic, epigenetic or metabolomic analyses to PA subjects. Studies involving serial analysis of gene expression and microarray, epigenetic studies with methylome analyses and micro-RNA expression profiles, and metabolomic studies focused on improving understanding of the regulation of autonomous aldosterone production in PA were all included. Results: In this review we summarize the main findings in this area and analyze the interplay between primary aldosteronism and several signaling pathways with differential regulation of the RNA and protein expression of several factors involved in, among others, steroidogenesis, calcium signaling, and nuclear, membrane and G-coupled protein receptors. Distinct transcriptomic and metabolomic patterns are also presented herein, depending on the mutational status of APAs. In particular, two partially opposite transcriptional and steroidogenic profiles appear to distinguish APAs carrying a *KCNJ5* mutation from all other APAs, which carry different mutations. Conclusions: These findings can substantially contribute to the development of personalized treatment in patients with PA.

Keywords: primary aldosteronism; transcriptomics; epigenetics; metabolomics

1. Introduction

Primary aldosteronism (PA) is the most common cause of endocrine hypertension, with a prevalence of approximately 10% in hypertensive subjects [1,2]. In addition to hypertension and occasionally hypokalemia, aldosterone excess significantly increases cardiovascular risk, stressing the need for better understanding of its pathophysiology for the optimization of treatment strategies [3]. There are two main clinical presentations of PA: aldosterone-producing adrenal adenoma (APA), and bilateral adrenal hyperplasia (BAH), whereas the clinical picture can rarely be attributed to an adrenocortical carcinoma [1]. Recently, both somatic and germline mutations have been identified as causative for the development of APAs; these also affect the clinical phenotype of the disease.

The most frequent genetic alteration in APAs, with a female predominance and a prevalence of 40–50% (and even higher in Asian populations), is a Potassium Inwardly Rectifying Channel Subfamily J Member 5 (*KCNJ5*) mutation which causes depolarization of the membrane of zona glomerulosa (ZG) cells, opening the voltage gated Ca^{2+} channels and increasing Ca^{2+} influx [4–7]. Acting in a similar way, identified mutations in the ATPase Plasma Membrane Ca^{2+} Transporting 3 (*ATP2B3*) and the Calcium Voltage-Gated Channel Subunit Alpha1 D (*CACNA1D*) genes act by increasing the intracellular Ca^{2+} and stimulating Cytochrome P450 Family 11 Subfamily B Member 2 (aldosterone synthase-*CYP11B2*) expression and subsequent aldosterone synthesis [8,9]. Mutations in the ATPase Na^+/K^+ Transporting Subunit Alpha 1 (*ATP1A1*) gene induce cellular acidification due to H^+ leakage, but the exact mechanism resulting in autonomous aldosterone secretion has not been elucidated yet [8,10]. β-catenin 1 (*CTNNB1*) mutations, identified in a small proportion of APAs, cause constitutive activation of β-catenin and are considered to directly promote CYP11B2 synthesis [11]. More recently, co-existence of *CTNNB1* with G Protein Subunit Alpha Q (*GNAQ*)/G Protein Subunit Alpha 11 (*GNA11*) mutations was documented in 59% of APAs [12]. Rarely, Protein Kinase cAMP-Activated Catalytic Subunit Alpha (*PRKACA*), sporadic Calcium Voltage-Gated Channel Subunit Alpha1 H (*CACNA1H*) and Chloride Voltage-Gated Channel 2 (*CLCN2*) mutations have also been identified in sporadic APAs [13–15].

In addition to the rather common somatic mutations responsible for sporadic PA cases, four rare familial forms of the disease associated with early-onset hypertension have been identified. In short, familial hyperaldosteronism type I is attributed to a hybrid Cytochrome P450 Family 11 Subfamily B Member 1 (*CYP11B1*)/*CYP11B2* gene inherited as an autosomal dominant characteristic where aldosterone synthesis is adrenocorticotropic hormone (ACTH)- and not angiotensin II-dependent [16]. Familial hyperaldosteronism type II is caused by a *CLCN2* mutation in chloride channels, clinically expressed as early-onset hypertension along with hypokalemia and was initially described in a population of PA individuals under the age of ten [17]. *KCNJ5* germline mutations are the genetic basis of familial hyperaldosteronism type III [4,18], whereas *CACNA1H* mutations result in a gain of function of the Ca^{2+} voltage gained channel, leading to familial hyperaldosteronism type IV [19,20].

However, the already complex genetic landscape of PA provides a trigger for the further understanding of the pathophysiology of this common endocrine form of hypertension caused by adrenal tumours and/or cancer. Gene expression profiling along with epigenetic and metabolomic studies can elucidate the mechanisms and signaling pathways which have a role in the pathogenesis of PA, enabling the identification of subgroups of PA with distinct clinical, histological, and molecular profiles.

2. Methodology

We performed a detailed web-based search of the PubMed and Cochrane database with the terms "Metabolomics"(Mesh) OR "Epigenomics"(Mesh) OR "DNA Methylation"(Mesh) OR "MicroRNAs"(Mesh) OR "Gene Expression"(Mesh) OR "Gene Expression Profiling"(Mesh) AND "Hyperaldosteronism"(Mesh), with the term hyperaldosteronism including "Aldosteronism", "Conn ('s) Syndrome" and "primary hyperaldosteronism", on 25 July 2021. The start date for the literature search was 1 January 1990, and the search was limited to articles written in English and to human studies. Reviews and case reports were excluded from the present analysis. The review was registered on the PROSPERO platform (CRD42021271111). The PRISMA flow diagram can be found in Figure 1.

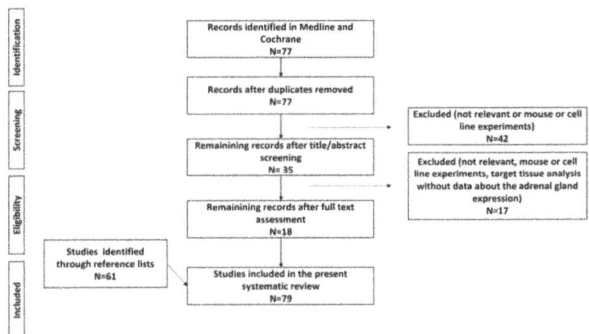

Figure 1. Flowchart for data collection.

3. Results

3.1. Clinical and Histological Traits of PA Patients

The first observations of the distinct characteristics of APAs carrying unique mutations can be obtained from their clinical and histological appearance. APAs carrying *KCNJ5* mutations are significantly larger in size, present lower pre-contrast Hounsfield units in abdominal computed tomography (CT) scans, and histologically display predominantly lipid-rich zona fasciculata (ZF)-like cells [21–23]. Further observations associate these tumors with young female patients and higher plasma aldosterone levels [7,24]. On the other hand, APA patients with ATPase mutations are frequently middle-aged men, with hypokalemia and low-renin hyperaldosteronism as well as increased aldosterone responsiveness upon ACTH stimulation, without large adrenal tumors upon CT scan but with histologically well-circumscribed tumors with compact eosinophilic cells and peritumoral hyperplasia [8,24,25]. ZF-like cells appear more typical for *KCNJ5* mutation-containing nodules, and ZG-like cells for *ATP1A1*, *ATP2B3* and *CACNA1D* mutations.

In normal human ZG, in situ hybridization shows focal *CYP11B2* expression with positive cell clusters that according to their size can be characterized as foci, megafoci and larger clusters and which, according to the present histopathology consensus for unilateral PA, are called aldosterone-producing micronodules or APM (formally known as aldosterone-producing cell clusters, or APCCs) [26–28]. The presence of APMs has been confirmed in several studies investigating the structure of normal adrenal glands. APMs are composed of both ZG-like and ZF-like cells; however, the ZF-like cells of APMs have high CYP11B2 expression and rather low CYP11B1 and CYP17A1 expression [27–29]. APMs do not typically present the cellular atypia seen in APAs [30]; however, a positive correlation between the total APM area and patient age has been documented [31]. In parallel, APMs produce increased levels of aldosterone and 18-oxocortisol, both steroids increased in APAs [32]. It has been suggested that with aging, when the physiological aldosterone production from ZG cells declines, APMs accumulate mutations that can lead to the transition to APAs [32].

Interestingly, APMs in normal adrenal glands are more frequent in women, without ethnic distribution but with a clear correlation with ageing, and often carry known APA mutations such as *CACNA1D* and *ATP1A1* [33]. PA patients with negative adrenal CT scans often present an increased number of APMs, predominantly carrying *CACNA1D* mutations; thus, a potential progression from APMs to micro-APAs can be postulated as part of a continuum in these cases [30,34]. However, in large APAs, which usually carry *KCNJ5* mutations, an APM origin does not seem to be a feasible progression mechanism [30]. Another study found transitional structures with a combination of subcapsular APM-like structure and an inner APA-like microstructure without well-defined borders, characterized by the presence of *KCNJ5* and *ATP1A1* mutations [35]. Recently, two further studies documented that APMs in the adrenals of patients with APAs carried mutations predominantly in *CACNA1D*, but also in *KCNJ5*, *ATP1A1*, *CACNA1H*, *PRKACA* and *CTNNB1*, weakening the hypothesis that *KCNJ5* mutations do not correlate with the APM-APA transition theory [36,37]. The presence of somatic mutations in APMs suggests that co-driver mutations are necessary in order to promote APA formation. In line with this two-hit theory, co-existence of *CTNNB1* with *GNAQ* or *GNA11* mutations was described in APAs, whereas solitary *GNAQ/GNA11* mutations were identified in the adjacent hyperplastic zona glomerulosa of the double mutant APAs [12]. Similarly, the occurrence of *KCNJ5* mutations in adrenals from patients with germline APC Regulator of WNT Signaling Pathway (*APC*) mutations has been previously described [38].

Histological examination of APAs without subtype classification reveals increased nodulation and reduced vascularization in the peritumoral tissues surrounding APAs [27]. The ZG adjacent to APAs appears continuous and thickened, with positive expression of CYP11B2 and Disabled 2 (Dab2), both markers of the ZG, and negative staining for CYP11B1, a typical marker of ZF responsible for cortisol synthesis. This finding is not in line with the observed staining in APMs, which was positive for CYP11B2 but negative for Dab2. Furthermore, the number of APMs in peritumoral adrenal tissues did not differ from control adrenals, whereas the number of megafoci was significantly increased in peritumoral adjacent tissues [27]. In another study, adrenal glands from APA patients presented positive CYP11B2 expression in only one dominant nodule, even in APA cases with histologically documented multinodularity. No conclusions about the correlation between a specific mutation and the multinodularity could be obtained in this study; however, the mutations were always located in the CYP11B2 positive nodules, with multiple positive nodules in the same adrenal gland occasionally carrying different mutations [39,40]. Furthermore, APMs and APAs share immunohistochemical overexpression of the endoplasmatic reticulum protein calmegin (CLGN) [41]. In summary, APMs have high CYP11B2 expression, present a ZG- and ZF-like appearance, and harbor APA-related mutations, all common characteristics with APAs. Still, as the mutational status of the principal nodule in APAs is not necessarily identical with the mutations found in secondary nodules, the theory of an APM to APA transition remains to be elucidated.

An increased number of APMs has been documented in a small cohort of adrenalectomized patients with BAH, predominantly carrying *CACNA1D* mutations [42]. In a different approach, in a very recent study adrenalectomized PA patients with partial or absent biochemical cure that displayed lower lateralization indexes histologically, frequently presented one or more APMs which frequently harbored *CACNA1D* mutations, suggesting common mechanisms in APA and BAH pathogenesis [43].

Furthermore, two-thirds of APAs exhibited positive immunohistochemical staining of G Protein Activated Inward Rectifier Potassium Channel 4 (GIRK4) and Dab2, both markers of the ZG, rendering these possible markers for the distinction of APAs from non-functioning adenomas. Additionally, APAs carrying KCNJ5 mutations exhibited lower GIRK4 expression in APA in comparison to the peritumoral ZG, allowing initial screening for the mutation status of these tumors using immunohistochemistry [44].

3.2. Transcriptomics

Gene expression profiles of APAs have increasingly been applied to shed light on the pathophysiology of PA. Either by microarray or serial analysis of gene expression (SAGE), the gene expression profile of APAs is routinely compared to that of adjacent adrenal glands or normal adrenal glands. Thus, an interplay between PA and a variety of signaling pathways can be documented. Among other factors, upon PA a differential expression of several molecules was observed, from classical enzymes involved in steroidogenesis, nuclear receptor transcription factors, ion channels, molecules involved in calcium signaling, and G-coupled proteins to molecules responsible for cell energy, mitochondrial function, protein binding, transcription factors, and oncogenes (Table 1 and Figure 2).

Table 1. Transcriptome-identified genes up- (↑) or downregulated (↓) in the following conditions: (a) in APAs versus normal adrenal tissue or other adrenal adenomas; (b) in two different subgroups of APAs: ZF-like (in some studies defined as carrying KCNJ5 mutations) versus ZG-like (in some studies defined as either WT or as carrying the ATP1A1, ATP2B3, CACNA1D or CTNNB1 mutations).

Genes	Description	Trend
	Steroidogenic enzymes	
CYP11B2	Cytochrome P450 Family 11 Subfamily B Member 2	↑(a), ↔ ↑(b)
CYP11B1	Cytochrome P450 Family 11 Subfamily B Member 1	↑(b)
CYP21A2	Cytochrome P450 Family 21 Subfamily A Member 2	↑(a)
HSD3B2	Hydroxy-Delta-5-Steroid Dehydrogenase, 3 Beta- And Steroid Delta-Isomerase 2	↑(a)
CYP17A1	Cytochrome P450 Family 17 Subfamily A Member 1	↓(a), ↑(b) *
CYP11A1	Cytochrome P450 Family 11 Subfamily A Member 1	↑(a)
AKR1C3	Aldo-Keto Reductase Family 1 Member C3	↓(a)
	Nuclear receptors/transcription factors	
NR4A2	Nuclear Receptor Subfamily 4 Group A Member 2 (NURR1)	↑(a), ↑(b)
NR4A1	Nuclear Receptor Subfamily 4 Group A Member 1 (NGF1B)	↑(a)
NR0B1	Nuclear Receptor Subfamily 0 Group B Member 1 (DAX1)	↑(a) *
NR5A1	Nuclear Receptor Subfamily 5 Group A Member 1 (Steroidogenic factor 1 _ SF1)	↑(a)
NR1B1	Retinoic Acid Receptor Alpha (RARα)	↓(a)
	Plasma membrane receptor	
SCARB1	Scavenger Receptor Class B Member 1 (CD36)	↑(a)
	Ion channels	
KCNK1	Potassium Two Pore Domain Channel Subfamily K Member 1 (TWIK-1)	↓(b)
KCNK5	Potassium Two Pore Domain Channel Subfamily K Member 5 (TASK-2)	↓(a)
SLC24A3	Solute Carrier Family 24 Member 3 (sodium calcium exchanger)	↓(b)
ANO4	Anoctamin 4 (calcium dependent chloride channel)	↓(a)
CACNA1A	Calcium Voltage-Gated Channel Subunit Alpha1 A	↑(a)
CACNA1C	Calcium Voltage-Gated Channel Subunit Alpha1 C	↑(a)
CACNA1E	Calcium Voltage-Gated Channel Subunit Alpha1 E	↑(a)
	Calcium signaling	
CALM2	Calmodulin 2	↑(a)
CALR	Calreticulin	↑(a)
CAMK1	Calcium/Calmodulin Dependent Protein Kinase I	↑(b)
CAMK2B	Calcium/Calmodulin Dependent Protein Kinase II Beta	↓(b)
CALN1	Calneuron 1	↑(a)
ATP2A3	ATPase Sarcoplasmic/Endoplasmic Reticulum Ca^{2+} Transporting 3 (SERCA3)	↑(a)
CLGN	Calmegin	↑(a)
PCP4	Purkinje Cell Protein 4	↑(a)
VSNL1	Visinin Like 1	↑(a), ↑(b)
GSTA1	Glutathione S-Transferase Alpha 1	↓(a), ↓(b)
	G-protein coupled receptors	
LHCGR	Luteinizing Hormone/Choriogonadotropin Receptor	↑(a) **
GNRHR	Gonadotropin Releasing Hormone Receptor	↑(a)
HTR2A	5-Hydroxytryptamine Receptor 2A	↑(a), ↑(b)
HTR4	5-Hydroxytryptamine Receptor 4	↑(a)
AGTR1	Angiotensin II Receptor Type 1 (AT1R)	↑(a), ↑(b)
PTGER1	Prostaglandin E Receptor 1	↑(a)
GRM3	Glutamate Metabotropic Receptor 3	↑(a)
EDNRB	Endothelin Receptor Type B	↑(a)
MC2R	Melanocortin 2 Receptor	↑(a), ↑(b)
AVPR1A	Arginin Vasopressin Receptor 1A	↓(a)
PTGFR	Prostaglandin F Receptor	↓(a)
GPER1	G-Protein-Coupled Estrogen Receptor 1	↑(a)

Table 1. Cont.

Genes	Description	Trend
Energy		
FDX1	Adrenodoxin	↑(a)
POR	Cytochrome P450 Oxidoreductase	↑(a)
CYB5	Cytochrome B5 Type A	↑(a)
ATAD3C	ATPase Family AAA Domain Containing 3C	↑(a)
ACSS3	Acyl-CoA Synthetase Short Chain Family Member 3	↑(b)
-	Genes related to lipid metabolism, glycolysis, and antioxidant systems	↑(a)
Protein binding		
NEFM	Neurofilament Medium Chain	↓(b)
NPNT	Nephronectin	↓(b)
MRAP	Melanocortin 2 Receptor Accessory Protein	↑(a), ↑(b)
PROM1	Prominin 1	↑(a)
SFRP2	Secreted Frizzled Related Protein 2	↓(a)
Cell growth/cell death		
COPS5	COP9 Signalosome Subunit 5 (JAB1)	↑(a)
MYC	MYC Proto-Oncogene, BHLH Transcription Factor	↑(a)
IGFBP2	Insulin Like Growth Factor Binding Protein 2	↑(a)
CCN3	Cellular Communication Network Factor 3 (IGFBP9 or NOV)	↑(a)
TDGF1	Teratocarcinoma-Derived Growth Factor 1	↑(a)
BID	BH3 Interacting Domain Death Agonist	↓(b) **
BIRC2	Baculoviral IAP Repeat Containing 2	↓(b) **
BIRC3	Baculoviral IAP Repeat Containing 3	↓(b) **
Immune response		
-	Genes related to inflammatory response, interferon-γ response, and IL-6, JAK/STAT3 signaling	↓(a)
DNA binding/RNA polymerase		
GATA6	GATA Binding Protein 6	↑(a)
PRRX1	Paired Related Homeobox 1	↑(a)
DACH1	Dachshund Family Transcription Factor 1	↓(a)
BEX1	Brain-Expressed X-Linked 1	↑(a), ↓(b)

* Ambiguous results, please see text for details. ** Higher expression in CTNNB1 tumors.

3.2.1. Steroidogenic Enzymes

As the rate limiting step for aldosterone synthesis, *CYP11B2* overexpression is present in a number of studies investigating gene expression profiles in APAs [14,45–54]. Interestingly, several studies have observed heterogeneity in *CYP11B2* expression in APAs, with one subgroup overexpressed and another group with either unchanged or even reduced CYP11B2 expression [47,55–57]. Several studies confirmed that *CYP11B2* expression was significantly higher in tumors carrying *ATP1A1*, *ATP2B3* or *CACNA1D* mutations than in tumors carrying *KCNJ5* mutations [47–49,58]. Kitamoto et al. found increased *CYP11B2* expression in *ATP2B3* tumors but not in *ATP1A1* tumors [59]. Another discrepancy in addition to this initial observation was described by Monticone et al., who documented increased *CYP11B2* expression in APAs with *KCNJ5* mutations [46].

In line with *CYP11B2* expression, differential expression of *CYP11B1*, responsible for cortisol synthesis, has been recognized in several studies. As a common observation, two different *CYP11B1* expression profiles were observed, with a subgroup of APAs presenting an overexpression of this steroidogenic enzyme and a second subgroup displaying very low expression [57]. Interestingly, *CYP11B1* expression was inversely correlated with *CYP11B2* expression. Thus, tumors carrying a *KCNJ5* mutation presented overexpression of *CYP11B1* and concomitant rather low *CYP11B2* levels, whereas *ATP1A1*, *ATP2B3* and *CACNA1D* mutant tumors had very low *CYP11B1* expression along with significant *CYP11B2* overexpression [22,37,49,59]. This pattern is suggestive of a particular biological behaviour of *KCNJ5* tumors, which also appear to co-secrete cortisol [60]. Unlike this rather common finding, a large European multicenter study did not document any significant *CYP11B1* expression differences among the different mutations of APAs [24].

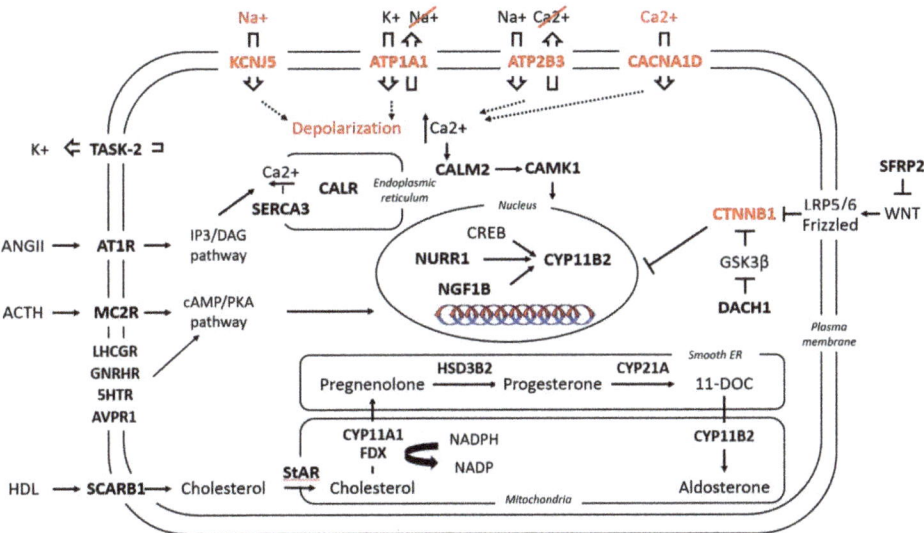

Figure 2. Simplified presentation of the main pathways involved in aldosterone regulation under physiological conditions and in APAs. In bold are the molecules involved in these pathways which have been found to be up-/down-regulated in APAs; in red are the five known mutant genes responsible for APAs and their aberrant cellular function. For nomenclature, the name of the respective genes and proteins have been used; for their respective abbreviations, see Table 1.

Differential expression of Cytochrome P450 Family 21 Subfamily A Member 2 (*CYP21A2*), the enzyme catalyzing the conversion of progesterone to 11-deoxycorticosterone (a precursor of aldosterone synthesis), is also well documented in PA, with APAs displaying a significant overexpression of this enzyme [48,53]. A concomitant increased expression of Hydroxy-Delta-5-Steroid Dehydrogenase, 3 Beta- And Steroid Delta-Isomerase 2 (*HSD3B2*), the enzyme converting pregnenolone to progesterone, has been documented in the majority of APAs [21,48,59,61]. Interestingly, Cytochrome P450 Family 17 Subfamily A Member 1 (*CYP17A1*) expression in APAs has thus far, shown contradictory trends. In one study, *CYP17A1*, responsible for the hydroxylation of pregnenolone and progesterone, was downregulated in the majority of APAs compared to adjacent adrenal tissue. However, this was not the case in tumors carrying *KCNJ5* mutations, which histologically presented more ZF-like characteristics [21]. Another study documented that *CYP17* expression was downregulated in APAs, without providing information about mutation status [51]. Furthermore, in the same study, Aldo-Keto Reductase Family 1 Member C3 (*AKR1C3*, 17β-hydroxysteroid dehydrogenase type 5) expression showed significantly lower transcript levels in APAs [51]. Finally, an upregulation of Cytochrome P450 Family 11 Subfamily A Member 1 (*CYP11A1*), the catalysator of cholesterol to pregnenolone, was documented in all investigated APAs [56]. For the main steps required for adrenocortical steroidogenesis, see also Figure 3.

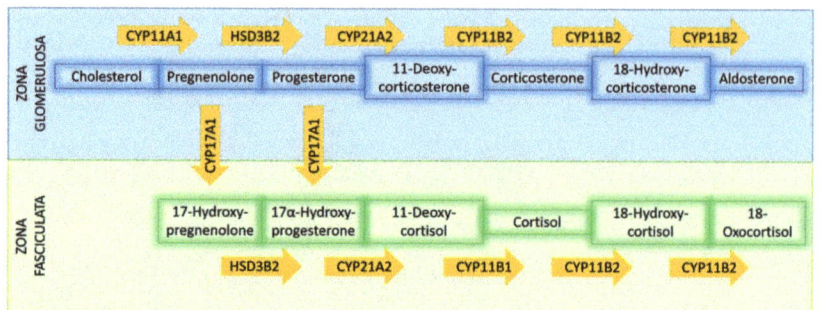

Figure 3. Simplified presentation of steroidogenesis in the zona glomerulosa and zona fasciculata; the yellow arrows represent the enzymes which catalyze the respective reactions.

3.2.2. Nuclear Receptor Transcription Factors

Several nuclear receptors, acting mainly as transcription factors, have been acknowledged as being involved in aldosterone secretion regulation. In line with these findings, several studies have presented an increase of the Nuclear Receptor Subfamily 4 Group A Member 2 (*NR4A2* or *NURR1*) and Nuclear Receptor Subfamily 4 Group A Member 1 (*NR4A1* or *NGF1B*) transcription factors in APAs [11,22,48], particularly KCNJ5 mutant APAs correlated with a pronounced *NURR1* increase [22,62]. Two further transcription factors play a role in both adrenal development and steroidogenesis, namely Nuclear Receptor Subfamily 5 Group A Member 1 (*NR5A1* or steroidogenic factor-1, *SF-1*) and Nuclear Receptor Subfamily 0 Group B Member 1 (*NR0B1* or dosage-sensitive sex reversal, *DAX-1*); both were found to be significantly increased in APAs [48,63]. In two older studies, however, lower *DAX-1* expression was documented in APAs compared to cortisol-producing or non-functioning adrenal adenomas [54,64]. Finally, in a recent study, the nuclear receptor Retinoic Acid Receptor α, (*RARα*) showed significantly lower expression in APAs compared to normal adrenal glands; the nodulation occurring in APAs was attributed to its downregulation, as this molecule is responsible for normal adrenal zonation [55].

3.2.3. Plasma Membrane Receptors

The single plasma membrane receptor identified so far with a role in APAs is the Scavenger Receptor Class B Member 1 (*SCARB1*), also known as CD36 antigen, responsible for the transport of high-density lipoprotein (HDL) into the ZG cells. In one study, the *SCARB1* expression, important for the cholesterol supplies in the adrenocortical cells, was found significantly upregulated in APAs compared to the adjacent adrenal glands [53].

3.2.4. Ion Channels

Little data is available concerning the differential expression of ion channels in APAs. Concomitant to the expression pattern of CYP11B1 in APAs, and depending on their mutation status as described above, the Potassium Two Pore Domain Channel Subfamily K Member 1 (*KCNK1* or *TWIK-1*) potassium channel and the Solute Carrier Family 24 Member 3 (*SLC24A3*) sodium/calcium exchanger show significant negative correlation with CYP11B1 expression in APAs [21]. The Potassium Two Pore Domain Channel Subfamily K Member 5 (*KCNK5* or *TASK2*) channel is also consistently less expressed in APAs compared to normal adrenal cortex [65]. Recently, Anoctamin 4 (*ANO4*), a calcium dependent chloride channel, was found to be significantly downregulated in APAs compared to normal ZG, independent of their respective mutation status [66]. Expression data on L-type and T-type voltage dependent calcium channels has demonstrated high CACNA1H expression in both normal adrenal glands and APAs, while CACNA1A, CACNA1C and CACNA1E expression was significantly upregulated in APAs [20].

3.2.5. Calcium Signaling

As one of the main pathways promoting physiological aldosterone secretion upon angiotensin II or potassium stimulation is calcium signaling, it is not a surprise that several molecules of the calcium signaling pathway are differentially regulated in APAs. Assié et al. documented an increased expression of Calmodulin 2 (*CALM2*), Calreticulin (*CALR*) and ATPase Sarcoplasmic/Endoplasmic Reticulum Ca^{2+} Transporting 3 (*ATP2A3*, or calcium adenosine triphosphatase 3, *SERCA3*) in APAs compared to the adjacent normal adrenal tissue [53]. Interestingly, in line with the already described heterogeneity of *CYP11B2* expression in two subgroups of APAs, one APA subgroup presents overexpression of Calcium/Calmodulin Dependent Protein Kinase I (*CAMK1*) in parallel with *CYP11B2* overexpression and Calcium/Calmodulin Dependent Protein Kinase II Beta (*CAMK2B*) underexpression, while another group presents the opposite profile [57]. Calneuron 1 (*CALN1*), localized in the endoplasmatic reticulum, binds calcium ions and positively correlates with the increased *CYP11B2* expression in APAs in comparison to non-functioning adrenal adenomas [67]. The endoplasmatic reticulum carrier Calmegin (*CLGN*) is also upregulated in APAs compared to non-functioning adenomas, with a clear positive correlation with *CYP11B2* expression [41,68]. Purkinje Cell Protein 4 (*PCP4*), a molecule modulating calcium binding by calmodulin, has been found to be significantly increased in APAs compared to the adjacent adrenal glands [51]. Finally, Vinisin like 1 (*VSNL1*), a neuronal calcium sensor protein functioning in the transduction of calcium signals, presents significantly higher expression in APAs compared to normal adrenals. Furthermore, *VSNL1* expression in APAs harboring KCNJ5 mutations is significantly higher than in wild-type tumors [52]. Glutathione S-Transferase Alpha 1 (*GSTA1*), an enzyme protecting cells from reactive oxygen species which also serving as transmitter of calcium signaling, presents significantly lower expression in APAs compared to non-aldosterone producing adenomas, while *KCNJ5* mutated APAs had significantly lower expression of this gene than did wild-type APAs [45,69].

3.2.6. G-Protein Coupled Receptors (GPCRs)

Several genes encoding G-protein coupled receptors have been identified as differentially expressed in APAs, whereas a clear interrelation between GPCRs and physiological aldosterone secretion is acknowledged for the Melanocortin 2 Receptor (*MC2R*) and the 5-Hydroxytryptamine Receptor (*5-HTR-4*). In several studies, Luteinizing Hormone/Choriogonadotropin Receptor (*LHCGR*), Gonadotropin Releasing Hormone Receptor (*GNRHR*), 5-HTRs 2A and 4, Angiotensin II Receptor Type 1 (*AGTR1* or *AT1R*), Glutamate Metabotropic Receptor 3 (*GRM3*), Endothelin Receptor Type B (*EDNRB*), *MC2R*, and Prostaglandin E Receptor 1 (*PTGER1*), among others, were all found to be significantly upregulated in APAs [50,70–72]. In one recent study, *MC2R* expression correlated positively with that of *AGTR1* in APAs harboring *KCNJ5* and *CACNA1D* mutations, whereas *MC2R* expression correlated positively with Melanocortin 2 Receptor Accessory Protein (*MRAP*) only in *ATP1A1*- and *ATP2B3*-mutated APAs [72]. Moreover, *LHCG*- and *GNRH*-receptor upregulation were both correlated with APAs harboring *CTNNB1* mutations [12,49]. On the contrary, Arginine vasopressin receptor 1A (*AVPR1A*) and Prostaglandin F Receptor (*PTGFR*) were significantly downregulated in APAs [70]. Furthermore, in an ex vivo study using primary cultures from APAs, predominant G-Coupled-Protein Estrogen Receptor 1 (*GPER1*) expression was documented in these tumors [73,74].

3.2.7. Energy

The cytochrome P450 steroidogenic enzymes require electrons to exert their catalytic activity on cholesterol during the various steps involved in the formation of aldosterone precursors. In accordance with this need, the expression of energy-providing enzymes such as Adrenodoxin (*FDX1*), Cytochrome P450 Oxidoreductase (*POR*), Cytochrome B5 (*CYB5*) have been found to be significantly upregulated in APAs compared to the adjacent ZG or normal adrenal glands [51,53,56]. ATPase Family AAA Domain Containing 3C

(*ATAD3C*), a mitochondrial membrane bound ATPase, showed the highest increase in APAs in one study [56], whereas Acyl-CoA Synthetase Short Chain Family Member 3 (*ACSS3*), a gene with acetate-CoA ligase activity, was the top gene upregulated in *KCNJ5* mutant APAs in comparison to wild types in another study [62]. In a recent study, transcriptome data analysis identified alterations in transcriptome signatures in pathways related to mitochondrial fatty acid β-oxidation and peroxisome proliferator receptor-α (*PPARα*), with suppression of ferroptosis suppressor genes and overexpression of genes related to glycolysis/glyconeogenesis in APAs. Furthermore, *KCNJ5* mutated APAs that have a higher proliferative index display increased expression of genes involved in glycolysis and lipid metabolism, an observation reminiscent of the well-characterized role of metabolic reprogramming in cancer progression [75].

3.2.8. Protein Binding

Neurofilament Medium (*NEFM*), which encodes a neurofilament subunit, was significantly upregulated in wild-type APAs for *KCNJ5* mutations (ZG-like APAs) compared to APAs carrying *KCNJ5* mutations (ZF-like APAs). Silencing of NEFM leads to a significant increase of aldosterone secretion in human adrenocortical cell cultures (H295R), suggesting a role of *NEFM* in the physiological negative regulation of aldosterone production [62,76].

Nephronectin (*NPNT*) is a secreted matrix protein with a role in calcium ion binding as well as in integrin binding. *NPNT* was found to be highly overexpressed in APAs with a ZG-like structure carrying *ATP1A1*, *ATP2B3* and *CTNNB1* mutations. *NPNT* production is regulated by the canonical Wnt/β-catenin signaling pathway and may upregulate aldosterone production [47,77].

PROM1 encodes a transmembrane protein with actinin- and cadherin-binding properties, which also binds cholesterol on the plasma membrane. Prominin 1 (*PROM1*) was found significantly upregulated in APAs when compared to normal adrenal glands [56].

A well-acknowledged mechanism for the development of PA is the constitutive activation of the wnt/β-catenin pathway. In accordance with this, Secreted Frizzled Related Protein 2 (*SFRP2*), a WNT inhibitor, was significantly downregulated in APAs compared to normal adrenal glands or non-functioning adrenal adenomas [11].

3.2.9. Cell Growth/Cell Death

In a SAGE study, although APAs are considered benign tumors, several oncogenes were identified as upregulated in comparison to normal adrenal glands, among others Jun-binding protein (*JAB1*), avian myelocytomatosis viral oncogene (*v-MYC*), IGF-binding protein-2 (*IGFBP2*), teratocarcinoma-derived growth factor (*TDGF1*), and nephroblastoma overexpressed gene (*NOV*). Although *v-MYC*, *IGFBP2* and *NOV* overexpression was not confirmed by in situ hybridization, no clear conclusions can be made on the mechanisms of tumorigenesis in APAs [53]. The Teratocarcinoma-Derived Growth Factor 1 (*TDGF1*) upregulation in APAs has, however, been confirmed in another microarray study [78]. The apoptosis inhibitors BH3 Interacting Domain Death Agonist (*BID*) and Baculoviral IAP Repeat Containing 2 (*BIRC2*) and 3 (*BIRC3*) were also found overexpressed in a subgroup of APAs harboring *CTNNB1* mutations [49]. Interestingly, the Wnt/β-Catenin pathway is also one of the most frequently altered pathways in adrenocortical carcinomas (ACC), mainly harboring alterations in *CTNNB1*, APC Regulator of WNT Signaling Pathway (*APC*), and Zinc and Ring Finger 3 (*ZNRF3*), suggesting that alterations in this pathway are, in part, shared events in both benign and malignant adrenocortical tumors [79,80].

3.2.10. Immune Response

In a very recent study, microarray analysis of APAs compared to adjacent adrenal cortex identified differentially expressed genes in a series of immune-related pathways, including inflammatory response, interferon-γ response, and IL-6, JAK/STAT3 signaling. APAs presented, in general, significant downregulation of immune related genes, with several of these genes belonging to pathways related to cellular response to oxidative stress, suggesting that oxidative stress may elicit an immune response in the adjacent adrenal cortex. On the contrary, adrenocortical tumor cells appeared to possess mechanisms for counteracting metabolic stress through upregulation of antioxidant systems. APAs were documented to display a high proportion of tumor cells, suggesting that their particular transcriptome profile enables them to escape from immune surveillance [75].

3.2.11. DNA Binding/RNA Polymerase

GATA Binding Protein 6 (*GATA6*), a gene with role in cellular differentiation via activation of HSD3B in the remodeled subcapsular adrenocortical zone, has shown pronounced upregulation in APAs compared to normal adrenals [48]. Paired Related Homeobox 1 (*PRRX1*), a gene related to tumorigenesis encoding a transcription co-activator, was found to be significantly overexpressed in APAs in a microarray study [51]. Dachshund Family Transcription Factor 1 (*DACH1*), a modulator of gene expression and mediator of steroidogenic responses with a role in the wnt/β-catenin pathway, is highly expressed in the ZG and has been identified as a ZG marker and a negative regulator of aldosterone secretion. *DACH1* expression was found to be downregulated in APAs in comparison to normal adrenal glands [56,81]. In functional analyses, it has been shown that DACH1 suppresses aldosterone production; thus, its downregulation is in line with APA development. Brain-Expressed X-Linked 1 (BEX1) is another gene with differential regulation in APAs. In particular, both micro-APAs and APAs present higher BEX1 expression with CACNA1D, ATP1A1 or non-KCNJ5 mutations. This gene is involved in ferroptosis, and it is hypothesized that increasing APA size leads to reduction of the need for anti-ferroptotic mechanisms [25,82].

3.3. Epigenetics

The complex regulation of autonomous aldosterone secretion not only includes an altered transcriptional regulation, but also involves further mechanisms such as DNA methylation and the effects of microRNAs.

In general, APAs present hypomethylation of several genes, in part already recognized as presenting transcriptional alterations. The gene with the most frequently hypomethylated promotor is *CYP11B2*, aldosterone synthase. In detail, the CpG island in the promotor region of *CYP11B2* has been found to be hypomethylated in APAs, but not in blood samples of the same patients [83]. Similarly, hypomethylation of *CYP11B2* was not observed in the adjacent adrenal tissue [84,85]. Additionally, the hypomethylated region of *CYP11B2* has not been proven to be induced by the *KCNJ5* or *ATP1A1* mutations [86]. *CYP11B2* hypomethylation in APAs with parallel hypercortisolemia was unchanged; however, these tumors also presented *CYP11B1* promoter hypomethylation, especially at two CpG sites near the Ad1/cAMP response element binding site [87]. Furthermore, lower methylation levels of *CYP11B2* are documented in APAs compared to APMs, suggesting a role of demethylation in a possible APM to APA transition [85].

In addition to these hypomethylated genes, APAs present hypomethylation in other differentially expressed genes, as presented above. In particular, the G-coupled-protein receptors *PCP4, HTR4, MC2R, PTGER1* showed hypomethylation in APAs [71,88]. *PCP4*, one of the genes highly expressed in APAs, presented as one of the most hypomethylated genes in APAs [88]. In a study applying integration of transcriptome and methylome analysis in APAs and the adjacent adrenal gland, 34 genes presented upregulation with parallel CpG hypomethylation. These include aldosterone-related genes (*CYP11B2, MC2R* and hemopexin (*HPX*)) as well as genes related to tumorigenesis (*PRRX*, member RAS oncogene family (*RAB38*), fibroblast activation protein alpha (*FAP*), Glucosaminyl (N-Acetyl) Transferase 2 (I Blood Group) (*GCNT2*)) and to differentiation (Calmodulin-like Protein 3 (*CALML3*)) [84]. Inversely, hypermethylation of *AVPR1* and Protein Kinase C alpha (*PRKCA*) has been observed in APAs in comparison to normal adrenal glands [83]. Thus, not only is *CYP11B2* hypomethylated in APAs, but several molecules related to *CYP11B2* expression present differential methylation levels as well.

Unlike APAs, ACCs present global hypomethylation when compared to normal and benign tissues. In comparison with benign samples, ACCs present differential methylation status of several CpG sites, including those associated with Insulin Like Growth Factor 2 (*IGF2*) and H19 Imprinted Maternally Expressed Transcript (*H19*), Tumor Protein P53 (*TP53*), and *CTNNB1*. Interestingly, hypermethylation in both ACCs and benign samples has been documented for genes involved in apoptosis and transcriptional and cell cycle control, in particular for Cyclin Dependent Kinase Inhibitor 2A (*CDKN2*), ATA Binding Protein 4 (*GATA4*), Histone Deacetylase 10 (*HDAC10*), PYD And CARD Domain Containing (*PYCARD*), and Secretoglobin Family 3A Member 1 (*SCGB3A1*) [89].

Several microRNAs were identified in APAs as modulators of *CYP11B2* expression and are responsible for the differential regulation of other aldosterone production relevant genes as well. Among others, miR-24 was significantly downregulated in APAs in comparison to normal adrenal glands [90], while its levels were found to be significantly lower in APAs with *KCNJ5* mutations than in those without. In parallel, a significant negative correlation of this microRNA with the expression levels of its target gene, Glutamate Receptor interacting protein 1 (*GRIP1*), has been demonstrated, possibly posing this gene as a candidate factor for aldosterone autonomy [91]. In another study, the expression of miR-375 was significantly downregulated in APAs, whereas the respective in vitro experiments implied a role in tumor suppression acting through the metadherin (MTDH)/Akt pathway [92]. miR-203 exerts an inhibitory action through its target gene, Wnt Family Member 5A (*WNT5A*), and controls aldosterone secretion. miR-203 demonstrated lower expression in APA samples than in adjacent adrenal glands. Interestingly, plasma levels of its target gene, WNT5A, in adrenal vein sampling were found to be useful in differentiating tumor localization and estimating postoperative cure [93]. In a further study, when compared to patients with APAs, patients with bilateral hyperplasia presented overexpression of circulating miR-30e-5p, miR-30d-5p, and miR-7-5p. However, possibly also due to heterogeneity at the microRNA expression level in the APA group, the diagnostic accuracy of these markers does not allow for their application in clinical practice. These findings suggest that APA and BAH form part of a spectrum leading to PA [94]. Finally, miR-23 and miR-34 were found to decrease expression of TASK2 in APAs, leading to an increase in aldosterone production [65].

3.4. Metabolomics

One of the oldest approaches to investigating metabolome differences in APAs began decades ago with the initial observation that a patient with APA had elevated C-18-oxygenated steroids [95]. Later studies confirmed the observation that patients with APAs had elevated 18-hydroxycortisol and 18-oxocortisol, while patients with BAH did not present this laboratory phenotype [96]. As a next step, the quantification of these two steroids in the adrenal veins of patients with PA undergoing adrenal vein sampling (AVS) took place and an elevated 18-oxocortisol/cortisol ratio was found, indicating the dominant site in the AVS and allowing differentiation of patients with APAs from patients with BAH [97]. In an attempt to develop a less invasive testing method, urinary 18-hydroxycortisol levels were used with sufficient diagnostic accuracy to distinguish APAs from BAHs [98]. Several metabolic adaptations have since been described in tumorigenesis, with tumor cells undergoing metabolic reprogramming in order to address increased metabolic demands and enhance progression. Characteristic examples include increased glucolysis in cancer cells (the Warburg effect) and the dysregulation of lipid oxidation with increased β-oxidation and subsequent increased NADPH (also critical for adrenal steroidogenesis) with enhancement of CYP11A1 and CYP11B2 activity, possibly leading to increased aldosterone synthesis [75].

The introduction of liquid chromatography with tandem mass spectrometry (LC-MS/MS) in the quantification of adrenal steroids confirmed the previous data, and additionally widened the spectrum of investigated steroids. In addition to the clear elevation of plasma 18-oxocortisol in APAs, increased levels of plasma cortisol, corticosterone, dehydroepiandrosterone (DHEA) and DHEA-S were documented in patients with BAH [99,100]. The combination of peripheral venous steroid profiles with the imaging data from CT or magnetic resonance imaging (MRI) has improved the diagnostic accuracy of correct subtype classification of PA. Lenders et al. observed that the secretion of 18-hydroxycortisol and 18-oxocortisol are highest in familial hyperaldosteronism type 1 and type 3, followed by APAs, whereas BAH patients had comparable levels of these two steroids to patients with essential hypertension [101]. Interestingly, in situ metabolomics has shown that the intratumoral levels of 18-oxocortisol and 18-hydroxycortisol negatively correlate with the CYP11B1 staining [102].

Recently, the steroid profiles of patients with APAs were correlated with their respective genotypes. It has been well documented that APAs carrying *KCNJ5* mutations present significantly higher levels of 18-oxocortisol in both adrenal vein and peripheral plasma samples than all other APAs; wild-type mutations of the *KCNJ5* gene and *KCNJ5* mutant APAs have higher lateralization ratios. In the same study, patients with APAs harboring ATPase mutations displayed the highest peripheral concentrations of aldosterone, cortisol, 11-deoxycorticosterone and corticosterone, while patients with *CACNA1D* mutated APAs had lower concentrations of aldosterone and corticosterone compared to all other groups [103]. In line with the previous observation, another study confirmed that *KCNJ5* carriers display significantly higher levels of 18-hydroxycortisol and 18-oxocortisol when compared to *CACNA1D* carriers. The levels of these hybrid steroids are negatively correlated with CYP11B2 expression, but not with aldosterone levels, and is positively correlated with CYP11B1 expression [37].

Furthermore, the use of peripheral venous plasma steroid profiling in combination with machine learning has not only enabled correct PA subtype classification, but also the correct prediction of APAs with *KCNJ5* mutations, with diagnostic sensitivities of 69% and 85% and specificities of 94% and 97%, respectively. This advance facilitates decision making in *KCNJ5* patients, who benefit most from surgical intervention [104].

Distinct patterns of urinary metabolites were observed in another study, enabling the grouping and distinguishing of essential hypertensives from PA patients and of APA from BAH patients. The identified metabolites include pyrimidine nucleoside and precursors, purine nucleotides and catabolites, and free amino acids [105].

Arlt et al. investigated the urinary steroid profiles of APA patients and documented, in parallel with tetrahydroaldosterone hypersecretion, an increase in glucocorticoid output which was not correlated with any known mutational status. The fact that glucocorticoid output in PA was comparable to that of patients with subclinical Cushing syndrome is particularly striking, suggesting glucocorticoid co-secretion in PA [106].

Targeted metabolomics of blood samples of patients with endocrine hypertension (PA, Cushing syndrome, pheochromocytoma/paraganglioma) and essential hypertension can distinguish between the two groups and has identified four metabolites as being common discriminators of the two disease groups, namely the long-chain acylcarnitines C18:1, C18:2, ornithine, and spermidine [107].

Murakami et al., performing in situ metabolomics, documented distinct molecular signatures between *KCNJ5*- and *CACNA1D*-mutated APAs involving metabolites of steroidogenesis as well as purine metabolism. Activation of purine metabolism was observed in *KCNJ5* mutant APAs, with a significant increase in adenosine monophosphate (AMP) and diphosphate (ADP), whereas these tumors displayed significantly higher 18-steroid intensities [102].

In another study, in situ metabolomics of APMs and APAs identified two distinct APM subgroups, only one of which shared some common characteristics with APAs. This subgroup presented metabolic traits supporting cell proliferation, with increased hexose phosphate and ribose phosphate, and increased purine and tryptophane metabolism. A correlation of these characteristics with respective known mutations was not possible in this study [108].

Finally, a proteomic and phosphoproteomic profiling of APAs in comparison to adjacent adrenal tissue demonstrated that increased steroidogenesis in APA positively correlates with the upregulation of the respective steroidogenic enzymes (*CYP11B2, CYP21A1, HSD3B2*) and their phosphorylation, without any increase in the mitochondrial enzymes providing the energy for the catalyzation of these reactions. Furthermore, the same study identified two distinct protein expression patterns, one common for *KCNJ5* tumors and their adjacent adrenal tissue and another for wild-type APAs for *KCNJ5* and their controls. This study also documented altered extracellular matrix composition in APAs and identified overexpression of Ras Homolog Family Member C (RHOC), an actin-organizing factor, in APAs along with deregulation of the mechanistic target of the rapamycin (mTOR) signaling pathway in these tumors [109].

4. Conclusions

In the present study, we have summarized the main findings of transcriptome, epigenetic and metabolomic studies investigating the pathogenesis of primary aldosteronism. One limitation of the present study is that we focused our search only on human studies. Animal and in vitro data, although always useful in elucidating pathophysiological mechanisms, were not included as the combined interpretation of in vivo and in vitro data with different backgrounds (i.e., immortalized cell lines or mouse models with, in part, deviating steroidogenesis patterns) could serve as confounding factors in this already complex pathomechanism.

Taken together, the application of new techniques has importantly contributed to the elucidation of aberrant mechanisms leading to pathological aldosterone production in PA. One main finding in this direction is the identification of APMs as possible APA precursors, as they share several common biological characteristics. However, an APM to APA transition is still a matter of debate. Furthermore, clearly distinct patterns of transcriptional, epigenetic and metabolomic profiling have now been attributed to APAs in comparison to BAHs, most importantly linking APAs with different causative mutations. In particular, two partially opposite transcriptional and steroidogenic profiles can distinguish APAs carrying a *KCNJ5* mutation from all other APAs, including those carrying a *CACNA1D*, *ATP1A1*, *ATP2B3* or even *CTNNB1* mutation. Interestingly, recent studies have analyzed the distinct metabolic signatures of these different mutations in depth. These findings can substantially contribute to the development of personalized treatments in patients with PA caused by adrenal neoplasms or hyperplasia. Although major progress has been made in understanding APAs, much remains to be done, as the molecular profiles and pathophysiological mechanisms underlying the development of BAH have not been sufficiently clarified yet.

Author Contributions: Conceptualization, K.I.A. and G.K.; methodology, A.S. and K.I.A.; investigation, A.S. and K.I.A.; writing—original draft preparation, A.S.; writing—review and editing, G.K., K.I.A. and G.P.P.; visualization, A.S. and K.I.A.; supervision, K.I.A. and G.K.; All authors have read and agreed to the published version of the manuscript.

Funding: This research received no external funding.

Institutional Review Board Statement: Not applicable.

Informed Consent Statement: Not applicable.

Data Availability Statement: Not applicable.

Conflicts of Interest: The authors declare no conflict of interest.

References

1. Funder, J.W.; Carey, R.M.; Mantero, F.; Murad, M.H.; Reincke, M.; Shibata, H.; Stowasser, M.; Young, W.F., Jr. The Management of Primary Aldosteronism: Case Detection, Diagnosis, and Treatment: An endocrine society clinical practice guideline. *J. Clin. Endocrinol. Metab.* **2016**, *101*, 1889–1916. [CrossRef] [PubMed]
2. Monticone, S.; Burrello, J.; Tizzani, D.; Bertello, C.; Viola, A.; Buffolo, F.; Gabetti, L.; Mengozzi, G.; Williams, T.A.; Rabbia, F.; et al. Prevalence and Clinical Manifestations of Primary Aldosteronism Encountered in Primary Care Practice. *J. Am. Coll. Cardiol.* **2017**, *69*, 1811–1820. [CrossRef] [PubMed]
3. Monticone, S.; D'Ascenzo, F.; Moretti, C.; Williams, T.A.; Veglio, F.; Gaita, F.; Mulatero, P. Cardiovascular events and target organ damage in primary aldosteronism compared with essential hypertension: A systematic review and meta-analysis. *Lancet Diabetes Endocrinol.* **2018**, *6*, 41–50. [CrossRef]
4. Choi, M.; Scholl, U.I.; Yue, P.; Bjorklund, P.; Zhao, B.; Nelson-Williams, C.; Ji, W.; Cho, Y.; Patel, A.; Men, C.J.; et al. K+ channel mutations in adrenal aldosterone-producing adenomas and hereditary hypertension. *Science* **2011**, *331*, 768–772. [CrossRef]
5. Okamura, T.; Nakajima, Y.; Katano-Toki, A.; Horiguchi, K.; Matsumoto, S.; Yoshino, S.; Yamada, E.; Tomaru, T.; Ishii, S.; Saito, T.; et al. Characteristics of Japanese aldosterone-producing adenomas with KCNJ5 mutations. *Endocr. J.* **2017**, *64*, 39–47. [CrossRef]
6. Azizan, E.A.; Murthy, M.; Stowasser, M.; Gordon, R.; Kowalski, B.; Xu, S.; Brown, M.J.; O'Shaughnessy, K.M. Somatic mutations affecting the selectivity filter of KCNJ5 are frequent in 2 large unselected collections of adrenal aldosteronomas. *Hypertension* **2012**, *59*, 587–591. [CrossRef]
7. Boulkroun, S.; Beuschlein, F.; Rossi, G.P.; Golib-Dzib, J.F.; Fischer, E.; Amar, L.; Mulatero, P.; Samson-Couterie, B.; Hahner, S.; Quinkler, M.; et al. Prevalence, clinical, and molecular correlates of KCNJ5 mutations in primary aldosteronism. *Hypertension* **2012**, *59*, 592–598. [CrossRef]
8. Beuschlein, F.; Boulkroun, S.; Osswald, A.; Wieland, T.; Nielsen, H.N.; Lichtenauer, U.D.; Penton, D.; Schack, V.R.; Amar, L.; Fischer, E.; et al. Somatic mutations in ATP1A1 and ATP2B3 lead to aldosterone-producing adenomas and secondary hypertension. *Nat. Genet.* **2013**, *45*, 440–444. [CrossRef]
9. Scholl, U.I.; Goh, G.; Stolting, G.; de Oliveira, R.C.; Choi, M.; Overton, J.D.; Fonseca, A.L.; Korah, R.; Starker, L.F.; Kunstman, J.W.; et al. Somatic and germline CACNA1D calcium channel mutations in aldosterone-producing adenomas and primary aldosteronism. *Nat. Genet.* **2013**, *45*, 1050–1054. [CrossRef]
10. Stindl, J.; Tauber, P.; Sterner, C.; Tegtmeier, I.; Warth, R.; Bandulik, S. Pathogenesis of Adrenal Aldosterone-Producing Adenomas Carrying Mutations of the Na(+)/K(+)-ATPase. *Endocrinology* **2015**, *156*, 4582–4591. [CrossRef]
11. Berthon, A.; Drelon, C.; Ragazzon, B.; Boulkroun, S.; Tissier, F.; Amar, L.; Samson-Couterie, B.; Zennaro, M.C.; Plouin, P.F.; Skah, S.; et al. WNT/beta-catenin signalling is activated in aldosterone-producing adenomas and controls aldosterone production. *Hum. Mol. Genet.* **2014**, *23*, 889–905. [CrossRef]
12. Zhou, J.; Azizan, E.A.B.; Cabrera, C.P.; Fernandes-Rosa, F.L.; Boulkroun, S.; Argentesi, G.; Cottrell, E.; Amar, L.; Wu, X.; O'Toole, S.; et al. Somatic mutations of GNA11 and GNAQ in CTNNB1-mutant aldosterone-producing adenomas presenting in puberty, pregnancy or menopause. *Nat. Genet.* **2021**, *53*, 1360–1372. [CrossRef]
13. Dutta, R.K.; Arnesen, T.; Heie, A.; Walz, M.; Alesina, P.; Soderkvist, P.; Gimm, O. A somatic mutation in CLCN2 identified in a sporadic aldosterone-producing adenoma. *Eur. J. Endocrinol.* **2019**, *181*, K37–K41. [CrossRef]
14. Rhayem, Y.; Perez-Rivas, L.G.; Dietz, A.; Bathon, K.; Gebhard, C.; Riester, A.; Mauracher, B.; Gomez-Sanchez, C.; Eisenhofer, G.; Schwarzmayr, T.; et al. PRKACA Somatic Mutations Are Rare Findings in Aldosterone-Producing Adenomas. *J. Clin. Endocrinol. Metab.* **2016**, *101*, 3010–3017. [CrossRef]
15. Nanba, K.; Blinder, A.R.; Rege, J.; Hattangady, N.G.; Else, T.; Liu, C.J.; Tomlins, S.A.; Vats, P.; Kumar-Sinha, C.; Giordano, T.J.; et al. Somatic CACNA1H Mutation as a Cause of Aldosterone-Producing Adenoma. *Hypertension* **2020**, *75*, 645–649. [CrossRef]
16. Lifton, R.P.; Dluhy, R.G.; Powers, M.; Rich, G.M.; Cook, S.; Ulick, S.; Lalouel, J.M. A chimaeric 11 beta-hydroxylase/aldosterone synthase gene causes glucocorticoid-remediable aldosteronism and human hypertension. *Nature* **1992**, *355*, 262–265. [CrossRef]
17. Scholl, U.I.; Stolting, G.; Schewe, J.; Thiel, A.; Tan, H.; Nelson-Williams, C.; Vichot, A.A.; Jin, S.C.; Loring, E.; Untiet, V.; et al. CLCN2 chloride channel mutations in familial hyperaldosteronism type II. *Nat. Genet.* **2018**, *50*, 349–354. [CrossRef]
18. Monticone, S.; Tetti, M.; Burrello, J.; Buffolo, F.; De Giovanni, R.; Veglio, F.; Williams, T.A.; Mulatero, P. Familial hyperaldosteronism type III. *J. Hum. Hypertens.* **2017**, *31*, 776–781. [CrossRef]
19. Scholl, U.I.; Stolting, G.; Nelson-Williams, C.; Vichot, A.A.; Choi, M.; Loring, E.; Prasad, M.L.; Goh, G.; Carling, T.; Juhlin, C.C.; et al. Recurrent gain of function mutation in calcium channel CACNA1H causes early-onset hypertension with primary aldosteronism. *elife* **2015**, *4*, e06315. [CrossRef]
20. Daniil, G.; Fernandes-Rosa, F.L.; Chemin, J.; Blesneac, I.; Beltrand, J.; Polak, M.; Jeunemaitre, X.; Boulkroun, S.; Amar, L.; Strom, T.M.; et al. CACNA1H Mutations Are Associated with Different Forms of Primary Aldosteronism. *EBioMedicine* **2016**, *13*, 225–236. [CrossRef]
21. Azizan, E.A.; Lam, B.Y.; Newhouse, S.J.; Zhou, J.; Kuc, R.E.; Clarke, J.; Happerfield, L.; Marker, A.; Hoffman, G.J.; Brown, M.J. Microarray, qPCR, and KCNJ5 sequencing of aldosterone-producing adenomas reveal differences in genotype and phenotype between zona glomerulosa- and zona fasciculata-like tumors. *J. Clin. Endocrinol. Metab.* **2012**, *97*, E819–E829. [CrossRef]
22. Monticone, S.; Castellano, I.; Versace, K.; Lucatello, B.; Veglio, F.; Gomez-Sanchez, C.E.; Williams, T.A.; Mulatero, P. Immunohistochemical, genetic and clinical characterization of sporadic aldosterone-producing adenomas. *Mol. Cell Endocrinol.* **2015**, *411*, 146–154. [CrossRef]

23. Scholl, U.I.; Healy, J.M.; Thiel, A.; Fonseca, A.L.; Brown, T.C.; Kunstman, J.W.; Horne, M.J.; Dietrich, D.; Riemer, J.; Kucukkoylu, S.; et al. Novel somatic mutations in primary hyperaldosteronism are related to the clinical, radiological and pathological phenotype. *Clin. Endocrinol.* **2015**, *83*, 779–789. [CrossRef]
24. Fernandes-Rosa, F.L.; Williams, T.A.; Riester, A.; Steichen, O.; Beuschlein, F.; Boulkroun, S.; Strom, T.M.; Monticone, S.; Amar, L.; Meatchi, T.; et al. Genetic spectrum and clinical correlates of somatic mutations in aldosterone-producing adenoma. *Hypertension* **2014**, *64*, 354–361. [CrossRef]
25. Azizan, E.A.; Poulsen, H.; Tuluc, P.; Zhou, J.; Clausen, M.V.; Lieb, A.; Maniero, C.; Garg, S.; Bochukova, E.G.; Zhao, W.; et al. Somatic mutations in ATP1A1 and CACNA1D underlie a common subtype of adrenal hypertension. *Nat. Genet.* **2013**, *45*, 1055–1060. [CrossRef]
26. Williams, T.A.; Gomez-Sanchez, C.E.; Rainey, W.E.; Giordano, T.J.; Lam, A.K.; Marker, A.; Mete, O.; Yamazaki, Y.; Zerbini, M.C.N.; Beuschlein, F.; et al. International Histopathology Consensus for Unilateral Primary Aldosteronism. *J. Clin. Endocrinol. Metab.* **2021**, *106*, 42–54. [CrossRef]
27. Boulkroun, S.; Samson-Couterie, B.; Dzib, J.F.; Lefebvre, H.; Louiset, E.; Amar, L.; Plouin, P.F.; Lalli, E.; Jeunemaitre, X.; Benecke, A.; et al. Adrenal cortex remodeling and functional zona glomerulosa hyperplasia in primary aldosteronism. *Hypertension* **2010**, *56*, 885–892. [CrossRef]
28. Nishimoto, K.; Nakagawa, K.; Li, D.; Kosaka, T.; Oya, M.; Mikami, S.; Shibata, H.; Itoh, H.; Mitani, F.; Yamazaki, T.; et al. Adrenocortical zonation in humans under normal and pathological conditions. *J. Clin. Endocrinol. Metab.* **2010**, *95*, 2296–2305. [CrossRef]
29. Omata, K.; Anand, S.K.; Hovelson, D.H.; Liu, C.J.; Yamazaki, Y.; Nakamura, Y.; Ito, S.; Satoh, F.; Sasano, H.; Rainey, W.E.; et al. Aldosterone-Producing Cell Clusters Frequently Harbor Somatic Mutations and Accumulate with Age in Normal Adrenals. *J. Endocr. Soc.* **2017**, *1*, 787–799. [CrossRef]
30. Omata, K.; Tomlins, S.A.; Rainey, W.E. Aldosterone-Producing Cell Clusters in Normal and Pathological States. *Horm. Metab. Res.* **2017**, *49*, 951–956. [CrossRef]
31. Nanba, K.; Vaidya, A.; Williams, G.H.; Zheng, I.; Else, T.; Rainey, W.E. Age-Related Autonomous Aldosteronism. *Circulation* **2017**, *136*, 347–355. [CrossRef] [PubMed]
32. Sugiura, Y.; Takeo, E.; Shimma, S.; Yokota, M.; Higashi, T.; Seki, T.; Mizuno, Y.; Oya, M.; Kosaka, T.; Omura, M.; et al. Aldosterone and 18-Oxocortisol Coaccumulation in Aldosterone-Producing Lesions. *Hypertension* **2018**, *72*, 1345–1354. [CrossRef] [PubMed]
33. Nishimoto, K.; Tomlins, S.A.; Kuick, R.; Cani, A.K.; Giordano, T.J.; Hovelson, D.H.; Liu, C.J.; Sanjanwala, A.R.; Edwards, M.A.; Gomez-Sanchez, C.E.; et al. Aldosterone-stimulating somatic gene mutations are common in normal adrenal glands. *Proc. Natl. Acad. Sci. USA* **2015**, *112*, E4591–E4599. [CrossRef] [PubMed]
34. Gomez-Sanchez, C.E.; Kuppusamy, M.; Reincke, M.; Williams, T.A. Disordered CYP11B2 Expression in Primary Aldosteronism. *Horm. Metab. Res.* **2017**, *49*, 957–962. [CrossRef]
35. Nishimoto, K.; Seki, T.; Kurihara, I.; Yokota, K.; Omura, M.; Nishikawa, T.; Shibata, H.; Kosaka, T.; Oya, M.; Suematsu, M.; et al. Case Report: Nodule Development from Subcapsular Aldosterone-Producing Cell Clusters Causes Hyperaldosteronism. *J. Clin. Endocrinol. Metab.* **2016**, *101*, 6–9. [CrossRef]
36. De Sousa, K.; Abdellatif, A.B.; Giscos-Douriez, I.; Meatchi, T.; Amar, L.; Fernandes-Rosa, F.L.; Boulkroun, S.; Zennaro, M.C. Colocalization of Wnt/beta-catenin and ACTH signaling pathways and paracrine regulation in aldosterone producing adenoma. *J. Clin. Endocrinol. Metab.* **2021**, dgab707. [CrossRef]
37. De Sousa, K.; Boulkroun, S.; Baron, S.; Nanba, K.; Wack, M.; Rainey, W.E.; Rocha, A.; Giscos-Douriez, I.; Meatchi, T.; Amar, L.; et al. Genetic, Cellular, and Molecular Heterogeneity in Adrenals with Aldosterone-Producing Adenoma. *Hypertension* **2020**, *75*, 1034–1044. [CrossRef]
38. Vouillarmet, J.; Fernandes-Rosa, F.; Graeppi-Dulac, J.; Lantelme, P.; Decaussin-Petrucci, M.; Thivolet, C.; Peix, J.L.; Boulkroun, S.; Clauser, E.; Zennaro, M.C. Aldosterone-Producing Adenoma with a Somatic KCNJ5 Mutation Revealing APC-Dependent Familial Adenomatous Polyposis. *J. Clin. Endocrinol. Metab.* **2016**, *101*, 3874–3878. [CrossRef]
39. Dekkers, T.; ter Meer, M.; Lenders, J.W.; Hermus, A.R.; Schultze Kool, L.; Langenhuijsen, J.F.; Nishimoto, K.; Ogishima, T.; Mukai, K.; Azizan, E.A.; et al. Adrenal nodularity and somatic mutations in primary aldosteronism: One node is the culprit? *J. Clin. Endocrinol. Metab.* **2014**, *99*, E1341–E1351. [CrossRef]
40. Nanba, K.; Chen, A.X.; Omata, K.; Vinco, M.; Giordano, T.J.; Else, T.; Hammer, G.D.; Tomlins, S.A.; Rainey, W.E. Molecular Heterogeneity in Aldosterone-Producing Adenomas. *J. Clin. Endocrinol. Metab.* **2016**, *101*, 999–1007. [CrossRef]
41. Itcho, K.; Oki, K.; Gomez-Sanchez, C.E.; Gomez-Sanchez, E.P.; Ohno, H.; Kobuke, K.; Nagano, G.; Yoshii, Y.; Baba, R.; Hattori, N.; et al. Endoplasmic Reticulum Chaperone Calmegin Is Upregulated in Aldosterone-Producing Adenoma and Associates with Aldosterone Production. *Hypertension* **2020**, *75*, 492–499. [CrossRef]
42. Omata, K.; Satoh, F.; Morimoto, R.; Ito, S.; Yamazaki, Y.; Nakamura, Y.; Anand, S.K.; Guo, Z.; Stowasser, M.; Sasano, H.; et al. Cellular and Genetic Causes of Idiopathic Hyperaldosteronism. *Hypertension* **2018**, *72*, 874–880. [CrossRef]
43. Hacini, I.; De Sousa, K.; Boulkroun, S.; Meatchi, T.; Amar, L.; Zennaro, M.C.; Fernandes-Rosa, F.L. Somatic mutations in adrenals from patients with primary aldosteronism not cured after adrenalectomy suggest common pathogenic mechanisms between unilateral and bilateral disease. *Eur. J. Endocrinol.* **2021**, *185*, 405–412. [CrossRef]
44. Fernandes-Rosa, F.L.; Amar, L.; Tissier, F.; Bertherat, J.; Meatchi, T.; Zennaro, M.C.; Boulkroun, S. Functional histopathological markers of aldosterone producing adenoma and somatic KCNJ5 mutations. *Mol. Cell Endocrinol.* **2015**, *408*, 220–226. [CrossRef]

45. Plaska, S.W.; Liu, C.J.; Lim, J.S.; Rege, J.; Bick, N.R.; Lerario, A.M.; Hammer, G.D.; Giordano, T.J.; Else, T.; Tomlins, S.A.; et al. Targeted RNAseq of Formalin-Fixed Paraffin-Embedded Tissue to Differentiate among Benign and Malignant Adrenal Cortical Tumors. *Horm. Metab. Res.* **2020**, *52*, 607–613. [CrossRef]
46. Monticone, S.; Hattangady, N.G.; Nishimoto, K.; Mantero, F.; Rubin, B.; Cicala, M.V.; Pezzani, R.; Auchus, R.J.; Ghayee, H.K.; Shibata, H.; et al. Effect of KCNJ5 mutations on gene expression in aldosterone-producing adenomas and adrenocortical cells. *J. Clin. Endocrinol. Metab.* **2012**, *97*, E1567–E1572. [CrossRef]
47. Akerstrom, T.; Willenberg, H.S.; Cupisti, K.; Ip, J.; Backman, S.; Moser, A.; Maharjan, R.; Robinson, B.; Iwen, K.A.; Dralle, H.; et al. Novel somatic mutations and distinct molecular signature in aldosterone-producing adenomas. *Endocr. Relat. Cancer* **2015**, *22*, 735–744. [CrossRef]
48. Bassett, M.H.; Mayhew, B.; Rehman, K.; White, P.C.; Mantero, F.; Arnaldi, G.; Stewart, P.M.; Bujalska, I.; Rainey, W.E. Expression profiles for steroidogenic enzymes in adrenocortical disease. *J. Clin. Endocrinol. Metab.* **2005**, *90*, 5446–5455. [CrossRef]
49. Backman, S.; Akerstrom, T.; Maharjan, R.; Cupisti, K.; Willenberg, H.S.; Hellman, P.; Bjorklund, P. RNA Sequencing Provides Novel Insights into the Transcriptome of Aldosterone Producing Adenomas. *Sci. Rep.* **2019**, *9*, 6269. [CrossRef]
50. Saner-Amigh, K.; Mayhew, B.A.; Mantero, F.; Schiavi, F.; White, P.C.; Rao, C.V.; Rainey, W.E. Elevated expression of luteinizing hormone receptor in aldosterone-producing adenomas. *J. Clin. Endocrinol. Metab.* **2006**, *91*, 1136–1142. [CrossRef]
51. Wang, T.; Satoh, F.; Morimoto, R.; Nakamura, Y.; Sasano, H.; Auchus, R.J.; Edwards, M.A.; Rainey, W.E. Gene expression profiles in aldosterone-producing adenomas and adjacent adrenal glands. *Eur. J. Endocrinol.* **2011**, *164*, 613–619. [CrossRef]
52. Williams, T.A.; Monticone, S.; Crudo, V.; Warth, R.; Veglio, F.; Mulatero, P. Visinin-like 1 is upregulated in aldosterone-producing adenomas with KCNJ5 mutations and protects from calcium-induced apoptosis. *Hypertension* **2012**, *59*, 833–839. [CrossRef]
53. Assie, G.; Auzan, C.; Gasc, J.M.; Baviera, E.; Balaton, A.; Elalouf, J.M.; Jeunemaitre, X.; Plouin, P.F.; Corvol, P.; Clauser, E. Steroidogenesis in aldosterone-producing adenoma revisited by transcriptome analysis. *J. Clin. Endocrinol. Metab.* **2005**, *90*, 6638–6649. [CrossRef]
54. Cao, C.X.; Yang, X.C.; Gao, Y.X.; Zhuang, M.; Wang, K.P.; Sun, L.J.; Wang, X.S. Expression of aldosterone synthase and adrenocorticotropic hormone receptor in adrenal incidentalomas from normotensive and hypertensive patients: Distinguishing subclinical or atypical primary aldosteronism from adrenal incidentaloma. *Int. J. Mol. Med.* **2012**, *30*, 1396–1402. [CrossRef]
55. El Zein, R.M.; Soria, A.H.; Golib Dzib, J.F.; Rickard, A.J.; Fernandes-Rosa, F.L.; Samson-Couterie, B.; Giscos-Douriez, I.; Rocha, A.; Poglitsch, M.; Gomez-Sanchez, C.E.; et al. Retinoic acid receptor alpha as a novel contributor to adrenal cortex structure and function through interactions with Wnt and Vegfa signalling. *Sci. Rep.* **2019**, *9*, 14677. [CrossRef]
56. Chu, C.; Zhao, C.; Zhang, Z.; Wang, M.; Zhang, Z.; Yang, A.; Ma, B.; Gu, M.; Cui, R.; Xin, Z.; et al. Transcriptome analysis of primary aldosteronism in adrenal glands and controls. *Int. J. Clin. Exp. Pathol.* **2017**, *10*, 10009–10018.
57. Lenzini, L.; Seccia, T.M.; Aldighieri, E.; Belloni, A.S.; Bernante, P.; Giuliani, L.; Nussdorfer, G.G.; Pessina, A.C.; Rossi, G.P. Heterogeneity of aldosterone-producing adenomas revealed by a whole transcriptome analysis. *Hypertension* **2007**, *50*, 1106–1113. [CrossRef]
58. Williams, T.A.; Monticone, S.; Schack, V.R.; Stindl, J.; Burrello, J.; Buffolo, F.; Annaratone, L.; Castellano, I.; Beuschlein, F.; Reincke, M.; et al. Somatic ATP1A1, ATP2B3, and KCNJ5 mutations in aldosterone-producing adenomas. *Hypertension* **2014**, *63*, 188–195. [CrossRef]
59. Kitamoto, T.; Suematsu, S.; Yamazaki, Y.; Nakamura, Y.; Sasano, H.; Matsuzawa, Y.; Saito, J.; Omura, M.; Nishikawa, T. Clinical and Steroidogenic Characteristics of Aldosterone-Producing Adenomas with ATPase or CACNA1D Gene Mutations. *J. Clin. Endocrinol. Metab.* **2016**, *101*, 494–503. [CrossRef]
60. Fallo, F.; Castellano, I.; Gomez-Sanchez, C.E.; Rhayem, Y.; Pilon, C.; Vicennati, V.; Santini, D.; Maffeis, V.; Fassina, A.; Mulatero, P.; et al. Histopathological and genetic characterization of aldosterone-producing adenomas with concurrent subclinical cortisol hypersecretion: A case series. *Endocrine* **2017**, *58*, 503–512. [CrossRef]
61. Bassett, M.H.; Suzuki, T.; Sasano, H.; De Vries, C.J.; Jimenez, P.T.; Carr, B.R.; Rainey, W.E. The orphan nuclear receptor NGFIB regulates transcription of 3beta-hydroxysteroid dehydrogenase. implications for the control of adrenal functional zonation. *J. Biol. Chem.* **2004**, *279*, 37622–37630. [CrossRef] [PubMed]
62. Zhou, J.; Lam, B.; Neogi, S.G.; Yeo, G.S.; Azizan, E.A.; Brown, M.J. Transcriptome Pathway Analysis of Pathological and Physiological Aldosterone-Producing Human Tissues. *Hypertension* **2016**, *68*, 1424–1431. [CrossRef] [PubMed]
63. Hu, D.; Ouyang, J.; Wu, Z.; Shi, T.; Wang, B.; Ma, X.; Li, H.; Wang, S.; Zhang, X. Elementary studies on elevated steroidogenic factor-1 expression in aldosterone-producing adenoma. *Urol. Oncol.* **2012**, *30*, 457–462. [CrossRef] [PubMed]
64. Reincke, M.; Beuschlein, F.; Lalli, E.; Arlt, W.; Vay, S.; Sassone-Corsi, P.; Allolio, B. DAX-1 expression in human adrenocortical neoplasms: Implications for steroidogenesis. *J. Clin. Endocrinol. Metab.* **1998**, *83*, 2597–2600. [CrossRef]
65. Lenzini, L.; Caroccia, B.; Campos, A.G.; Fassina, A.; Belloni, A.S.; Seccia, T.M.; Kuppusamy, M.; Ferraro, S.; Skander, G.; Bader, M.; et al. Lower expression of the TWIK-related acid-sensitive K+ channel 2 (TASK-2) gene is a hallmark of aldosterone-producing adenoma causing human primary aldosteronism. *J. Clin. Endocrinol. Metab.* **2014**, *99*, E674–E682. [CrossRef]
66. Maniero, C.; Scudieri, P.; Haris Shaikh, L.; Zhao, W.; Gurnell, M.; Galietta, L.J.V.; Brown, M.J. ANO4 (Anoctamin 4) Is a Novel Marker of Zona Glomerulosa That Regulates Stimulated Aldosterone Secretion. *Hypertension* **2019**, *74*, 1152–1159. [CrossRef]
67. Kobuke, K.; Oki, K.; Gomez-Sanchez, C.E.; Gomez-Sanchez, E.P.; Ohno, H.; Itcho, K.; Yoshii, Y.; Yoneda, M.; Hattori, N. Calneuron 1 Increased Ca(2+) in the Endoplasmic Reticulum and Aldosterone Production in Aldosterone-Producing Adenoma. *Hypertension* **2018**, *71*, 125–133. [CrossRef]

68. Oki, K.; Gomez-Sanchez, C.E. The landscape of molecular mechanism for aldosterone production in aldosterone-producing adenoma. *Endocr. J.* **2020**, *67*, 989–995. [CrossRef]
69. Li, X.; Wang, B.; Tang, L.; Zhang, Y.; Chen, L.; Gu, L.; Zhang, F.; Ouyang, J.; Zhang, X. GSTA1 Expression Is Correlated With Aldosterone Level in KCNJ5-Mutated Adrenal Aldosterone-Producing Adenoma. *J. Clin. Endocrinol. Metab.* **2018**, *103*, 813–823. [CrossRef]
70. Ye, P.; Mariniello, B.; Mantero, F.; Shibata, H.; Rainey, W.E. G-protein-coupled receptors in aldosterone-producing adenomas: A potential cause of hyperaldosteronism. *J. Endocrinol.* **2007**, *195*, 39–48. [CrossRef]
71. Itcho, K.; Oki, K.; Kobuke, K.; Yoshii, Y.; Ohno, H.; Yoneda, M.; Hattori, N. Aberrant G protein-receptor expression is associated with DNA methylation in aldosterone-producing adenoma. *Mol. Cell Endocrinol.* **2018**, *461*, 100–104. [CrossRef]
72. Lim, J.S.; Plaska, S.W.; Rege, J.; Rainey, W.E.; Turcu, A.F. Aldosterone-Regulating Receptors and Aldosterone-Driver Somatic Mutations. *Front. Endocrinol.* **2021**, *12*, 644382. [CrossRef]
73. Rossi, G.P.; Caroccia, B.; Seccia, T.M. Role of estrogen receptors in modulating aldosterone biosynthesis and blood pressure. *Steroids* **2019**, *152*, 108486. [CrossRef]
74. Caroccia, B.; Seccia, T.M.; Campos, A.G.; Gioco, F.; Kuppusamy, M.; Ceolotto, G.; Guerzoni, E.; Simonato, F.; Mareso, S.; Lenzini, L.; et al. GPER-1 and estrogen receptor-beta ligands modulate aldosterone synthesis. *Endocrinology* **2014**, *155*, 4296–4304. [CrossRef]
75. Gong, S.; Tetti, M.; Reincke, M.; Williams, T.A. Primary Aldosteronism: Metabolic Reprogramming and the Pathogenesis of Aldosterone-Producing Adenomas. *Cancers* **2021**, *13*, 3716. [CrossRef]
76. Maniero, C.; Garg, S.; Zhao, W.; Johnson, T.I.; Zhou, J.; Gurnell, M.; Brown, M.J. NEFM (Neurofilament Medium) Polypeptide, a Marker for Zona Glomerulosa Cells in Human Adrenal, Inhibits D1R (Dopamine D1 Receptor)-Mediated Secretion of Aldosterone. *Hypertension* **2017**, *70*, 357–364. [CrossRef]
77. Teo, A.E.; Garg, S.; Johnson, T.I.; Zhao, W.; Zhou, J.; Gomez-Sanchez, C.E.; Gurnell, M.; Brown, M.J. Physiological and Pathological Roles in Human Adrenal of the Glomeruli-Defining Matrix Protein NPNT (Nephronectin). *Hypertension* **2017**, *69*, 1207–1216. [CrossRef]
78. Williams, T.A.; Monticone, S.; Morello, F.; Liew, C.C.; Mengozzi, G.; Pilon, C.; Asioli, S.; Sapino, A.; Veglio, F.; Mulatero, P. Teratocarcinoma-derived growth factor-1 is upregulated in aldosterone-producing adenomas and increases aldosterone secretion and inhibits apoptosis in vitro. *Hypertension* **2010**, *55*, 1468–1475. [CrossRef]
79. Penny, M.K.; Finco, I.; Hammer, G.D. Cell signaling pathways in the adrenal cortex: Links to stem/progenitor biology and neoplasia. *Mol. Cell Endocrinol.* **2017**, *445*, 42–54. [CrossRef]
80. Tissier, F.; Cavard, C.; Groussin, L.; Perlemoine, K.; Fumey, G.; Hagnere, A.M.; Rene-Corail, F.; Jullian, E.; Gicquel, C.; Bertagna, X.; et al. Mutations of beta-catenin in adrenocortical tumors: Activation of the Wnt signaling pathway is a frequent event in both benign and malignant adrenocortical tumors. *Cancer Res.* **2005**, *65*, 7622–7627. [CrossRef]
81. Zhou, J.; Shaikh, L.H.; Neogi, S.G.; McFarlane, I.; Zhao, W.; Figg, N.; Brighton, C.A.; Maniero, C.; Teo, A.E.; Azizan, E.A.; et al. DACH1, a zona glomerulosa selective gene in the human adrenal, activates transforming growth factor-beta signaling and suppresses aldosterone secretion. *Hypertension* **2015**, *65*, 1103–1110. [CrossRef]
82. Yang, Y.; Tetti, M.; Vohra, T.; Adolf, C.; Seissler, J.; Hristov, M.; Belavgeni, A.; Bidlingmaier, M.; Linkermann, A.; Mulatero, P.; et al. BEX1 Is Differentially Expressed in Aldosterone-Producing Adenomas and Protects Human Adrenocortical Cells from Ferroptosis. *Hypertension* **2021**, *77*, 1647–1658. [CrossRef]
83. Howard, B.; Wang, Y.; Xekouki, P.; Faucz, F.R.; Jain, M.; Zhang, L.; Meltzer, P.G.; Stratakis, C.A.; Kebebew, E. Integrated analysis of genome-wide methylation and gene expression shows epigenetic regulation of CYP11B2 in aldosteronomas. *J. Clin. Endocrinol. Metab.* **2014**, *99*, E536–E543. [CrossRef]
84. Murakami, M.; Yoshimoto, T.; Nakabayashi, K.; Tsuchiya, K.; Minami, I.; Bouchi, R.; Izumiyama, H.; Fujii, Y.; Abe, K.; Tayama, C.; et al. Integration of transcriptome and methylome analysis of aldosterone-producing adenomas. *Eur. J. Endocrinol.* **2015**, *173*, 185–195. [CrossRef]
85. Di Dalmazi, G.; Morandi, L.; Rubin, B.; Pilon, C.; Asioli, S.; Vicennati, V.; De Leo, A.; Ambrosi, F.; Santini, D.; Pagotto, U.; et al. DNA Methylation of Steroidogenic Enzymes in Benign Adrenocortical Tumors: New Insights in Aldosterone-Producing Adenomas. *J. Clin. Endocrinol. Metab.* **2020**, *105*, e4605–e4615. [CrossRef]
86. Yoshii, Y.; Oki, K.; Gomez-Sanchez, C.E.; Ohno, H.; Itcho, K.; Kobuke, K.; Yoneda, M. Hypomethylation of CYP11B2 in Aldosterone-Producing Adenoma. *Hypertension* **2016**, *68*, 1432–1437. [CrossRef]
87. Kometani, M.; Yoneda, T.; Demura, M.; Aono, D.; Gondoh, Y.; Karashima, S.; Nishimoto, K.; Yasuda, M.; Horike, S.I.; Takeda, Y. Genetic and epigenetic analyses of aldosterone-producing adenoma with hypercortisolemia. *Steroids* **2019**, *151*, 108470. [CrossRef]
88. Kobuke, K.; Oki, K.; Gomez-Sanchez, C.E.; Ohno, H.; Itcho, K.; Yoshii, Y.; Yoneda, M.; Hattori, N. Purkinje Cell Protein 4 Expression Is Associated with DNA Methylation Status in Aldosterone-Producing Adenoma. *J. Clin. Endocrinol. Metab.* **2018**, *103*, 965–971. [CrossRef]
89. Ettaieb, M.; Kerkhofs, T.; van Engeland, M.; Haak, H. Past, Present and Future of Epigenetics in Adrenocortical Carcinoma. *Cancers* **2020**, *12*, 1218. [CrossRef]
90. Robertson, S.; MacKenzie, S.M.; Alvarez-Madrazo, S.; Diver, L.A.; Lin, J.; Stewart, P.M.; Fraser, R.; Connell, J.M.; Davies, E. MicroRNA-24 is a novel regulator of aldosterone and cortisol production in the human adrenal cortex. *Hypertension* **2013**, *62*, 572–578. [CrossRef]

91. Nakano, Y.; Yoshimoto, T.; Watanabe, R.; Murakami, M.; Fukuda, T.; Saito, K.; Fujii, Y.; Akashi, T.; Tanaka, T.; Yamada, T.; et al. miRNA299 involvement in CYP11B2 expression in aldosterone-producing adenoma. *Eur. J. Endocrinol.* **2019**, *181*, 69–78. [CrossRef] [PubMed]
92. He, J.; Cao, Y.; Su, T.; Jiang, Y.; Jiang, L.; Zhou, W.; Zhang, C.; Wang, W.; Ning, G. Downregulation of miR-375 in aldosterone-producing adenomas promotes tumour cell growth via MTDH. *Clin. Endocrinol.* **2015**, *83*, 581–589. [CrossRef] [PubMed]
93. Peng, K.Y.; Chang, H.M.; Lin, Y.F.; Chan, C.K.; Chang, C.H.; Chueh, S.J.; Yang, S.Y.; Huang, K.H.; Lin, Y.H.; Wu, V.C.; et al. miRNA-203 Modulates Aldosterone Levels and Cell Proliferation by Targeting Wnt5a in Aldosterone-Producing Adenomas. *J. Clin. Endocrinol. Metab.* **2018**, *103*, 3737–3747. [CrossRef] [PubMed]
94. Decmann, A.; Nyiro, G.; Darvasi, O.; Turai, P.; Bancos, I.; Kaur, R.J.; Pezzani, R.; Iacobone, M.; Kraljevic, I.; Kastelan, D.; et al. Circulating miRNA Expression Profiling in Primary Aldosteronism. *Front. Endocrinol.* **2019**, *10*, 739. [CrossRef]
95. Raman, P.B.; Sharma, D.C.; Dorfman, R.I.; Gabrilove, J.L. Biosynthesis of C-18-oxygenated steroids by an aldosterone-secreting human adrenal tumor. Metabolism of [4-14C] progesterone, [1,2-3H]11-deoxycorticosterone, and [4-14C] pregnenolone. *Biochemistry* **1965**, *4*, 1376–1385. [CrossRef]
96. Gordon, R.D.; Hamlet, S.M.; Tunny, T.J.; Gomez-Sanchez, C.E.; Jayasinghe, L.S. Distinguishing aldosterone-producing adenoma from other forms of hyperaldosteronism and lateralizing the tumour pre-operatively. *Clin. Exp. Pharm. Physiol.* **1986**, *13*, 325–328. [CrossRef]
97. Nakamura, Y.; Satoh, F.; Morimoto, R.; Kudo, M.; Takase, K.; Gomez-Sanchez, C.E.; Honma, S.; Okuyama, M.; Yamashita, K.; Rainey, W.E.; et al. 18-oxocortisol measurement in adrenal vein sampling as a biomarker for subclassifying primary aldosteronism. *J. Clin. Endocrinol. Metab.* **2011**, *96*, E1272–E1278. [CrossRef]
98. Mulatero, P.; di Cella, S.M.; Monticone, S.; Schiavone, D.; Manzo, M.; Mengozzi, G.; Rabbia, F.; Terzolo, M.; Gomez-Sanchez, E.P.; Gomez-Sanchez, C.E.; et al. 18-hydroxycorticosterone, 18-hydroxycortisol, and 18-oxocortisol in the diagnosis of primary aldosteronism and its subtypes. *J. Clin. Endocrinol. Metab.* **2012**, *97*, 881–889. [CrossRef]
99. Satoh, F.; Morimoto, R.; Ono, Y.; Iwakura, Y.; Omata, K.; Kudo, M.; Takase, K.; Seiji, K.; Sasamoto, H.; Honma, S.; et al. Measurement of peripheral plasma 18-oxocortisol can discriminate unilateral adenoma from bilateral diseases in patients with primary aldosteronism. *Hypertension* **2015**, *65*, 1096–1102. [CrossRef]
100. Eisenhofer, G.; Dekkers, T.; Peitzsch, M.; Dietz, A.S.; Bidlingmaier, M.; Treitl, M.; Williams, T.A.; Bornstein, S.R.; Haase, M.; Rump, L.C.; et al. Mass Spectrometry-Based Adrenal and Peripheral Venous Steroid Profiling for Subtyping Primary Aldosteronism. *Clin. Chem.* **2016**, *62*, 514–524. [CrossRef]
101. Lenders, J.W.M.; Williams, T.A.; Reincke, M.; Gomez-Sanchez, C.E. Diagnosis of endocrine disease: 18-Oxocortisol and 18-hydroxycortisol: Is there clinical utility of these steroids? *Eur. J. Endocrinol.* **2018**, *178*, R1–R9. [CrossRef]
102. Murakami, M.; Rhayem, Y.; Kunzke, T.; Sun, N.; Feuchtinger, A.; Ludwig, P.; Strom, T.M.; Gomez-Sanchez, C.; Knosel, T.; Kirchner, T.; et al. In situ metabolomics of aldosterone-producing adenomas. *JCI Insight* **2019**, *4*, e130356. [CrossRef]
103. Williams, T.A.; Peitzsch, M.; Dietz, A.S.; Dekkers, T.; Bidlingmaier, M.; Riester, A.; Treitl, M.; Rhayem, Y.; Beuschlein, F.; Lenders, J.W.; et al. Genotype-Specific Steroid Profiles Associated with Aldosterone-Producing Adenomas. *Hypertension* **2016**, *67*, 139–145. [CrossRef]
104. Eisenhofer, G.; Duran, C.; Cannistraci, C.V.; Peitzsch, M.; Williams, T.A.; Riester, A.; Burrello, J.; Buffolo, F.; Prejbisz, A.; Beuschlein, F.; et al. Use of Steroid Profiling Combined with Machine Learning for Identification and Subtype Classification in Primary Aldosteronism. *JAMA Netw. Open* **2020**, *3*, e2016209. [CrossRef]
105. Lana, A.; Alexander, K.; Castagna, A.; D'Alessandro, A.; Morandini, F.; Pizzolo, F.; Zorzi, F.; Mulatero, P.; Zolla, L.; Olivieri, O. Urinary Metabolic Signature of Primary Aldosteronism: Gender and Subtype-Specific Alterations. *Proteom. Clin. Appl.* **2019**, *13*, e1800049. [CrossRef]
106. Arlt, W.; Lang, K.; Sitch, A.J.; Dietz, A.S.; Rhayem, Y.; Bancos, I.; Feuchtinger, A.; Chortis, V.; Gilligan, L.C.; Ludwig, P.; et al. Steroid metabolome analysis reveals prevalent glucocorticoid excess in primary aldosteronism. *JCI Insight* **2017**, *2*, e93136. [CrossRef]
107. Erlic, Z.; Reel, P.; Reel, S.; Amar, L.; Pecori, A.; Larsen, C.K.; Tetti, M.; Pamporaki, C.; Prehn, C.; Adamski, J.; et al. Targeted Metabolomics as a Tool in Discriminating Endocrine from Primary Hypertension. *J. Clin. Endocrinol. Metab.* **2021**, *106*, 1111–1128. [CrossRef]
108. Sun, N.; Meyer, L.S.; Feuchtinger, A.; Kunzke, T.; Knosel, T.; Reincke, M.; Walch, A.; Williams, T.A. Mass Spectrometry Imaging Establishes 2 Distinct Metabolic Phenotypes of Aldosterone-Producing Cell Clusters in Primary Aldosteronism. *Hypertension* **2020**, *75*, 634–644. [CrossRef]
109. Swierczynska, M.M.; Betz, M.J.; Colombi, M.; Dazert, E.; Jeno, P.; Moes, S.; Pfaff, C.; Glatz, K.; Reincke, M.; Beuschlein, F.; et al. Proteomic Landscape of Aldosterone-Producing Adenoma. *Hypertension* **2019**, *73*, 469–480. [CrossRef]

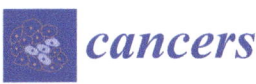

Review

Circulating microRNAs as Diagnostic Markers in Primary Aldosteronism

Scott M. MacKenzie [1,*], Hannah Saunders [1], Josie C. van Kralingen [1], Stacy Robertson [1], Alexandra Riddell [1], Maria-Christina Zennaro [2,3] and Eleanor Davies [1]

[1] British Heart Foundation Glasgow Cardiovascular Research Centre (BHF GCRC), Institute of Cardiovascular & Medical Sciences (ICAMS), University of Glasgow, Glasgow G12 8TA, UK; hannahsaunders1@sky.com (H.S.); Josie.VanKralingen@glasgow.ac.uk (J.C.v.K.); Stacy.Robertson@glasgow.ac.uk (S.R.); Alexandra.Riddell@glasgow.ac.uk (A.R.); eleanor.davies@glasgow.ac.uk (E.D.)
[2] Paris-Cardiovascular Research Center (PARCC), Institut National de la Santé et de la Recherche Médicale (INSERM), Université de Paris, 75015 Paris, France; maria-christina.zennaro@inserm.fr
[3] Assistance Publique-Hôpitaux de Paris, Hôpital Européen Georges Pompidou, Service de Génétique, 75015 Paris, France
* Correspondence: scott.mackenzie@glasgow.ac.uk

Simple Summary: Many patients remain at increased risk of primary aldosteronism (PA) and its consequences due to the difficulty of accurate diagnosis. MicroRNAs circulating in the bloodstream are emerging as biomarkers for disease, particularly specific forms of cancer. In this review article, we argue that they may also have a role in the diagnosis of PA, if observed changes in the microRNA profile of PA tissue are reflected in circulating microRNAs, which can be sampled and analysed readily in a clinical setting. However, for various practical reasons, studies of potential diagnostic circulating microRNAs have often proved difficult to reproduce consistently. We describe these problems and how they might be overcome using, as an example, our design of the circulating microRNA arm of the ongoing ENS@T-HT project, which is intended to confirm whether circulating microRNAs can serve as biomarkers for PA.

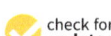

Citation: MacKenzie, S.M.; Saunders, H.; van Kralingen, J.C.; Robertson, S.; Riddell, A.; Zennaro, M.-C.; Davies, E. Circulating microRNAs as Diagnostic Markers in Primary Aldosteronism. *Cancers* **2021**, *13*, 5312. https://doi.org/10.3390/cancers13215312

Academic Editor: Peter Igaz

Received: 30 August 2021
Accepted: 15 October 2021
Published: 22 October 2021

Publisher's Note: MDPI stays neutral with regard to jurisdictional claims in published maps and institutional affiliations.

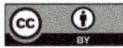

Copyright: © 2021 by the authors. Licensee MDPI, Basel, Switzerland. This article is an open access article distributed under the terms and conditions of the Creative Commons Attribution (CC BY) license (https://creativecommons.org/licenses/by/4.0/).

Abstract: Primary aldosteronism (PA) is a common and highly treatable condition, usually resulting from adrenocortical tumorous growth or hyperplasia. PA is currently underdiagnosed owing to its complex and protracted diagnostic procedures. A simplified biomarker-based test would be highly valuable in reducing cardiovascular morbidity and mortality. Circulating microRNAs are emerging as potential biomarkers for a number of conditions due to their stability and accessibility. PA is known to alter microRNA expression in adrenocortical tissue; if these changes or their effects are mirrored in the circulating miRNA profile, then this could be exploited by a diagnostic test. However, the reproducibility of studies to identify biomarker-circulating microRNAs has proved difficult for other conditions due to a series of technical challenges. Therefore, any studies seeking to definitively identify circulating microRNA biomarkers of PA must address this in their design. To this end, we are currently conducting the circulating microRNA arm of the ongoing ENS@T-HT study. In this review article, we present evidence to support the utility of circulating microRNAs as PA biomarkers, describe the practical challenges to this approach and, using ENS@T-HT as an example, discuss how these might be overcome.

Keywords: primary aldosteronism; microRNA; aldosterone; circulating; biomarker; adrenocortical

1. Introduction

The autonomous production of aldosterone by the adrenal gland, as observed in cases of primary aldosteronism (PA), adds significantly to the overall burden of cardiovascular risk, owing to the raised blood pressure and damage to vascular and other tissues that result from elevated circulating levels of the hormone. The majority of cases can be attributed to tumorous growth or hyperplasia of the adrenal cortex: the development of an aldosterone-producing adenoma (APA) on one gland results in lateralised oversecretion of aldosterone, while bilateral adrenal hyperplasia (BAH) causes elevated hormone production from both. These two subtypes account for ~90% of cases, with the remainder consisting of familial forms of PA or the less common unilateral form of hyperplasia [1]. Significant progress has been made in recent years to identify key mutations driving the pathogenesis of PA. APA are commonly found to have somatic mutations to the *KCNJ5* and *CACNA1D* genes or, less frequently, other genes including *ATP1A1*, *ATP2B3* and *CTNNB1* [2]. In cases of hyperplasia, there is now also strong evidence that mutation to certain of these same genes—particularly *CACNA1D*—could drive overproduction of aldosterone from small, distinct groups of cells within the cortex, termed aldosterone-producing cell clusters (APCC) [3].

Despite being acknowledged as the most common form of secondary hypertension, there is growing recognition that the currently accepted prevalence level of PA (5–10% of hypertensive patients) is likely to be a significant underestimation, with authorities in the field suggesting a true figure some 3 to 5 times higher [4]. That so many PA patients currently evade diagnosis is largely attributable to two main factors: firstly, the failure to refer hypertensive patients for PA screening tests and, secondly, the overly stringent and/or technically demanding nature of those same screening tests—and subsequent confirmatory tests—which limits throughput while also returning high rates of false negative results [5]. With a growing body of evidence showing that many PA cases may not be accompanied by an elevated aldosterone-renin ratio (ARR), hypokalaemia or even high blood pressure [6,7], accurate diagnosis of PA appears ever more difficult. Ongoing adaptations to existing tests that recognise, for example, the importance of 24 hr aldosterone measurement over a single spot test, or the impact of ACTH as well as the renin angiotensin system on aldosterone secretion, may result in some improvements to the situation, but diagnosis by these means will still remain highly demanding in terms of time, labour and cost. However, improving diagnosis to identify even a fraction of the currently undiagnosed cases would reap huge benefits, given that PA is highly responsive to treatment and its major consequences can be reduced or cured through adrenalectomy or administration of mineralocorticoid receptor antagonists (MRAs). The development of a simple high-throughput blood test for PA, utilising the measurement of one or more specific biomarkers, is therefore a highly attractive goal, albeit one that may previously have seemed somewhat remote.

A good biomarker should show high specificity and sensitivity for the intended disease state, be accessible through its presence in peripheral tissue or fluids (e.g., blood, saliva, urine, etc.) and be easily detected and/or quantified by robust, rapid and affordable assays. In light of the promise that circulating miRNA (c-miRNA) has shown as a biomarker in the diagnosis of other conditions, and the current evidence that PA results in changes to the levels of particular microRNAs, both in tissue and in the bloodstream, in this article, we discuss the prospect of using these molecules as the basis of a future PA diagnostic test. Additionally, given the common technical problems that have frustrated attempts to discover diagnostic c-miRNAs for other conditions, we examine how these might be addressed and hopefully overcome in the case of PA, with particular reference to our involvement in the ENS@T-HT project, an ongoing study that includes, among its aims, the identification of diagnostic c-miRNAs for PA and other forms of endocrine hypertension.

2. MicroRNA

MiRNA is a class of small, non-coding RNA (ncRNA) approximately 22 nucleotides long. The significant role of these molecules in gene expression was first identified in *C. elegans* some thirty years ago [8]. They are now known to have a crucial role in the development and regulation of key biological systems across all animals (and plants), with conservation of many of these processes across species. The current miRbase release (www.mirbase.org, accessed on 30 August 2021, v.22) from March 2018 lists 1115 different annotated mature human miRNAs, although a recent study estimates the true total number to be as high as 2300 [9]. The majority of miRNAs are transcribed from intra- and intergenic regions of DNA as pri-miRNAs, undergoing processing by RNAses to form pre-miRNAs and, finally, the mature miRNA itself. They generally act as repressors of gene expression, interacting through base complementarity with the 3′UTR of specific target messenger RNAs (mRNAs) to promote their degradation and prevent their translation [10]. This process is mediated via the RNA-induced silencing complex (RISC), a ribonucleoprotein complex that incorporates the miRNA alongside the Argonaute 2 (AGO2) protein to enable interaction with the mRNA. While instances have been reported of miRNAs interacting with other regions of the mRNA, and even of their stimulating gene expression, this repressive mode of miRNA action via the mRNA 3′UTR appears by far the most common. The interaction between the seed region of a miRNA (nucleotides 2–8) and its target mRNA is key, and this aspect of miRNA action has been exploited to develop specific bioinformatic algorithms that predict mRNA/gene targets, often on the basis of the miRNA seed sequence [11]. These predictions are far from perfect and are no substitute for experimental validation of miRNA action but can serve as useful tools in guiding such validation studies [12]. Given the short length of miRNAs, and the even shorter length of the seed region, an individual miRNA within a cell has the potential to target many different mRNA species that each harbour a complementary sequence within their 3′UTRs. Therefore, by producing just a single miRNA, the cell has the ability to target the expression of numerous genes simultaneously, making them a potentially powerful pleiotropic mediator of biological processes. Furthermore, given their post-transcriptional mode of action, a particular miRNA expressed in two or more different tissues may target a completely different array of mRNAs in each, due to differences in their respective transcriptomes. To fulfil their key regulatory role, production of miRNAs themselves must be tightly controlled so as to restrict their presence to particular tissues and/or specific biological conditions. Abnormal expression of miRNA—perhaps through loss of genetic or epigenetic control of pri-miRNA transcription, or faults in miRNA processing—can result in disease. Such changes in tissue levels of specific miRNAs within a tissue have been associated with various forms of cancer [13]. While such findings provide valuable insight into the mechanism and possible treatment of such conditions, the ability to detect, distinguish and quantify precisely the different miRNA species also means that they represent a potentially valuable diagnostic tool. For diagnostic purposes, it is irrelevant whether such changes in miRNA levels are the cause or the consequence of that condition. As with so many approaches based on diagnostic biomarkers, a major drawback to analysing tissue miRNAs is often the difficulty of obtaining tissue samples from the patient for analysis. In the case of miRNAs, however, this difficulty may be avoided due to their presence in extracellular fluids.

Low levels of miRNA have been detected in various bodily fluids, including serum, plasma, urine and breast milk. In plasma, they are found mostly in the form of RISC/AGO2 complexes, although they also associate with extracellular vesicles (EVs) or high-density lipoproteins; these structures apparently protect the miRNAs from RNase degradation [14,15]. The majority of extracellular miRNAs are thought to derive from the passive leakage of dead or apoptotic cell contents into the extracellular space and, to a lesser extent, from the packaging of miRNAs into EVs such as exosomes, microvesicles and apoptotic bodies, which are then actively secreted from the cell, possibly as a form of intercellular communication. Regardless of their source, the discovery of such miRNAs quickly prompted speculation that they might have value as circulating diagnostic biomarkers for specific disease states.

This hypothesis gained significant credibility following work by Mitchell et al. in 2008 [16]. Demonstrating the remarkable stability of these nucleic acids in clinical plasma and serum samples, they proposed miRNAs to be a novel class of blood-based cancer biomarkers well suited to that role given the common dysregulation of miRNA expression in cancers and the tissue-specific nature of such miRNA changes. To support their case, they detected an elevation of hsa-miR-141-3p levels in the serum of prostate cancer patients relative to healthy controls. Over subsequent years, numerous studies have emerged attempting to correlate c-miRNA profiles with particular diseases and, while different forms of cancer (including lung, breast, prostate, liver and ovarian) have undoubtedly been the main focus of such work, the principles underlying this concept can be expanded to encompass any disease affecting tissue miRNA expression, including diabetes, rheumatoid arthritis, Parkinson's disease, Alzheimer's disease and various forms of cardiovascular disease such as heart failure, coronary artery disease and stroke [17].

3. Adrenal miRNA in Adrenal Steroidogenesis and PA

The case for c-miRNAs as viable biomarkers for PA is supported by the regulatory role miRNAs play in the processes disrupted by PA—i.e., adrenal production of aldosterone—and the changes in adrenal miRNA expression that accompany this disruption. The main evidence of this nature comes from our own group, initially using the H295R human adrenocortical cell line. Using siRNA, we knocked down H295R expression of Dicer1, a key RNAseIII enzyme that generates miRNAs from their pre-miRNA precursors. This general reduction in miRNA levels effectively de-repressed cellular levels of specific messenger RNAs encoding key enzymes required for aldosterone biosynthesis, including *CYP11B2* (aldosterone synthase) [18]. Furthermore, Dicer1 knockdown also resulted in a 50% increase in cellular aldosterone levels, implying that adrenal miRNAs have a general inhibitory effect on aldosterone biosynthesis. More detailed analysis established that a specific miRNA, hsa-miR-24-5p (technically two miRNAs of identical sequence, hsa-miR-24-1-5p and hsa-miR-24-2-5p, transcribed from two different sites), was capable of binding *CYP11B2* mRNA, thereby repressing its expression; subsequently, we found miR-125a-5p and miR-125b-5p also repressed *CYP11B2* [19]. In our hands, we found no evidence that hsa-miR-10b-5p directly regulates *CYP11B2* [18], although Nusrin et al. reported contradictory findings using the same cell model, also showing expression of this miRNA to be induced under hypoxic conditions [20]. More recently, Zhang et al. also reported direct targeting of *CYP11B2* by hsa-mir-193-3p [21]. However, the influence of miRNA on the aldosterone steroidogenic pathway is not confined to *CYP11B2*; we have also shown significant effects on *CYP11A1* and *CYP21A2* [19], and it would seem likely that miRNAs are able to control this specific pathway at various stages, even before one considers their influence over the various regulatory mechanisms (primarily the renin–angiotensin system) that stimulate the adrenal cortex to produce aldosterone. Therefore, it seems likely that we have only scratched the surface of the numerous ways in which miRNAs intervene in the regulation, synthesis and action of aldosterone, either in the adrenal cortex or elsewhere [22–24].

In order to demonstrate that PA changes the levels of specific miRNAs in the adrenal glands of affected patients, we also undertook miRNA profiling that compared APA with nontumorous adrenal tissue. Due to the technologies available at the time, this study was small ($n = 4$ for each group) and current analytical methods are superior to the microarrays that were used (see below). Nevertheless, this study did show levels of many miRNAs to be highly correlated between the two tissue types, with several having significantly divergent expression, including the aforementioned hsa-mir-24-5p and hsa-mir-10b-5p, both of which were downregulated in APA relative to normal tissue [18]. A separate study by He et al. identified significant differential expression of 31 miRNAs in APA or unilateral adrenal hyperplasia tissue relative to normal adrenal cortex using microarray technology [25]. They confirmed downregulation of hsa-miR-375 by qRT-PCR and presented evidence that this miRNA may act as a suppressor of tumour growth through its repression of *MTDH* expression. Velázquez-Fernández et al. sought to distinguish subtypes of adrenocortical adenoma (ACA) on the basis of their tissue miRNA profiles. They detected and quantified miRNA in APA ($n = 9$), cortisol-producing adenoma (CPA, $n = 10$) and non-hyperfunctioning adenoma (NHFA) samples by microarray and were able to group these three subtypes according to their miRNA profiles [26]. Each subtype was also compared to "normal" adrenal reference samples and, relative to these, APAs were found to have eight miRNAs that were significantly over-expressed and four that were under-expressed in this subtype alone (although these miRNAs did not include hsa-mir-24-5p, hsa-mir-10b-5p or hsa-miR-375). More specifically, Lenzini et al. identified APA-expressed miRNAs likely to target directly the expression of TASK-2, a K⁺ channel whose downregulation is observed in APA and which apparently drives its pathogenic effects [27]. They found hsa-miR-23 and hsa-miR-34a to fulfil this role, modulating TASK-2 levels in APA in a manner likely to enhance aldosterone secretion through increased expression of *CYP11B2* and the steroidogenic acute regulatory protein (*STAR*). Peng et al. showed hsa-mir-203 to be downregulated in APA relative to adjacent adrenal tissue and confirmed that this miRNA targets *WNT5A*, a component of the Wnt/β-catenin pathway; by manipulating levels of miR-203 within APA cells, they could alter aldosterone production and cell proliferation [28]. These different studies not only provide insight into the miRNA-mediated mechanisms underlying aldosterone secretion, but also establish the possibility of identifying and distinguishing the tumorous APA tissue from normal adrenal tissue by their miRNA profiles due to the disruption of these same mechanisms.

Such changes between APA and non-diseased adrenocortical tissue, together with the knowledge that miRNAs participate in the control of aldosterone biosynthesis, are promising indicators that c-miRNA biomarkers for PA might exist. The simplest hypothesis would be that such adrenal changes in miRNA levels are reflected directly in the circulation, with levels of specific miRNAs rising or falling as they do in the adrenal cortex. However, it may not be a straightforward question of simply measuring these miRNAs in the bloodstream. For example, the quantities of a potential biomarker miRNA released from the adrenal gland may not be sufficient for it (or any changes in its quantity) to be measured reliably in the circulation. Alternatively, circulating quantities of that miRNA may be supplemented—or completely swamped—by release of the same miRNA from other tissues, preventing any detection of an adrenal-specific signal. Additionally, a viable c-miRNA biomarker for PA may not necessarily derive from the adrenal gland at all. Rather, PA could trigger miRNA changes in other affected tissues, such as the vasculature, which might be better candidate biomarkers than adrenal miRNAs. For these reasons, although studies of adrenal tissue are encouraging, identification of potential diagnostic miRNA biomarkers requires careful direct analysis of the miRNAs circulating in the bloodstreams of PA patients.

4. Circulating miRNA Studies of Hypertension and PA

A high-throughput biomarker-based diagnostic test that distinguishes PA patients from those with other forms of hypertension is clearly desirable. At present, we are unaware of any studies that have directly compared c-miRNA profiles of PA patients with those of essential hypertensives. Nevertheless, certain previous c-miRNA studies do provide useful insights.

The only major study to date examining c-miRNA profiles in the context of PA was published by Decmann et al. in 2019. Rather than attempting to diagnose PA as a single entity, they instead sought to distinguish the two principal forms of PA—BAH and APA—from one another on the basis of c-miRNA [29]. To this end, RNA-seq was first conducted on 30 plasma samples (16 APA and 14 BAH), identifying an initial list of 50 c-miRNAs that were significantly differentially expressed between groups. Attempted validation of the four most statistically significant of these by qRT-PCR in a further 93 samples confirmed differential expression of three c-miRNAs—hsa-miR-30e-5p, hsa-miR-30d-5p and hsa-miR-7-5p—all of which were upregulated in BAH relative to APA. Diagnostic performance of the three c-miRNAs, as assessed by ROC analysis, showed the specificities and sensitivities of each to be approximately 60% at the chosen (presumably optimal) cutoff points. While the authors correctly noted that this is poor in comparison to AVS (with sensitivity of 92.5% and specificity of 100%), the study findings are important in several respects. Firstly, the relatively large number of well-phenotyped samples analysed using RNA-seq provides a comprehensive survey of the c-miRNAs present in PA patients. Secondly, the great care taken in design and conduct of the study meant that, of just four miRNAs tested by qRT-PCR, three were successfully validated; there is therefore a strong possibility that levels of several more c-miRNAs are significantly altered between APA and BAH subjects.

Additionally, as the diagnostic utility of the three c-miRNAs was only assessed individually, it may be that combination of these miRNAs—plus other differentially expressed miRNAs yet to be validated—into a "signature" could significantly improve the performance of the test. Finally, as the investigators point out, adrenal glands in the bilateral form of disease are now known to harbour cell lesions with mutations that drive aldosterone production [3], blurring the boundary between BAH and APA. If the pathologies of these PA subtypes are really so closely related, then it is impressive that any consistent and significant difference was apparent at all and implies that the ostensibly simpler task of distinguishing PA (regardless of subtype) from essential hypertension might yield results of greater clinical relevance. Unfortunately, given that the study population was composed entirely of PA subjects, the findings of this study provide no indication of which individual c-miRNAs may be of diagnostic value in distinguishing PA from essential hypertension. It is also interesting to note that, for reasons unknown, patient samples contributed by different study centres were shown to differ significantly in their miRNA levels, as measured by qRT-PCR, underlining the need to standardise sample collection and storage in order to avoid bias even before sample processing.

Another recent study compared c-miRNA in the plasma of essential hypertensives and healthy (i.e., normotensive) individuals drawn from the Uyghur population of Northwest China. Initially, microarray was used to analyse a small number of samples ($n = 4$/group), identifying 257 differentially expressed c-miRNAs [30]. Of these, 161 were upregulated in hypertension, while 96 were downregulated; the upregulated miRNAs showed a much greater degree of fold change. Although it is tempting to conclude from this that the dysfunction associated with hypertension leads to large and readily detectable dynamic changes in levels of certain c-miRNAs, subsequent qRT-PCR validation found the fold changes to be far smaller and suggests such large observed shifts may be an artefact of microarray quantification. Just 4 of the most significant miRNAs were selected for qRT-PCR validation ($n = 15$/group), but all were confirmed, with hypertensives having significant upregulation of hsa-miR-198 and hsa-miR-1183, and downregulation of hsa-miR-144-3p and hsa-miR-30e-5p (note that this last c-miRNA was found to upregulated by Decmann et al. in BAH vs. APA [29]). The microarray data were used as the basis of Hierarchical Clustering analysis, which was able to group samples clearly into hypertensive and normotensive classes on the basis of increased and decreased levels of specific miRNAs. Clearly, it would be interesting to confirm whether this relationship is maintained using a larger study sample, more reliable quantitative data and other ethnic groups. It is to be hoped that improvements in methodology and greater standardisation of workflows will permit such replication but data from previous studies of c-miRNA in essential hypertension are not promising, with previous overviews of this topic highlighting the inconsistent study results [31].

In summary, while previous studies of PA and essential hypertension suggest disruption of the c-miRNA profile in a manner that might be exploited for diagnostic purposes, it is apparent that inconsistent methodologies present a significant obstacle, obscuring our ability to discern the true and specific effects, if any, of PA on the circulating miRnome.

5. Technical Challenges in the Design of Circulating miRNA Studies

Throughout the last decade, numerous studies have attempted to establish diagnostic c-miRNA profiles for a diverse range of conditions. Yet, even studies that analyse identical conditions have struggled to reach significant agreement in their findings. Such lack of reproducibility appears to be due mainly to differing methodological approaches [32]. This leads to variation in miRNA quantification and, ultimately, inconsistency in those individual miRNAs found to associate significantly with a particular disease. Therefore, any studies attempting to define diagnostic c-miRNA signatures, whether it be for PA or other conditions, must be designed in order to remove, or at least minimise, the impact of these confounding factors, which can affect every stage of the process. Additionally, any study that seeks to confirm or verify the findings of earlier work should seek to recreate that methodology as closely as is practical. Before discussing some of the existing c-miRNA studies relevant to PA, it is necessary to describe these confounding factors and how they influence good study design (see summary of factors in Table 1).

Table 1. Factors to be considered in the design of circulating miRNA analysis study protocols. These have the potential to affect outcome by influencing the number and identities of differentially expressed miRNAs detected.

Study Stage	Factors
Study population	Careful phenotyping and correct allocation to study groups
	Matching of groups for potentially confounding characteristics, e.g., sex, age, BMI, etc.
Sample type	Choice of cell-free or extracellular vesicle-bound miRNA
	Choice of biofluid, e.g., plasma or serum?
	Minimal haemolysis of serum/plasma samples
Sample storage	Avoidance of prolonged sample storage at room temperature
	Avoidance of freeze/thaw cycles
miRNA isolation method	Choice of miRNA isolation protocol/kit
	Consistent protocol to be maintained throughout study and across all centres
	Potential for operator effect?
Quantification method	Choice of methodology dictated by various factors including sample number, throughput, cost, accuracy/sensitivity, data analysis support
	Available methods include RNA-Seq, realtime qRT-PCR (incl. array plates), microarray.
Quality control/ data normalisation	Identification of poor quality/degraded samples
	Normalisation of data to account for variation across different centres, machine runs, operators, etc.
	Use of spike-in miRNAs at various points during sample analysis protocol
	Identification of stably expressed endogenous miRNAs that can be employed as normalisers (singly or in combination)
Data analysis	Standard statistical methodology to identify differential expression
	Establishment of optimal predictive/diagnostic miRNA combinations ('signatures') through multivariate analysis methods

5.1. Study Population

As with any clinical study, it is important to ensure that patient and control populations are carefully phenotyped in order to ensure their correct classification. In the case of a study seeking to distinguish PA patients from essential hypertensives, this is particularly difficult as, based on the emerging evidence of PA underdiagnosis, it is likely that any group of essential hypertensives will in fact harbour a significant proportion of undiagnosed PA subjects, which might frustrate attempts to clearly distinguish them from the diagnosed PA group on the basis of c-miRNA profile. Levels of c-miRNAs are known to associate with such characteristics as sex (e.g., hsa-miR-150-5p and hsa-miR-145-5p), age (e.g., hsa-miR-126-3p and hsa-miR-21-5p) and BMI (e.g., hsa-miR-122-5p, hsa-miR-148-3p and hsa-miR-505-3p), so any study populations must also be carefully matched for these if misleading conclusions are not to be drawn [33].

5.2. Sample Type

The analysis of cell-free miRNA (cfmiRNA) in the circulation requires the investigator to decide between plasma or serum as the sample medium of choice. Alternatively, investigators may choose instead to investigate c-miRNAs that have been secreted into extracellular vesicles (EVmiRNA). While it may appear obvious that cfmiRNA and EVmiRNA studies will significantly detect different arrays of miRNAs, reflecting their very different sources [34], it should be noted that plasma and serum might also yield broadly similar but different results despite both capturing the cfmiRNA fraction [35]. This underlines the fact that meaningful comparisons cannot necessarily be made between otherwise highly similar cfmiRNA studies that employ different sample media. There is also some evidence that the process of coagulation required for the preparation of serum leads to contamination of the sample with haemolysis-derived miRNAs, implying plasma may be the superior biofluid [35]. Comparisons between EVmiRNA studies are even more problematic, as different protocols will isolate EVs of differing properties (e.g., size, density, solubility) and, consequently, different miRNA composition [36].

5.3. Sample Storage and Quality

High-quality cfmiRNA samples should suffer minimal degradation prior to analysis and should also not be contaminated with cellular miRNAs that might skew results. Therefore, plasma or serum samples should not be significantly haemolysed and might be excluded on the basis of visual/spectrophotometric inspection or high levels of miRNAs thought to be of erythrocyte or platelet origin [37]. Heparin should be avoided as it has been shown to interfere with downstream miRNA detection [38]. It is desirable to isolate miRNA from blood samples immediately upon collection, although this may not always be possible in a clinical setting. Instead, plasma/serum should be prepared from whole blood as soon as possible after sampling (<2 h) in order to minimise haemolysis, before freezing, preferably at $-80\ °C$. MiRNA stability under such storage conditions is very good—and superior to that in whole blood—but multiple freeze/thaw cycles should be avoided [39]. Post-isolation from plasma or serum, miRNA itself appears highly stable for many years at ultra-low temperature and through multiple freeze/thaw cycles [40].

5.4. miRNA Isolation Method

A diverse variety of methods are available for the isolation of miRNA from plasma/serum, varying in such key factors as their use of filter columns and/or phenol for extraction. Numerous studies have demonstrated the significant impact of different RNA isolation protocols on the quantified levels of serum/plasma miRNAs, emphasising that consistent methodology must be employed throughout individual studies [41]. In addition to protocol differences, operator variability may also be a factor. For example, Kloten et al. compared the performance of seven different protocols for the extraction of cfmiRNA and EVmiRNA from plasma. Analysis of the resulting RNA samples by real-time qRT-PCR and NGS showed clear differences in the measured quantities of specific miRNAs, which were attributed mainly to the variable efficiency of each miRNA extraction method. However, given that each method was performed at one of six different centres, operator variability was possibly also a factor [42].

5.5. Quantification Method

The choice of method employed to quantify miRNAs extracted from liquid biopsy samples is determined to a large degree by the range of miRNAs one wishes to detect, the accuracy of quantification one wants to achieve and overall cost. The pros and cons of different methods have been well reviewed elsewhere [41] but it is worth summarising the main options here in order to draw attention to the challenges of accurately quantifying the diverse range of c-miRNA species accurately. Added to this are the different requirements of initial screening studies that aim to survey as much of the c-miRNA transcriptome as possible versus those of a final diagnostic test, designed to quantify only a select number of miRNA species accurately and reproducibly.

Initial studies of c-miRNA species tended to use microarray technology, which enabled detection of several hundred miRNAs simultaneously in a single sample. The main drawback to this method is its semi-quantitative nature: while useful for initial identification of shifts in miRNA levels, any such changes required validation using a fully quantitative method such as realtime quantitative RT-PCR (RT-qPCR). Given that such validation often fails to confirm the microarray results, presentation of microarray data without this supporting evidence should be treated with caution. This confirms the status of RT-qPCR as the gold standard for quantitative measurement of miRNA, although the protocol for small RNAs is not so straightforward as for mRNA. MiRNAs must be enzymatically treated prior to reverse transcription (RT) in order to attach additional linker sequences that provide sufficient length for the annealing of PCR primers. This can introduce bias into the RT stage due to the variable efficiency of linker attachment. PCR assays themselves are generally sensitive and specific, although there is a risk of false positive results where a given assay fails to distinguish two highly similar miRNA species. Specificity can be improved through the use of locked nucleic acid (LNA) primers, which have greater binding stability than DNA, enabling the use of shorter sequences. The greatest drawback of RT-qPCR is the need to perform a separate assay for each individual miRNA species which, at least in the early discovery stages of a study, may be highly intensive in terms of operator time, cost and template RNA. The inconvenience of this can be reduced by the use of array plates (e.g., QIAGEN LNA miRNA Focus PCR panels), which assemble numerous different qPCR assays on to a 384-well plate format. On the other hand, a distinctive miRNA diagnostic "signature" consisting of, for example, five or six different miRNAs, would not be such an issue, and qRT-PCR would be by far the most practical, efficient and reliable method for such assays.

Finally, there is RNA-Seq which, due to significant reduction in the costs of next-generation (NGS) sequencing technology over the last decade, has become a much more viable tool for discovery studies that wish to survey the whole of the c-miRNA transcriptome, though still expensive and requiring a great deal of downstream data analysis. The major advantage of RNA-Seq is its ability to detect the presence of novel or unexpected miRNAs in a sample, as opposed to microarray and RT-qPCR where measurement is confined to known miRNA species selected in advance (and to the capacity of the plate/chip, although several hundred miRNAs can potentially be assayed in a single run). NGS requires the assembly of a library from the original RNA sample, and this can be the source of considerable bias and variability, as can batch effects where technical variability between machine runs makes comparison of samples across larger studies challenging. Additionally, as for microarray, RT-qPCR validation of any quantitative shifts is necessary. However, this area of technology is developing rapidly, and RNA-Seq is likely to be the main tool, at least for large-scale analysis of diverse miRNAs, in the future. Relative to the other technologies, it should be borne in mind that RNA-seq produces large datasets requiring a great deal of operator and computer time to process, using workflows that are not yet fully standardised in order to map sequencing reads to genomic databases of miRNA sequences [41]. This, again, is an important practical consideration to take into account when designing c-miRNA studies.

5.6. Quality Control/Normalisation of Data

Variation in the quality and quantity of starting RNA and also in the efficiencies of the various stages of the quantitation process—RNA isolation, RT, PCR—mean that data derived from multiple samples must be normalised to a common reference. However, at present, there is no standard normalisation procedure for c-miRNA and such data correction must be applied carefully if it is not to produce misleading results [43]. Exogenous reference miRNAs (also known as spike-in controls) can be introduced in known quantities to the sample at various stages. In human studies, these tend to be synthetic sequences that mimic miRNAs from other species such as *C. elegans* that have no human counterpart, in order to avoid confusion with endogenous sequences. An alternative approach has been to separately amplify known concentrations of exogenous miRNAs, in synthetic form, alongside the study samples. Standard curves can then be constructed that enable quantification of these specific miRNAs in the samples [44]. These are highly useful ways of confirming the efficiencies of the various technical stages, thereby maintaining quality control and ensuring the consistency of these processes across an entire study. However, they do not permit normalisation for variation in the quality and quantity of the original RNA sample, for which an endogenous miRNA (or miRNAs) is required to act as reference. Unfortunately, there is no consensus as to which c-miRNAs, if any, are sufficiently stable to serve as a reference in all situations, enabling normalisation of data on the basis of minor shifts in RNA quality/quantity, and also flagging outlying samples containing RNA that is degraded or at a concentration outside acceptable limits. At present, it is therefore necessary to quantify a number of endogenous miRNAs across all samples and then identify those which show the most stable expression on the basis of the delta Ct method or using specialist software such as NormFinder, geNorm or BestKeeper. These packages also permit multiple miRNAs to be used as normalisers, reducing error due to small fluctuations in a single reference and enhancing the robustness of data normalisation. Although this approach has identified certain c-miRNAs that are stably expressed in biofluids in multiple studies (e.g., hsa-miR-16-5p, hsa-miR-93-5p, hsa-miR-191-5p), it is doubtful that any one of these could be used universally [45]. So, at least for the immediate future, normalising c-miRNAs must be identified on a study-by-study basis.

5.7. Data Analysis

Standard statistical analysis can be used to highlight those c-miRNAs present at readily detectable levels in patient and/or control samples as well as identifying those that are significantly differentially expressed between the two. While this is a valid approach to identifying candidate diagnostic c-miRNAs on an individual basis, it is suboptimal when trying to establish the optimal combination of biomarker c-miRNAs into a diagnostic "signature" of high sensitivity and specificity. Such analysis requires the use of multivariate methods. c-miRNA studies can benefit from the lead taken by proteomic biomarker studies in this regard, where a variety of both unsupervised pattern recognition methods (e.g., principal component analysis, hierarchical clustering) and unsupervised methods (e.g., Bayesian methods and machine learning) have been employed [46]. Clearly, such work requires close collaboration with specialised statistical experts.

6. Study Design and the ENS@T-HT Project

The previous section serves to emphasise the numerous choices faced in the development of c-miRNA studies and while many of these options may not be objectively superior to their alternative, it is apparent that they could have significant impact on the study findings. Therefore, we should perhaps not be surprised that there has been such apparent lack of correlation even between superficially similar c-miRNA studies given that their methodologies are likely to have diverged in significant ways. Evidently, to determine whether a c-miRNA-based diagnostic test for PA is viable, we require a comprehensive study to be conducted utilising, as far as is practicable, the best and most consistent methods for quantifying and analysing c-miRNAs so as to develop an identifying signature. This signature can then be tested in an independent population using the same methodology as confirmation of consistent and reproducible shifts in c-miRNA levels.

This is the thinking behind ENS@T-HT, an EU-funded Horizon 2020 research and innovation project designed to develop diagnostic signatures for various forms of endocrine hypertension—including PA, Cushing's syndrome (CS) and phaeochromocytoma/functional paraganglioma (PPGL)—on the basis of patient profiles that have been defined using various "-omics" approaches (www.ensat-ht.eu, accessed on 30 August 2021). These omics include measurements of steroids, small metabolites and metanephrines in plasma, as well as urinary steroids, and—most relevant here—c-miRNAs. The ultimate aim is to combine the most informative measurements from these various omics into an optimal multiomic signature that would form the basis of a single high-throughput diagnostic test that could be performed readily at non-specialist clinical centres. The study consists of two distinct stages—the retrospective phase and the prospective phase—each of which involves the analysis of a completely separate and independent study population; as these names imply, the samples analysed during the retrospective phase were collected over a period of years prior to the study ($n = 357$, plus normotensive volunteers as comparators), while the prospective phase analyses samples collected specifically for ENS@T-HT ($n > 1000$). The intention is first to define a diagnostic signature in the retrospective population that can then be validated in the prospectively collected subjects. Our group has led the c-miRNA arm of this project and has therefore been required to make several key decisions regarding the c-miRNA quantification/analysis pipeline that must balance several occasionally conflicting considerations. Furthermore, during our design of the retrospective study, we were mindful of the ultimate purpose of the project, which is to develop a diagnostic assay that can be rapidly and reproducibly employed in non-specialist healthcare centres using commonly available laboratory equipment. These considerations are summarised below and in Figure 1.

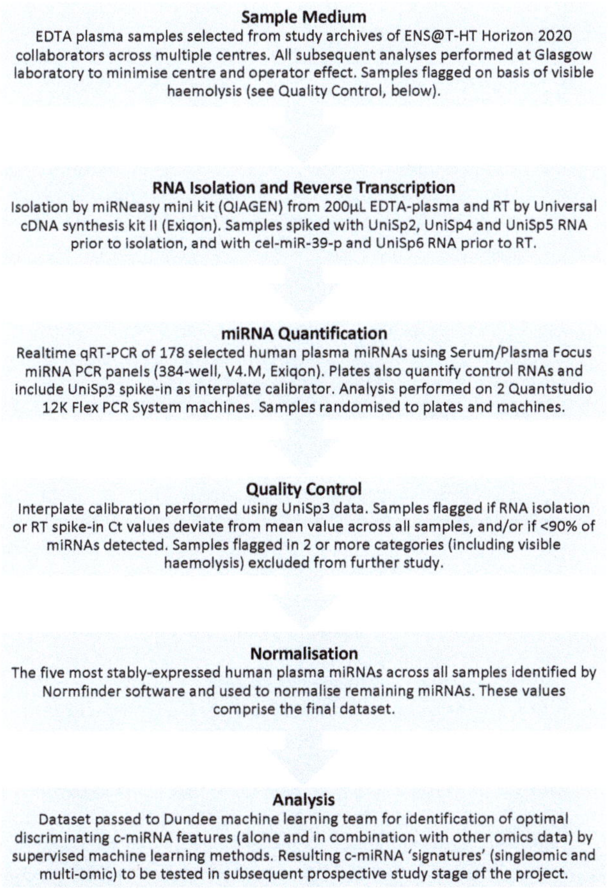

Sample Medium
EDTA plasma samples selected from study archives of ENS@T-HT Horizon 2020 collaborators across multiple centres. All subsequent analyses performed at Glasgow laboratory to minimise centre and operator effect. Samples flagged on basis of visible haemolysis (see Quality Control, below).

RNA Isolation and Reverse Transcription
Isolation by miRNeasy mini kit (QIAGEN) from 200µL EDTA-plasma and RT by Universal cDNA synthesis kit II (Exiqon). Samples spiked with UniSp2, UniSp4 and UniSp5 RNA prior to isolation, and with cel-miR-39-p and UniSp6 RNA prior to RT.

miRNA Quantification
Realtime qRT-PCR of 178 selected human plasma miRNAs using Serum/Plasma Focus miRNA PCR panels (384-well, V4.M, Exiqon). Plates also quantify control RNAs and include UniSp3 spike-in as interplate calibrator. Analysis performed on 2 Quantstudio 12K Flex PCR System machines. Samples randomised to plates and machines.

Quality Control
Interplate calibration performed using UniSp3 data. Samples flagged if RNA isolation or RT spike-in Ct values deviate from mean value across all samples, and/or if <90% of miRNAs detected. Samples flagged in 2 or more categories (including visible haemolysis) excluded from further study.

Normalisation
The five most stably-expressed human plasma miRNAs across all samples identified by Normfinder software and used to normalise remaining miRNAs. These values comprise the final dataset.

Analysis
Dataset passed to Dundee machine learning team for identification of optimal discriminating c-miRNA features (alone and in combination with other omics data) by supervised machine learning methods. Resulting c-miRNA 'signatures' (singleomic and multi-omic) to be tested in subsequent prospective study stage of the project.

Figure 1. Summary of workflow for c-miRNA analysis in the retrospective ENSAT-HT study.

6.1. Study Subjects

For the retrospective study, samples from >350 patients (male or female, aged 11–78y) have been studied, each allocated to one of the four groups: PA, CS, PPGL and primary hypertension (PHT). Although secondary hypertension had been ruled out as a factor in some of the PHT subjects within the retrospective phase, the possibility does remain that a minority of the PHT group may include either "pre-PA" or undiagnosed PA subjects. This possible confounder in the identification of diagnostic biomarkers for PA is unfortunate but largely unavoidable owing to the shortcomings in PA diagnosis that we aim to address. We depend upon our study size and analytical methods to reduce the impact of this effect.

6.2. Sample Medium

EDTA-plasma has been used as the biofluid of choice throughout this project, as it was judged that this would be the simplest medium to collect, store and process in a "real-world" clinical environment (as opposed to the more complex procedures for serum and microvesicles) and would, therefore, reduce inter-sample variability.

6.3. miRNA Quantification Method

The use of RNAseq for this large number of subjects was deemed impractical due to practical considerations (e.g., the considerable amount of data generated) and the prohibitive cost. For this reason, we instead settled on using a realtime qRT-PCR array plate system (Exiqon Serum/Plasma Focus microRNA PCR Panels), which would offer robust quantitative data across 178 endogenous circulating miRNAs, as well as the necessary exogenous control miRNAs. While this approach does not permit the identification of novel c-miRNAs, it does remove the need for subsequent validation of quantitative data, as would be required for RNAseq or microarray analysis. Additionally, quantification can be performed on standard realtime thermal cyclers (we used the QuantStudio 12K Flex Real-Time PCR System, Thermo-Fisher, Waltham, MA, USA), which is common laboratory equipment likely to be available in the diagnostic laboratories that are the intended end-users of this test. Therefore, this approach provides further insight into whether measurement on this type of equipment is sufficiently sensitive to be practical in a clinical setting.

6.4. RNA Isolation Method/RT/Quality Control/Normalisation Methods

The choice of quantification method dictated to some degree the RNA isolation and RT methodologies used (QIAGEN miRNeasy mini kit and Exiqon Universal cDNA synthesis kit II, respectively), as it was necessary to ensure all were compatible and provided sufficient yield, purity, etc., for quantification. Total RNA was isolated from 200 microlitres of total plasma in all cases and subsequent volumes carried over for RNA elution, cDNA synthesis, etc., were standardised throughout the process to minimise as far as possible any inter-sample variation. In addition, plasma samples were seeded with three different spike-in miRNAs (UniSp2, UniSp4 and UniSp5), and an additional two miRNAs (cel-miR-39-3p and UniSp6) were added to RNA prior to cDNA synthesis, thereby providing measures for efficiency of RNA isolation and reverse transcription. The order in which samples were run on the QuantStudio equipment was randomised in order to reduce possible batch effects that might emerge over the course of the project. Prior to normalisation, outlier samples were excluded from further analysis; these included samples where levels of spike-in control miRNAs deviated significantly from the mean and samples where >10% of endogenous c-miRNAs were not detected. In addition, c-miRNAs that were not detected in >50% of all samples were not subjected to further analysis. Remaining miRNA data from samples that had passed these quality control thresholds were subjected to normalisation using Normfinder, which is proven to offer robust correction of minor variation in such quantitative measurements [47,48]. As mentioned previously, Normfinder is a software package that identifies the most stably expressed c-miRNAs across all analysed samples and uses these to normalise the levels of the remaining endogenous miRNAs. Using this software, we have used a combination of five stably expressed c-miRNAs to normalise the quantification data.

6.5. Analytical Methods

Given the complex multivariate analyses required to evaluate the numerous molecules measured by each omic approach within the ENS@T-HT project (as well as the combination of each omic into a single signature), a machine learning approach has been implemented to define each endocrine hypertension disease signature relative to an essential hypertensive group. While it is anticipated that this multiomic approach will yield the most informative signature for each condition, individual omics (i.e., singleomics, including c-miRNA) are also being analysed separately to assess their diagnostic utility. The role that significant factors might play in disease aetiology will also be investigated.

To date, miRNA measurement and analysis has been completed for the retrospective population, providing a reduced list of potential biomarker c-miRNAs that have now also been quantified in the prospective population using the same methodologies as for the retrospective phase. Analysis of these data by machine learning methods is ongoing. Despite spending several years in freezer storage, the quality of miRNA isolated from retrospective study samples was generally high and not appreciably different from that of the prospective samples, which had been frozen for only a few months, at most.

The above is intended to give some insight into the potential confounders of consistent measurement that we have sought to address and minimise during a large project designed to discover c-miRNA biomarkers. It is obviously our hope that there will be significant correlation between the findings of the retrospective and prospective studies, providing reproducible evidence for the first time that c-miRNAs can serve as diagnostic molecules for various forms of endocrine hypertension, including PA, either as a singleomic signature or, more likely, as components of a multiomic signature that also encompasses other types of molecules, including steroids, small metabolites and metanephrines.

7. Conclusions

Improved diagnosis of PA would yield significant benefits, reducing cardiovascular morbidity and mortality through the early diagnosis and treatment of the many hypertensives whose underlying pathology is presently unidentified. Here, we have described the role that miRNAs play in regulating steroidogenic processes within the adrenal cortex and the disruption to its miRNA transcriptome that occurs in PA. This lends compelling support to the hypothesis that such changes in adrenal tissue (and elsewhere) may be reflected in the array of c-miRNAs in the bloodstream. Molecular laboratory methods have now reached the point where such c-miRNAs can be routinely and accurately quantified using commonly available laboratory equipment. The development of a rapid diagnostic test for PA utilising c-miRNAs that could be performed routinely in non-specialist centres is, therefore, a highly desirable and potentially achievable goal. However, as is apparent from previous studies of c-miRNAs in the context of numerous conditions over the past decade or so, there is still some doubt as to whether circulating levels of miRNAs linked to particular diseases show sufficient specificity and sensitivity to be employed as effective biomarkers. It is the belief of ourselves and others that a great deal of the observed variability and lack of reproducibility are the result of inconsistent and non-standardised practices at various stages of the c-miRNA quantification procedure. Therefore, we argue that the validity of c-miRNAs as PA biomarkers should be tested in two independent populations using identical methodology. We are currently engaged in conducting such a study under the umbrella of the ENS@T-HT project. The design of this study has been carefully considered in order to minimise confounding variability in c-miRNA quantification, while also utilising approaches that can be easily performed in a non-specialist clinical setting. The full data from this study are now undergoing final analysis. It is our hope that its findings will establish a firm evidence base for the use of c-miRNAs as diagnostic biomarkers for PA.

Author Contributions: Conceptualisation: S.M.M., J.C.v.K., S.R., A.R., M.-C.Z., E.D.; writing—original draft preparation, S.M.M. and H.S.; writing—review and editing, S.M.M. and E.D. All authors have read and agreed to the published version of the manuscript.

Funding: The ENS@T-HT project (http://www.ensat-ht.eu, accessed on 30 August 2021) has received funding from the European Union's Horizon 2020 research and innovation programme under Grant Agreement No. 633983.

Conflicts of Interest: The authors declare no conflict of interest.

References

1. Young, W.F. Diagnosis and Treatment of Primary Aldosteronism: Practical Clinical Perspectives. *J. Intern. Med.* **2019**, *285*, 126–148. [CrossRef]
2. Zennaro, M.-C.; Boulkroun, S.; Fernandes-Rosa, F.L. Pathogenesis and Treatment of Primary Aldosteronism. *Nat. Rev. Endocrinol.* **2020**, *16*, 578–589. [CrossRef]
3. Omata, K.; Satoh, F.; Morimoto, R.; Ito, S.; Yamazaki, Y.; Nakamura, Y.; Anand, S.K.; Guo, Z.; Stowasser, M.; Sasano, H.; et al. Cellular and Genetic Causes of Idiopathic Hyperaldosteronism. *Hypertension* **2018**, *72*, 874–880. [CrossRef]
4. Funder, J. Primary Aldosteronism. *Trends Cardiovas. Med.* **2021**. [CrossRef] [PubMed]
5. Yozamp, N.; Hundemer, G.L.; Moussa, M.; Underhill, J.; Fudim, T.; Sacks, B.; Vaidya, A. Intraindividual Variability of Aldosterone Concentrations in Primary Aldosteronism: Implications for Case Detection. *Hypertension* **2021**, *77*, 891–899. [CrossRef]
6. Brown, J.M.; Siddiqui, M.; Calhoun, D.A.; Carey, R.M.; Hopkins, P.N.; Williams, G.H.; Vaidya, A. The Unrecognized Prevalence of Primary Aldosteronism: A Cross-Sectional Study. *Ann. Intern. Med.* **2020**, *173*, 10–20. [CrossRef]
7. Baudrand, R.; Guarda, F.J.; Fardella, C.; Hundemer, G.; Brown, J.; Williams, G.; Vaidya, A. Continuum of Renin-Independent Aldosteronism in Normotension. *Hypertension* **2017**, *69*, 950–956. [CrossRef]
8. Lee, R.C.; Feinbaum, R.L.; Ambros, V. The C. Elegans Heterochronic Gene Lin-4 Encodes Small RNAs with Antisense Complementarity to Lin-14. *Cell* **1993**, *75*, 843–854. [CrossRef]
9. Alles, J.; Fehlmann, T.; Fischer, U.; Backes, C.; Galata, V.; Minet, M.; Hart, M.; Abu-Halima, M.; Grässer, F.A.; Lenhof, H.-P.; et al. An Estimate of the Total Number of True Human MiRNAs. *Nucleic Acids Res.* **2019**, *47*, gkz097. [CrossRef]
10. O'Brien, J.; Hayder, H.; Zayed, Y.; Peng, C. Overview of MicroRNA Biogenesis, Mechanisms of Actions, and Circulation. *Front. Endocrinol.* **2018**, *9*, 402. [CrossRef] [PubMed]
11. Quillet, A.; Saad, C.; Ferry, G.; Anouar, Y.; Vergne, N.; Lecroq, T.; Dubessy, C. Improving Bioinformatics Prediction of MicroRNA Targets by Ranks Aggregation. *Front. Genet.* **2020**, *10*, 1330. [CrossRef]
12. Riolo, G.; Cantara, S.; Marzocchi, C.; Ricci, C. MiRNA Targets: From Prediction Tools to Experimental Validation. *Methods Protoc.* **2020**, *4*, 1. [CrossRef] [PubMed]
13. Syeda, Z.A.; Langden, S.S.S.; Munkhzul, C.; Lee, M.; Song, S.J. Regulatory Mechanism of MicroRNA Expression in Cancer. *Int. J. Mol. Sci.* **2020**, *21*, 1723. [CrossRef] [PubMed]
14. Geekiyanage, H.; Rayatpisheh, S.; Wohlschlegel, J.A.; Brown, R.; Ambros, V. Extracellular MicroRNAs in Human Circulation Are Associated with MiRISC Complexes That Are Accessible to Anti-AGO2 Antibody and Can Bind Target Mimic Oligonucleotides. *Proc. Nat. Acad. Sci. USA* **2020**, *117*, 24213–24223. [CrossRef]
15. Bayraktar, R.; Roosbroeck, K.V.; Calin, G.A. Cell-to-cell Communication: MicroRNAs as Hormones. *Mol. Oncol.* **2017**, *11*, 1673–1686. [CrossRef]
16. Mitchell, P.S.; Parkin, R.K.; Kroh, E.M.; Fritz, B.R.; Wyman, S.K.; Pogosova-Agadjanyan, E.L.; Peterson, A.; Noteboom, J.; O'Briant, K.C.; Allen, A.; et al. Circulating MicroRNAs as Stable Blood-Based Markers for Cancer Detection. *Proc. Natl. Acad. Sci. USA* **2008**, *105*, 10513–10518. [CrossRef] [PubMed]
17. Wu, Y.; Li, Q.; Zhang, R.; Dai, X.; Chen, W.; Xing, D. Circulating MicroRNAs: Biomarkers of Disease. *Clin. Chim. Acta* **2021**, *516*, 46–54. [CrossRef]
18. Robertson, S.; MacKenzie, S.M.; Alvarez-Madrazo, S.; Diver, L.A.; Lin, J.; Stewart, P.M.; Fraser, R.; Connell, J.M.; Davies, E. MicroRNA-24 Is a Novel Regulator of Aldosterone and Cortisol Production in the Human Adrenal Cortex. *Hypertension* **2013**, *62*, 572–578. [CrossRef]
19. Robertson, S.; Diver, L.A.; Alvarez-Madrazo, S.; Livie, C.; Ejaz, A.; Fraser, R.; Connell, J.M.; MacKenzie, S.M.; Davies, E. Regulation of Corticosteroidogenic Genes by MicroRNAs. *Int. J. Endocrinol.* **2017**, *2017*, 2021903–2021911. [CrossRef]
20. Nusrin, S.; Tong, S.K.H.; Chaturvedi, G.; Wu, R.S.S.; Giesy, J.P.; Kong, R.Y.C. Regulation of CYP11B1 and CYP11B2 Steroidogenic Genes by Hypoxia-Inducible MiR-10b in H295R Cells. *Mar. Pollut. Bull.* **2014**, *85*, 344–351. [CrossRef] [PubMed]
21. Zhang, G.; Zou, X.; Liu, Q.; Xie, T.; Huang, R.; Kang, H.; Lai, C.; Zhu, J. MiR-193a-3p Functions as a Tumour Suppressor in Human Aldosterone-Producing Adrenocortical Adenoma by down-Regulating CYP11B2. *Int. J. Exp. Pathol.* **2018**, *99*, 77–86. [CrossRef] [PubMed]
22. Butterworth, M.B. Role of MicroRNAs in Aldosterone Signaling. *Curr. Opin. Nephrol. Hypertens.* **2018**, *27*, 390–394. [CrossRef]
23. Butterworth, M.B. MicroRNAs and the Regulation of Aldosterone Signaling in the Kidney. *Am. J. Physiol. Cell Physiol.* **2015**, *308*, C521–C527. [CrossRef] [PubMed]
24. Tömböl, Z.; Turai, P.; Decmann, Á.; Igaz, P. MicroRNAs and Adrenocortical Tumors: Where Do We Stand on Primary Aldosteronism? *Horm. Metab. Res.* **2020**, *52*, 394–403. [CrossRef]
25. He, J.; Cao, Y.; Su, T.; Jiang, Y.; Jiang, L.; Zhou, W.; Zhang, C.; Wang, W.; Ning, G. Downregulation of MiR-375 in Aldosterone-Producing Adenomas Promotes Tumor Cell Growth via MTDH. *Clin. Endocrinol.* **2015**, *83*, 581–589. [CrossRef] [PubMed]
26. Velazquez-Fernandez, D.; Caramuta, S.; Ozata, D.M.; Lu, M.; Höög, A.; Bäckdahl, M.; Larsson, C.; Lui, W.-O.; Zedenius, J. MicroRNA Expression Patterns Associated with Hyperfunctioning and Non-Hyperfunctioning Phenotypes in Adrenocortical Adenomas. *Eur. J. Endocrinol. Eur. Fed. Endocr. Soc.* **2014**, *170*, 583–591. [CrossRef] [PubMed]
27. Lenzini, L.; Caroccia, B.; Campos, A.G.; Fassina, A.; Belloni, A.S.; Seccia, T.M.; Kuppusamy, M.; Ferraro, S.; Skander, G.; Bader, M.; et al. Lower Expression of the TWIK-Related Acid-Sensitive K^+ Channel 2 (TASK-2) Gene Is a Hallmark of Aldosterone-Producing Adenoma Causing Human Primary Aldosteronism. *J. Clin. Endocrinol. Metab.* **2014**, *99*, E674–E682. [CrossRef]

28. Peng, K.-Y.; Chang, H.-M.; Lin, Y.-F.; Chan, C.-K.; Chang, C.-H.; Chueh, S.-C.J.; Yang, S.-Y.; Huang, K.-H.; Lin, Y.-H.; Wu, V.-C.; et al. MicroRNA-203 Modulates Aldosterone Levels and Cell Proliferation by Targeting Wnt5a in Aldosterone-Producing Adenomas. *J. Clin. Endocrinol. Metab.* **2018**, *103*, 3737. [CrossRef]
29. Decmann, A.; Nyírö, G.; Darvasi, O.; Turai, P.; Bancos, I.; Kaur, R.J.; Pezzani, R.; Iacobone, M.; Kraljevic, I.; Kastelan, D.; et al. Circulating MiRNA Expression Profiling in Primary Aldosteronism. *Front. Endocrinol.* **2019**, *10*, 739. [CrossRef] [PubMed]
30. Ye, Y.; Yang, J.; Lv, W.; Lu, Y.; Zhang, L.; Zhang, Y.; Musha, Z.; Fan, P.; Yang, B.; Zhou, X.; et al. Screening of Differentially Expressed MicroRNAs of Essential Hypertension in Uyghur Population. *Lipids Health Dis.* **2019**, *18*, 98. [CrossRef]
31. Romaine, S.P.; Charchar, F.J.; Samani, N.J.; Tomaszewski, M. Circulating MicroRNAs and Hypertension—From New Insights into Blood Pressure Regulation to Biomarkers of Cardiovascular Risk. *Curr. Opin. Pharmacol.* **2016**, *27*, 1–7. [CrossRef] [PubMed]
32. Witwer, K.W. Circulating MicroRNA Biomarker Studies: Pitfalls and Potential Solutions. *Clin. Chem.* **2015**, *61*, 56–63. [CrossRef] [PubMed]
33. Ameling, S.; Kacprowski, T.; Chilukoti, R.K.; Malsch, C.; Liebscher, V.; Suhre, K.; Pietzner, M.; Friedrich, N.; Homuth, G.; Hammer, E.; et al. Associations of Circulating Plasma MicroRNAs with Age, Body Mass Index and Sex in a Population-Based Study. *BMC Med. Genom.* **2015**, *8*, 61. [CrossRef]
34. Endzeliņš, E.; Berger, A.; Melne, V.; Bajo-Santos, C.; Soboļevska, K.; Ābols, A.; Rodriguez, M.; Šantare, D.; Rudņickiha, A.; Lietuvietis, V.; et al. Detection of Circulating MiRNAs: Comparative Analysis of Extracellular Vesicle-Incorporated MiRNAs and Cell-Free MiRNAs in Whole Plasma of Prostate Cancer Patients. *BMC Cancer* **2017**, *17*, 730. [CrossRef]
35. Wang, K.; Yuan, Y.; Cho, J.-H.; McClarty, S.; Baxter, D.; Galas, D.J. Comparing the MicroRNA Spectrum between Serum and Plasma. *PLoS ONE* **2012**, *7*, e41561. [CrossRef]
36. Buschmann, D.; Kirchner, B.; Hermann, S.; Märte, M.; Wurmser, C.; Brandes, F.; Kotschote, S.; Bonin, M.; Steinlein, O.K.; Pfaffl, M.W.; et al. Evaluation of Serum Extracellular Vesicle Isolation Methods for Profiling MiRNAs by Next-generation Sequencing. *J. Extracell. Vesicles* **2018**, *7*, 1481321. [CrossRef]
37. Kirschner, M.B.; Edelman, J.J.B.; Kao, S.C.-H.; Vallely, M.P.; van Zandwijk, N.; Reid, G. The Impact of Hemolysis on Cell-Free MicroRNA Biomarkers. *Front. Genet.* **2013**, *4*, 94. [CrossRef] [PubMed]
38. Wu, C.-S.; Lin, F.-C.; Chen, S.-J.; Chen, Y.-L.; Chung, W.-J.; Cheng, C.-I. Optimized Collection Protocol for Plasma MicroRNA Measurement in Patients with Cardiovascular Disease. *Biomed. Res. Int.* **2016**, *2016*, 1–12. [CrossRef]
39. Glinge, C.; Clauss, S.; Boddum, K.; Jabbari, R.; Jabbari, J.; Risgaard, B.; Tomsits, P.; Hildebrand, B.; Kääb, S.; Wakili, R.; et al. Stability of Circulating Blood-Based MicroRNAs—Pre-Analytic Methodological Considerations. *PLoS ONE* **2017**, *12*, e0167969. [CrossRef]
40. Matias-Garcia, P.R.; Wilson, R.; Mussack, V.; Reischl, E.; Waldenberger, M.; Gieger, C.; Anton, G.; Peters, A.; Kuehn-Steven, A. Impact of Long-Term Storage and Freeze-Thawing on Eight Circulating MicroRNAs in Plasma Samples. *PLoS ONE* **2020**, *15*, e0227648. [CrossRef]
41. Valihrach, L.; Androvic, P.; Kubista, M. Circulating MiRNA Analysis for Cancer Diagnostics and Therapy. *Mol. Asp. Med.* **2019**, *72*, 100825. [CrossRef]
42. Kloten, V.; Neumann, M.H.D.; Pasquale, F.D.; Sprenger-Haussels, M.; Shaffer, J.M.; Schlumpberger, M.; Herdean, A.; Betsou, F.; Ammerlaan, W.; Hällström, T.A.; et al. Multicenter Evaluation of Circulating Plasma MicroRNA Extraction Technologies for the Development of Clinically Feasible Reverse Transcription Quantitative PCR and Next-Generation Sequencing Analytical Work Flows. *Clin. Chem.* **2019**, *65*, 1132–1140. [CrossRef]
43. Schwarzenbach, H.; da Silva, A.M.; Calin, G.; Pantel, K. Data Normalization Strategies for MicroRNA Quantification. *Clin. Chem.* **2015**, *61*, 1333–1342. [CrossRef]
44. Ying, L.; Du, L.; Zou, R.; Shi, L.; Zhang, N.; Jin, J.; Xu, C.; Zhang, F.; Zhu, C.; Wu, J.; et al. Development of a Serum MiRNA Panel for Detection of Early Stage Non-Small Cell Lung Cancer. *Proc. Natl. Acad. Sci. USA* **2020**, *117*, 25036–25042. [CrossRef]
45. Donati, S.; Ciuffi, S.; Brandi, M.L. Human Circulating MiRNAs Real-Time QRT-PCR-Based Analysis: An Overview of Endogenous Reference Genes Used for Data Normalization. *Int. J. Mol. Sci.* **2019**, *20*, 4353. [CrossRef]
46. Manfredi, E.R.M. Biomarkers Discovery through Multivariate Statistical Methods: A Review of Recently Developed Methods and Applications in Proteomics. *J. Proteom. Bioinform.* **2014**, *2015*, 3. [CrossRef]
47. Andersen, C.L.; Jensen, J.L.; Ørntoft, T.F. Normalization of Real-Time Quantitative Reverse Transcription-PCR Data: A Model-Based Variance Estimation Approach to Identify Genes Suited for Normalization, Applied to Bladder and Colon Cancer Data Sets. *Cancer Res.* **2004**, *64*, 5245–5250. [CrossRef]
48. Sundaram, V.K.; Sampathkumar, N.K.; Massaad, C.; Grenier, J. Optimal Use of Statistical Methods to Validate Reference Gene Stability in Longitudinal Studies. *PLoS ONE* **2019**, *14*, e0219440. [CrossRef] [PubMed]

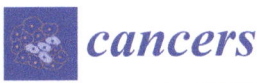

Article

Identifying New Potential Biomarkers in Adrenocortical Tumors Based on mRNA Expression Data Using Machine Learning

André Marquardt [1,2,3,4,*], Laura-Sophie Landwehr [5], Cristina L. Ronchi [5,6], Guido di Dalmazi [7], Anna Riester [8], Philip Kollmannsberger [9], Barbara Altieri [5], Martin Fassnacht [1,5] and Silviu Sbiera [5,*]

1. Comprehensive Cancer Center Mainfranken, University Hospital, University of Würzburg, 97080 Würzburg, Germany; Fassnacht_M@ukw.de
2. Institute of Pathology, University of Würzburg, 97080 Würzburg, Germany
3. Interdisciplinary Center for Clinical Research, University Hospital Würzburg, 97080 Würzburg, Germany
4. Bavarian Cancer Research Center (BZKF), 97080 Würzburg, Germany
5. Division of Endocrinology and Diabetes, University Hospital, University of Würzburg, 97080 Würzburg, Germany; Landwehr_L@ukw.de (L.-S.L.); C.L.Ronchi@bham.ac.uk (C.L.R.); Altieri_B@ukw.de (B.A.)
6. Institute of Metabolism and Systems Research, University of Birmingham, Birmingham B15 2TT, UK
7. Endocrinology Unit, Department of Medical and Surgical Sciences, University of Bologna, 40138 Bologna, Italy; guido.didalmazi@unibo.it
8. Department of Endocrinology, Medizinische Klinik und Poliklinik IV, Ludwig-Maximilians-University, 80336 Munich, Germany; Anna.Riester@med.uni-muenchen.de
9. Center for Computational and Theoretical Biology, University of Würzburg, 97074 Würzburg, Germany; Philip.Kollmannsberger@uni-wuerzburg.de
* Correspondence: Marquardt_A@ukw.de (A.M.); Sbiera_S@ukw.de (S.S.)

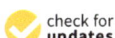

Citation: Marquardt, A.; Landwehr, L.-S.; Ronchi, C.L.; di Dalmazi, G.; Riester, A.; Kollmannsberger, P.; Altieri, B.; Fassnacht, M.; Sbiera, S. Identifying New Potential Biomarkers in Adrenocortical Tumors Based on mRNA Expression Data Using Machine Learning. *Cancers* **2021**, *13*, 4671. https://doi.org/10.3390/cancers13184671

Academic Editor: Peter Igaz

Received: 6 September 2021
Accepted: 10 September 2021
Published: 17 September 2021

Publisher's Note: MDPI stays neutral with regard to jurisdictional claims in published maps and institutional affiliations.

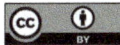

Copyright: © 2021 by the authors. Licensee MDPI, Basel, Switzerland. This article is an open access article distributed under the terms and conditions of the Creative Commons Attribution (CC BY) license (https://creativecommons.org/licenses/by/4.0/).

Simple Summary: Using a visual-based clustering method on the TCGA RNA sequencing data of a large adrenocortical carcinoma (ACC) cohort, we were able to classify these tumors in two distinct clusters largely overlapping with previously identified ones. As previously shown, the identified clusters also correlated with patient survival. Applying the visual clustering method to a second dataset also including benign adrenocortical samples additionally revealed that one of the ACC clusters is more closely located to the benign samples, providing a possible explanation for the better survival of this ACC cluster. Furthermore, the subsequent use of machine learning identified new possible biomarker genes with prognostic potential for this rare disease, that are significantly differentially expressed in the different survival clusters and should be further evaluated.

Abstract: Adrenocortical carcinoma (ACC) is a rare disease, associated with poor survival. Several "multiple-omics" studies characterizing ACC on a molecular level identified two different clusters correlating with patient survival (C1A and C1B). We here used the publicly available transcriptome data from the TCGA-ACC dataset (*n* = 79), applying machine learning (ML) methods to classify the ACC based on expression pattern in an unbiased manner. UMAP (uniform manifold approximation and projection)-based clustering resulted in two distinct groups, ACC-UMAP1 and ACC-UMAP2, that largely overlap with clusters C1B and C1A, respectively. However, subsequent use of random-forest-based learning revealed a set of new possible marker genes showing significant differential expression in the described clusters (e.g., *SOAT1*, *EIF2A1*). For validation purposes, we used a secondary dataset based on a previous study from our group, consisting of 4 normal adrenal glands and 52 benign and 7 malignant tumor samples. The results largely confirmed those obtained for the TCGA-ACC cohort. In addition, the ENSAT dataset showed a correlation between benign adrenocortical tumors and the good prognosis ACC cluster ACC-UMAP1/C1B. In conclusion, the use of ML approaches re-identified and redefined known prognostic ACC subgroups. On the other hand, the subsequent use of random-forest-based learning identified new possible prognostic marker genes for ACC.

Keywords: adrenocortical carcinoma; in silico analysis; machine learning; bioinformatic clustering; biomarker prediction

1. Introduction

Adrenocortical carcinoma (ACC) is a rare endocrine malignancy with an incidence rate of approximately 0.7–2.0 per million [1] and is characterized by high aggressiveness, which leads to poor prognosis. The 5 year overall survival rate ranges from 16% to 47% and is particularly poor in patients with metastatic disease [2]. Complete surgical resection is the treatment of choice in localized ACC and is virtually the only option to achieve a cure. As recurrence is frequent, adjuvant therapy is recommended in most patients [3,4]. Despite continuous development in therapeutic concepts of ACC, the improvements brought to patient survival remain modest [5,6]. Preliminary studies on the molecular events leading to tumorigenesis in ACC [7] led to the first molecular targeted therapies, such as IGF1R (insulin-like growth factor 1 receptor) [8] and VEGF (vascular endothelial growth factor) [9] inhibitors, which all proved disappointing [10]. Given the situation only five years ago, it was even pessimistically asserted that a breakthrough might not be in sight for the next 10 to 15 years [11]. Therefore, detailed information about the molecular and genetic background of tumorigenesis in ACC is still as needed as before. In more recent years, with the advent of affordable next generation sequencing and through concerted efforts of international consortia, several pan-genomic studies were performed in adrenocortical tumors with the goal to better understand the mechanisms that lead to adrenal tumorigenesis and are linked to worse clinical outcome [12–15].

In the first integrated genomics study on ACC, Assié et al. [12] uncovered several novel molecular features by performing a multi-omics profiling of germline and somatic exomes, copy number variations, DNA methylation, as well as mRNA and miRNA expression in 45 ACC tissues. Among other things, the authors confirmed that somatic copy number alterations (gains and losses) are common in ACC as shown by prior single nucleotide polymorphism array studies [16]. While also confirming previously identified alterations in *CTNNB1*, *TP53*, *CDKN2A*, *RB1*, and *MEN1*, the authors also identified novel somatic alterations in *ZNRF3*, *DAXX*, *TERT*, and *MED12*. The gene most frequently targeted for somatic alteration was *ZNRF3*, altered in 21% of ACC and mutually exclusive with mutations in *CTNNB1*. This alteration suggests that Wnt ligands may be implicated in the tumorigenesis of a subset of ACC [17]. The authors also identified a unique miRNA signature associated with an imprinted *DLK1-MEG3* cluster downregulated in a subset of ACC that the group identified earlier and named C1B [18]. Importantly, they also showed a higher mutation rate and higher incidence of recurrent mutations in the other subset, called C1A, which was also associated with a poorer prognosis. These data were partly validated by Juhlin et al. [14], who performed whole-exome sequencing and copy number variations screening in a cohort of 41 ACC tissues.

In 2016, the largest multiplatform study on adrenocortical carcinoma to date followed as part of the consortium of genomic cancer studies—The Cancer Genome Atlas project (TCGA-ACC) [15]. The involvement of TCGA enabled the inclusion of 91 international ACC samples in the study. However, the number of samples analyzed varied for each method: whole-exome sequencing ($n = 90$), mRNA sequencing ($n = 79$), miRNA sequencing ($n = 79$), DNA copy number via SNP arrays ($n = 89$), DNA methylation via DNA methylation arrays ($n = 79$), and targeted proteome from reverse phase protein array (RPPA; $n = 45$). Compared to Assié et al., TCGA-ACC identified additional recurrent somatic alterations in *PRKAR1A*, *RPL22*, *TERF2*, and *CCNE1*, and somatic alterations in epigenetic modifiers including MLL family members, *SETD2*, *TET1*, and *SMARCA4*. Somatic mutations observed in ACC affected in ~45% of cases the cell cycle, in ~40% the Wnt pathway, and in ~20% epigenetic modifiers. Looking at the copy number alterations, TCGA-ACC identified three recurrent profiles: quiet (diploid tumor genome), chromosomal (frequent whole chromosome loss of heterozygosity and hypodiploidy in a subset of tumors), and noisy (frequent focal gains and losses). A subset of the "noisy" and "chromosomal" tumors was also characterized by whole genome doubling, associated with TERT overexpression. "Chromosomal" tumors with genome doubling and "noisy" tumors in general were also associated with worse prognosis [15].

TCGA-ACC identified that ACCs can also be classified in steroid-low/immune-high (low expression of steroidogenic markers and high-expression markers associated with an activated immune response) and steroid-high (high-expression of steroidogenic markers). Both categories can be further subdivided considering cell-cycle activation markers. Steroid-low/low proliferation tumors were associated with the previously identified "good prognosis" C1B cluster, whereas steroid-high/high-proliferation signature was associated with the "poor prognosis" C1A cluster. Combining all the data from all the different approaches, ACC-TCGA divided the ACCs into three distinct molecular subtypes, referred to as cluster of clusters (COC) 1, COC2, and COC3, directly correlating with patient prognosis: COC1 tumors—best prognosis, COC2 tumors—intermediate prognosis, and patients with COC3 tumors had the worst prognosis, with rapid disease progression [15].

What all these above-mentioned studies [13–15] have in common is the use of multi-platform molecular profiling and clustering of genome wide data into several prognostic relevant clusters. However, the multi-platform nature of these studies makes them also very costly and unpractical to be routinely used in patient stratification in a clinical setting. Furthermore, while defining the clustering analyses as unsupervised, the authors perform several adjustments to the datasets—for example, quantification cut-offs, selection of adrenal cortex specific markers and assisted combinations at different levels, which are introducing a scientist-biased component into the analysis, making it even harder to adapt the retrospective analysis into clinical everyday life. In this study, we present a new, simple, unsupervised, machine-learning-based method that is delivering the same clustering power for the adrenocortical tumors as the original complex analysis, based only on the mRNA expression dataset from the ACC-TCGA study and validated in a separate cohort of adrenocortical tumors that was previously evaluated by RNA-seq [19].

2. Materials and Methods

2.1. Patient Cohorts

In this work, we used the RNA-sequencing data provided by the TCGA-ACC consortium consisting of 79 ACC samples [20] (accessed on 8 August 2019). For our analyses, we used the fragments per kilobase per million (FPKM) files as input. For independent confirmation, we additionally used a dataset published recently by the ENSAT consortium [19] after being granted access to the sequencing results and clinical data. This dataset containing RNA-sequencing results, consists of ACC (n = 7) samples, but mainly of non-malignant forms: normal adrenal glands (NAG, n = 4) and adrenocortical adenomas (ACA; n = 52), differentiating between endocrine inactive adenomas (EIA; ns = 9), adenomas with mild autonomous cortisol secretion (MACS-CPA; n = 17) and Cushing syndrome cortisol producing adenomas (CS-CPA; n = 26). As this study is only an in silico reanalysis of previously published data, no ethic committee approval was needed.

2.2. Bioinformatics Analyses

A Jupyter Notebook environment (version 7.5.0) was used to perform all bioinformatic steps using Python version 3.6.9, scikit-learn version 0.22.1 [20], SciPy version 1.3.0 [21] and pandas version 0.24.2 [21,22]. The notebook for the unsupervised UMAP clustering is available upon request.

2.2.1. Uniform Manifold Approximation and Projection (UMAP) Clustering

For UMAP clustering and plotting, we used euclidean_distances from the sklearn.metrics.pairwise module to determine the squared pairwise Euclidean distance between samples of the initial data set, on which the local connectivity parameter rho, together with the first nearest neighbor, is based. For each entry of the distance matrix, the sum of probabilities in the high-dimensional space is calculated. The nearest neighbors and the probabilities for each entry determine the entropy and, based on a binary search the optimal rho for a fixed number of the 15 nearest neighbors is computed. To satisfy the symmetry condition of the UMAP algorithm we used a simplified calculation: instead of subtracting the product of the probability and the transposed probability from the sum of the probability and the transposed probability, we divided the sum by 2. For the subsequent building of low-dimensional probabilities we used mind_dist = 0.25. As a cost function, we used cross-entropy—with a normalized Q parameter. The gradient of it was used in the gradient descent learning—using the regular instead of the stochastic one with 2 dimensions and 50 neighbors.

Based on the results of the UMAP, we manually curated the data, determined the clusters for subsequent analysis and deleted three outliers (TCGA-OR-A5J8, TCGA-OR-A5JB, and TCGA-P6-A5OG—Table S1). Two of these three outliers (TCGA-OR-A5J8 and TCGA-OR-A5JB) have been classified as sarcomatoid samples in the original publication and were, therefore, expected to be outliers. The last datapoint (TCGA-P6-A5OG) was not described at all in the original work but, as all three samples cluster closely together, is most probably also a sarcomatoid sample. We then again performed the described UMAP plotting with the curated data for better cluster representation, obtaining two distinct clusters, which we named ACC-UMAP1 and ACC-UMAP2 according to their position in the given UMAP.

2.2.2. Random Forest Learning

Based on the obtained clusters, we trained a supervised random forest (RF) classifier (RandomForestClassifier of the sklearn.ensemble module) to specify the transcriptional differences—based on unprocessed FPKM values—between the two identified clusters. For training our model, we used a 50/50 split, letting the model learn on 50% of the data and evaluating it on the other 50%, with 1000 trees in the forest (n_estimators = 1000). We trained 100 models and determined the 100 features—representing the ensemble gene IDs—with the highest impact on the model using the according "feature values", which imply the importance of the corresponding feature. For each feature, we counted its occurrence in the top 100 for each of the 100 trained models, creating a form of ensemble technique. For subsequent analysis, the combined top 100 genes—according to the number of appearances in the top 100 of each individual model and the calculated mean rank—from these, 100 different models were used, adapted from a previous analysis [23]. For the 100 trained models, the minimum testing accuracy is 81.58%, the maximum testing accuracy is 100%, and the mean testing accuracy over all different models is 95.5%. Within these 100 trained models, 18 had a testing accuracy of 100%. The 5-fold cross-fold validation yielded a mean accuracy of 96.00% ± 5.33%.

2.2.3. Mutation Analysis

For further insight into the differences between the determined clusters, we also investigated common mutations for ACC, namely *TP53*, *CTNNB1*, *NF1*, *APC*, *ZNRF3*, *MEN1*, *GNAS*, and *ATRX*. The information on the mutational status of the samples were obtained from cbioportal (https://www.cbioportal.org/ accessed on 2 September 2020) [24,25].

2.2.4. Plots and Statistical Analysis

Box and scatter plots were generated using matplotlib. For survival analysis, Kaplan Meier (KM) plots were generated using the lifelines module (version 0.23.1) [26]. If not stated otherwise, the statistical tests for clinical characteristics and mutation analysis were performed using Kruskal–Wallis-Test—using scipy.stats module including indicated significances in the box and scatter plots, for which we used the statannot module for python (version 0.2.2). For the analysis of further interactions and relations between the identified top 100 genes, we used a network generated by StringDB [27] showing a close relation of the genes used for further analysis. Kaplan–Meier followed by Cox regression analysis was used to estimate overall survival (OS) using IBM SPSS v 26 for Windows.

3. Results

3.1. An UMAP Clustering Approach Is Able to Generate Two Distinct Clusters of ACC Samples That Largely Confirm Previously Published Clusters and Correlate with Patient Survival

In a first UMAP clustering approach of the log transformed FPKM values of the whole TCGA-ACC dataset, most of the samples were attributed to two large clusters, with only three samples not fitting in these clusters (Figure S1A). After curating the dataset by eliminating these outliers from the analysis (see Table S1), the subsequent UMAP provided two distinct clusters, which we named "ACC-UMAP1" (the left cluster) and "ACC-UMAP2" (the right cluster) (Figure 1A). We correlated the samples from these two clusters with the different clustering characteristics that were attributed to these samples in the original description by Zheng et al. [15] and, interestingly, the clusters generated by our UMAP approach overlapped very well with several clusters published before (Table S1). Most importantly, the clusters identified this way overlapped nearly completely with the clusters C1A and C1B from the Zheng et al. study (Figure 1B), with only 9 samples (11.84%) not directly matching our cluster assignment. As clusters C1A and C1B were already shown to tightly correlate with patient prognosis [12], it was no surprise that the two ACC-UMAP clusters also correlated very well with the overall survival of the patients (12.46 (95%CI 11.43–13.48) vs. 7.38 (95%CI 5.48–9.27) years, hazard ratio for death 6.27 (95%CI 2.34–16.77, $p = 0.000029$) (Figure 1C). Cluster ACC-UMAP1, mostly overlapping with the C1B cluster, is associated with a better prognosis, while ACC-UMAP2 is associated with a poorer prognosis, as previously described. The ACC-UMAP clusters also correlated very well with other clusters from Zheng et al., like the steroid and immune phenotype with only 11 samples (14.47%) off (Figure S1B), and with the COC with only 9 samples (11.84%) that clustered differently (Figure S1D). In contrast, the genomic doubling clusters from Zheng et al. were distributed independently over the two described UMAP clusters (Figure S1C).

We applied the same UMAP approach to a dataset published recently by the ENSAT consortium [19] which contained only 7 ACCs but many other adrenocortical tissues, either from normal adrenal glands or from different benign adrenocortical tumors, as previously described [19]. Interestingly, the obtained clusters for the ACC samples show a similar clustering to the ACC-TCGA samples, with an ACC-UMAP1 cluster on the left side and an ACC-UMAP2 on the right side, even though the sample numbers are comparatively low (Figure 1D). Additionally, the number of samples per cluster with roughly 50% each (4 left, 3 right) is comparable to the ACC-TCGA results (40 left, 36 right). Due to the low number of ACC samples in this dataset, we could not perform a statistically relevant analysis regarding patient survival, however, we observed that 2 out 3 (66.7%) ACC of the ACC-UMAP2 cluster died (median survival was 7.25 years), whereas none of the ACC patients of the ACC-UMAP1 cluster died due to the disease during the time interval of the study. Another interesting cluster is the one containing nearly all of the benign tumor samples, which is close to the ACC-UMAP1 cluster, showing a closer relation between these two (Figure 1D).

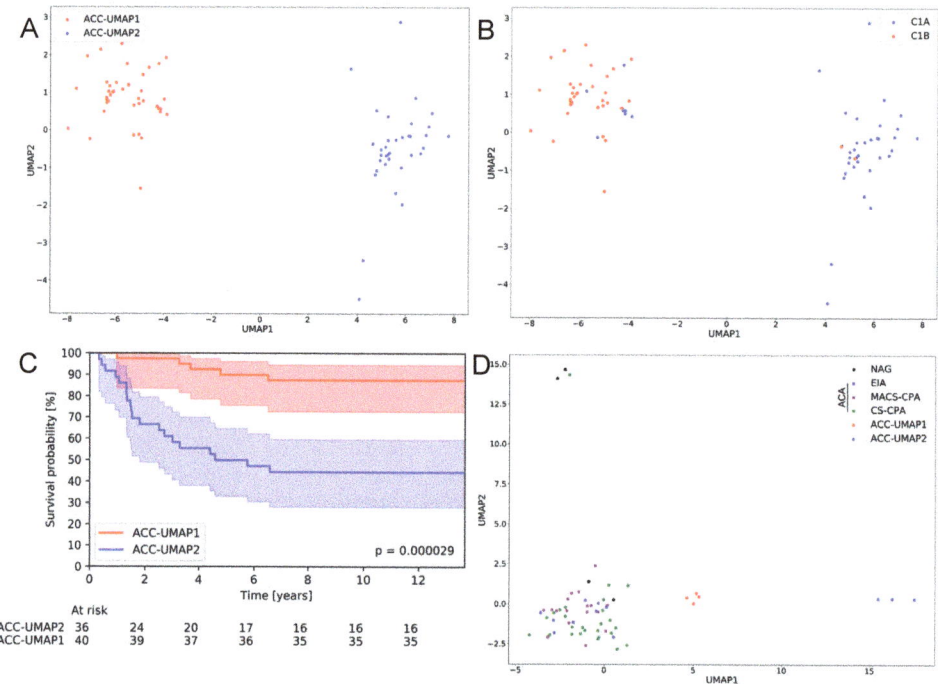

Figure 1. UMAP cluster representation of different mRNA expression patterns. Representation of the UMAP (uniform manifold approximation and projection) clustering of the ACC-TCGA dataset without outliers (**A**) and the overlap with C1A/C1B clustering from the original publication of Zheng et al. [15] (**B**). Kaplan–Meier curve of overall survival of ACC-TCGA patients assigned to the two clusters by UMAP. Shaded area: confidence interval with alpha = 0.05 (**C**). Representation of the UMAP clustering of the ENSAT dataset [19] (**D**). NAG = normal adrenal gland; EIA = endocrine inactive adenoma; MACS-CPA = mild autonomous cortisol secretion adenoma-cortisol producing adenoma; CS-CPA = Cushing syndrome-cortisol producing adenoma which together make the ACA = adrenocortical adenoma; ACC = adrenocortical carcinoma.

3.2. Random Forest Analysis Identifies 100 Genes That Are Differentially Expressed in Cluster ACC-UMAP2, but Most of These Genes Have Not Yet Been Associated with Adrenocortical Tumorigenesis

Being able to recreate already established ACC clusters with our UMAP approach, we were interested in the molecular differences between the identified clusters. Applying RF learning, we were able to determine the 100 genes with the most influence in distinguishing our clusters (Figure S2). Further analyses revealed that 98 of these 100 genes were overexpressed in the ACC-UMAP2 cluster as compared to the ACC-UMAP1 cluster of the ACC-TCGA data (Figure 2, Table S2). The only two exceptions were *CSGALNACT1*, encoding for chondroitin sulfate N-acetylgalactosaminyltransferase 1, an enzyme usually associated with cartilage development and *KLRB1*, encoding for the killer-cell lectin-like receptor B1, a type II membrane protein known to play an inhibitory role on natural killer cell cytotoxicity (Figure S2). Surprisingly, the vast majority of the 100 genes identified by the RF analysis have little known connection with the adrenocortical function and tumorigenesis. Notably, among the known genes we found the solute carrier family 2 member 1/glucose transporter 1 (*SLC2A1/GLUT1*) (Figure 2A), an important, stage independent predictor of ACC patient outcome [28] as well as those encoding for the sterol-O acyltransferase (*SOAT1*) (Figure 2B) and eukaryotic translation initiation factor 2 α (*EIF2S1*) (Figure 2C), both known to be involved in endoplasmic reticulum stress processes in the adrenocortical tissues associated with mitotane treatment and also having an influence on ACC patient outcome [29,30]. There were also other interesting genes overexpressed in the poor survival cluster ACC-UMAP2 that were already reported in the context of adrenal function disturbances, such as the proto-oncogene *MYC* (Figure 2D) [31] the TGF-β signal transducer *SMAD2* (Sma—and mad-related protein 2) (Figure 2E) [32], the mitotic checkpoint gene *BUB3* (udding uninhibited by benzimidazoles 3 homolog) (Figure 2F) [33] and *ASB4* (ankyrin repeat and SOCS box containing 4) (Figure 2G) [20]. *MED27* (mediator complex subunit 27) (Figure 2H), a cofactor involved in the transcriptional initiation by the RNA polymerase II apparatus was shown to be involved in adrenal cortical carcinogenesis by targeting the Wnt/β-catenin signaling pathway and the epithelial-mesenchymal transition process [34]. *FSCN1* (Figure 2I), a fascin family member, was recently shown to be associated with tumor invasiveness in ACC [35] and *GNAI3* (guanine nucleotide binding protein (G protein), alpha inhibiting activity polypeptide 3) (Figure 2J) was shown to be increased in nutrient starved adrenal glands in $RGS4_{ko}$ mice [36].

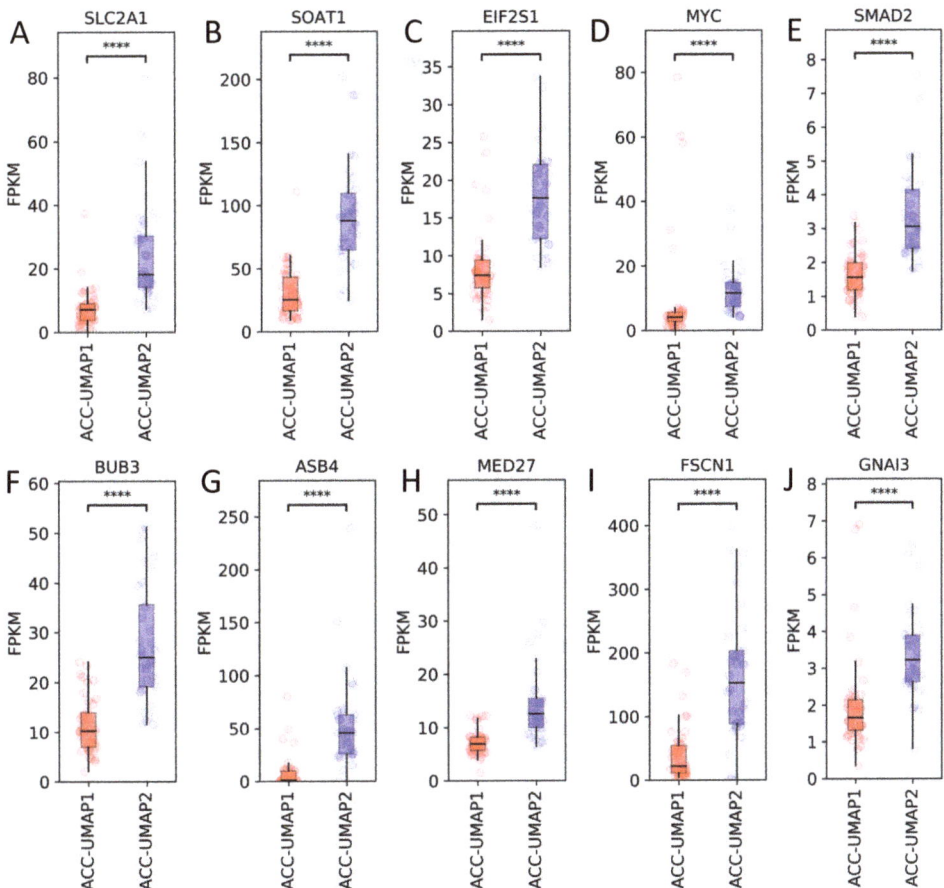

Figure 2. Selection of mRNA expression pattern of 10 genes from the TCGA-ACC dataset, as identified by RF analysis, that were previously shown to be involved in adrenal function. *SLC2A1*: solute carrier family 2 member 1 (**A**), *SOAT1*: sterol-O acyltransferase (**B**), *EIF2S1*: eukaryotic translation initiation factor 2 α (**C**), *MYC* proto-oncogene MYC (**D**), *SMAD2*: sma—and mad-related protein 2 (**E**), *BUB3* budding uninhibited by benzimidazoles 3 homolog (**F**), *ASB4*: ankyrin repeat And SOCS box containing 4 (**G**), *MED27*: mediator complex subunit 27 (**H**), *FSCN1*: fascin actin-bundling protein 1 (**I**), *GNAI3*: guanine nucleotide binding protein (G protein), alpha inhibiting activity polypeptide 3 (**J**). ns, not significant. **** $p < 0.0001$. Y-axis units: FPKM.

Looking at the mRNA expression of the same factors in the validation dataset, it became obvious that, while some of the genes followed the same pattern of expression as in the ACC-TCGA dataset, some differed (Figure S3A). Furthermore, in the validation cohort we observed only a tendency of overexpression in most of the genes, without significant differences (Table S3), probably due to the low number of ACC cases in this dataset. However, more interesting are the differences in expression between the two ACC clusters and the normal adrenal glands and adrenocortical adenomas (Figures S3A and 3). For example, while the expression of *SLC2A1* (GLUT-1) is higher in ACC than in NAG and adenomas and highest in the ACC-UMAP2 cluster (Figure 3A), the expression of *MYC* for example is significantly lower in both ACC clusters when compared to the NAG (Figure 3D). This is in conformity with previously published data that shows low *MYC* expression in adrenocortical tumors [31,37]. We performed these analyses while also considering the different ACA entities (EIA, MACS-CPA and CS-CPA) separately (Figure S3B, Table S4), however, as there were no significant differences between the three subgroups, we pooled all ACAs together for the main analysis.

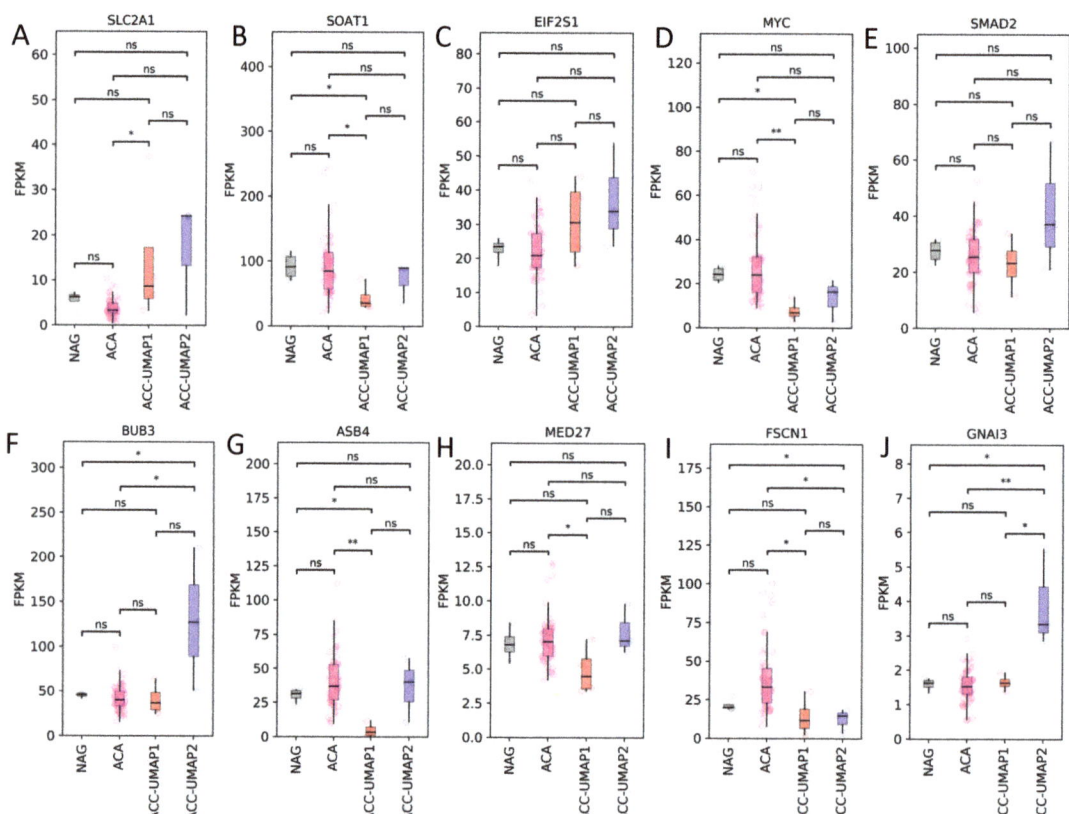

Figure 3. Selection of mRNA expression pattern of 10 genes from the validation dataset, as identified by RF analysis, that were previously shown to be involved in adrenal function. *SLC2A1*: solute carrier family 2 member 1 (**A**), *SOAT1*: sterol-O acyltransferase (**B**), *EIF2S1*: eukaryotic translation initiation factor 2 α (**C**), *MYC*: proto-oncogene MYC (**D**), *SMAD2*: sma—and mad-related protein 2 (**E**), *BUB3*: budding uninhibited by benzimidazoles 3 homolog (**F**), *ASB4*: ankyrin repeat and SOCS box containing 4 (**G**), *MED27*: mediator complex subunit 27 (**H**), *FSCN1*: fascin actin-bundling protein 1 (**I**), *GNAI3*: guanine nucleotide binding protein (G protein), alpha inhibiting activity polypeptide 3 (**J**). NAG = normal adrenal gland; ACA = adrenocortical adenoma; ACC = adrenocortical carcinoma. ns, not significant. * $p < 0.05$, ** $p < 0.01$, ns, not significant. Y-axis units: FPKM.

To gain further insight into possible connections of the identified genes, we performed a network analysis, showing that overall, half of the top 100 genes is interconnected in a large network that is involved in both cell division and transcription control.

3.3. Mutational Analysis Reveals CTNNB1 and TP53 as the Only Known Differentially Mutated Genes

Previous studies have already shown the close relation between the C1A/C1B clusters and mutation status. To further confirm our used approach, we additionally looked at driver mutations and their impact on cluster affiliation. Analysis of known driver mutations in ACC, including TP53, CTNNB1, NF1, APC, ZNRF3, MEN1, GNAS, and ATRX, show that there is only a small proportion of genes that are significantly altered within the UMAP identified clusters. For NF1, APC, ZNRF3, GNAS, and ATRX, no significance could be observed. Only for the genes TP53 (ACC-UMAP2 vs. ACC-UMAP1: 11 vs. 1 sample, $p = 0.042$) and CTNNB1 (ACC-UMAP2 vs. ACC-UMAP1: 12 vs. 1 sample, $p = 0.00026$) were significant results present with a higher proportion of mutated samples in the right cluster. For MEN1 a tendency was observable ($p = 0.058$), also with more mutated samples in the right cluster. As such, these analyses confirm our used approach and confirm the cluster ACC-UMAP2 as the worse cluster regarding both survival and distribution of mutated genes.

4. Discussion

In comparison to Zheng et al. [15], our approach considers only the mRNA expression, as it was performed previously by de Reyniès et al., in 2009 [18]. At that time, a gene signature was determined on the basis of mRNA from microarrays, based on hierarchical clustering methods [7], which identified the two groups C1A/C1B. Compared to Zheng et al., who performed a pre-selection of genes before the clustering analysis (only considering the genes that are expressed in more than 25% of the samples and then only the 5000 most variable genes), we do not limit the amount of data in our approach using all possible 60.483 transcripts provided by TCGA for our analysis, which is also the strength of our study. Despite this difference, we can almost completely confirm the grouping according to C1A and C1B, just as Zheng et al. had in their "K2" approach, who already showed the separability into these two groups in their data. When we split the clusters further to take into consideration the samples that clustered differently between the C1A/B system and our ACC-UMAP1/2 system, it became clear that the unbiased UMAP clustering system is more robust in clustering together samples with similar expression patterns. This is shown by the fact that in the majority of the split cases the differences between the different UMAP sub-clusters were non-significant while this was not the case for the C1A/B sub-clusters.

The subsequent use of a RF to identify the transcriptomic differences between the two groups shows great differences between the two approaches. While Zheng et al. name 151 genes in their K4 approach and de Reyniès et al. can limit their overall survival prediction to only 2 genes (*BUB1B* and *PINK1*) [18], we show 100 genes that are most likely to separate the two clusters found. Because of the unbiased consideration of all possible transcripts, it is not surprising that the top 100 genes identified are mostly unknown in the field of tumorigenesis or adrenocortical function, because preselection of variable genes was widely used before the era of machine learning. This might be considered a weakness of our method and leads to apparently strange results. For example, the overlap of the top 100 genes of our approach compared to the K4 approach of Zheng et al. is just one gene—*ASB4*. It is also striking that 98 genes are overexpressed in one of the clusters and only two in the other cluster. However, this is solely a representation of the approach, which represents the most influential genes for the learned models. Despite this, we could still find at least 10 genes among the top 100 that were previously reported in the context of the adrenal function, underlining their importance in the adrenocortical disease progression, also strengthening the results and the approach. The prognostic role of some of these genes was reported before, as in the case of *SLC2A1/GLUT1* [28] or *FSCN1* [35]. In other cases, such as with *GNAI3*, an increase in gene expression was reported in nutrient starved adrenal glands in a mouse model [36], starvation that is often observed in adrenal cancer. The fact that GNAI3 expression is highest in the poor prognosis cluster ACC-UMAP2 and low in ACC-UMAP1 and benign adrenal tissues show that this gene has high prognostic potential. Nevertheless, a gene does not have to already be reported in the context of adrenal disease to be considered a good prognostic candidate. Just to take one example, while not yet analyzed in adrenal cancer, *CBX3* (Chrombox 3) has a similar expression pattern between the different clusters with low expression in normal and benign adrenocortical tissues and high expression in ACC, especially in the poor prognosis cluster ACC-UMAP2. While it has no obvious connection with adrenal function, it is a gene that is involved in histone methylation and was associated with other types of cancer [38]. We are confident that the future analysis of the RF generated top 100 list of genes will bring to light several new prognostic markers for ACC.

Our results also show that for the known mutations, *CTNNB1* and *TP53* both cluster significantly differently between the two ACC-UMAP clusters. Combining these results with the tendency observed for *MEN1* (1 mutated sample in the left and 5 in the right cluster) and the significant survival differences between the two clusters, it can be indirectly assumed that these mutations do have an impact on patient survival.

Here we show a novel, completely unbiased way to clusters the TCGA-ACC dataset without limiting the input data. We were able to clarify and maybe even refine the already established and well-known ACC subgroups C1A and C1B described by TCGA-ACC. Also, the novel differentially expressed genes discovered by our approach should be further investigated and verified in future work regarding their potential role as prognostic biomarkers.

5. Conclusions

In the present work, we applied machine-learning methods to a published ACC dataset generated by the TCGA consortium and validated it in an ENSAT generated dataset. First, we applied UMAP, a standard clustering method in single-cell sequencing analysis, to identify possible clusters within the data. This approach yielded two clusters that match to a large extent (>80%) the already published and well-known ACC clusters (C1A/C1B). Subsequent survival analyses confirmed the clusters found by our approach and show a significant survival advantage for the ACC-UMAP1 cluster (corresponding to the already described C1A cluster). Examination of known mutations distribution within the clusters showed a significant accumulation of mutations of the *CTNNB1* and *TP53* genes in the poorer survival cluster (ACC-UMAP2). The subsequent use of a RF learning revealed the 100 genes that have the greatest influence on the separation of the two clusters and could potentially serve as new biomarkers or novel targets for therapeutic approaches. Taken together, we were able to show the capabilities of machine-learning-based methods by identifying and redefining the already well-known C1A and C1B cluster of the TCGA-ACC cohort and opening up their further evaluation and use in sub-group identification research also for other entities.

Supplementary Materials: The following are available online at https://www.mdpi.com/article/10.3390/cancers13184671/s1, Table S1. Clinical characteristics and different associated clustering of the ACC samples in the ACC-TCGA cohort; Table S2. Differential mRNA expression levels of the 100 genes selected by random forest in the ACC-TCG) cohort; Table S3. Differential mRNA expression levels of the 100 genes selected by random forest in the validation (ENSAT) cohort considering all the ACA subgroups together; Table S4. Differential mRNA expression levels of the 100 genes selected by random forest in the validation (ENSAT) cohort considering all the ACA subgroups separately; Figure S1. Various UMAP (Uniform Manifold Approximation and Projection) cluster representations for the TCGA-ACC dataset. Representation of the UMAP of the. (A) ACC-TCCA dataset and the overlap with different molecular clustering from the original publication of Zheng et al. [15] without outliers: steroid phenotype (B), genome doubling (gd; (C)) and cluster of clusters (COC; (D)).; Figure S2. mRNA expression pattern of all top 100 genes, in alphabetical order, from the validation dataset, considering the different ACA entities separately, as identified by random forest. NAG = normal adrenal gland; EIA = endocrine inactive adrenocortical adenoma; MACS-CPA = mild autonomous cortisol secreting adrenocortical adenoma; CS-CPA = Cushing syndrome cortisol producing adenoma; ACC = adrenocortical carcinoma. ns, not significant. $p < 0.05$, * $p < 0.01$, *** $p < 0.0001$. Y-axis units: FPKM; Figure S3. STRING-DB network (https://string-db.org/, accessed on 8 August 2019) analysis of known interactions between the top 100 genes as identified by random forest learning to separate the ACC-TCGA dataset in clusters.

Author Contributions: Conceptualization, A.M. and S.S.; Data curation, A.M. and B.A.; Funding acquisition, C.L.R., A.R., M.F. and S.S.; Investigation, A.M., L.-S.L. and S.S.; Project administration, A.M. and S.S.; Resources, M.F. and S.S.; Software, A.M.; Supervision, P.K., M.F. and S.S.; Validation, A.M., L.-S.L., C.L.R., G.d.D., A.R., P.K., B.A. and S.S.; Visualization, A.M. and S.S.; Writing—original draft, A.M. and S.S.; Writing—review and editing, A.M., L.-S.L., C.L.R., G.d.D., A.R., P.K., B.A., M.F. and S.S. All authors have read and agreed to the published version of the manuscript.

Funding: This research was funded by the Else Kröner-Fresenius-Stiftung, grant 2016_A96 to S.S., Deutsche Krebshilfe, project number 70112969 to C.L.R. and M.F. and several grants of the German Research Foundation/DFG, grant FA-466/4-2 and FA-466/8-1 to M.F., SB52/1-1 to S.S., and RO-5435/3-1 to C.L.R. and project 314061271- TRR 205 to A.R., M.F. and S.S. A.M. was funded by a grant of the Central Unit for Precision Oncology, Grant Z-14, Interdisciplinary Center for Clinical Research, University Hospital Würzburg, Germany. The APC was partially funded by the Open Access Publication Fund of the University of Würzburg.

Institutional Review Board Statement: Ethical review and approval were waived for this study, due to the fact that this study is an in silico analysis of previously published data. The original studies have been individually approved by the respective ethical committees, this information can be found in the original publications.

Informed Consent Statement: Patient consent was waived due to the fact that this study is an in silico analysis of previously published data. Patient consent was obtained for the original studies, this information can be found in the original publications.

Data Availability Statement: The results shown here are based upon data generated by the TCGA Research Network: https://www.cancer.gov/tcga (accessed on 8 August 2019) and the European Network for the Study of Adrenal Tumors/ENSAT (ensat.org, accessed on 8 August 2019). The original data can be explored through the Broad Institute GDAC FireBrowse portal (http://firebrowse.org/?cohort=ACC, accessed on 8 August 2019) and the platform EGA (https://www.ebi.ac.uk/ega/home, accession number EGAS00001004533), respectively.

Acknowledgments: The results shown here are based upon data generated by the TCGA Research Network.

Conflicts of Interest: The authors declare no conflict of interest. The funders had no role in the design of the study; in the collection, analyses, or interpretation of data; in the writing of the manuscript, or in the decision to publish the results.

References

1. Erickson, L.A.; Rivera, M.; Zhang, J. Adrenocortical Carcinoma: Review and Update. *Adv. Anat. Pathol.* **2014**, *21*, 151–159. [CrossRef]
2. Stigliano, A.; Cerquetti, L.; Lard, P.; Petrangeli, E.; Toscano, V. New insights and future perspectives in the therapeutic strategy of adrenocortical carcinoma (Review). *Oncol. Rep.* **2017**, *37*, 1301–1311. [CrossRef]
3. Fassnacht, M.; Dekkers, O.M.; Else, T.; Gaudin, E.; Berruti, A.; de Krijger, R.R.; Haak, H.R.; Mihail, R.; Assie, G.; Terzolo, M. European Society of Endocrinology Clinical Practice Guidelines on the management of adrenocortical carcinoma in adults, in collaboration with the European Network for the Study of Adrenal Tumors. *Eur. J. Endocrinol.* **2018**, *179*, G1–G46. [CrossRef] [PubMed]
4. Fassnacht, M.; Assie, G.; Baudin, E.; Eisenhofer, G.; de la Fouchardiere, C.; Haak, H.R.; de Krijger, R.; Porpiglia, F.; Terzolo, M.; Berruti, A.; et al. Adrenocortical carcinomas and malignant phaeochromocytomas: ESMO-EURACAN Clinical Practice Guidelines for diagnosis, treatment and follow-up. *Ann. Oncol.* **2020**, *31*, 1476–1490. [CrossRef]
5. Jasim, S.; Habra, M.A. Management of Adrenocortical Carcinoma. *Curr. Oncol. Rep.* **2019**, *21*, 273–287. [CrossRef]
6. Varghese, J.; Habra, M.A. Update on adrenocortical carcinoma management and future directions. *Curr. Opin. Endocrinol.* **2017**, *24*, 208–214. [CrossRef] [PubMed]

7. Giordano, T.J.; Kuick, R.; Else, T.; Gauger, P.G.; Vinco, M.; Bauersfeld, J.; Sanders, D.; Thomas, D.G.; Doherty, G.; Hammer, G. Molecular Classification and Prognostication of Adrenocortical Tumors by Transcriptome Profiling. *Clin. Cancer Res.* **2009**, *15*, 668–676. [CrossRef]
8. Fassnacht, M.; Berruti, A.; Baudin, E.; Demeure, M.J.; Gilbert, J.; Haak, H.; Kroiss, M.; Quinn, D.I.; Hesseltine, E.; Ronchi, C.L.; et al. Linsitinib (OSI-906) versus placebo for patients with locally advanced or metastatic adrenocortical carcinoma: A double-blind, randomised, phase 3 study. *Lancet Oncol.* **2015**, *16*, 426–435. [CrossRef]
9. Wortmann, S.; Quinkler, M.; Ritter, C.; Kroiss, M.; Johanssen, S.; Hahner, S.; Allolio, B.; Fassnacht, M. Bevacizumab plus capecitabine as a salvage therapy in advanced adrenocortical carcinoma. *Eur. J. Endocrinol.* **2010**, *162*, 349–356. [CrossRef]
10. Altieri, B.; Ronchi, C.L.; Kroiss, M.; Fassnacht, M. Next-generation therapies for adrenocortical carcinoma. *Best Pract. Res. Clin. Endocrinol. Metab.* **2020**, *34*, 101434. [CrossRef] [PubMed]
11. Creemers, S.G.; Hofland, L.J.; Korpershoek, E.; Franssen, G.J.H.; van Kemenade, F.J.; de Herder, W.W.; Feelders, R.A. Future directions in the diagnosis and medical treatment of adrenocortical carcinoma. *Endocr.-Relat. Cancer* **2016**, *23*, R43–R69. [CrossRef]
12. Assie, G.; Letouze, E.; Fassnacht, M.; Jouinot, A.; Luscap, W.; Barreau, O.; Omeiri, H.; Rodriguez, S.; Perlemoine, K.; Rene-Corail, F.; et al. Integrated genomic characterization of adrenocortical carcinoma. *Nat. Genet.* **2014**, *46*, 607–612. [CrossRef] [PubMed]
13. Assie, G.; Jouinot, A.; Fassnacht, M.; Libe, R.; Garinet, S.; Jacob, L.; Hamzaoui, N.; Neou, M.; Sakat, J.; de La Villeon, B.; et al. Value of Molecular Classification for Prognostic Assessment of Adrenocortical Carcinoma. *JAMA Oncol.* **2019**, *5*, 1440–1447. [CrossRef]
14. Juhlin, C.C.; Goh, G.; Healy, J.M.; Fonseca, A.L.; Scholl, U.I.; Stenman, A.; Kunstman, J.W.; Brown, T.C.; Overton, J.D.; Mane, S.M.; et al. Whole-Exome Sequencing Characterizes the Landscape of Somatic Mutations and Copy Number Alterations in Adrenocortical Carcinoma. *J. Clin. Endocr. Metab.* **2015**, *100*, E493–E502. [CrossRef] [PubMed]
15. Zheng, S.Y.; Cherniack, A.D.; Dewal, N.; Moffitt, R.A.; Danilova, L.; Murray, B.A.; Lerario, A.M.; Else, T.; Knijnenburg, T.A.; Ciriello, G.; et al. Comprehensive Pan-Genomic Characterization of Adrenocortical Carcinoma. *Cancer Cell* **2016**, *29*, 723–736. [CrossRef]
16. Ronchi, C.L.; Sbiera, S.; Leich, E.; Henzel, K.; Rosenwald, A.; Allolio, B.; Fassnacht, M. Single Nucleotide Polymorphism Array Profiling of Adrenocortical Tumors—Evidence for an Adenoma Carcinoma Sequence? *PLoS ONE* **2013**, *8*, e73959. [CrossRef] [PubMed]
17. Hao, H.X.; Xie, Y.; Zhang, Y.; Charlat, O.; Oster, E.; Avello, M.; Lei, H.; Mickanin, C.; Liu, D.; Ruffner, H.; et al. ZNRF3 promotes Wnt receptor turnover in an R-spondin-sensitive manner. *Nature* **2012**, *485*, 195–200. [CrossRef] [PubMed]
18. de Reynies, A.; Assie, G.; Rickman, D.S.; Tissier, F.; Groussin, L.; Rene-Corrail, F.; Dousset, B.; Bertagna, X.; Clauser, E.; Bertherat, J. Gene Expression Profiling Reveals a New Classification of Adrenocortical Tumors and Identifies Molecular Predictors of Malignancy and Survival. *J. Clin. Oncol.* **2009**, *27*, 1108–1115. [CrossRef]
19. Di Dalmazi, G.; Altieri, B.; Scholz, C.; Sbiera, S.; Luconi, M.; Waldman, J.; Kastelan, D.; Ceccato, F.; Chiodini, I.; Arnaldi, G.; et al. RNA Sequencing and Somatic Mutation Status of Adrenocortical Tumors: Novel Pathogenetic Insights. *J. Clin. Endocrinol. Metab.* **2020**, *105*, e4459–e4473. [CrossRef]
20. Murakami, M.; Yoshimoto, T.; Nakabayashi, K.; Tsuchiya, K.; Minami, I.; Bouchi, R.; Izumiyama, H.; Fujii, Y.; Abe, K.; Tayama, C.; et al. Integration of transcriptome and methylome analysis of aldosterone-producing adenomas. *Eur. J. Endocrinol.* **2015**, *173*, 185–195. [CrossRef]
21. Reback, J.; McKinney, W.; Augspurger, T.; Cloud, P.; Roeschke, M.; Hawkins, S.; Tratner, J.; She, C.; Ayd, W.; Petersen, T.; et al. pandas-dev/pandas: Pandas 1.0.3. 2020. Available online: Available online: https://doi.org/10.5281/ZENODO.3715232 (accessed on 6 September 2021).
22. McKinney, W. Data structures for statistical computing in python. In Proceedings of the 9th Python in Science Conference, Austin, TX, USA, 28 June–8 July 2010; Volume 56, pp. 51–56. [CrossRef]
23. Marquardt, A.; Solimando, A.G.; Kerscher, A.; Bittrich, M.; Kalogirou, C.; Kubler, H.; Rosenwald, A.; Bargou, R.; Kollmannsberger, P.; Schilling, B.; et al. Subgroup-Independent Mapping of Renal Cell Carcinoma-Machine Learning Reveals Prognostic Mitochondrial Gene Signature Beyond Histopathologic Boundaries. *Front. Oncol.* **2021**, *11*, 621278. [CrossRef] [PubMed]
24. Cerami, E.; Gao, J.; Dogrusoz, U.; Gross, B.E.; Sumer, S.O.; Aksoy, B.A.; Jacobsen, A.; Byrne, C.J.; Heuer, M.L.; Larsson, E.; et al. The cBio cancer genomics portal: An open platform for exploring multidimensional cancer genomics data. *Cancer Discov.* **2012**, *2*, 401–404. [CrossRef]
25. Gao, J.; Aksoy, B.A.; Dogrusoz, U.; Dresdner, G.; Gross, B.; Sumer, S.O.; Sun, Y.; Jacobsen, A.; Sinha, R.; Larsson, E.; et al. Integrative analysis of complex cancer genomics and clinical profiles using the cBioPortal. *Sci. Signal.* **2013**, *6*, 11. [CrossRef]
26. Davidson-Pilon, C.; Kalderstam, J.; Zivich, P.; Kuhn, B.; Williamson, M.; Fiore-Gartland, A.; Moneda, L.; WIlson, D.; Parij, A.; Stark, K.; et al. CamDavidsonPilon/lifelines: v0.21.3. 2019. Available online: Available online: http://doi.org/10.5281/zenodo.3240536 (accessed on 6 September 2021).
27. Szklarczyk, D.; Gable, A.L.; Lyon, D.; Junge, A.; Wyder, S.; Huerta-Cepas, J.; Simonovic, M.; Doncheva, N.T.; Morris, J.H.; Bork, P.; et al. STRING v11: Protein-protein association networks with increased coverage, supporting functional discovery in genome-wide experimental datasets. *Nucleic. Acids. Res.* **2019**, *47*, D607–D613. [CrossRef]
28. Fenske, W.; Volker, H.U.; Adam, P.; Hahner, S.; Johanssen, S.; Wortmann, S.; Schmidt, M.; Morcos, M.; Muller-Hermelink, H.K.; Allolio, B.; et al. Glucose transporter GLUT1 expression is an stage-independent predictor of clinical outcome in adrenocortical carcinoma. *Endocr. Relat. Cancer* **2009**, *16*, 919–928. [CrossRef]

29. Weigand, I.; Altieri, B.; Lacombe, A.M.F.; Basile, V.; Kircher, S.; Landwehr, L.S.; Schreiner, J.; Zerbini, M.C.N.; Ronchi, C.L.; Megerle, F.; et al. Expression of SOAT1 in Adrenocortical Carcinoma and Response to Mitotane Monotherapy: An ENSAT Multicenter Study. *J. Clin. Endocrinol. Metab.* **2020**, *105*, 2642–2653. [CrossRef] [PubMed]
30. Sbiera, S.; Leich, E.; Liebisch, G.; Sbiera, I.; Schirbel, A.; Wiemer, L.; Matysik, S.; Eckhardt, C.; Gardill, F.; Gehl, A.; et al. Mitotane Inhibits Sterol-O-Acyl Transferase 1 Triggering Lipid-Mediated Endoplasmic Reticulum Stress and Apoptosis in Adrenocortical Carcinoma Cells. *Endocrinology* **2015**, *156*, 3895–3908. [CrossRef] [PubMed]
31. Pennanen, M.; Hagstrom, J.; Heiskanen, I.; Sane, T.; Mustonen, H.; Arola, J.; Haglund, C. C-myc expression in adrenocortical tumours. *J. Clin. Pathol.* **2018**, *71*, 129–134. [CrossRef]
32. Parviainen, H.; Schrade, A.; Kiiveri, S.; Prunskaite-Hyyrylainen, R.; Haglund, C.; Vainio, S.; Wilson, D.B.; Arola, J.; Heikinheimo, M. Expression of Wnt and TGF-beta pathway components and key adrenal transcription factors in adrenocortical tumors: Association to carcinoma aggressiveness. *Pathol. Res. Pract.* **2013**, *209*, 503–509. [CrossRef] [PubMed]
33. Subramanian, C.; Cohen, M.S. Over expression of DNA damage and cell cycle dependent proteins are associated with poor survival in patients with adrenocortical carcinoma. *Surgery* **2019**, *165*, 202–210. [CrossRef] [PubMed]
34. He, H.; Dai, J.; Yang, X.; Wang, X.; Sun, F.; Zhu, Y. Silencing of MED27 inhibits adrenal cortical carcinogenesis by targeting the Wnt/beta-catenin signaling pathway and the epithelial-mesenchymal transition process. *Biol. Chem.* **2018**, *399*, 593–602. [CrossRef] [PubMed]
35. Poli, G.; Ruggiero, C.; Cantini, G.; Canu, L.; Baroni, G.; Armignacco, R.; Jouinot, A.; Santi, R.; Ercolino, T.; Ragazzon, B.; et al. Fascin-1 Is a Novel Prognostic Biomarker Associated With Tumor Invasiveness in Adrenocortical Carcinoma. *J. Clin. Endocrinol. Metab.* **2019**, *104*, 1712–1724. [CrossRef]
36. Bastin, G.; Dissanayake, K.; Langburt, D.; Tam, A.L.C.; Lee, S.H.; Lachhar, K.; Heximer, S.P. RGS4 controls Galphai3-mediated regulation of Bcl-2 phosphorylation on TGN38-containing intracellular membranes. *J. Cell Sci.* **2020**, *133*, jcs241034. [CrossRef] [PubMed]
37. Szabo, P.M.; Racz, K.; Igaz, P. Underexpression of C-myc in adrenocortical cancer: A major pathogenic event? *Horm. Metab. Res.* **2011**, *43*, 297–299. [CrossRef]
38. van Wijnen, A.J.; Bagheri, L.; Badreldin, A.A.; Larson, A.N.; Dudakovic, A.; Thaler, R.; Paradise, C.R.; Wu, Z. Biological functions of chromobox (CBX) proteins in stem cell self-renewal, lineage-commitment, cancer and development. *Bone* **2021**, *143*, 115659. [CrossRef] [PubMed]

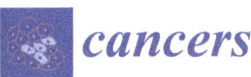

Article

Tissue miRNA Combinations for the Differential Diagnosis of Adrenocortical Carcinoma and Adenoma Established by Artificial Intelligence

Péter István Turai [1,2,3], Zoltán Herold [4], Gábor Nyirő [1,3,5], Katalin Borka [6], Tamás Micsik [7], Judit Tőke [1,2], Nikolette Szücs [1,2], Miklós Tóth [1,2], Attila Patócs [5,8,9] and Peter Igaz [1,2,3,*]

1. Department of Endocrinology, ENS@T Research Center of Excellence, Faculty of Medicine, Semmelweis University, H-1083 Budapest, Hungary; turai.peter_istvan@semmelweis-univ.hu (P.I.T.); nyiro.gabor1@med.semmelweis-univ.hu (G.N.); toke.judit@med.semmelweis-univ.hu (J.T.); szucs.nikolette@med.semmelweis-univ.hu (N.S.); toth.miklos@med.semmelweis-univ.hu (M.T.)
2. Department of Internal Medicine and Oncology, Faculty of Medicine, Semmelweis University, H-1083 Budapest, Hungary
3. MTA-SE Molecular Medicine Research Group, Eötvös Loránd Research Network, H-1083 Budapest, Hungary
4. Division of Oncology, Department of Internal Medicine and Oncology, Faculty of Medicine, Semmelweis University, H-1083 Budapest, Hungary; herold.zoltan@med.semmelweis-univ.hu
5. Department of Laboratory Medicine, Faculty of Medicine, Semmelweis University, H-1089 Budapest, Hungary; patocs.attila@med.semmelweis-univ.hu
6. 2nd Department of Pathology, Semmelweis University, H-1091 Budapest, Hungary; borka.katalin@med.semmelweis-univ.hu
7. 1st Department of Pathology and Experimental Cancer Research, Semmelweis University, H-1088 Budapest, Hungary; micsik.tamas@med.semmelweis-univ.hu
8. MTA-SE Hereditary Tumors Research Group, Eötvös Loránd Research Network, H-1122 Budapest, Hungary
9. Department of Molecular Genetics, National Institute of Oncology, H-1122 Budapest, Hungary
* Correspondence: igaz.peter@med.semmelweis-univ.hu; Tel.: +36-1-266-0816

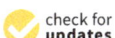

Citation: Turai, P.I.; Herold, Z.; Nyirő, G.; Borka, K.; Micsik, T.; Tőke, J.; Szücs, N.; Tóth, M.; Patócs, A.; Igaz, P. Tissue miRNA Combinations for the Differential Diagnosis of Adrenocortical Carcinoma and Adenoma Established by Artificial Intelligence. *Cancers* **2022**, *14*, 895. https://doi.org/10.3390/cancers14040895

Academic Editor: Guido Alberto Massimo Tiberio

Received: 11 January 2022
Accepted: 7 February 2022
Published: 11 February 2022

Publisher's Note: MDPI stays neutral with regard to jurisdictional claims in published maps and institutional affiliations.

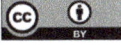

Copyright: © 2022 by the authors. Licensee MDPI, Basel, Switzerland. This article is an open access article distributed under the terms and conditions of the Creative Commons Attribution (CC BY) license (https://creativecommons.org/licenses/by/4.0/).

Simple Summary: The histological differential diagnosis of adrenocortical adenoma and carcinoma is difficult and requires great expertise. MiRNAs were shown to be useful for the differential diagnosis of benign and malignant tumors of several organs, and several findings have suggested their utility in adrenocortical tumors as well. Here, we have selected tissue miRNAs based on the literature search, and used machine learning to identify novel clinically applicable miRNA combinations. Combinations with high sensitivity and specificity (both over 90%) have been identified that could be promising for clinical use. Besides being a useful adjunct to histological examination, these miRNA combinations could enable preoperative adrenal biopsy in patients with adrenal tumors suspicious for malignancy.

Abstract: The histological analysis of adrenal tumors is difficult and requires great expertise. Tissue microRNA (miRNA) expression is distinct between benign and malignant tumors of several organs and can be useful for diagnostic purposes. MiRNAs are stable and their expression can be reliably reproduced from archived formalin-fixed, paraffin-embedded (FFPE) tissue blocks. Our purpose was to assess the potential applicability of combinations of literature-based miRNAs as markers of adrenocortical malignancy. Archived FFPE tissue samples from 10 adrenocortical carcinoma (ACC), 10 adrenocortical adenoma (ACA) and 10 normal adrenal cortex samples were analyzed in a discovery cohort, while 21 ACC and 22 ACA patients were studied in a blind manner in the validation cohort. The expression of miRNA was determined by RT-qPCR. Machine learning and neural network-based methods were used to find the best performing miRNA combination models. To evaluate diagnostic applicability, ROC-analysis was performed. We have identified three miRNA combinations (hsa-miR-195 + hsa-miR-210 + hsa-miR-503; hsa-miR-210 + hsa-miR-375 + hsa-miR-503 and hsa-miR-210 + hsa-miR-483-5p + hsa-miR-503) as unexpectedly good predictors to determine adrenocortical malignancy with sensitivity and specificity both of over 90%. These miRNA panels can supplement the histological examination of removed tumors and could even be performed from small volume adrenal biopsy samples preoperatively.

Keywords: adrenocortical carcinoma; adenoma; adrenal; tissue; microRNA; biomarker; artificial intelligence; neural network

---

1. Introduction

Adrenal tumors are relatively frequent with a prevalence of 4.2% in high-resolution abdominal imaging studies [1]. Among adrenocortical tumors, adrenocortical carcinoma (ACC) has a poor prognosis, as less than a third of the patients survive at least 5 years [2–4]. Although ACC is the rarest among adrenal tumors, with an annual incidence of 0.7–2/million, it is included in the differential diagnosis of any incidentally discovered adrenal mass [3]. Adrenocortical adenoma (ACA) is the most frequent diagnosis (49–69% in surgical series) among adrenal tumors [5]. In addition to tumors of the adrenal cortex, myelolipoma, which is invariably benign and contains fat and bone marrow elements, and pheochromocytoma, of an adrenal medullary origin causing severe blood pressure fluctuations, may also occur [5]. Adrenal glands often harbor metastasis from distinct malignancies; moreover, adrenocortical hyperplasia, adrenal cyst, adrenal hemorrhage, and, very rarely, adrenal lymphoma and adrenal tuberculosis should also be kept in mind as potential adrenal pathologies [6]. The differentiation of adrenocortical adenoma and carcinoma is often challenging.

Medical imaging is especially helpful in establishing the diagnosis of adrenocortical malignancy. Tumor size, density, heterogeneity, irregular borders and necrosis are assessed on CT (computed tomography), and there are also options for further imaging, e.g., washout CT, MRI (magnetic resonance imaging) or ^{18}FDG-PET-CT (^{18}fluorodeoxyglucose-positron emission tomography-CT) [5]. Still there is no preoperative blood-borne molecular marker of malignancy. Urinary steroid metabolomics can be helpful [7], but it is not widely available.

The histological examination of adrenal tumors (including the Weiss-score and modified Weiss-score) is difficult and requires great expertise. Moreover, significant interobserver variability and a lack of accuracy in borderline cases are known limitations [8]. Mainly due to the difficulty of histological examinations, a biopsy of adrenal tumors is not recommended in routine practice and according to the current guidelines [3,5], as it would be difficult to determine malignancy from a small amount of tissue obtained, and there is a potential risk of complications (bleeding, pneumothorax) and maybe tumor dissemination as well [9,10]. The risk of complications linked to adrenal biopsy is not very high (2.5%), but it has only a sensitivity of 70% for diagnosing ACC [11,12].

For all these reasons there is a great need for additional markers that can help determine the biological behavior of adrenocortical tumors.

MicroRNAs (miRNA, miR) have long been one of the cornerstones of biomarker research [13]. MiRNAs are 19–25 nucleotide long evolutionary conserved single stranded non-coding RNA molecules, most often encoded by their own genes. MiRNAs are the epigenetic regulators of RNA interference as they regulate up to 30–60% of human genes at the post-transcriptional level—without altering the very sequence of DNA [14].

miRNAs exert their inhibitory functions on translation via binding to the 3′ untranslated region (UTR) of their target mRNA in the cytoplasm [15]. Besides, it was shown that miRNAs might act within the cell nucleus by the modification of histone proteins and transcription itself [16]. Biological functions of miRNAs have been characterized from abundant sources [17–19]. In tumors, both overexpressed (oncogenic) and underexpressed (tumor suppressor), miRNAs are known for acting in a tissue specific fashion [20–22]. From a biomarker research point of view the two most important features of miRNAs are their exceptional stability and reproducibility from fresh frozen tissue, FFPE (formalin-fixed, paraffin-embedded) samples or even from biofluids (e.g., from blood), and their marked tissue/cell and disease specificity [23,24]. Currently, there are about 2500 known human miRNAs and only a minor part of them has been described in the pathogenesis of adrenocortical tumors [25–29].

The long-lasting quest for a legit biomarker of adrenocortical carcinoma set our research group to design novel miRNA combination panels as markers of malignancy. Based on the current literature and bolstered by the state-of-art biostatistics tools, such as artificial intelligence (AI) implemented through machine learning and neural networks, our aim was to establish miRNA models with high sensitivity and specificity applicable for clinical use.

2. Materials and Methods

2.1. Tissue Collection and Ethics Approval

A total of 31 ACC, 32 ACA (Table 1) and 10 normal adrenal cortex (NAC) FFPE samples were recruited in the study. NAC samples were included only to investigate whether there are differences in the expression of the selected microRNAs between normal, benign, and malignant adrenocortical tissues. All samples were histologically confirmed by adrenal expert pathologists. Only specific parts of the blocks were dissected for RNA isolation. NAC samples were obtained from patients undergoing total nephrectomy for kidney tumors (females: 5, males: 5, mean age: 36.2 and 55.8, respectively). The discovery cohort was comprised of 10 ACA, 10 ACC, 10 NAC and the independent validation cohort contained another 21 ACC and 22 ACA FFPE samples (Table S1).

Table 1. Clinical and main pathological characteristics of the tumor samples included. F: female, M: male, NF: non-functioning, DHEAS: dehydroepiandrosterone sulfate, DOC: 11-Deoxycorticosterone, ND: no data.

Cohort/Samples	Sex	Mean Age at Sample Taking (Years)	Mean Tumor Size (mm)	Ki-67 (%)	ENSAT Stage	Hormonal Activity
Discovery ACA	10 F	47.5	33.9	-	-	7 cortisol 3 NF
Discovery ACC	6 F 4 M	45.2	96.2	10–15 (1–40)	5 II 5 III	3 cortisol 5 NF 1 DOC 1 DOC + cortisol + estradiol
Validation ACA	17 F 5 M	53.9	35	-	-	11 cortisol 10 NF 1 DHEAS
Validation ACC	14 F 7 M	55.4	102	25–30 (8–50)	1 I 4 II 5 III 11 IV	7 cortisol 11 NF 2 cortisol + DHEAS 1 cortisol + androgen

The study was approved by the Ethical Committee of the Hungarian Health Council. All experiments were performed in accordance with applicable guidelines and regulations and informed consent was obtained from the involved patients.

2.2. Literature Search

Literature search was performed in the PubMed database (https://pubmed.ncbi.nlm.nih.gov/) using the following search terms: adrenocortical carcinoma; adrenocortical cancer; adrenal cancer; adrenal tumor; and microRNA. Only original articles were selected. Most microRNAs included have been described as differentially expressed by multiple studies. We have selected 16 differentially expressed miRNAs to be included in our study (Table 2).

Table 2. List of selected, differentially expressed miRNAs based on literature search that were included in our study.

miRNAs	Expression in ACC	References
hsa-miR-7	Down-regulated	[30,31]
hsa-miR-9	Up-regulated	[32,33]
hsa-miR-21	Up-regulated	[34,35]
hsa-miR-195	Down-regulated	[30,34,36–39]
hsa-miR-205	Down-regulated	[40,41]
hsa-miR-210	Up-regulated	[34,39,42,43]
hsa-miR-214	Down-regulated	[38,42,44]
hsa-miR-335	Down-regulated	[36,38,45]
hsa-miR-375	Down-regulated	[42]
hsa-miR-431	Down-regulated	[44,46]
hsa-miR-483-3p	Up-regulated	[34,38,47,48]
hsa-miR-483-5p	Up-regulated	[30,34,36,38,39,49–51]
hsa-miR-497	Down-regulated	[34,38]
hsa-miR-503	Up-regulated	[38,42]
hsa-miR-508	Up-regulated	[36,44,52]
hsa-miR-511	Down-regulated	[42,44,53]

This list includes miRNAs that are extensively described in the literature to be important in adrenocortical tumor pathogenesis or differential diagnosis (such as *hsa-miR-195* or *hsa-miR-483-5p, or hsa-miR-503*) [30,34,36–39,42,49–51], and also miRNAs where there is only limited evidence of pathogenic relevance. By including more miRNAs to be tested by artificial intelligence, we aimed to increase the chance of finding well-performing miRNA combinations.

2.3. Sample Processing and RNA Isolation

Total RNA was isolated by RecoverAll Total Nucleic Acid Isolation Kit for FFPE (catalog number: AM1975, Thermo Fisher Scientific, Waltham, MA, USA). As a spike-in control for isolation efficiency we used 1 µL of 0.002 fmol/µL *syn-cel-miR-39-3p* according to the manufacturer's protocol for miRCURY LNA RNA Spike-in kit (Qiagen GmbH, Hilden, Germany, catalog number: 339390) and was added before the nucleic acid isolation step. Total RNA quantity was measured by NanoDrop 2000 Spectrophotometer (Thermo Fisher Scientific, Waltham, MA, USA) after isolation and Qubit 4 Fluorometer with Qubit™ hsRNA Assay Kit (Thermo Fisher Scientific, Waltham, MA, USA) before reverse transcription. Total RNA was stored at $-80\,°C$ until further processing.

2.4. Analysis of the miRNA Panel Expression by Real-Time RT-qPCR

A 2-step process for RT-qPCR was used. Each sample was processed separately for all miRNA targets. Ten nanograms of isolated total RNA was used in individual RT reactions.

First, TaqMan miRNA Reverse Transcription Kit (catalog number: 4366596, Thermo Fisher Scientific, Waltham, MA, USA) and individual TaqMan MiRNA Assay primer mixes (catalog number: 4427975, Thermo Fisher Scientific, Waltham, MA, USA) were used to reverse-transcribe total RNA. The expression of *hsa-miR-7* (ID: 000386), *hsa-miR-9* (ID: 000583), *hsa-miR-21* (ID: 000397), *hsa-miR-195* (ID: 000494), *hsa-miR-205* (ID: 000509), *hsa-miR-210* (ID: 000512), *hsa-miR-214* (ID: 002306), *hsa-miR-335* (ID: 000546), *hsa-miR-375* (ID: 000564), *hsa-miR-431* (ID: 001979), *hsa-miR-483-3p* (ID: 002339), *hsa-miR-483-5p* (ID: 002338), *hsa-miR-497* (ID: 001043), *hsa-miR-503* (ID: 001048), *hsa-miR-508* (ID: 001052), and *hsa-miR-511* (ID: 001111) were measured, and as an internal control *RNU48* (ID: 001006) along with *cel-miR-39* (ID: 000200) as an external control were used.

For quantification, TaqMan Fast Advanced Master Mix (catalog number: 4444963, Thermo Fisher Scientific, Waltham, MA, USA), with the matching probe mixes on a Quantstudio 7 Flex Real-Time PCR System (Thermo Fisher Scientific, Waltham, MA, USA) according to the manufacturer's protocol, was used. Negative control reactions contained no cDNA templates, and all samples were measured in triplicate. We used 0,67 μL of undiluted cDNA as template.

After analysis of the miRNA panel expression by real-time RT-qPCR on the discovery cohort, we proceeded to validate our best performing combinations by carrying out another set of real-time RT-qPCR measurements on an independent validation cohort, but with a further refined group of miRNAs: *hsa-miR-9* (ID: 000583), *hsa-miR-195* (ID: 000494), *hsa-miR-210* (ID: 000512), *hsa-miR-375* (ID: 000564), *hsa-miR-483-3p* (ID: 002339), *hsa-miR-483-5p* (ID: 002338), *hsa-miR-497* (ID: 001043), *hsa-miR-503* (ID: 001048), and *hsa-miR-508* (ID: 001052).

2.5. Statistical Analysis

Statistical analysis was carried out with R for Windows version 4.1.1 (R Foundation for Statistical Computing, 2021, Vienna, Austria). Normalization of miRNAs was performed with the ΔCt method, in which geometric means of intrinsic "housekeeping gene" (*RNU48*) and extrinsic spike-in (*cel-miR-39*) served as controls (R package NormqPCR). Down-regulated miRNAs, when presented with no measurable Ct values, were omitted. The order of miRNAs that played prominent role in the group classification of the samples was determined by the random forest method, using the importance measure 'mean decrease in accuracy' (R package randomForest), which was used to strengthen relationships already known from the literature [54]. The possibility of automatic classification of samples into ACA or ACC groups was tested by machine learning methods (R packages nnet and caret) [55,56]. The classification efficiency of possible miRNA combinations was examined by neural network-based, 90–10% random learner-tester cross validation consisting of 10-10-10 known ACC, ACA, and NAC samples. A hidden-layer neural network-based statistical model was created that randomly selected 9-9-9 samples per group from 10-10-10 histological specimens (learner data set). Classification efficacy of the model was tested on the remaining 1-1-1 samples (tester data set). By repeating this step 1000 times, we were able to determine the miRNA combinations, which had high specificity and sensitivity for group classification. The analysis was also performed both on all 30 samples from all three groups and on the 20 samples from benign and malignant adrenal tumors alone as well. Twenty-four models with at least 90% classification capability were selected for validation of subsequent machine learning-based classification (Table 3).

During validation, the same ACA and ACC samples were used as previously, and the 43 unknown samples were classified individually, with 10,000 iterations each. The final estimated group classification of the sample was determined by selecting the most common value (>50%) from the 10,000 estimates.

Sensitivity and specificity for each model were determined—after revealing the benign or malignant histological diagnosis of each sample—by comparing the estimated and the actual groupings from the models. At this point, as a technical step, the ACA group was designated as the "control" group and the ACC group as the "patient" group. Based on the differences between the two classifications, we determined the number of correct results (true positives and negatives), false positive (benign tumor instead of malignant tumor) and false negative (malignant tumor instead of benign tumor) results.

The percentage of correct classifications in the ACA group and the correct classification were compared and plotted by ROC analysis (R package pROC) [57]. Additional epidemiological measures (e.g., area under curve) were determined using the true group classifications and the percentages of the estimated classification in the ROC analysis.

Table 3. The 24 miRNA combination models used in the validation cohort.

Model Number	miRNA Combination
1	hsa-miR-9 + hsa-miR-375
2	hsa-miR-9 + hsa-miR-503
3	hsa-miR-375 + hsa-miR-503
4	hsa-miR-210 + hsa-miR-503
5	hsa-miR-375 + hsa-miR-497
6	hsa-miR-483-3p + hsa-miR-503
7	hsa-miR-503 + hsa-miR-508
8	hsa-miR-195 + hsa-miR-503 + hsa-miR-508
9	hsa-miR-195 + hsa-miR-210 + hsa-miR-503
10	hsa-miR-9 + hsa-miR-195 + hsa-miR-503
11	hsa-miR-9 + hsa-miR-210 + hsa-miR-503
12	hsa-miR-9 + hsa-miR-375 + hsa-miR-503
13	hsa-miR-9 + hsa-miR-483-3p + hsa-miR-503
14	hsa-miR-9 + hsa-miR-497 + hsa-miR-503
15	hsa-miR-195 + hsa-miR-375 + hsa-miR-497
16	hsa-miR-210 + hsa-miR-375 + hsa-miR-503
17	hsa-miR-210 + hsa-miR-483-5p + hsa-miR-503
18	hsa-miR-375 + hsa-miR-503 + hsa-miR-508
19	hsa-miR-375 + hsa-miR-483-3p + hsa-miR-503
20	hsa-miR-9 + hsa-miR-195 + hsa-miR-375 + hsa-miR-503
21	hsa-miR-9 + hsa-miR-210 + hsa-miR-483-5p + hsa-miR-503
22	hsa-miR-210 + hsa-miR-375 + hsa-miR-503 + hsa-miR-508
23	hsa-miR-375 + hsa-miR-483-5p + hsa-miR-503 + hsa-miR-508
24	hsa-miR-375 + hsa-miR-497 + hsa-miR-503 + hsa-miR-508

3. Results

3.1. miRNA Expression in the Discovery Cohort by RT-qPCR

RT-qPCR was performed on 10-10-10 known ACA, ACC, NAC FFPE tissue samples in the discovery cohort. The list of selected miRNAs is presented in Table 2. Random forest results revealed that hsa-miR-503, hsa-miR-483_3p, hsa-miR-195, hsa-miR-375 and hsa-miR-483_5p were the top 5 miRNAs to properly group the 30 samples into their respective groups. (Figure 1 presents box plots representing the expression of these five miRNA in ACA and ACC.) The best performing miRNA combinations (statistical models) were selected by neural network-based, 90–10% random learner-tester cross validation. Twenty-four statistical models (Table 3) with at least 90% grouping capability were selected for validation. These 24 models contain the following miRNAs: hsa-*miR-9, hsa-miR-195, hsa-miR-210, hsa-miR-375, hsa-miR-483-3p, hsa-miR-483-5p, hsa-miR-497, hsa-miR-503,* and *hsa-miR-508*.

3.2. Diagnostic Performance of the miRNA Models by RT-qPCR

In total, 43 independent FFPE samples (22 ACA and 21 ACC) were measured in the validation cohort by RT-qPCR to establish the utility of selected miRNA combinations as markers of malignancy. Table 4 presents the sensitivity, specificity, area under curve, positive and negative predictive values of the 24 models. Among these, 3 models yielded sensitivity and specificity both over 90%: model 9 (*hsa-miR-195 + hsa-miR-210 + hsa-miR-503*), model 16 (*hsa-miR-210 + hsa-miR-375 + hsa-miR-503*) and model 17 (*hsa-miR-210 + hsa-miR-483-5p + hsa-miR-503*) (Figure 2). False negative (V14, V19) and false positive (V33) samples are marked in Table S1. These samples were commonly missed by the three best performing models, whereas Sample V38 has been recognized by Model 17, and not by the two other models. We could not find common or peculiar features in the falsely classified samples. The values for individual miRNAs are presented in Table 5. These combination-based predictions are clearly superior to the diagnostic performance of individual miRNAs.

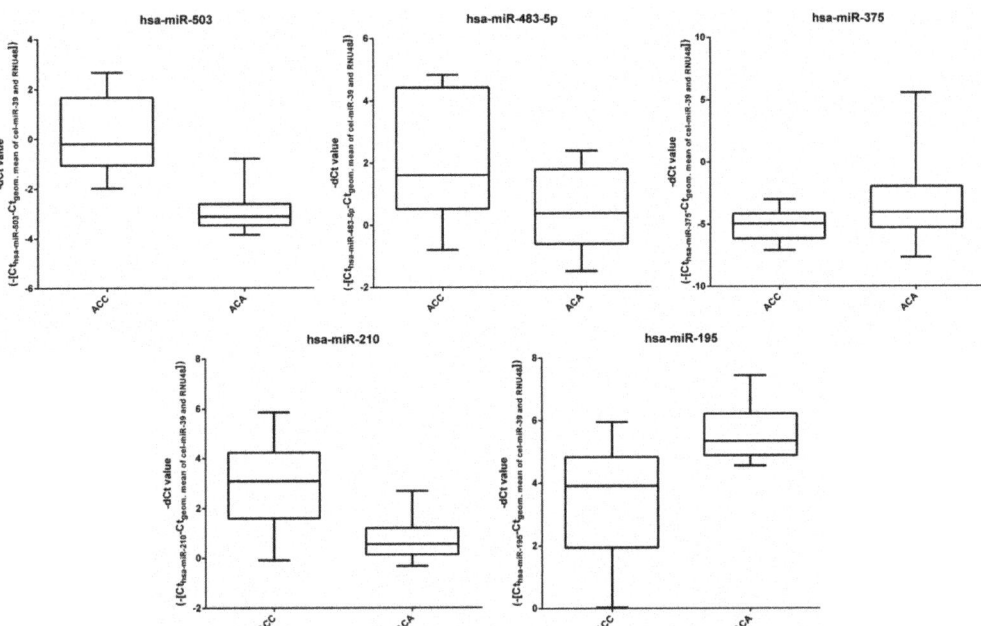

Figure 1. Box plots representing the expression of the top five miRNAs relative to the geometric means of cel-miR-39 and RNU48 in ACA and ACC samples. The top 5 selected miRNAs contributing to the best performing three models were determined based on artificial intelligence.

Table 4. Diagnostic performance of the 24 miRNA combination models. The best performing three models are highlighted in bold.

Model Number	Sensitivity	Specificity	Area under Curve (AUC)	Negative Predictive Value	Positive Predictive Value
1	72.73%	42.86%	56.49%	57.14%	60.00%
2	72.73%	85.71%	81.17%	84.21%	75.00%
3	90.91%	85.71%	90.04%	86.96%	90.00%
4	86.36%	90.48%	88.42%	90.48%	86.36%
5	86.36%	66.67%	76.52%	73.08%	82.35%
6	72.73%	95.24%	86.15%	94.12%	76.92%
7	81.82%	90.48%	85.93%	90.00%	82.61%
8	86.36%	85.71%	87.34%	86.36%	85.71%
9	**90.91%**	**90.48%**	**90.69%**	**90.91%**	**90.48%**
10	68.18%	85.71%	78.90%	83.33%	72.00%
11	86.36%	85.71%	88.10%	86.36%	85.71%
12	86.36%	80.95%	83.66%	82.61%	85.00%
13	68.18%	90.48%	82.47%	88.24%	73.08%
14	77.27%	85.71%	80.84%	85.00%	78.26%
15	86.36%	66.67%	76.52%	73.08%	82.35%
16	**90.91%**	**90.48%**	**90.69%**	**90.91%**	**90.48%**
17	**90.91%**	**95.24%**	**92.86%**	**95.24%**	**90.91%**
18	90.91%	85.71%	90.04%	86.96%	90.00%
19	77.27%	90.48%	85.61%	89.47%	79.17%
20	86.36%	80.95%	85.50%	82.61%	85.00%
21	86.36%	80.95%	85.71%	82.61%	85.00%
22	90.91%	85.71%	90.04%	86.96%	90.00%
23	90.91%	85.71%	88.31%	86.96%	90.00%
24	90.91%	85.71%	89.39%	86.96%	90.00%

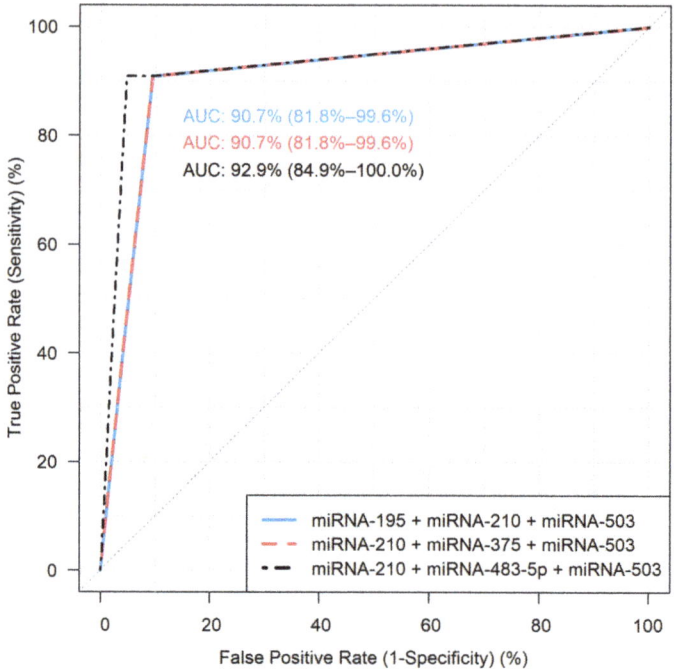

Figure 2. ROC curves of the best performing three miRNA combinations. Model 9: *hsa-miR-195 + hsa-miR-210 + hsa-miR-503* (left upper corner), model 16: *hsa-miR-210 + hsa-miR-375 + hsa-miR-503* (right upper corner), model 17: *hsa-miR-210 + hsa-miR-483-5p + hsa-miR-503* (down). AUC: area under curve.

Table 5. Individual diagnostic performance of the miRNAs included in the 24 miRNA combination models.

miRNA	Sensitivity	Specificity	Area under Curve (AUC)	Negative Predictive Value	Positive Predictive Value
hsa-miR-9	54.55%	61.90%	59.52%	60.00%	56.52%
hsa-miR-195	86.36%	71.43%	78.90%	76.00%	83.33%
hsa-miR-210	68.18%	80.95%	76.41%	78.95%	70.83%
hsa-miR-375	81.82%	23.81%	53.68%	52.94%	55.56%
hsa-miR-483-3p	54.55%	90.48%	74.57%	85.71%	65.52%
hsa-miR-483-5p	81.82%	90.48%	86.15%	90.00%	82.61%
hsa-miR-497	86.36%	80.95%	83.66%	82.61%	85.00%
hsa-miR-503	81.82%	90.48%	86.15%	90.00%	82.61%
hsa-miR-508	59.09%	52.38%	58.33%	56.52%	55.00%

4. Discussion

The histological diagnosis of adrenocortical tumors is challenging. In this study, we assessed the applicability for various miRNA combinations established by an artificial intelligence approach (machine learning and neural networks) that could reliably be utilized as markers of adrenocortical malignancy.

Sixteen miRNAs were included in our study, based on the literature search, but the established miRNA combinations include only 5 of these (*hsa-miR-195, hsa-miR-210, hsa-miR-375, hsa-miR-483-5p,* and *hsa-miR-503*). Not surprisingly, this 5-miRNA set includes the miRNAs that have been described in most adrenocortical tumor studies as differentially expressed between benign and malignant tumors.

Hsa-miR-195 was shown to be underexpressed in ACC compared to ACA in various studies [30,34,36–39]. Furthermore, the underexpression of *hsa-miR-195* was associated with poor outcome, and lower circulating levels of *hsa-miR-195* tended to be correlated with a larger tumor size [30,36,38]. On the other hand, the up-regulation of *hsa-miR-195* decreased cell proliferation in human NCI-H295R ACC cells [34]. The gene for *hsa-miR-195* is located within the genomic region of 17p13, that was shown to be frequently lost in adrenocortical tumors [58].

Hsa-miR-210 is a general hypoxamiR as it was shown to be involved in tumor hypoxia, thereby, the overexpression of *hsa-miR-210* seems to be a common event in various tumors [59]. *Hsa-miR-210* is regulated by the hypoxia-inducible factor 1α (HIF1α), an important factor in antitumoral therapy resistance [60–62]. It was shown to be overexpressed in ACC compared to ACA and NAC in multiple studies [34,39,42,43], and also significantly overexpressed in ACC with distant metastases [38]. High expression of *hsa-miR-210* was associated with poor prognosis [47].

Hsa-miR-375 was shown to be significantly underexpressed in ACC and ACA compared to NAC in our previous study [42]. It targets certain oncogenes, such as *AEG-1/MTDH, PDK1, YWHAZ/14-3-3ζ, YAP* and *JAK2*, in multiple types of carcinomas [63–67]. Reciprocal action between Wnt–β-catenin signaling and *hsa-miR-375* has been proposed [68]. The Wnt–β-catenin pathway is an important factor in the pathogenesis of ACC [69,70]. It was surprising that this miRNA has been included in the models by artificial intelligence, and even in one of the best performing combinations (Model 16).

Overexpressed *hsa-miR-483-5p* is considered to be the best marker of adrenocortical malignancy [26,31,33,35,36,41,47–49,69,70]. However, we have recently shown its limitation in the differentiation of ACC and adrenal myelolipoma [71]. *Hsa-miR-483-5p* is coexpressed with the insulin-like growth factor 2 (*IGF2*) from the same locus at 11p15.5 [37]. Overexpression of *IGF2* mRNA is a main feature of ACC [72,73]. N-myc downstream-regulated gene family members 2 and 4 (*NDRG2* and *NDRG4*) were identified as targets of *miR-483-5p*, and their expression was inversely correlated with *miR-483-5p* [74]. *Hsa-miR-483-5p* is also an interesting example of miRNA's tissue and disease specificity as it has been shown to be down-regulated in Wilms tumors and glioma cells, suggesting its tumor suppressor activity in these tumors and tissues [75,76].

Hsa-miR-503 has also been described in several adrenal tumor studies [34,36,38,42,43]. Its pathogenic role was also proposed in other malignancies [77,78]. A larger tumor size has been shown to correlate with the overexpression of *hsa-miR-503*, and also, a significant correlation with Weiss-criteria, clinical outcome and survival was revealed [34,38]. *Hsa-miR-503* has previously been described as a direct cell cycle and differentiation regulator in different cell lines [79,80].

The three best-performing miRNA combinations yielded clearly superior sensitivity and specificity values than the individual miRNAs included in the combinations (Table 4 vs. Table 5.) and also than the previous literature data for individual miRNAs (e.g., sensitivity–specificity: 68.7–93.7; 73.7–100 for *hsa-miR-195* and for *hsa-miR-483-5p*, respectively [33]). Some literature data, however, show comparable, or even better diagnostic performance data than our combinations. For example, in our previous study, the combination of *hsa-miR-511* and *hsa-miR-503* was associated with 100% sensitivity and 97% specificity [42], and in Feinmesser's study a 100% sensitivity and 96% specificity of the *hsa-miR-497* and *hsa-miR-34a* combination was noted [38]. In most previous studies, however, smaller cohorts were included, (e.g., only 7 and 17 ACC samples included in the two above mentioned studies, respectively [38,42]). Different cohort compositions, platforms and statistical methods might also be accounted for these differences.

Our study certainly has limitations. These include the limited set of miRNAs examined and the sizes of the cohorts that are larger than in most previous studies but should still be augmented to assess the clinical utility of the markers identified. Moreover, we performed our measurements on FFPE samples in a retrospective setup, hence the clinical utility of these miRNA combinations should further be examined on fresh frozen samples in a prospective manner.

Using small sample sizes in machine learning techniques can lead to biased machine learning performance estimates. To overcome this type of bias, it is recommended to use a different, new dataset for validation. In our study, both the baseline and validation cohorts consist of different patients; therefore, our results do not suffer from this type of bias.

Another type of bias can be introduced from using specific types of cross validation. It was previously reported that using nested types of cross-validation produce unbiased and robust results [81]. The 90%–10% random learner-tester cross-validation used in our study belongs to the nested cross-validation family.

The sensitivity and specificity values of the three best performing biomarker combinations appear to be promising for clinical introduction. Besides a useful adjunct to histological analysis of surgically resected tumor specimens, the possible testing of these microRNA panels on adrenal biopsy samples might also be envisaged. Adrenal biopsy is currently not recommended in the work-up of adrenal tumors, only in exceptional cases, mainly due to the difficulties of histological analysis, but there are also some possible complications [3,5,11,12]. If the diagnosis of malignancy could be reliably established by using these microRNA panels from small biopsy samples, this might even broaden the use of adrenal biopsy in preoperative diagnosis and the current recommendations might be revisited.

5. Conclusions

In this study, novel miRNA marker combinations have been established by artificial intelligence-based methods showing high sensitivity and specificity that could aid in the differential diagnosis of benign and malignant adrenocortical tissue specimens. The clinical utility of these biomarkers should be further validated in even larger sample cohorts, and their potential use on biopsy samples might also be evaluated. Prospective analysis on fresh frozen samples is also warranted. These miRNA combinations could help postoperative histological diagnosis.

6. Patents

Claims for patenting the three best performing biomarker combinations have been submitted to the Hungarian Intellectual Property Office (P2200007).

Supplementary Materials: The following supporting information can be downloaded at: https://www.mdpi.com/article/10.3390/cancers14040895/s1, Table S1: Clinical and main pathological characteristics of the tumor samples

Author Contributions: Conceptualization: P.I.; methodology: P.I.T., Z.H., G.N.; biostatistics: Z.H.; validation: P.I.T., G.N.; clinical management of patients; P.I., N.S., J.T., M.T.; pathology/histology: K.B., T.M.; writing—original draft preparation: P.I.T.; writing—review and editing: P.I.T., P.I., A.P.; supervision, P.I.; funding acquisition, P.I. All authors have read and agreed to the published version of the manuscript.

Funding: This research was funded by Hungarian National Research, Development and Innovation Office (NKFIH) grant K134215 to Dr. Peter Igaz. The study was also financed by the Higher Education Institutional Excellence Program— of the Ministry of Human Capacities in Hungary, within the framework of the molecular biology thematic program of the Semmelweis University and by the ÚNKP-21-3 New National Excellence Program of the Ministry of Human Capacities.

Institutional Review Board Statement: The study was conducted according to the guidelines of the Declaration of Helsinki and approved by the Ethical Board of the Hungarian Health Science Council (ETT-TUKEB) (24441-2/2016/EKU).

Informed Consent Statement: Informed consent was obtained from all subjects involved in the study.

Data Availability Statement: Data are contained within the article or supplementary material. The data presented in this study are available in Table S1.

Conflicts of Interest: The authors declare no conflict of interest. The funders had no role in the design of the study; in the collection, analyses, or interpretation of data; in the writing of the manuscript, or in the decision to publish the results.

References

1. Bovio, S.; Cataldi, A.; Reimondo, G.; Sperone, P.; Novello, S.; Berruti, A.; Borasio, P.; Fava, C.; Dogliotti, L.; Scagliotti, G.V.; et al. Prevalence of adrenal incidentaloma in a contemporary computerized tomography series. *J. Endocrinol. Investig.* **2006**, *29*, 298–302. [CrossRef]
2. Libé, R.; Borget, I.; Ronchi, C.L.; Zaggia, B.; Kroiss, M.; Kerkhofs, T.; Bertherat, J.; Volante, M.; Quinkler, M.; Chabre, O.; et al. Prognostic factors in stage III–IV adrenocortical carcinomas (ACC): An European Network for the Study of Adrenal Tumor (ENSAT) study. *Ann. Oncol.* **2015**, *26*, 2119–2125. [CrossRef] [PubMed]
3. Fassnacht, M.; Dekkers, O.M.; Else, T.; Baudin, E.; Berruti, A.; De Krijger, R.R.; Haak, H.R.; Mihai, R.; Assie, G.; Terzolo, M. European Society of Endocrinology Clinical Practice Guidelines on the management of adrenocortical carcinoma in adults, in collaboration with the European Network for the Study of Adrenal Tumors. *Eur. J. Endocrinol.* **2018**, *179*, G1–G46. [CrossRef] [PubMed]
4. Terzolo, M.; Daffara, F.; Ardito, A.; Zaggia, B.; Basile, V.; Ferrari, L.; Berruti, A. Management of adrenal cancer: A 2013 update. *J. Endocrinol. Investig.* **2014**, *37*, 207–217. [CrossRef] [PubMed]
5. Fassnacht, M.; Arlt, W.; Bancos, I.; Dralle, H.; Newell-Price, J.; Sahdev, A.; Tabarin, A.; Terzolo, M.; Tsagarakis, S.; Dekkers, O.M. Management of adrenal incidentalomas: European Society of Endocrinology Clinical Practice Guideline in collaboration with the European Network for the Study of Adrenal Tumors. *Eur. J. Endocrinol.* **2016**, *175*, G1–G34. [CrossRef]
6. Lattin, G.E.; Sturgill, E.D.; Tujo, C.A.; Marko, J.; Sanchez-Maldonado, K.W.; Craig, W.D.; Lack, E.E. From the radiologic pathology archives: Adrenal tumors and tumor-like conditions in the adult: Radiologic-pathologic correlation. *Radiographics* **2014**, *34*, 805–829. [CrossRef]
7. Bancos, I.; Arlt, W. Diagnosis of a malignant adrenal mass: The role of urinary steroid metabolite profiling. *Curr. Opin. Endocrinol. Diabetes Obes.* **2017**, *24*, 200–207. [CrossRef]
8. Viëtor, C.L.; Creemers, S.G.; van Kemenade, F.J.; van Ginhoven, T.M.; Hofland, L.J.; Feelders, R.A. How to Differentiate Benign from Malignant Adrenocortical Tumors? *Cancers* **2021**, *13*, 4383. [CrossRef]
9. Mazzaglia, P.J.; Monchik, J.M. Limited Value of Adrenal Biopsy in the Evaluation of Adrenal Neoplasm: A Decade of Experience. *Arch. Surg.* **2009**, *144*, 465–470. [CrossRef]
10. Williams, A.R.; Hammer, G.D.; Else, T. Transcutaneous Biopsy of Adrenocortical Carcinoma is rarely helpful in diagnosis, potentially harmful, but does not affect patient outcome. *Eur. J. Endocrinol.* **2014**, *170*, 829. [CrossRef]
11. Zhang, C.D.; Delivanis, D.A.; Eiken, P.W.; Atwell, T.D.; Bancos, I. Adrenal biopsy: Performance and use. *Minerva Endocrinol.* **2019**, *44*, 288–300. [CrossRef]
12. Bancos, I.; Tamhane, S.; Shah, M.; Delivanis, D.A.; Alahdab, F.; Arlt, W.; Fassnacht, M.; Murad, M.H. DIAGNOSIS OF ENDOCRINE DISEASE: The diagnostic performance of adrenal biopsy: A systematic review and meta-analysis. *Eur. J. Endocrinol.* **2016**, *175*, R65–R80. [CrossRef]
13. Condrat, C.E.; Thompson, D.C.; Barbu, M.G.; Bugnar, O.L.; Boboc, A.; Cretoiu, D.; Suciu, N.; Cretoiu, S.M.; Voinea, S.C. miRNAs as Biomarkers in Disease: Latest Findings Regarding Their Role in Diagnosis and Prognosis. *Cells* **2020**, *9*, 276. [CrossRef]
14. Gebert, L.F.R.; MacRae, I.J. Regulation of microRNA function in animals. *Nat. Rev. Mol. Cell Biol.* **2018**, *20*, 21–37. [CrossRef]
15. Krol, J.; Loedige, I.; Filipowicz, W. The widespread regulation of microRNA biogenesis, function and decay. *Nat. Rev. Genet.* **2010**, *11*, 597–610. [CrossRef]
16. Ritland Politz, J.C.; Hogan, E.M.; Pederson, T. MicroRNAs with a nucleolar location. *RNA* **2009**, *15*, 1705. [CrossRef]
17. O'Brien, J.; Hayder, H.; Zayed, Y.; Peng, C. Overview of microRNA biogenesis, mechanisms of actions, and circulation. *Front. Endocrinol.* **2018**, *9*, 402. [CrossRef]
18. Peng, Y.; Croce, C.M. The role of MicroRNAs in human cancer. *Signal Transduct. Target. Ther.* **2016**, *1*, 1–9. [CrossRef]
19. Hayes, J.; Peruzzi, P.P.; Lawler, S. MicroRNAs in cancer: Biomarkers, functions and therapy. *Trends Mol. Med.* **2014**, *20*, 460–469. [CrossRef]
20. Igaz, I.; Igaz, P. Tumor surveillance by circulating microRNAs: A hypothesis. *Cell. Mol. Life Sci.* **2014**, *71*, 4081–4087. [CrossRef]
21. Ma, Y.; She, X.; Ming, Y.Z.; Wan, Q. quan miR-24 promotes the proliferation and invasion of HCC cells by targeting SOX7. *Tumor Biol.* **2014**, *35*, 10731–10736. [CrossRef]
22. Yin, Y.; Zhong, J.; Li, S.W.; Li, J.Z.; Zhou, M.; Chen, Y.; Sang, Y.; Liu, L. TRIM11, a direct target of miR-24-3p, promotes cell proliferation and inhibits apoptosis in colon cancer. *Oncotarget* **2016**, *7*, 86755. [CrossRef]
23. Weber, J.A.; Baxter, D.H.; Zhang, S.; Huang, D.Y.; Huang, K.H.; Lee, M.J.; Galas, D.J.; Wang, K. The MicroRNA Spectrum in 12 Body Fluids. *Clin. Chem.* **2010**, *56*, 1733–1741. [CrossRef]

24. Hall, J.S.; Taylor, J.; Valentine, H.R.; Irlam, J.J.; Eustace, A.; Hoskin, P.J.; Miller, C.J.; West, C.M.L. Enhanced stability of microRNA expression facilitates classification of FFPE tumour samples exhibiting near total mRNA degradation. *Br. J. Cancer* **2012**, *107*, 684–694. [CrossRef]
25. Kozomara, A.; Birgaoanu, M.; Griffiths-Jones, S. miRBase: From microRNA sequences to function. *Nucleic Acids Res.* **2019**, *47*, D155. [CrossRef]
26. Igaz, P.; Igaz, I.; Nagy, Z.; Nyíro, G.; Szabó, P.M.; Falus, A.; Patócs, A.; Rácz, K. MicroRNAs in adrenal tumors: Relevance for pathogenesis, diagnosis, and therapy. *Cell. Mol. Life Sci.* **2014**, *72*, 417–428. [CrossRef]
27. Decmann, A.; Perge, P.; Turai, P.I.; Patócs, A.; Igaz, P. Non-Coding RNAs in Adrenocortical Cancer: From Pathogenesis to Diagnosis. *Cancers* **2020**, *12*, 461. [CrossRef]
28. Chehade, M.; Bullock, M.; Glover, A.; Hutvagner, G.; Sidhu, S. Key MicroRNA's and Their Targetome in Adrenocortical Cancer. *Cancers* **2020**, *12*, 2198. [CrossRef]
29. Singh, P.; Soon, P.S.H.; Feige, J.J.; Chabre, O.; Zhao, J.T.; Cherradi, N.; Lalli, E.; Sidhu, S.B. Dysregulation of microRNAs in adrenocortical tumors. *Mol. Cell. Endocrinol.* **2012**, *351*, 118–128. [CrossRef]
30. Soon, P.S.H.; Tacon, L.J.; Gill, A.J.; Bambach, C.P.; Sywak, M.S.; Campbell, P.R.; Yeh, M.W.; Wong, S.G.; Clifton-Bligh, R.J.; Robinson, B.G.; et al. miR-195 and miR-483-5p Identified as Predictors of Poor Prognosis in Adrenocortical Cancer. *Clin. Cancer Res.* **2009**, *15*, 7684–7692. [CrossRef]
31. Glover, A.R.; Zhao, J.T.; Gill, A.J.; Weiss, J.; Mugridge, N.; Kim, E.; Feeney, A.L.; Ip, J.C.; Reid, G.; Clarke, S.; et al. microRNA-7 as a tumor suppressor and novel therapeutic for adrenocortical carcinoma. *Oncotarget* **2015**, *6*, 36675. [CrossRef] [PubMed]
32. Faria, A.M.; Sbiera, S.; Ribeiro, T.C.; Soares, I.C.; Mariani, B.M.P.; Freire, D.S.; De Sousa, G.R.V.; Lerario, A.M.; Ronchi, C.L.; Deutschbein, T.; et al. Expression of LIN28 and its regulatory microRNAs in adult adrenocortical cancer. *Clin. Endocrinol.* **2015**, *82*, 481–488. [CrossRef] [PubMed]
33. Khafaei, M.; Rezaie, E.; Mohammadi, A.; Shahnazi Gerdehsang, P.; Ghavidel, S.; Kadkhoda, S.; Zorrieh Zahra, A.; Forouzanfar, N.; Arabameri, H.; Tavallaie, M. miR-9: From function to therapeutic potential in cancer. *J. Cell. Physiol.* **2019**, *234*, 14651–14665. [CrossRef] [PubMed]
34. Özata, D.M.; Caramuta, S.; Velázquez-Fernández, D.; Akçakaya, P.; Xie, H.; Höög, A.; Zedenius, J.; Bäckdahl, M.; Larsson, C.; Lui, W.O. The role of microRNA deregulation in the pathogenesis of adrenocortical carcinoma. *Endocr. Relat. Cancer* **2011**, *18*, 643–655. [CrossRef]
35. Romero, D.G.; Plonczynski, M.W.; Carvajal, C.A.; Gomez-Sanchez, E.P.; Gomez-Sanchez, C.E. Microribonucleic Acid-21 Increases Aldosterone Secretion and Proliferation in H295R Human Adrenocortical Cells. *Endocrinology* **2008**, *149*, 2477. [CrossRef]
36. Chabre, O.; Libé, R.; Assie, G.; Barreau, O.; Bertherat, J.; Bertagna, X.; Feige, J.J.; Cherradi, N. Serum miR-483-5p and miR-195 are predictive of recurrence risk in adrenocortical cancer patients. *Endocr. Relat. Cancer* **2013**, *20*, 579–594. [CrossRef]
37. Patterson, E.E.; Holloway, A.K.; Weng, J.; Fojo, T.; Kebebew, E. MicroRNA profiling of adrenocortical tumors reveals miR-483 as a marker of malignancy. *Cancer* **2011**, *117*, 1630. [CrossRef]
38. Feinmesser, M.; Benbassat, C.; Meiri, E.; Benjamin, H.; Lebanony, D.; Lebenthal, Y.; De Vries, L.; Drozd, T.; Spector, Y. Specific microRNAs differentiate adrenocortical adenomas from carcinomas and correlate with weiss histopathologic system. *Appl. Immunohistochem. Mol. Morphol.* **2015**, *23*, 522–531. [CrossRef]
39. Szabó, D.R.; Luconi, M.; Szabó, P.M.; Tóth, M.; Szücs, N.; Horányi, J.; Nagy, Z.; Mannelli, M.; Patócs, A.; Rácz, K.; et al. Analysis of circulating microRNAs in adrenocortical tumors. *Lab. Investig.* **2013**, *94*, 331–339. [CrossRef]
40. Wu, Y.; Wang, W.; Hu, W.; Xu, W.; Xiao, G.; Nie, Q.; Ouyang, K.; Chen, S. MicroRNA-205 suppresses the growth of adrenocortical carcinoma SW-13 cells via targeting Bcl-2. *Oncol. Rep.* **2015**, *34*, 3104–3110. [CrossRef]
41. Pereira, S.S.; Monteiro, M.P.; Antonini, S.R.; Pignatelli, D. Apoptosis regulation in adrenocortical carcinoma. *Endocr. Connect.* **2019**, *8*, R91. [CrossRef]
42. Tömböl, Z.; Szabó, P.M.; Molnár, V.; Wiener, Z.; Tölgyesi, G.; Horányi, J.; Riesz, P.; Reismann, P.; Patócs, A.; Likó, I.; et al. Integrative molecular bioinformatics study of human adrenocortical tumors: MicroRNA, tissue-specific target prediction, and pathway analysis. *Endocr. Relat. Cancer* **2009**, *16*, 895–906. [CrossRef]
43. Koperski, L.; Kotlarek, M.; Swierniak, M.; Kolanowska, M.; Kubiak, A.; Górnicka, B.; Jazdzewski, K.; Wójcicka, A. Next-generation sequencing reveals microRNA markers of adrenocortical tumors malignancy. *Oncotarget* **2017**, *8*, 49191. [CrossRef]
44. Assié, G.; Letouzé, E.; Fassnacht, M.; Jouinot, A.; Luscap, W.; Barreau, O.; Omeiri, H.; Rodriguez, S.; Perlemoine, K.; René-Corail, F.; et al. Integrated genomic characterization of adrenocortical carcinoma. *Nat. Genet.* **2014**, *46*, 607–612. [CrossRef]
45. Schmitz, K.J.; Helwig, J.; Bertram, S.; Sheu, S.Y.; Suttorp, A.C.; Seggewiß, J.; Willscher, E.; Walz, M.K.; Worm, K.; Schmid, K.W. Differential expression of microRNA-675, microRNA-139-3p and microRNA-335 in benign and malignant adrenocortical tumours. *J. Clin. Pathol.* **2011**, *64*, 529–535. [CrossRef]
46. Kwok, G.T.Y.; Zhao, J.T.; Glover, A.R.; Gill, A.J.; Clifton-Bligh, R.; Robinson, B.G.; Ip, J.C.Y.; Sidhu, S.B. microRNA-431 as a Chemosensitizer and Potentiator of Drug Activity in Adrenocortical Carcinoma. *Oncologist* **2019**, *24*, e241. [CrossRef]
47. Duregon, E.; Rapa, I.; Votta, A.; Giorcelli, J.; Daffara, F.; Terzolo, M.; Scagliotti, G.V.; Volante, M.; Papotti, M. MicroRNA expression patterns in adrenocortical carcinoma variants and clinical pathologic correlations. *Hum. Pathol.* **2014**, *45*, 1555–1562. [CrossRef]
48. Veronese, A.; Lupini, L.; Consiglio, J.; Visone, R.; Ferracin, M.; Fornari, F.; Zanesi, N.; Alder, H.; D'Elia, G.; Gramantieri, L.; et al. Oncogenic Role of miR-483-3p at the IGF2/483 Locus. *Cancer Res.* **2010**, *70*, 3140. [CrossRef]

49. Perge, P.; Butz, H.; Pezzani, R.; Bancos, I.; Nagy, Z.; Pálóczi, K.; Nyíro, G.; Decmann, Á.; Pap, E.; Luconi, M.; et al. Evaluation and diagnostic potential of circulating extracellular vesicle-associated microRNAs in adrenocortical tumors. *Sci. Rep.* **2017**, *7*, 5474. [CrossRef]
50. Salvianti, F.; Canu, L.; Poli, G.; Armignacco, R.; Scatena, C.; Cantini, G.; Di Franco, A.; Gelmini, S.; Ercolino, T.; Pazzagli, M.; et al. New insights in the clinical and translational relevance of miR483-5p in adrenocortical cancer. *Oncotarget* **2017**, *8*, 65525. [CrossRef]
51. Decmann, A.; Bancos, I.; Khanna, A.; Thomas, M.A.; Turai, P.; Perge, P.; Pintér, J.Z.; Tóth, M.; Patócs, A.; Igaz, P. Comparison of plasma and urinary microRNA-483-5p for the diagnosis of adrenocortical malignancy. *J. Biotechnol.* **2019**, *297*, 49–53. [CrossRef]
52. Zheng, S.; Cherniack, A.D.; Dewal, N.; Moffitt, R.A.; Danilova, L.; Murray, B.A.; Lerario, A.M.; Else, T.; Knijnenburg, T.A.; Ciriello, G.; et al. Comprehensive Pan-Genomic Characterization of Adrenocortical Carcinoma. *Cancer Cell* **2016**, *29*, 723. [CrossRef]
53. Goh, G.; Scholl, U.I.; Healy, J.M.; Choi, M.; Prasad, M.L.; Nelson-Williams, C.; Kuntsman, J.W.; Korah, R.; Suttorp, A.C.; Dietrich, D.; et al. Recurrent activating mutation in PRKACA in cortisol-producing adrenal tumors. *Nat. Genet.* **2014**, *46*, 613. [CrossRef]
54. Liaw, A.; Wiener, M. Classification and Regression by randomForest. *R News* **2002**, *2*, 18–22.
55. Modern Applied Statistics with S. Available online: https://link.springer.com/book/10.1007/978-0-387-21706-2 (accessed on 7 December 2021).
56. Caret: Classification and Regression Training R Package Version 6.0-90. Available online: https://CRAN.R-project.org/package=caret (accessed on 7 December 2021).
57. Robin, X.; Turck, N.; Hainard, A.; Tiberti, N.; Lisacek, F.; Sanchez, J.C.; Müller, M. pROC: An open-source package for R and S+ to analyze and compare ROC curves. *BMC Bioinform.* **2011**, *12*, 77. [CrossRef]
58. Soon, P.S.H.; Libe, R.; Benn, D.E.; Gill, A.; Shaw, J.; Sywak, M.S.; Groussin, L.; Bertagna, X.; Gicquel, C.; Bertherat, J.; et al. Loss of heterozygosity of 17p13, with possible involvement of ACADVL and ALOX15B, in the pathogenesis of adrenocortical tumors. *Ann. Surg.* **2008**, *247*, 157–164. [CrossRef]
59. Bavelloni, A.; Ramazzotti, G.; Poli, A.; Piazzi, M.; Focaccia, E.; Blalock, W.; Faenza, I. MiRNA-210: A Current Overview. *Anticancer Res.* **2017**, *37*, 6511–6521.
60. Pouysségur, J.; Dayan, F.; Mazure, N.M. Hypoxia signalling in cancer and approaches to enforce tumour regression. *Nature* **2006**, *441*, 437–443. [CrossRef]
61. Semenza, G.L. Targeting HIF-1 for cancer therapy. *Nat. Rev. Cancer* **2003**, *3*, 721–732. [CrossRef]
62. Grosso, S.; Doyen, J.; Parks, S.K.; Bertero, T.; Paye, A.; Cardinaud, B.; Gounon, P.; Lacas-Gervais, S.; Noël, A.; Pouysségur, J.; et al. MiR-210 promotes a hypoxic phenotype and increases radioresistance in human lung cancer cell lines. *Cell Death Dis.* **2013**, *4*, e544. [CrossRef]
63. Nohata, N.; Hanazawa, T.; Kikkawa, N.; Mutallip, M.; Sakurai, D.; Fujimura, L.; Kawakami, K.; Chiyomaru, T.; Yoshino, H.; Enokida, H.; et al. Tumor suppressive microRNA-375 regulates oncogene AEG-1/MTDH in head and neck squamous cell carcinoma (HNSCC). *J. Hum. Genet.* **2011**, *56*, 595–601. [CrossRef] [PubMed]
64. Tsukamoto, Y.; Nakada, C.; Noguchi, T.; Tanigawa, M.; Nguyen, L.T.; Uchida, T.; Hijiya, N.; Matsuura, K.; Fujioka, T.; Seto, M.; et al. MicroRNA-375 Is Downregulated in Gastric Carcinomas and Regulates Cell Survival by Targeting PDK1 and 14-3-3ζ. *Cancer Res.* **2010**, *70*, 2339–2349. [CrossRef] [PubMed]
65. Liu, A.M.; Poon, R.T.P.; Luk, J.M. MicroRNA-375 targets Hippo-signaling effector YAP in liver cancer and inhibits tumor properties. *Biochem. Biophys. Res. Commun.* **2010**, *394*, 623–627. [CrossRef] [PubMed]
66. Ding, L.; Xu, Y.; Zhang, W.; Deng, Y.; Si, M.; Du, Y.; Yao, H.; Liu, X.; Ke, Y.; Si, J.; et al. MiR-375 frequently downregulated in gastric cancer inhibits cell proliferation by targeting JAK2. *Cell Res.* **2010**, *20*, 784–793. [CrossRef]
67. Li, X.; Lin, R.; Li, J. Epigenetic silencing of microRNA-375 regulates PDK1 expression in esophageal cancer. *Dig. Dis. Sci.* **2011**, *56*, 2849–2856. [CrossRef]
68. Ladeiro, Y.; Couchy, G.; Balabaud, C.; Bioulac-Sage, P.; Pelletier, L.; Rebouissou, S.; Zucman-Rossi, J. MicroRNA profiling in hepatocellular tumors is associated with clinical features and oncogene/tumor suppressor gene mutations. *Hepatology* **2008**, *47*, 1955–1963. [CrossRef]
69. Tissier, F.; Cavard, C.; Groussin, L.; Perlemoine, K.; Fumey, G.; Hagneré, A.M.; René-Corail, F.; Jullian, E.; Gicquel, C.; Bertagna, X.; et al. Mutations of β-Catenin in Adrenocortical Tumors: Activation of the Wnt Signaling Pathway Is a Frequent Event in both Benign and Malignant Adrenocortical Tumors. *Cancer Res.* **2005**, *65*, 7622–7627. [CrossRef]
70. Berthon, A.; Martinez, A.; Bertherat, J.; Val, P. Wnt/β-catenin signalling in adrenal physiology and tumour development. *Mol. Cell. Endocrinol.* **2012**, *351*, 87–95. [CrossRef]
71. Decmann, A.; Perge, P.; Nyíro, G.; Darvasi, O.; Likó, I.; Borka, K.; Micsik, T.; Tóth, Z.; Bancos, I.; Pezzani, R.; et al. MicroRNA Expression Profiling in Adrenal Myelolipoma. *J. Clin. Endocrinol. Metab.* **2018**, *103*, 3522–3530. [CrossRef]
72. Soon, P.S.H.; Gill, A.J.; Benn, D.E.; Clarkson, A.; Robinson, B.G.; McDonald, K.L.; Sidhu, S.B. Microarray gene expression and immunohistochemistry analyses of adrenocortical tumors identify IGF2 and Ki-67 as useful in differentiating carcinomas from adenomas. *Endocr. Relat. Cancer* **2009**, *16*, 573–583. [CrossRef]
73. De Fraipont, F.; El Atifi, M.; Cherradi, N.; Le Moigne, G.; Defaye, G.; Houlgatte, R.; Bertherat, J.; Bertagna, X.; Plouin, P.F.; Baudin, E.; et al. Gene Expression Profiling of Human Adrenocortical Tumors Using Complementary Deoxyribonucleic Acid

Microarrays Identifies Several Candidate Genes as Markers of Malignancy. *J. Clin. Endocrinol. Metab.* **2005**, *90*, 1819–1829. [CrossRef]
74. Agosta, C.; Laugier, J.; Guyon, L.; Denis, J.; Bertherat, J.; Libé, R.; Boisson, B.; Sturm, N.; Feige, J.J.; Chabre, O.; et al. MiR-483-5p and miR-139-5p promote aggressiveness by targeting N-myc downstream-regulated gene family members in adrenocortical cancer. *Int. J. Cancer* **2018**, *143*, 944–957. [CrossRef]
75. Wang, L.; Shi, M.; Hou, S.; Ding, B.; Liu, L.; Ji, X.; Zhang, J.; Deng, Y. MiR-483–5p suppresses the proliferation of glioma cells via directly targeting ERK1. *FEBS Lett.* **2012**, *586*, 1312–1317. [CrossRef]
76. Liu, K.; He, B.; Xu, J.; Li, Y.; Guo, C.; Cai, Q.; Wang, S. miR-483-5p Targets MKNK1 to Suppress Wilms' Tumor Cell Proliferation and Apoptosis In Vitro and In Vivo. *Med. Sci. Monit.* **2019**, *25*, 1459. [CrossRef]
77. Zhao, J.J.; Yang, J.; Lin, J.; Yao, N.; Zhu, Y.; Zheng, J.; Xu, J.; Cheng, J.Q.; Lin, J.Y.; Ma, X. Identification of miRNAs associated with tumorigenesis of retinoblastoma by miRNA microarray analysis. *Child's Nerv. Syst.* **2009**, *25*, 13–20. [CrossRef]
78. Corbetta, S.; Vaira, V.; Guarnieri, V.; Scillitani, A.; Eller-Vainicher, C.; Ferrero, S.; Vicentini, L.; Chiodini, I.; Bisceglia, M.; Beck-Peccoz, P.; et al. Differential expression of microRNAs in human parathyroid carcinomas compared with normal parathyroid tissue. *Endocr. Relat. Cancer* **2010**, *17*, 135–146. [CrossRef]
79. Sarkar, S.; Dey, B.K.; Dutta, A. MiR-322/424 and -503 Are Induced during Muscle Differentiation and Promote Cell Cycle Quiescence and Differentiation by Down-Regulation of Cdc25A. *Mol. Biol. Cell* **2010**, *21*, 2138. [CrossRef]
80. Forrest, A.R.R.; Kanamori-Katayama, M.; Tomaru, Y.; Lassmann, T.; Ninomiya, N.; Takahashi, Y.; De Hoon, M.J.L.; Kubosaki, A.; Kaiho, A.; Suzuki, M.; et al. Induction of microRNAs, mir-155, mir-222, mir-424 and mir-503, promotes monocytic differentiation through combinatorial regulation. *Leukemia* **2009**, *24*, 460–466. [CrossRef]
81. Vabalas, A.; Gowen, E.; Poliakoff, E.; Casson, A.J. Machine learning algorithm validation with a limited sample size. *PLoS ONE* **2019**, *14*, e0224365. [CrossRef]

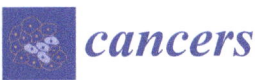

Article

Newborn Screening for the Detection of the *TP53* R337H Variant and Surveillance for Early Diagnosis of Pediatric Adrenocortical Tumors: Lessons Learned and Way Forward

Karina C. F. Tosin [1], Edith F. Legal [2], Mara A. D. Pianovski [3], Humberto C. Ibañez [2], Gislaine Custódio [4], Denise S. Carvalho [1], Mirna M. O. Figueiredo [4], Anselmo Hoffmann Filho [2], Carmem M. C. M. Fiori [5], Ana Luiza M. Rodrigues [3], Rosiane G. Mello [2,6], Karin R. P. Ogradowski [2,6], Ivy Z. S. Parise [2], Tatiana E. J. Costa [7], Viviane S. Melanda [8], Flora M. Watanabe [9], Denise B. Silva [7], Heloisa Komechen [2,4], Henrique H. L. Laureano [2], Edna K. Carboni [9], Ana P. Kuczynski [9], Gabriela C. F. Luiz [9], Leniza Lima [10], Tiago Tormen [10], Viviane K. Q. Gerber [11], Tania H. Anegawa [12], Sylvio G. A. Avilla [9], Renata B. Tenório [9], Elaine L. Mendes [9], Rayssa D. Fachin Donin [4], Josiane Souza [9], Vanessa N. Kozak [3], Gisele S. Oliveira [3], Deivid C. Souza [3], Israel Gomy [6,9], Vinicius B. Teixeira [2], Helena H. L. Borba [13], Nilton Kiesel Filho [9], Guilherme A. Parise [4], Raul C. Ribeiro [14,*] and Bonald C. Figueiredo [1,2,4,6,*]

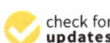

Citation: Tosin, K.C.F.; Legal, E.F.; Pianovski, M.A.D.; Ibañez, H.C.; Custódio, G.; Carvalho, D.S.; Figueiredo, M.M.O.; Hoffmann Filho, A.; Fiori, C.M.C.M.; Rodrigues, A.L.M.; et al. Newborn Screening for the Detection of the *TP53* R337H Variant and Surveillance for Early Diagnosis of Pediatric Adrenocortical Tumors: Lessons Learned and Way Forward. *Cancers* 2021, 13, 6111. https://doi.org/10.3390/cancers13236111

Academic Editor: Peter Igaz

Received: 31 August 2021
Accepted: 1 November 2021
Published: 3 December 2021

Publisher's Note: MDPI stays neutral with regard to jurisdictional claims in published maps and institutional affiliations.

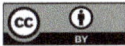

Copyright: © 2021 by the authors. Licensee MDPI, Basel, Switzerland. This article is an open access article distributed under the terms and conditions of the Creative Commons Attribution (CC BY) license (https://creativecommons.org/licenses/by/4.0/).

1. Departamento de Saúde Coletiva, Federal University of Paraná, Rua Padre Camargo, 260, Centro, Curitiba 80.060-240, PR, Brazil; karinacfraguas@gmail.com (K.C.F.T.); denisecarvalho@ufpr.br (D.S.C.)
2. Instituto de Pesquisa Pelé Pequeno Príncipe, Silva Jardim, 1532, Curitiba 80.250-060, PR, Brazil; eamfalcon@gmail.com (E.F.L.); humberto.ibanez@gmail.com (H.C.I.); anselmohoffmannf@gmail.com (A.H.F.); rosiane.mello@fpp.edu.br (R.G.M.); karin.persegona@fpp.edu.br (K.R.P.O.); ivyparise@gmail.com (I.Z.S.P.); heloisakomechen@gmail.com (H.K.); henriquelaureano@outlook.com (H.A.L.); viniciusbiology@hotmail.com (V.B.T.)
3. Oncologia Pediátrica, Hospital Erasto Gaertner, R. Dr. Ovande do Amaral, 201, Jardim das Américas, Curitiba 81.520-060, PR, Brazil; mpianovski@erastinho.com.br (M.A.D.P.); analuizademelorodrigues@gmail.com (A.L.M.R.); vanessakosak@hotmail.com (V.N.K.); giselesantosdeoliveira@gmail.com (G.S.O.); deivid.genetica@gmail.com (D.C.S.)
4. Centro de Genética Molecular e Pesquisa do Câncer em Crianças (CEGEMPAC-APACN), Avenida Agostinho Leão Jr., 400, Curitiba 80.030-110, PR, Brazil; custodio.gislaine@gmail.com (G.C.); mirnafigueiredo@hotmail.com (M.M.O.F.); rayssadf@icloud.com (R.D.F.P.); gaparise@gmail.com (G.A.P.)
5. Hospital do Câncer, UOPECCAN, R. Itaquatiaras, 769, Santo Onofre, Cascavel 85.806-300, PR, Brazil; carmem.fiori@uopeccan.org.br
6. Faculdades Pequeno Príncipe, Av. Iguaçu, 333, Rebouças, Curitiba 80.230-020, PR, Brazil; isgomy@gmail.com
7. Hospital Infantil Joana de Gusmão, R. Rui Barbosa, 152, Agronômica, Florianópolis 88.025-301, SC, Brazil; tatianaeljaick@gmail.com (T.E.J.C.); denisebousfielddasilva@gmail.com (D.B.S.)
8. Secretaria do Estado da Saúde do Paraná, R. Piquiri, 170, Rebouças, Curitiba 80.230-140, PR, Brazil; vivianes@sesa.pr.gov.br
9. Hospital Pequeno Príncipe, Silva Jardim, 1532, Curitiba 80.250-060, PR, Brazil; flora.watanabe@hpp.org.br (F.M.W.); edna.kakitani@gmail.com (E.K.C.); anapkuczynski@hotmail.com (A.P.K.); Gabriela.luiz@hpp.org.br (G.C.F.L.); silvio.avila@hpp.org.br (S.G.A.A.); renatabtenorio@gmail.com (R.B.T.); laine_med@yahoo.com.br (E.L.M.); jositwin@gmail.com (J.S.); niltonkiesel@terra.com.br (N.K.F.)
10. Oncologia Pediátrica, Hospital de Clínicas da Universidade Federal do Paraná, R. Gen. Carneiro, 181, Alto da Glória, Curitiba 80.060-900, PR, Brazil; lenizacll@hotmail.com (L.L.); tiago@tormen.com (T.T.)
11. Departamento de Enfermagem, Universidade Estadual do Centro-Oeste, UNICENTRO, Rua Padre R. Salvatore Renna, 875-Santa Cruz, Guarapuava 85.015-430, PR, Brazil; vivianekg@yahoo.com.br
12. Oncologia Pediátrica, Campus Universitário, Universidade Estadual de Londrina, Rodovia Celso Garcia Cid—Pr 445 Km 380, Londrina 86.057-970, PR, Brazil; tanegawa@uel.br
13. Departamento de Ciências Farmacêuticas, Federal University of Paraná, Av. Prefeito Lothário Meissner, 632-Jardim Botanico, Curitiba 80.210-170, PR, Brazil; Helena.hlb@gmail.com
14. Leukemia and Lymphoma Division, Department of Oncology, St. Jude Children's Research Hospital, Memphis, TN 38105, USA
* Correspondence: raul.ribeiro@stjude.org (R.C.R.); bonaldf@yahoo.com.br or bonald@ufpr.br (B.C.F.)

Simple Summary: Adrenocortical tumor (ACT) is rare in children and fatal if not detected early. Children who inherit a mutation of the *TP53* gene tend to develop ACT early in life. In the 1990s, scientists revealed that a *TP53* variant (R337H) was frequent in South Brazil. Therefore, the incidence of ACT in children is 20 times higher in this region than in other countries. We reviewed the records of 16 children with ACT treated in a pediatric hospital in Parana state (southern Brazil) and 134 children registered in the state public registry data. We found a high number of cases with advanced disease, leading to an unacceptable number of deaths. These observations contradict newborn R337H screening and surveillance data, showing that surgical intervention in early cases of ACT is associated with a 100% cure. Newborn screening/surveillance should be implemented in regions with a high frequency of the R337H variant.

Abstract: The incidence of pediatric adrenocortical tumors (ACT) is high in southern Brazil due to the founder *TP53* R337H variant. Neonatal screening/surveillance (NSS) for this variant resulted in early ACT detection and improved outcomes. The medical records of children with ACT who did not participate in newborn screening (non-NSS) were reviewed (2012–2018). We compared known prognostic factors between the NSS and non-NSS cohorts and estimated surveillance and treatment costs. Of the 16 non-NSS children with ACT carrying the R337H variant, the disease stages I, II, III, and IV were observed in five, five, one, and five children, respectively. The tumor weight ranged from 22 to 608 g. The 11 NSS children with ACT all had disease stage I and were alive. The median tumor weight, age of diagnosis, and interval between symptoms and diagnosis were 21 g, 1.9 years, and two weeks, respectively, for the NSS cohort and 210 g, 5.2 years, and 15 weeks, respectively, for the non-NSS cohort. The estimated surveillance/screening cost per year of life saved is US$623/patient. NSS is critical for improving the outcome of pediatric ACT in this region. Hence, we strongly advocate for the inclusion of R337H in the state-mandated universal screening and surveillance.

Keywords: *TP53* R337H; genetic testing; adrenocortical tumor; neonatal screening; surveillance

1. Introduction

The incidence of pediatric adrenocortical tumors (ACT) is approximately 20 times higher in southern Brazil [1–3] than in other regions of the world [4–6]. The presence of a founder *TP53* R337H variant in the population accounts for the increased number of cases of ACT, and other pediatric tumors [4,5]. The co-occurrence of germline *TP53* and activating mutations in β-catenin *(CTNNB1)* is rare in pediatric ACT. In a study using two different cohorts and methods (71 pediatric cases of ACT), activating β-catenin mutations ($n = 13$) were detected only in the tumors of individuals with wild-type *TP53* ($n = 35$) and none of those with germline *TP53* mutations ($n = 36$) [6]. The availability of a reliable and inexpensive genetic test to detect the *TP53* R337H heterozygote in the blood makes newborn screening a reasonable approach for the identification of R337H carriers [7]. Neonatal screening/surveillance (NSS) of R337H carriers consisting of close clinical observation, adrenal cortical hormone blood level monitoring, and scheduled imaging studies was associated with an excellent outcome, revealing the efficacy of surveillance for early diagnosis and intervention [1]. The cumulative risk of ACT is approximately 4% in the first decade of life and gradually declines. This cumulative incidence is 25 times higher than that of children with any type of cancer in this age group in the general population [8]. The risk of other cancers, especially choroid plexus carcinoma [7,9], neuroblastoma, and osteosarcoma [9], is slightly higher in children carrying the R337H variant than in the general population [1,7]. Late-onset (adult) tumors are more common than pediatric tumors in R337H-carrier families [10]. Whether the surveillance of ACT would help in the early diagnosis of other pediatric tumors in this age group remains unknown. Furthermore, surveillance is complex and expensive, requiring frequent hospital visits and blood draws for hormonal testing and imaging studies [1]. Although rare, surveillance test results can be false positive or false negative in Li-Fraumeni syndrome. However, it is important to consider this possibility in large longitudinal studies [11]. Indirect effects of intense surveillance on the condition of carriers include pain and discomfort for participants due to frequent blood draws, imaging studies, travel to clinical visits, missing school time, disruption of routine activities, and psychological harm [12].

Since almost all children carrying the R337H variant who develop ACT show conspicuous clinical findings associated with the overproduction of adrenal cortex hormones early in tumor formation, we simplified the surveillance process by focusing on early parental education to recognize the physical changes caused by excess androgen and cortisol, and scheduled periodic telephone interactions with a health agent to provide ongoing education for parents. We reasoned that repeatedly teaching parents to recognize the first clinical signs associated with excess hormones would have a similar efficacy to that of our previous intense surveillance approach [1]. The second neonatal screening followed by a simplified surveillance protocol of 122 families of newborns carrying R337H revealed that this simplified surveillance was also highly effective [2]. Newborn screening for R337H may be continued with pending approval of the government for the inclusion of R337H in the Parana State universal newborn screening panel, followed by this simplified NSS strategy. Given the identified similarities (prevalence of newborns R337H carriers and ACT incidence) in Santa Catarina State [2], the evaluation shifted from Paraná to the federal government. Other southern and southeastern Brazilian states may also have a high prevalence of R337H and incidence of pediatric ACT in the population. For example, the first cluster of pediatric ACT was reported in a charity hospital in the city of Sao Paulo [13]. In another study involving 35,000 newborns in the city of Campinas, Sao Paulo, the prevalence of R337H was 0.21% [14], which is slightly inferior to that in Santa Catarina (0.24%) and Parana state (0.30%) [2]. There has been no systematic analysis of R337H in other Brazilian states or interest in pursuing universal newborn screening. Individuals in these Brazilian states raised concerns associated with the psychological burden for the families of R337H carriers and the potentially high intervention costs. However, early-onset ACT has a unique clinical presentation and natural history in children. When managed at the time of the first clinical signs of virilization or Cushing, the cure rate approaches 100%, whereas death is almost certain in children with advanced stage ACT.

In this study, we described a retrospective analysis of the children with ACT admitted for treatment to the largest children's hospital in Curitiba, the capital of Paraná. These children were found to carry the R337H variant at the time of ACT diagnosis but did not participate in newborn screening or surveillance (non-NSS). We compared the tumor weight and stage, and interval from the first signs and symptoms to the diagnosis of ACT, according to when the R337H variant had been detected, through the NSS or at the time of ACT diagnosis. We combined the data of both surveillance protocols in the analysis. In addition, we estimated variations in treatment costs according to disease stage using different data sources.

2. Materials and Methods

2.1. Subjects

The medical records of unrelated children diagnosed with R337H-associated ACT admitted to the Pequeno Principe Hospital were analyzed for age, disease stage, tumor weight, and interval between the initial clinical signs of virilization or Cushing and the diagnosis of ACT. Children with ACT from families known to carry the R337H mutation were excluded. Targeted *TP53* R337H analysis was performed using the polymerase chain reaction-restriction fragment length polymorphism test assay (PCR-RFLP) for R337H [7]. Patients were classified into disease stages I–IV according to their initial and post-surgical features [15]. Stage I patients were managed with surgery alone. Patients with stage III and IV received a combination of cisplatin, doxorubicin, and etoposide (CDE) plus oral mitotane [15–18]. Some patients with completely resected large stage II tumors received mitotane [15–17].

The goal of surveillance of newborns tested positive for the *TP53* R337H variant is to detect early-onset ACT and provide timely intervention. We mainly focused on ACT during the first five years of life because ACT accounts for about 95% of all R337H-associated malignancies in this age group and can be easily suspected. Most importantly, if ACT is detected early, the cure rate is close to 100%. Other tumors such as choroid plexus carcinoma and neuroblastoma are rarely identified. During our first visit with the parents of an infant carrier, we provide a booklet describing the signs and symptoms associated with ACT (virilization and Cushing syndrome signs). The booklet also describes the signs and symptoms of choroid plexus tumors (irritability, altered feedings, seizure, and persistent crying), and neuroblastoma (weight loss, irritability, poor oral intake, abdominal distention and pain, and skin and subcutaneous lesions). However, whether NSS of ACT would be effective in early diagnosis of other pediatric tumors in this age group remains unknown. The parents are also informed of the increased risk of late-onset (adult) cancer associated with this mutation, but do not engage in active surveillance of children above five years or adults. Nonetheless, parents are encouraged to contact our center to discuss any enquiries regarding signs or symptoms that could be suggestive of a malignancy.

The most important contribution of the identification of R337H in newborns is the education of parents on the pattern of inheritance of the variant and the health consequences of carrying R337H. Free testing for the variant is offered to the parents, siblings of newborns, and all relatives of the parental side segregating the R337H. Counseling is focused on the importance of adopting a healthy lifestyle, the risk of developing other pediatric or adult-onset cancers, and information on established preventive routine procedures (Figure 1). Finally, symptomatic individuals who tested positive for R337H are referred to hospitals.

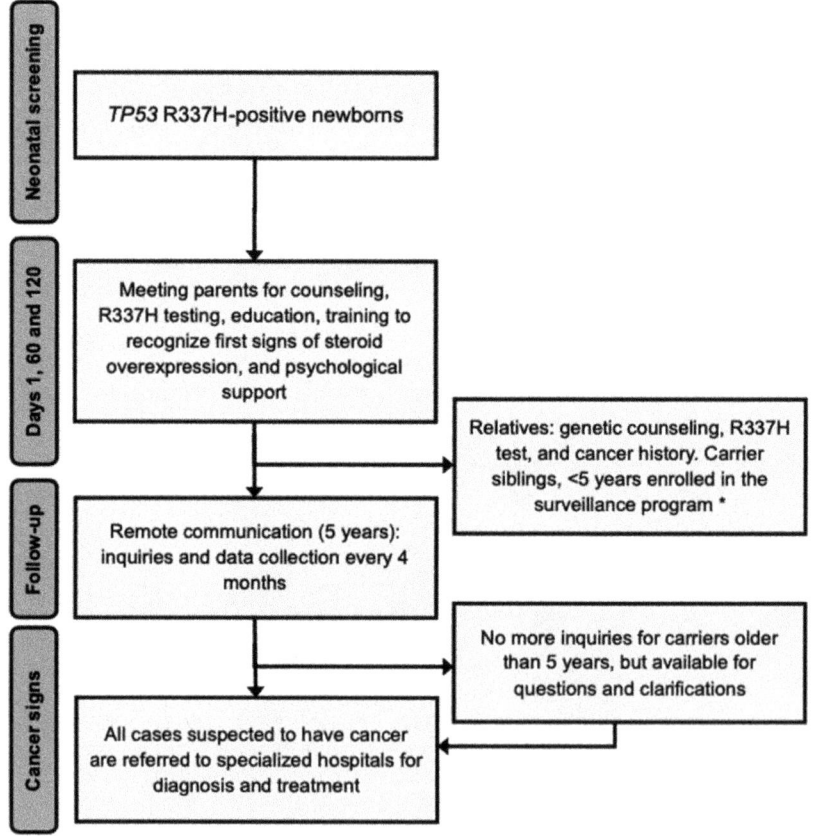

Figure 1. Follow-up flowchart for R337H screening and ACT treatment. * Provided at the study center or at another center closest to the participant home address.

2.2. Newborn Screening and Surveillance Database of Pele Pequeno Principe Research Institute/Pequeno Principe Hospital

In 2005–2010 and 2015–2018, two NSS pilot studies were conducted [1,2]. Briefly, the first study involved identification of the R337H variant from neonatal blood (heel prick) and inviting the families of the children who tested positive for the variant to participate in a surveillance program, consisting of regularly occurring visits to outpatient clinics, imaging studies, and monitoring the blood levels of androgens and cortisol. Information about the clinical manifestations of ACT, treatment, and outcome were provided at the time of the newborn screening consent and reporting of the testing results, and during the clinical visits. In the second study, the surveillance protocol was changed to replace frequent contact with the parents with emphasis on the early detection of the signs and symptoms resulting from an excess of dehydroepiandrosterone sulfate (DHEA-S) and cortisol produced by ACT. Instead of frequent outpatient clinical visits and extensive laboratory evaluations, the families were contacted by phone by an advanced practice nurse. Laboratory evaluations were triggered by suspicious clinical features. In the current report, we updated the data on newborn screening and surveillance of the two previously reported studies. The study was approved by the Ethics Committee of Pequeno Príncipe Hospital and National Research Ethics Committee (CAAE number (Curitiba, Paraná state, Brazil, under the ethical codes CAA: 0023.0.208.000-05 (2005), CAAE 0612.0.015.000-08 (2009, 2012, and 2015).

2.3. Costs

Estimating the cost of pediatric cancer in Brazil is very complex. We used different sources to estimate the average costs of treating patients with limited or advanced disease. First, we analyzed data from the Brazilian Public Health System (SUS), which is a constitutionally approved universal health system that guarantees free medical access to the population. In this health system, reimbursement is based on fixed costs established by the federal government. However, the reimbursement for pediatric cancer treatment is insufficient. Therefore, it is subsidized by nongovernment foundations. We reviewed and analyzed the DATASUS registry data of patients with ACT less than 18 years of age registered and treated in any of the Parana State public hospitals between 2006 and 2019. Data collected included the number of independent patients, hospital admissions, and disease stage. We estimated government expenses with chemotherapy based on purchase prices (2019 and 2020) listed in the Management System for Procedures, Drugs and Orthoses, Prostheses, and Special Materials of SUS [19] and Medications Market Regulation Chamber [20]. The chemotherapy regimen typically recommended for patients with stage III or IV disease throughout Paraná State is based on the Children's Oncology Group ARAR0332 [18]. We assumed that patients with stage III or IV disease received a total of eight courses of cisplatin, doxorubicin, and etoposide. We obtained actual reimbursement data from eight patients with advanced-stage disease treated in a pediatric cancer center (Hospital Erasto Gaertner (Curitiba, Brazil)) throughout their clinical course.

2.4. Statistical Analysis

The proportion of patients within each characteristic group was compared using Fisher's exact test, when appropriate. The median tumor weights between the screening and surveillance groups were compared using the Kruskal–Wallis test. The age at ACT diagnosis for different groups was visualized through a transformation of survival curves, called cumulative events. Its distributions were compared through the log-rank test [21]. The marginal (least-squares) means of the staging between the groups were estimated in the emmeans package [22] and the Tukey test was used for the multiple comparison of means. The level of statistical significance was set at $p < 0.05$ and all computations were performed within the R language [23].

3. Results

3.1. Single Hospital Cohort vs. Newborn Screening and Surveillance Cohorts

Between 2011 and 2019, 16 children with newly diagnosed ACT were admitted to the Pequeno Príncipe Hospital. All of them were heterozygous for the TP53 R337H variant. The median age of the 16 patients was 4.0 years (range, 0.7–16.1 years). The median interval between the first symptoms noted by the parents and the diagnosis was 15 weeks (range, 3–48 weeks). Five patients had completely resected small tumors without evidence of metastasis. Thus, they were classified as having stage I. Five patients without evidence of microscopic residual microscopic tumor were classified as stage II due to the large tumor sizes. The median tumor weight was 296 g (range, 18–608 g). Finally, six patients had advanced-stage disease, one with stage III and five with stage IV (Table 1). The management of ACT in these cases consisted of surgery only for patients with disease stages I and II. At the discretion of the primary attending, some patients with stage II disease received mitotane. Patients with stage IV disease were individualized and typically received intensive chemotherapy before or after surgery, following the previously reported guidelines [15,17,18].

Table 1. Upper: features of cases admitted to a single hospital between 2011 and 2019 (non-NSS); Lower: features of participants in newborn screening and who had tumor detected by surveillance (NSS).

ID	Age at Diagnosis (Years)	Stage	Interval between Symptoms and Diagnosis (Weeks)	Tumor Weight (g)	Treatment
1	2.0	I	32	38	Surgery
2	5.7	I	3	43	Surgery
3	0.7	I	4	18	Surgery
4	1.0	I	12	70	Surgery
5	6.1	I	32	22	Surgery
6	4.0	II	32	318	Surgery/Mitotane
7	4.8	II	24	258	Surgery/Mitotane
8	2.0	II	4	298	Surgery/Mitotane
9	1.0	II	12	126	Surgery
10	2.0	II	24	178	Surgery/Chemo
11	3.1	III	16	376	Surgery/Chemo/Mitotane
12	5.7	IV	8	264	Surgery/Chemo/Mitotane
13	4.0	IV	16	608	Surgery/Chemo
14	7.0	IV	12	242	Surgery/Chemo/Mitotane
15	16.1	IV	40	140	Surgery/Chemo
16	5.0	IV	48	250	Surgery/Chemo/Mitotane
Median	5.2	-	15	210	
1	2.3	I	<3	30	Surgery
2	1.9	I	<3	35	Surgery
3	0.2	I	<3	45	Surgery
4	1.2	I	<3	20	Surgery
5	2.3	I	<3	22	Surgery
6	1.9	I	<3	17	Surgery
7	1.8	I	<3	1	Surgery
8	6.2	I	<3	14	Surgery
9 *	0.9	I	<3	21	Surgery
10 *	2.8	I	<3	54	Surgery
11 *	1.8	I	<3	12	Surgery
Median	1.9	-	<3	21	-

Abbreviations: Chemo, chemotherapy; NSS, newborn screening and surveillance. * Patients participants in the second pilot study; follow-up (years) ranged from 0.5–14.8 years.

Of the 171,649 newborns tested in the first screening, 461 (0.27%) newborns and their 238 siblings aged <15 years were found to be carriers during the first newborn screening pilot study ($n = 699$), but only 347 (49.6%) participated in the surveillance program. Of the 42,438 newborns tested in the second screening, 159 (0.37%) newborns were carriers, but only 122 (76.7%) were confirmed to participate and were from Paraná state, and included in the surveillance program. The reasons for the surveillance rejection included personal reasons, preference for private clinics, and being born but not raised in Paraná state, among others. As of June 2021, 11 children who participated in one of the two NSS studies developed ACT. The median age of the 11 patients was 1.8 years (range, two months to 6.2 years). All of them had stage I disease, and the tumor weight ranged from 1 to 54 g (median, 20 g). The interval between endocrine signs and symptoms was less than three weeks in all cases (Table 1). All these patients are alive and disease-free at follow-up period ranging from 0.5 to 14.8 years. None of the patients developed a second malignancy. The 12th stage I ACT from screening was not included in the present analysis because it was a rare R337H/R337H homozygous case of a 9.3-year-old boy, who died after the fifth recurrence. This genotype may occur every other year. Although the observation time of the second pilot study was short, the first three cases of ACT were diagnosed early in the course (<3 weeks), and the tumor weights were 12 g, 21 g, and 54 g, respectively. This observation suggests that both surveillance strategies are similarly effective in detecting early ACT (<100 g). Hence, the results of the two studies were combined for comparative analysis.

Since tumor weight is an independent prognostic indicator in pediatric ACT, we compared the impact of NSS on tumor weight. Among children with ACT from both NSS cohorts, all had tumor weights less than 100 g, whereas only about 35% of those who did not participate in the surveillance ($p = 0.0005$, Supplementary Table S1) did. Parents who participated in the first newborn screening but refused to sign consent for surveillance received information about ACT at time of consent for newborn screening and at time of reporting of testing results. The age at diagnosis of the 10 patients ranged from six months to 7.3 years (median, 1.2 years), three patients were diagnosed with stage I disease and one patient with stage IV disease. The remaining patients were classified as having stage II or III disease. The outcome and follow-up data were incomplete for these patients. Supplementary Table S2 shows the analysis of tumor weights according to NSS. Disease stage is also a critical prognostic indicator in pediatric ACT. Patients with stage I disease have an excellent prognosis, whereas stage IV disease have a dismal prognosis. The impact of stages II and III on outcomes is less established. Surveillance was significantly associated with stage I disease ($p = 0.0008$; Table S3).

We did not observe a significant difference in age at diagnosis, surveillance, or non-surveillance ($p = 0.12$; Figure S1). In addition, we examined the distribution of disease stage according to age. We noted that in the non-surveillance group, patients with stage I disease were typically diagnosed under two years of age, whereas those with stage IV disease were older than three years of age. Conversely, in those who participated in the surveillance, stage I disease was observed up to six years of age. Age at diagnosis, tumor size, and disease stage can also be influenced by the interval between the first symptom and diagnosis (Supplementary Table S4). Our analysis showed a strong association between symptom duration before diagnosis and NSS. In children participating in the surveillance, diagnoses were made within three months from the start of symptoms of virilization and/or Cushing syndrome, whereas the median duration of symptoms in non-participants was 17 months (range, 3–53; $p < 0.00002$). The median tumor weight, age of diagnosis, and interval between symptoms and diagnosis were 21 g, 1.9 years, and <3 weeks, respectively, for the NSS cohort and 210 g, 5.2 years, and 15 weeks, respectively, for the non-NSS cohort.

3.2. DATASUS Registry Cohort and Neonatal Screening and Surveillance Costs

Between 2006 and 2019, 134 cases of pediatric ACT were registered in the government DATASUS registry (mean, 11 per year). This number does not include most pediatric ACT cases from private hospitals (approximately 20%) and may fail to register other cases from SUS (public hospitals). The number of admissions for each patient in the DATASUS-covered hospitals varied from 1 to 17. As expected, there was an association between the number of admissions for patients with stage III and IV (Table 2).

Table 2. DATASUS registry data of children diagnosed with ACT between 2006 and 2019 admitted to public hospitals in Parana State.

Patients N (%)	Disease Stage [1]	Number of Admissions	Surgery and/or Adjuvant Therapy [2] (US$)	Lives Saved [3]	Years of Life Lost [4]
20 (14.9%)	I	20	50,460	20	none
22 (16.4%)	II	32	80,763	15	420
92 (68.6%)	III or IV	427	1,581,948	27	3900
134 (100%)	-	479	1,713,171	62	4320

[1] Staging criteria [15]. [2] Costs associated with hospitalizations or other supportive care medications is not included. [3] Assume survival of 100%, 80% and 30% for patients with disease stage I, II and III/IV, respectively. [4] Assuming 60 years of life lost per patient who dies from the disease.

Twenty hospital admissions were required for 20 patients with stage I, 32 hospital admissions were required for stage II, whereas 427 admissions were required for 92 children with stage III or IV disease ($p < 0.00001$ for stage I and/or II vs. III and IV). The reasons for multiple hospital admissions include surgeries for metastases or recurrences, chemotherapy cycles, and management of treatment-related toxicity.

The estimated amount paid by SUS to the different hospitals for surgery and chemotherapy agents was US$ 1,713,171 during the study period or about US$ 12,784 per patient. This amount did not include coverage for expenses during hospitalization and those incurred from the loss of parents' workdays, transportation, meals, and lodging. Furthermore, because 70% of the patients had advanced-stage ACT, the mortality rates and years of life lost were high among these patients (Table 2). To illustrate the burdensome complexity in managing advanced-stage ACT, we analyzed the reimbursed costs of eight patients admitted to a public charity pediatric cancer center in the Paraná state. The amount reimbursed by SUS corresponds to approximately 60% of the actual care cost, which is supplemented by the Hospital Foundation. It is common that the care of patients with metastatic disease at diagnosis, many of whom eventually succumb to the disease, may extend for several years. Therefore, prolonged suffering is frequent during the management of advanced-stage ACT.

The estimated cost of the first neonatal screening in Paraná state followed by surveillance has been reported [1]. Because of the complexity and high cost of this approach, surveillance has been simplified. We estimated that the cost of surveillance featuring only three visits to the hospital and frequent periodic remote contacts with families would substantially reduce costs compared with the previous. Using data from the simplified NSS study, we estimated that the costs for neonatal screening and surveillance per year for the public system of the Paraná state are approximately US$ 802,880 per year or US$ 50,180 per patient per year. Without the simplified NSS intervention, the expected cost per patient is at least US$ 12,784. Thus, the screening/surveillance costs an additional US$ 37,396 per patient. Considering the life expectancy of these children to be about 60 years, the cost per year of life saved is US$623 (Figure 2).

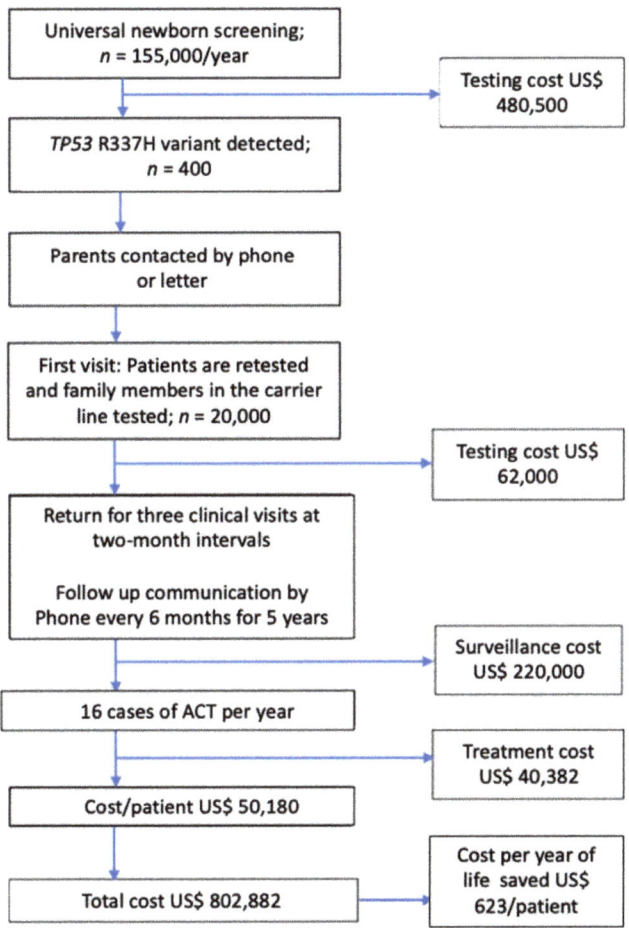

Figure 2. Cost of screening and surveillance. Considering a life expectancy of 60 years, the cost per year of life saved is US$623 per patient.

4. Discussion

In this study, we demonstrated that the outcome of children with ACT continues to be dismal in the Paraná state. Between 2011 and 2019, only 30% of the 16 children referred to the largest pediatric hospital in Curitiba, the state capital, had stage I ACT. These data are corroborated by the analysis of 134 pediatric ACT cases registered between 2006 and 2019 in the Parana State Public Database (DATASUS), which includes cases from rural and urban areas, showing that only 15% of cases had stage I ACT. The extent of disease at diagnosis is the single most important variable associated with the outcome of ACT after surgery [24]. Patients with stage I ACT (complete resected tumors weighing < 100 g) have high probability of disease-free survival, which approached 100% for tumors < 50 g [24]. Conversely, patients with metastatic (stage IV) or residual disease after surgery (stage III) have a high rate of disease progression and poor prognosis [24]. Finally, patients who are classified as stage II have increased relapse rates, but can still be cured with additional surgery and intensive chemotherapy [24]. The low rate of cases with stage I disease identified at Pequeno Príncipe Hospital and other hospitals of Paraná state is surprising given the existing knowledge on the biology and presenting signs of this type of pediatric cancer in Paraná and surrounding states [25–31]. The delay in diagnosis is associated with higher proportions of stages II, III, and IV, and is in part because children with ACT appear to be healthy and energetic in the early phases of tumor development due to the increased somatic growth of these children, which together may confound untrained parents as precocious puberty. These signs are sometimes ignored or not appropriately investigated, mainly due to the parents' unawareness, usually with a low education level. When overt signs and symptoms associated with the overproduction of androgens (virilization) or cortisol (Cushing syndrome) are noted, the tumor has already progressed beyond stage I. Almost all ACT weighing < 50 g produce hormones that cause clinical manifestations, which are easily observed by trained parents, as documented in the simplified surveillance study [2]. These tumors are often completely resected and eradicated [24]. Moreover, many children with early signs of virilization and Cushing are suspected to have more common endocrinopathies, and may undergo extensive laboratory investigations that might further delay the diagnosis of ACT. Finally, because of the rarity of pediatric ACT, healthcare providers at the point of care do not consider this tumor in the differential diagnosis.

In the late 1990s, the discovery that children with ACT in this geographic region carried a mutation in the *TP53* (R337H variant) [3], which could be detected in the blood by a simple and inexpensive restriction fragment polymorphism enzymatic test [7], created the opportunity for NSS of carriers. A study of newborns who tested positive for R337H at birth and whose parents provided consent for participation in a surveillance program for early detection of ACT showed that all participants who developed ACT had post-surgical stage I disease. Moreover, no recurrence has been noted among members of this cohort, who had been alive for more than 10 years from diagnosis. This observation proved that a small ACT can be eradicated with surgery alone. The *TP53* R337H variant is considered to have low penetrance for cancer [2,31], and in many families, pediatric ACT is the first clinical manifestation of this variant. During the first 17 years of life, ACT accounts for approximately 90% of all cancers in R337H carriers, whereas ACT accounts for only 12% of pediatric cancers in *TP53* carriers with classic Li-Fraumeni syndrome (LFS) [32]. The lifetime risk of cancer is also lower in R337H carriers than in carriers of classic LFS variants [32,33]. Finally, about 80% of ACT survivors carrying classic LFS *TP53* variants develop a secondary cancer within 30 years from the diagnosis of ACT [32], whereas ACT survivors carrying the R337H variant rarely develop secondary cancers during the first four decades of life [10]. Therefore, most children with post-surgical stage I ACT are expected to have medical conditions comparable to those in the general population. However, the cost and complexity of the surveillance precluded the introduction of R337H testing in the Parana state universal newborn screening. The main argument against the implementation of universal NSS was the relatively low cumulative incidence of ACT in R337H carriers (4%), suggesting that approximately 95% of the children undergoing surveillance do not develop ACT. Therefore, the number of imaging studies and repeated blood draws to test for abnormal levels of adrenal cortex hormones was beneficial only for less than 5% of the carriers. A subsequent retrospective analysis of the first surveillance program [1] revealed that the early recognition of the physical changes associated with overproduction of adrenal cortex hormones could substitute for blood levels and imaging studies to identify children with tumors <100 g. Based on these observations, the simplified surveillance program was designed focusing on education and training of parents to recognize early physical changes associated with overproduction of adrenal cortex hormones [2]. The program consisted of three visits at two-month intervals to the clinic for counseling and education, followed by phone contact by healthcare professionals. A feasibility surveillance study of 122 children positive for the R337H variant using this approach detected three cases with clinical findings suspicious for an ACT (two of them in the present study), where all of them were found to have post-surgical stage I disease.

The most compelling reason to implement the universal newborn screening and simplified surveillance for R337H is that without this intervention, the mortality and morbidity of children who develop ACT are unacceptably high. Despite the inclusion of specific information on pediatric ACT and the medical consequences of the founder R337H variant in the curriculum of the local medical schools and pediatric residency programs, there has been no evidence that the frequency of cases with stage I ACT has substantially increased over the past several years. Similarly, among ACT cases in families who agreed to participate in the newborn screening and were informed of the clinical implications of a positive test but declined to participate in the surveillance program, only 30% of children had stage I disease, suggesting that the information was not retained or was incorrectly interpreted in most cases.

The cost–benefit analysis also strongly supports the surveillance program. The estimated cost without surveillance is US$ 12,784 per patient. These estimates are based on the DATASUS registry, which does not consider the costs associated with nonmedical expenses, which can substantially increase the overall cost. A study found that nonmedical expenses accounted for about 46% of the monthly household income of parents from rural areas and 22% of those from urban areas. Out-of-pocket expenses include travel, accommodation (lodging), food, communication, and work disruption [34]. Moreover, the management of advanced-stage ACT is associated with prolonged exposure to toxic chemotherapy and multiple surgeries. As illustrated in Table S5, many patients without stage I disease are treated for several years, requiring different chemotherapy regimens and surgical procedures. Therefore, without intervention, the potential for loss of life, suffering, and psychological distress for patients and families are substantial. Whether the risk for second cancers is increased in heavily treated patients remains to be determined.

Conversely, surveillance is highly effective in detecting patients with stage I disease, which is highly curable with surgery alone and a short hospital admission. The surgical cost of eradicating the disease is negligible. The nonmedical costs for neonatal screening and infrastructure to run the surveillance are estimated to be US$50,180 per patient over five years of follow-up. Although the monetary cost per patient in the intervention program is higher than the alternative, the number of lives saved and quality life years are much higher among children undergoing surveillance. Considering that these patients would live for at least 60 years with good quality, the cost-effectiveness ratio is US$623 per quality life-year gained. In pediatrics, a medical intervention that costs less than US$50,000 per year of life saved is considered justifiable [35].

The ethical issues that arise regarding the genetic testing and screening of children have been addressed for other diseases [36,37], but they are not yet clear for hereditary cancer [38,39], such as *TP53* R337H in Southern Brazil. Despite advances in genomic research associated with the *TP53* R337H variant [40], with an increased cure rate with genetic testing and different surveillance protocols [1,2], it is necessary to examine the ethics of this matter. The R337H variant is almost always inherited and is associated with early and late-onset cancers [10,40,41]. A newborn positive case triggers a chain of events such as cancer surveillance of the infant and testing of the siblings younger than ten years of age, parents, and other relatives in the affected parental line. To address the psychological and ethical concerns, the parents of a newborn who tested positive are invited for medical visits to discuss the findings, including confirmatory testing, information on the implications of positive testing, genetic counseling, testing relatives, and age-adapted surveillance for carriers (Figure 3). Counseling is focused on the importance of adopting a healthy lifestyle, the types of adolescent and adult neoplasms associated with this mutation, and preventive routine procedures. However, we do not offer systematic surveillance for late-onset cancers beyond being available to discuss with family members any medical event and to facilitate referral to a medical center. Figure 3 summarizes the estimates from the expected 400 R337H-carrier newborns among 155,000 births per year in the state of Paraná. The simplified protocol protects 16 infants and young children with ACT (4%). Parents are encouraged to consider their autonomy in accepting confirmatory testing, surveillance, and expanded family testing. In this context, vulnerabilities and cultural and socioeconomic conditions are considered. The critical points in this process are to save the lives of children younger than five years of age, avoid suffering associated with intensive chemotherapy, and empower the parents through an education program to make informed decisions.

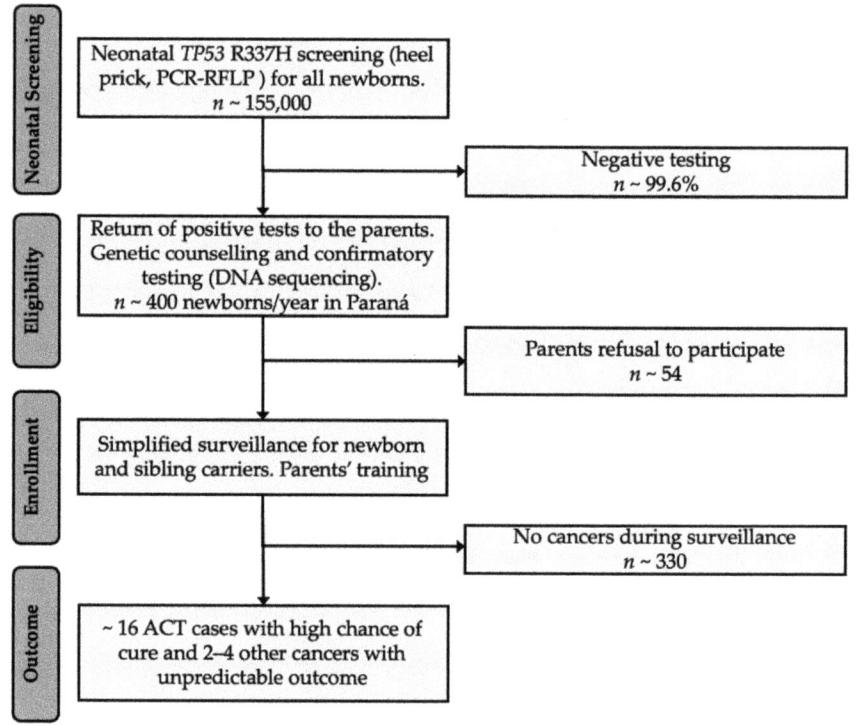

Figure 3. A neonatal and surveillance proposal for the state of Paraná (and state of Santa Catarina with approximately 50% of the projected numbers for Paraná). First step (neonatal screening) expected to be included in the universal Parana and Santa Catarina's state panel, and provided free of charge. Subsequent steps (eligibility/enrollment) would require the parents' consent and acceptance to be trained to detect and report early signs and symptoms of ACT.

The ethical impact of whether it is worthwhile to pursue non-intense measures to detect ~14–16 stage I ACTs/year among R337H-carrier children younger than five years, or whether we should avoid psychological exposure of ~95% of the unaffected carrier children, remains unclear. It is also worth noting that *TP53* R337H neonatal screening will ultimately disclose one of the parents and all consenting carrier relatives on the same side of the family, and they all should be monitored as a low cancer risk p53 variant [2]. The neonatal test, if mandatory, should also preserve the interest and privacy of the parents, as illustrated in Figure 3, and only they should decide whether to disclose the result and be enrolled in the surveillance program. Article 10 of the International Declaration of Human Genetic Data [42] could also be understood as "a right" of the parents to ignore the neonatal positive R337H results and reject surveillance.

5. Conclusions

The high incidence of pediatric ACT in southern Brazil is a consequence of the population's high frequency of the germline TP53 R337H variant. The inclusion of R337H in newborn screening is in the best interests of all children born in this geographic region because surveillance of R337H carriers reduces the mortality and suffering of young children who develop ACT. The entire process should have public governance to protect the children as a group and the autonomy of their parents. Therefore, we strongly advocate for the inclusion of R337H in the state-mandated universal newborn screening, surveillance for the children during the years of highest tumor incidence, and education and psychosocial support for the parents of the affected children.

Supplementary Materials: The following are available online at https://www.mdpi.com/article/10.3390/cancers13236111/s1, Figure S1: (A) There is no significant difference between age at diagnosis of pediatric ACT according to participation in the surveillance. (B) Age at diagnosis is strongly associated with tumor weight. The number of children with tumor weight <100 g is significantly higher in the surveillance group than that of children who did not participate in the surveillance; Table S1: Features at diagnosis of children with ACT in newborn screening, but not surveillance; Table S2: Analysis of tumor weight according to newborn screening and surveillance; Table S3: Analysis of disease stage according to newborn screening and surveillance; Table S4: Analysis of duration of symptoms according to newborn screening and surveillance; Table S5: Cost with chemotherapy or surgery for patients with advanced-stage disease.

Author Contributions: Conceptualization and formal analysis, B.C.F., R.C.R., M.A.D.P. and K.C.F.T.; writing—original draft; K.C.F.T.; investigation and editing, all authors, reviewed the literature, and approved the final manuscript; methodology, B.C.F., R.C.R., M.A.D.P. and K.C.F.T.; supervision and visualization, B.C.F. and R.C.R.; writing—review and editing, B.C.F., R.C.R. and M.A.D.P. All authors have read and agreed to the published version of the manuscript.

Funding: This research received no external funding.

Institutional Review Board Statement: The study was conducted according to the guidelines of the Declaration of Helsinki, and approved by the Ethics Committee of Pequeno Príncipe Hospital and National Research Ethics Committee (CAAE number (Curitiba, Paraná state, Brazil, under the ethical codes CAA: 0023.0.208.000-05 (2005), CAAE 0612.0.015.000-08 (2009, 2012, and 2015).

Informed Consent Statement: Informed consent was obtained from all subjects involved in screening and surveillance [1,2]. Patient consent was waived for other types of data (staging, costs, age, sex, and duration of clinical signs before diagnosis).

Data Availability Statement: The datasets used during the current study are available from the corresponding authors upon request.

Acknowledgments: We would like to thank all the families that participated in the study. Raul C. Ribeiro is partially funded by NCI grant CA21765 and by the American Lebanese and Syrian Associated Charities (ALSAC). The content is solely the responsibility of the authors and does not necessarily represent the official views of the National Institutes of Health.

Conflicts of Interest: The authors declare no conflict of interest.

References

1. Custódio, G.; Parise, G.A.; Kiesel Filho, N.; Komechen, H.; Sabbaga, C.C.; Rosati, R.; Grisa, L.; Parise, I.Z.; Pianovski, M.A.; Fiori, C.M.; et al. Impact of Neonatal Screening and Surveillance for the TP53 R337H Mutation on Early Detection of Childhood Adrenocortical Tumors. *J. Clin. Oncol.* **2013**, *31*, 2619–2626. [CrossRef]
2. Costa, T.E.J.; Gerber, V.K.Q.; Ibañez, H.C.; Melanda, V.S.; Parise, I.Z.S.; Watanabe, F.M.; Pianovski, M.A.D.; Fiori, C.M.C.M.; Fabro, A.L.M.R.; Silva, D.B.D.; et al. Penetrance of the TP53 R337H Mutation and Pediatric Adrenocortical Carcinoma Incidence Associated with Environmental Influences in a 12-Year Observational Cohort in Southern Brazil. *Cancers* **2019**, *11*, 1804. [CrossRef]
3. Ribeiro, R.C.; Sandrini, F.; Figueiredo, B.; Zambetti, G.P.; Michalkiewicz, E.; Lafferty, A.R.; DeLacerda, L.; Rabin, M.; Cadwell, C.; Sampaio, G.; et al. An Inherited p53 Mutation That Contributes in a Tissue-Specific Manner to Pediatric Adrenal Cortical carcinoma 2001. *Proc. Natl. Acad. Sci. USA* **2001**, *98*, 9330–9335. [CrossRef]
4. Kerkhofs, T.M.; Ettaieb, M.H.; Verhoeven, R.H.; Kaspers, G.J.; Tissing, W.J.; Loeffen, J.; Van den Heuvel-Eibrink, M.M.; De Krijger, R.R.; Haak, H.R. Adrenocortical carcinoma in children: First population-based clinicopathological study with long-term follow-up. *Oncol. Rep.* **2014**, *32*, 2836–2844. [CrossRef]
5. McAteer, J.P.; Huaco, J.A.; Gow, K.W. Predictors of survival in pediatric adrenocortical carcinoma: A Surveillance, Epidemiology, and End Results (SEER) program study. *J. Pediatr. Surg.* **2013**, *48*, 1025–1031. [CrossRef]
6. Pinto, E.M.; Chen, X.; Easton, J.; Finkelstein, D.; Liu, Z.; Pounds, S.; Rodriguez-Galindo, C.; Lund, T.C.; Mardis, E.R.; Wilson, R.K.; et al. Genomic landscape of pediatric adrenocortical tumors. *Nat. Commun.* **2015**, *6*, 6302. [CrossRef]
7. Custodio, G.; Taques, G.R.; Figueiredo, B.C.; Gugelmin, E.S.; Oliveira Figueiredo, M.M.; Watanabe, F.; Pontarolo, R.; Lalli, E.; Torres, L.F. Increased Incidence of Choroid Plexus Carcinoma due to the Germline TP53 R337H Mutation in Southern Brazil. *PLoS ONE* **2011**, *6*, e18015. [CrossRef]

8. Howlader, N.; Noone, A.M.; Krapcho, M.; Brest, A.; Yu, M.; Ruhl, J.; Tatalovich, Z.; Mariotto, A.; Lewis, D.R.; Chen, H.S.; et al. *SEER Cancer Statistics Review, 1975–2017*; National Cancer Institute: Bethesda, MD, USA, 2020.
9. Seidinger, A.L.; Mastellaro, M.J.; Paschoal Fortes, F.; Godoy Assumpção, J.; Aparecida Cardinalli, I.; Aparecida Ganazza, M.; Correa Ribeiro, R.; Brandalise, S.R.; Dos Santos Aguiar, S.; Yunes, J.A. Association of the Highly Prevalent TP53 R337H Mutation with Pediatric Choroid Plexus Carcinoma and Osteosarcoma in Southeast Brazil. *Cancer* **2011**, *117*, 2228–2235. [CrossRef]
10. Mastellaro, M.J.; Seidinger, A.L.; Kang, G.; Abrahão, R.; Miranda, E.C.M.; Pounds, S.B.; Cardinalli, I.A.; Aguiar, S.S.; Figueiredo, B.C.; Rodriguez-Galindo, C.; et al. Contribution of the TP53 R337H mutation to the cancer burden in southern Brazil: Insights from the study of 55 families of children with adrenocortical tumors. *Cancer* **2017**, *123*, 3150–3158. [CrossRef]
11. Kumar, P.; Gill, R.M.; Phelps, A.; Tulpule, A.; Matthay, K.; Nicolaides, T. Surveillance Screening in Li-Fraumeni Syndrome: Raising Awareness of False Positives. *Cureus* **2018**, *10*, e2527. [CrossRef]
12. Lammens, C.R.; Aaronson, N.K.; Wagner, A.; Sijmons, R.H.; Ausems, M.G.; Vriends, A.H.; Ruijs, M.W.; van Os, T.A.; Spruijt, L.; Gómez García, E.B.; et al. Genetic testing in Li-Fraumeni syndrome: Uptake and psychosocial consequences. *J. Clin. Oncol.* **2010**, *28*, 3008–3014. [CrossRef]
13. Marigo, C.; Muller, H.; Davies, J.N.P. Survey of cancer in children admitted to a Brazilian charity hospital. *Natl. Cancer Inst.* **1969**, *43*, 1231–1240. [CrossRef]
14. Caminha, I.P. Prevalence of TP53 Germline Mutation p. R337H in the Metropolitan Region of Campinas and Surrounding Cities. Ph.D. Thesis, Universidade Estadual de Campinas, Campinas, Brazil, 2015.
15. Rodriguez-Galindo, C.; Figueiredo, B.C.; Zambetti, G.P.; Ribeiro, R.C. Biology, Clinical Characteristics, and Management of Adrenocortical Tumors in Children. *Pediatr. Blood Cancer* **2005**, *45*, 265–273. [CrossRef]
16. Berruti, A.; Terzolo, M.; Pia, A.; Angeli, A.; Dogliotti, L. Mitotane associated with etoposide, doxorubicin, and cisplatin in the treatment of advanced adrenocortical carcinoma. Italian Group for the Study of Adrenal Cancer. *Cancer* **1998**, *83*, 2194–2200. [CrossRef]
17. Zancanella, P.; Pianovski, M.A.; Oliveira, B.H.; Ferman, S.; Piovezan, G.C.; Lichtvan, L.L.; Voss, S.Z.; Stinghen, S.T.; Callefe, L.G.; Parise, G.A.; et al. Mitotane associated with cisplatin, etoposide, and doxorubicin in advanced childhood adrenocortical carcinoma: Mitotane monitoring and tumor regression. *J. Pediatr. Hematol. Oncol.* **2006**, *28*, 513–524. [CrossRef] [PubMed]
18. Rodriguez-Galindo, C.; Krailo, M.D.; Pinto, E.M.; Pashankar, F.; Weldon, C.B.; Huang, L.; Caran, E.M.; Hicks, J.; McCarville, M.B.; Malkin, D.; et al. Treatment of Pediatric Adrenocortical Carcinoma With Surgery, Retroperitoneal Lymph Node Dissection, and Chemotherapy: The Children's Oncology Group ARAR0332 Protocol. *J. Clin. Oncol.* **2021**, *39*, 2463–2473. [CrossRef]
19. Ministry of Health. Management System for Procedures, Drugs and Orthoses, Prostheses, and Special Materials of SUS 2020. Available online: http://sigtap.datasus.gov.br/tabela-unificada/app/sec/inicio.jsp (accessed on 3 October 2020).
20. National Health Surveillance Agency (ANVISA). 2020. Available online: https://www.gov.br/anvisa/pt-br/assuntos/medicamentos/cmed/precos/arquivos/lista-conformidade-2020-09 (accessed on 3 June 2021).
21. Kassambara, A.; Kosinski, M.; Biecek, P.; Fabian, S. Survminer: Drawing Survival Curves Using 'ggplot2'. R Package Version 0.4.9. 2021. Available online: https://CRAN.R-project.org/package=survminer (accessed on 4 June 2021).
22. Lenth, R.V. Emmeans: Estimated Marginal Means, aka Least-Squares Means. R Package Version 1.5.0. 2020. Available online: https://CRAN.R-project.org/package=emmeans (accessed on 4 June 2021).
23. R Core Team. *R: A Language and Environment for Statistical Computing*; R Foundation for Statistical Computing: Vienna, Austria, 2021.
24. Michalkiewicz, E.; Sandrini, R.; Figueiredo, B.; Miranda, E.C.; Caran, E.; Oliveira-Filho, A.G.; Marques, R.; Pianovski, M.A.; Lacerda, L.; Cristofani, L.M.; et al. Clinical and Outcome Characteristics of Children with Adrenocortical Tumors: A Report from the International Pediatric Adrenocortical Tumor Registry. *J. Clin. Oncol.* **2004**, *22*, 838–845. [CrossRef]
25. Doghman, M.; Karpova, T.; Rodrigues, G.A.; Arhatte, M.; De Moura, J.; Cavalli, L.R.; Virolle, V.; Barbry, P.; Zambetti, G.P.; Figueiredo, B.C.; et al. Increased Steroidogenic factor-1 Dosage Triggers Adrenocortical Cell Proliferation and Cancer. *Mol. Endocrinol.* **2007**, *21*, 2968–2987. [CrossRef]
26. Rosati, R.; Cerrato, F.; Doghman, M.; Pianovski, M.A.; Parise, G.A.; Custódio, G.; Zambetti, G.P.; Ribeiro, R.C.; Riccio, A.; Figueiredo, B.C.; et al. High Frequency of Loss of Heterozygosity at 11p15 and IGF2 Overexpression Are Not Related to Clinical Outcome in Childhood Adrenocortical Tumors Positive for the R337H TP53 Mutation. *Cancer Genet. Cytogenet.* **2008**, *186*, 19–24. [CrossRef] [PubMed]
27. Leal, L.F.; Mermejo, L.M.; Ramalho, L.Z.; Martinelli, C.E., Jr.; Yunes, J.A.; Seidinger, A.L.; Mastellaro, M.J.; Cardinalli, I.A.; Brandalise, S.R.; Moreira, A.C.; et al. Wnt/Beta-Catenin Pathway Deregulation in Childhood Adrenocortical Tumors. *J. Clin. Endocrinol. Metab.* **2011**, *96*, 3106–3114. [CrossRef]
28. Letouzé, E.; Rosati, R.; Komechen, H.; Doghman, M.; Marisa, L.; Flück, C.; de Krijger, R.R.; van Noesel, M.M.; Mas, J.C.; Pianovski, M.A.; et al. SNP array profiling of childhood adrenocortical tumors reveals distinct pathways of tumorigenesis and highlights candidate driver genes. *J. Clin. Endocrinol. Metab.* **2012**, *97*, 1284–1293. [CrossRef] [PubMed]
29. Parise, I.Z.S.; Parise, G.A.; Noronha, L.; Surakhy, M.; Woiski, T.D.; Silva, D.B.; Costa, T.E.B.; Del-Valle, M.H.C.P.; Komechen, H.; Rosati, R.; et al. The Prognostic Role of CD8+ T Lymphocytes in Childhood Adrenocortical Carcinomas Compared to Ki-67, PD-1, PD-L1, and the Weiss Score. *Cancers* **2019**, *11*, 1730. [CrossRef]
30. Sandrini, R.; Raul, R.; DeLacerda, L. Childhood Adrenocortical Tumors. *J. Clin. Endocrinol. Metab.* **1997**, *82*, 2027–2031. [CrossRef] [PubMed]

31. Figueiredo, B.C.; Sandrini, R.; Zambetti, G.P.; Pereira, R.M.; Cheng, C.; Liu, W.; Lacerda, L.; Pianovski, M.A.; Michalkiewicz, E.; Jenkins, J.; et al. Penetrance of Adrenocortical Tumours Associated with the Germline TP53 R337H Mutation. *J. Med. Genet.* **2006**, *43*, 91–96. [CrossRef] [PubMed]
32. Mai, P.L.; Best, A.F.; Peters, J.A.; DeCastro, R.; Khincha, P.P.; Loud, J.T.; Bremer, R.C.; Rosenberg, P.S.; Savage, S.A. Risks of first and subsequent cancers among TP53 mutation-carriers in the NCI LFS cohort. *Cancer* **2016**, *122*, 3673–3681. [CrossRef] [PubMed]
33. Wasserman, J.D.; Novokmet, A.; Eichler-Jonsson, C.; Ribeiro, R.C.; Rodriguez-Galindo, C.; Zambetti, G.P.; Malkin, D. Prevalence and Functional Consequence of TP53 Mutations in Pediatric Adrenocortical Carcinoma: A Children's Oncology Group Study. *J. Clin. Oncol.* **2015**, *33*, 602–609. [CrossRef]
34. Santacroce, S.J.; Tan, K.R.; Killela, M.K. A Systematic Scoping Review of the Recent Literature (~2011–2017) About the Costs of Illness to Parents of Children Diagnosed with Cancer. *Eur. J. Oncol. Nurs.* **2018**, *35*, 22–32. [CrossRef]
35. Grosse, S.D. Assessing cost-effectiveness in healthcare: History of the $50,000 per QALY threshold. *Expert Rev. Pharmacoecon. Outcomes Res.* **2008**, *8*, 165–178. [CrossRef]
36. Ross, L.F.; Saal, H.M.; David, K.L.; Anderson, R.R. American Academy of Pediatrics; American College of Medical Genetics and Genomics. Technical report: Ethical and policy issues in genetic testing and screening of children. *Gene Med.* **2013**, *15*, 234–245. [CrossRef] [PubMed]
37. Borry, P.; Goffin, T.; Nys, H.; Dierickx, K. Predictive genetic testing in minors for adult-onset genetic diseases. *Mt. Sinai J. Med.* **2008**, *75*, 287–296. [CrossRef]
38. Parker, M. Genetic testing in children and young people. *Fam. Cancer* **2010**, *9*, 15–18. [CrossRef] [PubMed]
39. Gilbar, R. Genetic testing of children for familial cancers: A comparative legal perspective on consent, communication of information, and confidentiality. *Fam. Cancer* **2010**, *9*, 75–87. [CrossRef] [PubMed]
40. Pinto, E.M.; Zambetti, G.P. What 20 years of research has taught us about the TP53 p.R337H mutation. *Cancer* **2020**, *126*, 4678–4686. [CrossRef] [PubMed]
41. Mathias, C.; Bortoletto, S.; Centa, A.; Komechen, H.; Lima, R.S.; Fonseca, A.S.; Sebastião, A.P.; Urban, C.A.; Soares, E.W.S.; Prando, C.; et al. Frequency of the TP53 R337H variant in sporadic breast cancer and its impact on genomic instability. *Sci. Rep.* **2020**, *10*, 16614. [CrossRef] [PubMed]
42. UNESCO. Records of the General Conference, 32nd Session, Paris, 29 September to 17 October, 2003, v. 1: Resolutions. International Declaration on Human Genetic Data Article 10—The Right to Decide Whether to be Informed about Research Results. Available online: https://unesdoc.unesco.org/ark:/48223/pf0000133171.page=45 (accessed on 17 November 2020).

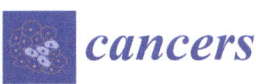

Review

Molecular Mechanisms of Mitotane Action in Adrenocortical Cancer Based on In Vitro Studies

Marco Lo Iacono, Soraya Puglisi *, Paola Perotti, Laura Saba, Jessica Petiti, Claudia Giachino, Giuseppe Reimondo † and Massimo Terzolo †

Department of Clinical and Biological Sciences, San Luigi Gonzaga Hospital, University of Turin, Orbassano, 10043 Turin, Italy; marco.loiacono@unito.it (M.L.I.); paola.perotti@unito.it (P.P.); laura.saba@unito.it (L.S.); jessica.petiti@unito.it (J.P.); claudia.giachino@unito.it (C.G.); giuseppe.reimondo@unito.it (G.R.); massimo.terzolo@unito.it (M.T.)
* Correspondence: soraya.puglisi@unito.it
† Joint senior author.

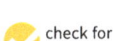

Citation: Lo Iacono, M.; Puglisi, S.; Perotti, P.; Saba, L.; Petiti, J.; Giachino, C.; Reimondo, G.; Terzolo, M. Molecular Mechanisms of Mitotane Action in Adrenocortical Cancer Based on In Vitro Studies. *Cancers* **2021**, *13*, 5255. https://doi.org/10.3390/cancers13215155

Academic Editors: Peter Igaz and Maurizio Iacobone

Received: 17 September 2021
Accepted: 16 October 2021
Published: 20 October 2021

Publisher's Note: MDPI stays neutral with regard to jurisdictional claims in published maps and institutional affiliations.

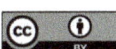

Copyright: © 2021 by the authors. Licensee MDPI, Basel, Switzerland. This article is an open access article distributed under the terms and conditions of the Creative Commons Attribution (CC BY) license (https://creativecommons.org/licenses/by/4.0/).

Simple Summary: Mitotane is the only approved drug for the treatment of advanced adrenocortical carcinoma and for postoperative adjuvant therapy. It is known that mitotane destroys the adrenal cortex impairing steroidogenesis, although its exact molecular mechanism is still unclear. However, confounding factors affecting in vitro experiments could reduce the relevance of the studies. In this review, we explore in vitro studies on mitotane effects, highlighting how different experimental conditions might contribute to the controversial findings. On this basis, it may be necessary to re-evaluate the experiments taking into account their potential confounding factors such as cell strains, culture serum, lipoprotein concentration, and culture passages, which could hide important molecular results. As a consequence, the identification of novel pharmacological molecular pathways might be used in the future to implement personalized therapy, maximizing the benefit of mitotane treatment while minimizing its toxicity.

Abstract: Mitotane is the only approved drug for the treatment of advanced adrenocortical carcinoma and is increasingly used for postoperative adjuvant therapy. Mitotane action involves the deregulation of cytochromes P450 enzymes, depolarization of mitochondrial membranes, and accumulation of free cholesterol, leading to cell death. Although it is known that mitotane destroys the adrenal cortex and impairs steroidogenesis, its exact mechanism of action is still unclear. The most used cell models are H295-derived cell strains and SW13 cell lines. The diverging results obtained in presumably identical cell lines highlight the need for a stable in vitro model and/or a standard methodology to perform experiments on H295 strains. The presence of several enzymatic targets responsive to mitotane in mitochondria and mitochondria-associated membranes causes progressive alteration in mitochondrial structure when cells were exposed to mitotane. Confounding factors of culture affecting in vitro experiments could reduce the significance of any molecular mechanism identified in vitro. To ensure experimental reproducibility, particular care should be taken in the choice of culture conditions: aspects such as cell strains, culture serum, lipoproteins concentration, and culture passages should be carefully considered and explicated in the presentation of results. We aimed to review in vitro studies on mitotane effects, highlighting how different experimental conditions might contribute to the controversial findings. If the concerns pointed out in this review will be overcome, the new insights into mitotane mechanism of action observed in-vitro could allow the identification of novel pharmacological molecular pathways to be used to implement personalized therapy.

Keywords: mitotane; adrenocortical carcinoma; H295 strains

1. Introduction

Mitotane, 1,1-(o,p′-Dichlorodiphenyl)-2,2-dichloroethane (o,p′-DDD), commercially available as Lysodren® (HRA Pharma Rare Diseases, Paris, France), is a parent compound of the insecticide dichlorodiphenyltrichloroethane (DDT). o,p′-DDD is metabolized by the mitochondria of adrenal cells in DDE (1,1-(o,p′-Dichlorodiphenyl)-2,2 dichloroethene) and DDA (1,1-(o,p′-Dichlorodiphenyl) acetic acid) through α-hydroxylation and β-hydroxylation, respectively. In addition, the unstable precursor of DDA, o,p′-dichlorodiphenyl acyl chloride (DDAC), obtained through cytochrome P540 (CYP450), could covalently bind to mitochondrial macromolecules of adrenal cells or can be metabolized by CYP2B6 in the liver or intestine, reducing its bioavailability [1]. Mitotane is the reference drug for the treatment of advanced adrenocortical carcinoma (ACC) either alone or in combination with chemotherapy [2,3] and is increasingly used for postoperative adjuvant therapy [1–5].

Although mitotane can exert its effects on the gonads and pituitary gland [6–9], it acts primarily on the adrenal cortex leading to cell destruction and impairment of steroidogenesis [10–12]. Indeed, mitotane produces dose-related cellular toxicity causing the rupture of mitochondrial membranes mainly on the zona fasciculata and reticularis, whereas a minimal effect on the zona glomerulosa has been observed [13]. This differential action explains why aldosterone secretion is less affected by mitotane treatment [14,15]. It is generally accepted that circulating levels of mitotane should be maintained between 14 and 20 mg/L (approximately 40–60 µM), the therapeutic window, to obtain the anti-tumoral effect while avoiding severe neurological toxicity [3,16]. Indeed, several retrospective analyzes have shown that mitotane blood concentrations $\geq$14 mg/L are associated with a disease response in both advanced and adjuvant ACC treatment [17–22]. The upper limits are more uncertain; in fact, central neurological toxicity has been more frequently associated with elevated mitotane concentrations (>20 mg/L), but mild symptoms can be observed even with lower plasma levels [17,23]. Studies, however, have suggested that inhibition of steroid secretion could be obtained even with lower mitotane levels [24,25]. Mitotane accumulates in lipoproteins and is stored in adipose tissue, although little is known about how this distribution affects its effectiveness [26].

Nevertheless, the mechanism of action of mitotane remains poorly defined at a molecular level due to controversial results generated by in vitro studies addressing its anticancer effect. Here, we will review these in vitro studies on mitotane action highlighting how different experimental conditions might contribute to the controversial results. Further elucidation of mitotane action after a reappraisal of the in vitro experimental conditions may contribute to the implementation of patient-tailored treatment.

2. In Vitro Cell Models of ACC

The need to develop appropriate cell models that mimic adrenal physiology or pathology has led to the development of different immortalized ACC cell lines because several issues have limited the use of primary adrenal cells as in vitro models. The most common limitations were (1) the need for fresh tissue, (2) the difficulty in isolating a sufficient number of cells with the adrenocortical phenotype, (3) the difficulty in identifying the cancerous lesions as either primary tumors or metastases from other organs, and (4) the great variability in clones obtained from different human donors, which make their comparison difficult. The variability of primary adrenal cells in terms of drug resistance, hormone production, and gene and protein expression has also recently been reported by van Koetsveld et al. [27]. To overcome these problems, many groups have attempted to establish cell lines from human ACCs, as previously reviewed by Tao Wang and William E. Rainey [28]. For this scope, cells derived from human ACCs were subsequently amplified in vitro with culture media supplemented with different serum additives. For the "in vitro" anti-cancer drugs' analysis, particularly for studies on mitotane, the most widely used cell models included H295-derived cell strains and SW13 cell lines.

In particular, the H295 cell line was established from a female patient with ACC whose tumor was extracted, defragmented, and maintained in culture media for one year [29]. The selected cells, called NCI-H295, appear to act as pluripotent adrenal cells capable of producing each of the zone-specific steroids [28]. The parental H295 has a poorly adherent phenotype and a relatively long population doubling time. To address this issue, alternative culture conditions and different commercial sera (Nu-Serum™ type 1, Ultroser™, and Cosmic Calf™ serum) were used to generate three H295R sub-strains. In comparison to the original H295 cell line, the H295R sub-strains showed a tightly adherent phenotype and a reduction in doubling time from five to two days [30]. Cell strains, culture medium, and passaging have a critical impact on the cellular response, growth rate, and steroid production [31,32]. Furthermore, the angiotensin II limited responder strain, H295A, was obtained with a similar strategy, removing nonattached cells during passaging. The H295 progenitor cell line produces more glucocorticoids compared with the H295R and H295A sub-strains, which produce more androgens and mineralocorticoids, respectively [28,31]. Furthermore, in 2008, it was demonstrated, by the SNP array analysis, that the HAC13 and the HAC15 cell lines were not ACC-independent cell models but were monoclonal sub-strains from H295R cells, probably isolated from a sample contaminated with this cell line [33].

The other in vitro human model often utilized in mitotane experiments is the SW13 cell line. These cells were isolated and amplified from a 55-year-old female with a small cell type carcinoma excised from the adrenal cortex [34]. Given their unusual histology and lack of steroidogenic potential, it is unclear whether SW13 cell lines are primary adrenocortical carcinoma or resulting from adrenal cortex metastases [28]. This latter scenario is also supported by studies showing that the SW13 cell model, unlike H295R cells, is responsive to a drug that is mainly effective on lung metastases [35]. Interestingly, mitotane does not appear to be effective on tumor cell lines that originated from the lung [36]. Despite the controversy about the SW13 origin, this cell line has often been used in studies on mitotane as the archetype of a mitotane-resistant cell line.

Recently, to increase the availability of ACC cell models in vitro, some protocols have been developed to extract cells from in vivo patient-derived tumor xenografts (PDTXs). PDTXs have been established for a wide range of cancer types maintaining the original tumor characteristics. However, these tumors often have low growth capacity, limiting the applicability of PDTXs in preclinical studies. This derived cell models could be useful to overtake this limitation [37,38]. The first adult ACC PDTX and the corresponding cell line MUC-1 were recently developed from a 24-year-old male patient with supraclavicular ACC metastasis by Hantel et al. MUC-1 cells maintain hormonal activity in vitro and, even after several passages, the specific phenotypic characteristics for ACC. Furthermore, MUC-1 cells appear to be resistant to routine drug treatment [37]. With a similar approach, Kiseljak-Vassiliades et al. generated two independent ACC cell models: CU-ACC1 and CU-ACC2 [38]. The CU-ACC1 models were derived from a 66-year-old patient who initially presented hypertension and hypokalemia, whereas CU-ACC2 models were developed by liver metastases from a 26-year-old patient with Lynch syndrome. CU-ACC1 and CU-ACC2 share some peculiar characteristics of progenitor tumors. In particular, CU-ACC1 possess a mutation in exon 3 of *CTNNB1* gene despite the allele frequency being higher than both patient-derived tumor and PDTX [38]. CU-ACC2 shares with the PDTX and the patient tumor a deletion of exons 1–6 in *MSH2* gene, which is a deletion often associated with Lynch syndrome [38].

All available ACC cell lines, in animals or humans, show a loss of function of the p53 protein. In particular, a large homozygous deletion of exons 8 and 9 in the *TP53* gene has been identified in cellular strains derived from H295, while a single nucleotide variant that alters the *TP53* coding sequence has been observed in SW13 [39]. MUC1 carry a frameshift deletion of one guanidine on *TP53* gene [37], while p.G245S protein mutation has been identified in CU-ACC2. Although its functional significance has not yet been elucidated, it could affect p53 DNA binding, which has also been reported in other adrenocortical carcinoma samples [38]. In contrast, mutations in *TP53* gene have not been identified in CU-ACC1, despite the drastically reduced p53 protein expression compared to the CU-ACC2 cell line [38]. This situation could partly explain the peculiar cell model characteristics, such as a reduction in corticosteroid production, an altered gene expression, and a different cell doubling time, observed by increasing the culture passages. In fact, it is plausible that the accumulation of mutations over time, favored by the p53 functional lack, leads to the development of different cellular subpopulations with altered drug resistance and/or with different steroidogenic potential [40].

3. Mitotane Effects on Mitochondrial Membrane and Gene Expression

Mitotane seems to act selectively on the adrenal cortex affecting steroidogenesis. This specificity for the adrenal cortex could be related to the massive presence in these cells of enzymes involved in steroidogenesis and/or cholesterol metabolism that could interact directly with mitotane (Figure 1). Indeed, mitotane shares characteristics with other endocrine disruptors and may affect steroidogenesis by binding to steroid receptors, mimicking the action of steroids [41]. A binding between mitotane and cytochrome P450 has been directly observed [42–44]. Interestingly, this interaction inhibits CYP11A1-mediated metabolic transformation regardless of the presence of the CYP11A1 substrate or its inhibitor. This result may indicate that either CYP11A1 is not the mitotane activator or that mitotane activation is not required to destroy CYP enzyme function. Indeed, the formation of adducts can affect the endogenous function of critical target proteins and thus directly causes toxicity or binds to non-essential proteins and thus constitutes an exposure biomarker [45]. Similar behavior was observed in murine corticosterone-producing Y1 cell line [42]. Furthermore, mitotane-induced protein adducts could also explain the altered transcriptomic profile, with varying degrees of post-translational modifications, identified by Stigliano et al. [12].

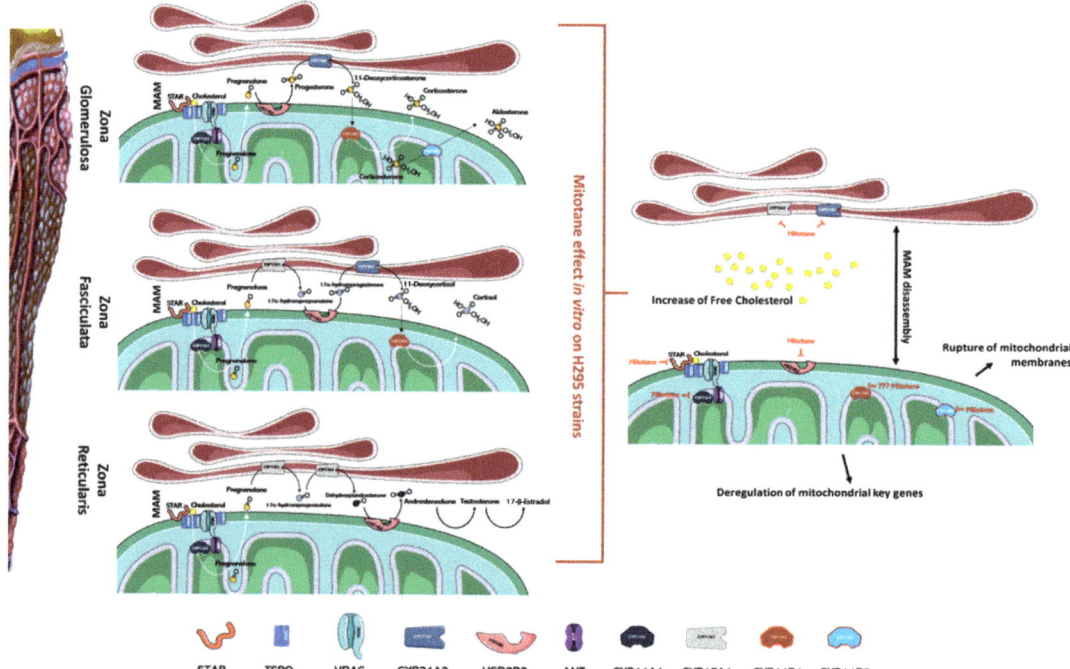

Figure 1. Mitotane impairs the function of the adrenal cortex. In the left part of the figure, the different zones of the adrenal cortex are schematized; the main enzymes involved in the biosynthesis of steroid hormones are also indicated. As depicted in the right part of figure, mitotane action, identified by in vitro experiments, involves several mechanisms ranging from the deregulation of mitochondrial key genes at a transcriptional and functional level, to the MAMs dissociation, the rupture of mitochondrial membranes, and altered cholesterol transports/metabolism. Mitotane action for each enzyme is indicated by a red mark. Figures have been created modifying an image set from Servier Medical Art (SMART) http://smart.servier.com/ (19 July 2021).

Several articles have reported that mitochondria are the organelles primarily involved in mitotane susceptibility in adrenal cells. This action involves several mechanisms ranging from the deregulation of mitochondrial key genes to the rupture of mitochondrial membranes (Figure 1). Mitotane affects mitochondrial enzymes at a transcriptional and functional level and significantly decreases the expression of the protein that transports cholesterol into mitochondria and of its related gene *STAR* [26,31,46]. Inside of mitochondria, cholesterol is converted to pregnenolone by CYP11A1 and, as indicated previously, mitotane mediates functional and transcriptional CYP11A1 inhibition [26,31,46–50]. Further, mitotane-related downregulation of steroidogenic enzymes *HSD3B2*, encoding for 3β-hydroxysteroid dehydrogenase/Δ5-4 isomerase, and *CYP21A2*, encoding for steroid 21-hydroxylase, was also observed [46,51]. Contrasting results were obtained for the *CYP11B1* gene, encoding for the enzyme 11b-hydroxylase, which catalyzes the transformation of 11-deoxycorticosterone and 11-deoxycortisol into corticosterone and cortisol, respectively [31,51–54]. As for CYP11A1, the CYP11B1 enzyme has also been indicated as an activator of mitotane, but much experimental evidence may suggest that its involvement is not essential in mitotane-induced mitochondrial dysfunction: (1) mitotane interacts with CYP11B1, creating an irreversible bond and decreasing both cortisol and aldosterone secretion in a concentration-dependent manner, yet metyrapone, a known inhibitor of CYP11B1, is unable to modify mitotane-induced effects [1,42]; (2) cells that do not express CYP11B1, or cells that express it, are likewise affected by treatment with mitotane [51]; (3) CYP11B1 modulation in H295R cells, by either chemical or molecular inhibition, is not able to affect mitotane action [54]. At the transcriptional level, depending on the model cell line in the study and/or experimental conditions, *CYP11B1* was observed as either downmodulated [51,53,54] or upmodulated by mitotane treatment [31,52]. To complete the intra-mitochondrial aldosterone synthesis, the enzyme aldosterone synthase, codified by the *CYP11B2* gene, was transcriptionally inhibited by mitotane in vitro [51]. All these enzyme inhibitions, mediated by mitotane, generate mitochondrial dysfunction that correlates with alterations in the ATP/ADP ratio, which is a critical factor to control nuclear gene expression.

SF-1 protein, identified independently by two laboratories in 1992, is the major nuclear factor that determines the cell-specific expression of P450 steroidogenic enzymes in gonads and adrenal glands [55,56]. SF1 activates adenylate cyclase by acting via G protein-coupled receptors, such as ACTH, and thereby increasing cAMP levels. The cAMP response elements (CRE) present in the proximal promoter of all P450 steroidogenic enzymes respond to increased cAMP levels by initiating the synthesis of P450 steroidogenic enzymes. Mitotane blocks the ACTH/cAMP-related signaling, although contrasting results due to specific human cell models have been observed. In particular, H295A are non-responsive, whereas H295R respond to this hormone depending on subclones and culture conditions [28]. The response of the H295 progenitor cell line is not so clear; it is often indicated as ACTH-unresponsive [28] but probably follows the same behavior of H295R cells. Indeed, Lin et al. showed that H295 responds to increasing ACTH concentration by increasing cortisol secretion and that mitotane was able to completely abolish this response [31].

Mitotane could also affect the angiotensin II/K+ related signaling principally responsible for CYP11B2 transcription. All H295R strains, including the subclone HAC15, respond to this molecular signaling pathway, in contrast to H295A, which are selected as not responder cells. No indication of angiotensin II/K+ signaling was obtained for the H295 progenitor cell line [28]. Although all studies agree on the blocking action of mitotane on corticosteroid synthesis, conflicting results in molecular pathways and in the deregulation of specific genes or enzymes could support the hypothesis that specific cell line characteristics and variable experimental conditions have an important impact on mitotane action and should be carefully considered for a meaningful assessment of in vitro studies on mitotane.

4. Physiological Regulation of Cholesterol Uptake, Synthesis, and Steroidogenesis and the Proposed Mitotane Effect/Mechanism of Action

Mitochondria-associated membranes (MAM) are reversible contact points between the mitochondria and the endoplasmic reticulum (ER) membrane and are involved in the mitochondrial import of certain lipids, such as cholesterol. The presence of several enzymatic targets responsive to mitotane in mitochondria and MAM caused a progressive alteration in mitochondrial structure and the number of normal mitochondria when H295R were exposed to mitotane (Figures 1 and 2). In addition, a more punctiform pattern, as a sign of mitochondrial fragmentation, was frequently observed [51,57]. Further, mitotane exposure alters the MAM integrity, reducing the interactions between mitochondria and ER in H295R [49]. These results could be related to a progressive depolarization of the mitochondrial membrane, also due to the functional block of COX enzymes, with consequent interruption of the respiratory system and MAM disassembly [49,51]. Sterol O-acyltransferase enzymes, SOAT1 and SOAT2, are located within MAM and catalyze cholesteryl esters formation from cholesterol. Sbiera et al. identified SOAT1 as the key molecular target of mitotane and showed a correlation between SOAT1 expression and the outcome of adjuvant mitotane treatment [58], whereas Lacombe et al. found that SOAT1 expression is a prognostic marker in combination with the Ki67 index [59]. Unfortunately, the hypothesis that SOAT1 expression could be a clinically useful marker for predicting treatment response to mitotane has not been confirmed by further studies [27,60]. Weigand et al. retrospectively analyzed data of 231 patients with ACC treated with mitotane in 12 reference centers and did not find any significant differences between tumors with high or low SOAT1 expression in terms of recurrence-free survival (in 158 patients treated with adjuvant mitotane), progression-free survival (in 73 patients with advanced ACC), or disease-specific survival (in both settings) [60].

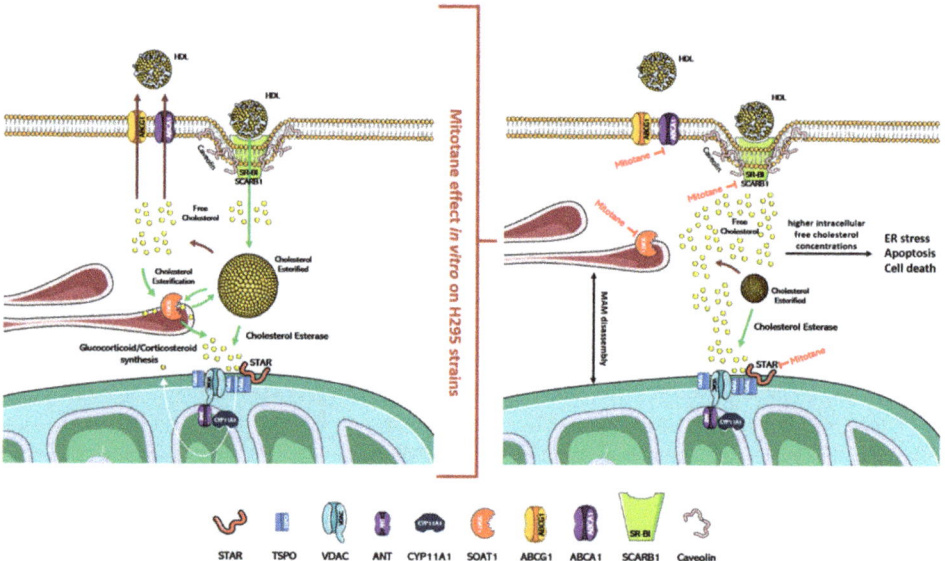

Figure 2. Physiological regulation of cholesterol uptake, synthesis, and steroidogenesis and proposed mitotane effect/mechanism of action. In the left part of the figure is indicated the physiological mechanism that regulates the absorption/synthesis of cholesterol and steroidogenesis. As depicted in the right part of the figure, mitotane induces in vitro the dissociation of MAMs and the blockade of cholesterol transport/synthesis and steroidogenesis. Accumulation of free cholesterol in cells causes ER stress, apoptosis, and cell death. The action of mitotane for each enzyme is indicated by a red mark. Figures were created modifying an image set from SMART http://smart.servier.com/ (19 July 2021).

In vitro, mitotane induces ER stress through inhibition of SOAT1, which leads to the blockade of cholesterol synthesis and steroidogenesis, and this accumulation of free cholesterol rapidly becomes toxic to the cells (Figure 2) [58,61]. Furthermore, mitotane in H295R subclones reduces the expression of ABCA1, which is involved in the cellular efflux of cholesterol [62], and of *SCARB1*, which encodes for scavenger receptor B1 (SR-BI), the most important transporter for adrenal cholesterol uptake [46,63]. The adrenal cortex has critical enzymes and substrates necessary for ferroptosis, a form of iron-dependent cell death associated with increased lipid peroxidation. Curiously, despite the strong induction of lipid peroxidation, mitotane does not induce ferroptosis [64,65]. Since mitotane increases free cholesterol in cells and oxysterols, such as 27-hydroxycholesterol, which could reduce this process [66], the cholesterol metabolism could be an interesting druggable pathway to counteract mitotane resistance in ACC. On these bases, the introduction of LXRα and PCSK9 inhibitors as future therapeutic approaches could be a promising tool to reduce mitotane resistance and/or to optimize its therapeutic dose [46,66]. In the adrenal gland, the role of LXRα and its oxysterol ligands are critically important in the fine regulation of cholesterol efflux since the excess free cholesterol in cells is converted into oxysterols through the action of enzymes, such as CYP27A1. Pharmacological inhibition of LXRα significantly reduces the expression of the cholesterol efflux pump (ABCA1 and ABCG1) and is accompanied by higher intracellular free cholesterol concentrations, ER stress, apoptosis, and cell death markers expression. This effect is complementary to mitotane-induced lipotoxicity, and, using a combined therapeutic approach, lower doses of mitotane can be expected to be used, resulting in reduced toxicity [66].

5. Culture Conditions and Mitotane Cytotoxicity: A Need for Reappraisal

The close relationship between cholesterol and mitotane's chemical structure could also justify the conflicting results obtained in the last decade in evaluating the effect of mitotane in vitro. Since the creation of the original H295 strain, several laboratories have explored the cytotoxic ability of mitotane with mixed success. The IC50 of mitotane, at different time intervals, in the H295 and H295R subclones ranged from the therapeutic dose of about 40–60 μM up to over 100–200 μM (the most relevant experimental conditions are summarized in Table 1). Intriguingly, the work of Hescot et al. seems to throw light on this question by identifying an opposite correlation between the effect mediated by mitotane and the lipoprotein concentration in culture media. In particular, mitotane was more efficient in exerting its toxic effect when cells were grown in a lipoprotein-free medium, indicating that HDL and LDL sequester mitotane, reducing its actions. Furthermore, a similar blocking effect was also observed for bovine serum albumin (BSA) [26]. Lipoproteins and BSA are the most abundant proteins in culture serum, and, except for Lin et al. who used an uncommon medium, there seems to be an opposite relationship between mitotane effect and serum concentration of these proteins in culture media (Table 1). This hypothesis was apparently also confirmed by other authors, who observed that mitotane action was strongly influenced by the culture conditions, the sub-strain selected, and the growth under different serum conditions [32,46,62]. Note that most ACC cell models, such as SW13, MUC1, CU-ACC1, and ACC2, reported in vitro as more resistant to mitotane respect H295 cell strains, which are maintained in high serum/BSA conditions (5–10% FBS) [64–67]. Intriguingly, mitotane treatment in patients induces hypercholesterolemia via an incompletely understood mechanism that also increases lipoproteins synthesis. This effect is of particular importance as it could potentially self-promote drug resistance [1,26]. On this basis, several in vitro and clinical studies were recently conducted to evaluate how to counteract resistance to mitotane by lowering lipoprotein levels through, for example, statins or PCSK9 inhibitors [61,62,68]. In a recent clinical case, the strategy of targeting the PCSK9 gene [68], which encodes an enzyme expressed mainly in the liver and intestine with an important role in lipid metabolism, was reported. PCSK9 binds to the LDL receptor favoring its degradation with the effect of increasing circulating LDL. Therefore, the inhibition of PCSK9 by monoclonal antibodies leads to an increase in the levels of LDL receptors in the cell surface that bind LDL particles and thus circulating LDL is decreased. Tsakiridou et al. reported the case of a patient with drug-resistant hypercholesterolemia induced by mitotane, in which the administration of evolocumab, a PCSK9 inhibitor, led to a reduction in circulating LDL levels by 36%. This effect allowed to increase the dose of mitotane and to reach therapeutic plasma levels. These data indicate that treatment with PCSK9 inhibitors should be considered in patients who develop mitotane-related hypercholesterolemia that cannot be managed with conventional lipid-lowering treatment [68].

Table 1. Mitotane cytotoxicity and in vitro culture conditions.

Author	Year	IC50 (µM)	Serum in Experimental Conditions
Chia-Wen Lin [31]	2012	Cell viability not significantly affected by 5–40 µM for 24 h, or 48 µM for 72 h	RPMI1640 supplemented with hydrocortisol (10 pM), β-estradiol (10 pM), no serum in experiments
Poli [57]	2013	10–20 µM (72–48 h)	1% FBS for all the experiments (10% FBS in culture)
Doghman [69]	2013	22.8 µM (144 h)	2% Nu-Serum^{TM}
Zsippai [41]	2012	10–100 µM (72–48 h)	2.5% Nu-Serum^{TM}
Germano [70]	2015	30.6 µM (72 h)	2.5% Nu-Serum^{TM}
Germano [67]	2014	30.62 µM (72 h)	2.5% Nu-Serum^{TM}
Sbiera [58]	2015	18.1 µM (24 h)	2.5% FCS (by article doi:10.3389/fendo.2011.00027)
Hescot [26]	2015	40 µM (lipoprotein-free medium) 140 µM (control lipoprotein conditions)	Different experimental conditions [10% FCS in culture]
Hescot [51]	2013	100 µM (45% of cells dead at 48 h)	10% FBS
Hescot [53]	2014	100 µM (48 h) (95% inhibition when treated with 200 and 300 µM)	10% FBS
Boulate [62]	2019	50 µM did not affect cell viability (24–48 h)	10% FBS
Goyzueta Mamani [71]	2021	20–50 µM did not affect cell viability (24 h)	10% FBS

6. Conclusions

This review collected several in vitro studies assessing the mechanisms of mitotane action and pointed out the search for new molecular pathways that could define mitotane sensitivity. Mitotane appears to act selectively on the adrenal cortex by influencing steroidogenesis. Several molecular mechanisms have been identified in vitro and involve: deregulation of key mitochondrial genes, such as those encoding the P450 family of cytochromes, both at the transcriptional and functional level; depolarization and rupture of mitochondrial membranes; reduction in interactions between mitochondria and endoplasmic reticulum by altering the integrity of MAMs; reduction in the expression of proteins, such as STAR and SOAT1, involved in cellular uptake and cholesterol metabolism leading to the accumulation of free cholesterol and cell death. The divergent results obtained in presumably identical cell lines highlight the need for a stable in vitro model and/or a standard methodology to perform experiments on H295 strains. To ensure experimental reproducibility, particular care should be given to the choice of culture conditions: aspects such as cell strains, culture serum, lipoproteins and BSA concentration, and culture passages should be carefully considered and explicated in the presentation of results. Specific attention should be paid to the use of fetal bovine serum (FBS) or fetal calf serum (FCS) during cell culture as they represent poorly defined supplements and, therefore, unpredictable experimental variability factors. Indeed, different serum lots show quantitative and qualitative composition variations, and this variability introduces a possible confounder making the experiments difficult to reproduce [72]. In light of these considerations, it might be necessary to re-evaluate the experiments on mitotane to clean them of any confounding factors that could hide important molecular findings. In addition to that, another important aspect to evaluate is the heterogeneity of ACC tumors. This scenario stimulates scientists to create different ACC cell lines to have multiple models resembling variability observed in patients. The concept is fundamental to explain mechanisms of drug resistance that could be subsequentially evaluate in patients; however, it is mandatory that cell line experiments be conducted in a neutral milieu, where only the genetic/molecular characteristics of the model may influence the results, in the absence of other confounding factors. Molecular characterization of ACC achieved using in vitro experiments is a powerful tool that expands knowledge in mitotane molecular mechanism. If these concerns are overcome in future, the new insights into mitotane mechanism of action could allow the identification of novel pharmacological molecular pathways to be used to implement personalized therapy, maximizing the benefit of mitotane treatment and minimizing its toxicity.

Author Contributions: M.L.I. and S.P. searched for the literature and wrote the first draft; P.P., L.S., J.P., C.G., G.R. and M.T. reviewed and edited the manuscript; supervision was performed by G.R. and M.T. All authors have read and agreed to the published version of the manuscript.

Funding: This research was funded by Associazione Italiana per la Ricerca sul Cancro, grant number IG2019-23069 to Massimo Terzolo.

Conflicts of Interest: S.P. received a grant for scientific writing from HRA Pharma; M.T. received research grants from HRA Pharma and advisory board honoraria from HRA Pharma and Corcept Therapeutics; the other authors stated explicitly that there are no conflicts of interest in connection with this article. The funders had no role in the design of the study; in the collection, analyses, or interpretation of data; in the writing of the manuscript; or in the decision to publish the results.

References

1. Corso, C.R.; Acco, A.; Bach, C.; Bonatto, S.J.R.; de Figueiredo, B.C.; de Souza, L.M. Pharmacological profile and effects of mitotane in adrenocortical carcinoma. *Br. J. Clin. Pharmacol.* **2021**, *87*, 2698–2710. [CrossRef] [PubMed]
2. Fassnacht, M.; Terzolo, M.; Allolio, B.; Baudin, E.; Haak, H.; Berruti, A.; Welin, S.; Schade-Brittinger, C.; Lacroix, A.; Jarzab, B.; et al. Combination chemotherapy in advanced adrenocortical carcinoma. *N. Engl. J. Med.* **2012**, *366*, 2189–2197. [CrossRef] [PubMed]
3. Puglisi, S.; Calabrese, A.; Basile, V.; Pia, A.; Reimondo, G.; Perotti, P.; Terzolo, M. New perspectives for mitotane treatment of adrenocortical carcinoma. *Best Pract. Res. Clin. Endocrinol. Metab.* **2020**, *34*, 101415. [CrossRef] [PubMed]
4. Terzolo, M.; Zaggia, B.; Allasino, B.; De Francia, S. Practical treatment using mitotane for adrenocortical carcinoma. *Curr. Opin. Endocrinol. Diabetes Obes.* **2014**, *21*, 159–165. [CrossRef] [PubMed]
5. Bedrose, S.; Daher, M.; Altameemi, L.; Habra, M.A. Adjuvant Therapy in Adrenocortical Carcinoma: Reflections and Future Directions. *Cancers* **2020**, *12*, 508. [CrossRef] [PubMed]
6. Gentilin, E.; Tagliati, F.; Terzolo, M.; Zoli, M.; Lapparelli, M.; Minoia, M.; Ambrosio, M.R.; Degli Uberti, E.C.; Zatelli, M.C. Mitotane reduces human and mouse ACTH-secreting pituitary cell viability and function. *J. Endocrinol.* **2013**, *218*, 275–285. [CrossRef]
7. Reimondo, G.; Puglisi, S.; Zaggia, B.; Basile, V.; Saba, L.; Perotti, P.; De Francia, S.; Volante, M.; Zatelli, M.C.; Cannavo, S.; et al. Effects of mitotane on the hypothalamic-pituitary-adrenal axis in patients with adrenocortical carcinoma. *Eur. J. Endocrinol.* **2017**, *177*, 361–367. [CrossRef] [PubMed]
8. Innocenti, F.; Cerquetti, L.; Pezzilli, S.; Bucci, B.; Toscano, V.; Canipari, R.; Stigliano, A. Effect of mitotane on mouse ovarian follicle development and fertility. *J. Endocrinol.* **2017**, *234*, 29–39. [CrossRef]
9. Chortis, V.; Johal, N.J.; Bancos, I.; Evans, M.; Skordilis, K.; Guest, P.; Cullen, M.H.; Porfiri, E.; Arlt, W. Mitotane treatment in patients with metastatic testicular Leydig cell tumor associated with severe androgen excess. *Eur. J. Endocrinol.* **2018**, *178*, K21–K27. [CrossRef]
10. Fang, V.S. Cytotoxic activity of 1-(o-chlorophenyl)-1-(p-chlorophenyl)-2,2-dichloroethane (mitotane) and its analogs on feminizing adrenal neoplastic cells in culture. *Cancer Res.* **1979**, *39*, 139–145.
11. Martz, F.; Straw, J.A. Metabolism and covalent binding of 1-(o-chlorophenyl)-1-(p-chlorophenyl)-2,2-dichloroethane (o,p,'-DDD). Correlation between adrenocorticolytic activity and metabolic activation by adrenocortical mitochondria. *Drug Metab. Dispos.* **1980**, *8*, 127–130.
12. Stigliano, A.; Cerquetti, L.; Borro, M.; Gentile, G.; Bucci, B.; Misiti, S.; Piergrossi, P.; Brunetti, E.; Simmaco, M.; Toscano, V. Modulation of proteomic profile in H295R adrenocortical cell line induced by mitotane. *Endocr. Relat. Cancer* **2008**, *15*, 1–10. [CrossRef] [PubMed]

13. Hart, M.M.; Reagan, R.L.; Adamson, R.H. The effect of isomers of DDD on the ACTH-induced steroid output, histology and ultrastructure of the dog adrenal cortex. *Toxicol. Appl. Pharmacol.* **1973**, *24*, 101–113. [CrossRef]
14. Daffara, F.; De Francia, S.; Reimondo, G.; Zaggia, B.; Aroasio, E.; Porpiglia, F.; Volante, M.; Termine, A.; Di Carlo, F.; Dogliotti, L.; et al. Prospective evaluation of mitotane toxicity in adrenocortical cancer patients treated adjuvantly. *Endocr. Relat. Cancer* **2008**, *15*, 1043–1053. [CrossRef]
15. Basile, V.; Puglisi, S.; Calabrese, A.; Pia, A.; Perotti, P.; Berruti, A.; Reimondo, G.; Terzolo, M. Unwanted Hormonal and Metabolic Effects of Postoperative Adjuvant Mitotane Treatment for Adrenocortical Cancer. *Cancers* **2020**, *12*, 2615. [CrossRef]
16. Fassnacht, M.; Dekkers, O.M.; Else, T.; Baudin, E.; Berruti, A.; de Krijger, R.; Haak, H.R.; Mihai, R.; Assie, G.; Terzolo, M. European Society of Endocrinology Clinical Practice Guidelines on the management of adrenocortical carcinoma in adults, in collaboration with the European Network for the Study of Adrenal Tumors. *Eur. J. Endocrinol.* **2018**, *179*, G1–G46. [CrossRef] [PubMed]
17. Baudin, E.; Leboulleux, S.; Al Ghuzlan, A.; Chougnet, C.; Young, J.; Deandreis, D.; Dumont, F.; Dechamps, F.; Caramella, C.; Chanson, P.; et al. Therapeutic management of advanced adrenocortical carcinoma: What do we know in 2011? *Horm. Cancer* **2011**, *2*, 363–371. [CrossRef] [PubMed]
18. Haak, H.R.; Hermans, J.; van de Velde, C.J.; Lentjes, E.G.; Goslings, B.M.; Fleuren, G.J.; Krans, H.M. Optimal treatment of adrenocortical carcinoma with mitotane: Results in a consecutive series of 96 patients. *Br. J. Cancer* **1994**, *69*, 947–951. [CrossRef]
19. Hermsen, I.G.; Fassnacht, M.; Terzolo, M.; Houterman, S.; den Hartigh, J.; Leboulleux, S.; Daffara, F.; Berruti, A.; Chadarevian, R.; Schlumberger, M.; et al. Plasma concentrations of o,p′DDD, o,p′DDA, and o,p′DDE as predictors of tumor response to mitotane in adrenocortical carcinoma: Results of a retrospective ENS@T multicenter study. *J. Clin. Endocrinol. Metab.* **2011**, *96*, 1844–1851. [CrossRef]
20. Megerle, F.; Herrmann, W.; Schloetelburg, W.; Ronchi, C.L.; Pulzer, A.; Quinkler, M.; Beuschlein, F.; Hahner, S.; Kroiss, M.; Fassnacht, M.; et al. Mitotane Monotherapy in Patients With Advanced Adrenocortical Carcinoma. *J. Clin. Endocrinol. Metab.* **2018**, *103*, 1686–1695. [CrossRef]
21. Terzolo, M.; Baudin, A.E.; Ardito, A.; Kroiss, M.; Leboulleux, S.; Daffara, F.; Perotti, P.; Feelders, R.A.; deVries, J.H.; Zaggia, B.; et al. Mitotane levels predict the outcome of patients with adrenocortical carcinoma treated adjuvantly following radical resection. *Eur. J. Endocrinol.* **2013**, *169*, 263–270. [CrossRef]
22. Puglisi, S.; Calabrese, A.; Basile, V.; Ceccato, F.; Scaroni, C.; Altieri, B.; Della Casa, S.; Loli, P.; Pivonello, R.; De Martino, M.C.; et al. Mitotane Concentrations Influence Outcome in Patients with Advanced Adrenocortical Carcinoma. *Cancers* **2020**, *12*, 740. [CrossRef] [PubMed]
23. Kasperlik-Zaluska, A.A. Clinical results of the use of mitotane for adrenocortical carcinoma. *Braz. J. Med. Biol. Res.* **2000**, *33*, 1191–1196. [CrossRef] [PubMed]
24. Puglisi, S.; Perotti, P.; Pia, A.; Reimondo, G.; Terzolo, M. Adrenocortical Carcinoma with Hypercortisolism. *Endocrinol. Metab. Clin. N. Am.* **2018**, *47*, 395–407. [CrossRef]
25. Tritos, N.A. Adrenally Directed Medical Therapies for Cushing Syndrome. *J. Clin. Endocrinol. Metab.* **2021**, *106*, 16–25. [CrossRef]
26. Hescot, S.; Seck, A.; Guerin, M.; Cockenpot, F.; Huby, T.; Broutin, S.; Young, J.; Paci, A.; Baudin, E.; Lombes, M. Lipoprotein-Free Mitotane Exerts High Cytotoxic Activity in Adrenocortical Carcinoma. *J. Clin. Endocrinol. Metab.* **2015**, *100*, 2890–2898. [CrossRef] [PubMed]
27. Van Koetsveld, P.M.; Creemers, S.G.; Dogan, F.; Franssen, G.J.H.; de Herder, W.W.; Feelders, R.A.; Hofland, L.J. The Efficacy of Mitotane in Human Primary Adrenocortical Carcinoma Cultures. *J. Clin. Endocrinol. Metab.* **2020**, *105*, 407–417. [CrossRef]
28. Wang, T.; Rainey, W.E. Human adrenocortical carcinoma cell lines. *Mol. Cell Endocrinol.* **2012**, *351*, 58–65. [CrossRef]
29. Gazdar, A.F.; Oie, H.K.; Shackleton, C.H.; Chen, T.R.; Triche, T.J.; Myers, C.E.; Chrousos, G.P.; Brennan, M.F.; Stein, C.A.; La Rocca, R.V. Establishment and characterization of a human adrenocortical carcinoma cell line that expresses multiple pathways of steroid biosynthesis. *Cancer Res.* **1990**, *50*, 5488–5496.
30. Rainey, W.E.; Saner, K.; Schimmer, B.P. Adrenocortical cell lines. *Mol. Cell Endocrinol.* **2004**, *228*, 23–38. [CrossRef]
31. Lin, C.W.; Chang, Y.H.; Pu, H.F. Mitotane exhibits dual effects on steroidogenic enzymes gene transcription under basal and cAMP-stimulating microenvironments in NCI-H295 cells. *Toxicology* **2012**, *298*, 14–23. [CrossRef] [PubMed]
32. Kurlbaum, M.; Sbiera, S.; Kendl, S.; Martin Fassnacht, M.; Kroiss, M. Steroidogenesis in the NCI-H295 Cell Line Model is Strongly Affected By Culture Conditions and Substrain. *Exp. Clin. Endocrinol. Diabetes* **2020**, *128*, 672–680. [CrossRef] [PubMed]
33. Parmar, J.; Key, R.E.; Rainey, W.E. Development of an adrenocorticotropin-responsive human adrenocortical carcinoma cell line. *J. Clin. Endocrinol. Metab.* **2008**, *93*, 4542–4546. [CrossRef] [PubMed]
34. Leibovitz, A.; McCombs, W.M., 3rd; Johnston, D.; McCoy, C.E.; Stinson, J.C. New human cancer cell culture lines. I. SW-13, small-cell carcinoma of the adrenal cortex. *J. Natl. Cancer Inst.* **1973**, *51*, 691–697. [PubMed]
35. Pezzani, R.; Rubin, B.; Bertazza, L.; Redaelli, M.; Barollo, S.; Monticelli, H.; Baldini, E.; Mian, C.; Mucignat, C.; Scaroni, C.; et al. The aurora kinase inhibitor VX-680 shows anti-cancer effects in primary metastatic cells and the SW13 cell line. *Investig. New Drugs* **2016**, *34*, 531–540. [CrossRef] [PubMed]
36. Volante, M.; Terzolo, M.; Fassnacht, M.; Rapa, I.; Germano, A.; Sbiera, S.; Daffara, F.; Sperone, P.; Scagliotti, G.; Allolio, B.; et al. Ribonucleotide reductase large subunit (RRM1) gene expression may predict efficacy of adjuvant mitotane in adrenocortical cancer. *Clin. Cancer Res.* **2012**, *18*, 3452–3461. [CrossRef] [PubMed]

37. Hantel, C.; Shapiro, I.; Poli, G.; Chiapponi, C.; Bidlingmaier, M.; Reincke, M.; Luconi, M.; Jung, S.; Beuschlein, F. Targeting heterogeneity of adrenocortical carcinoma: Evaluation and extension of preclinical tumor models to improve clinical translation. *Oncotarget* **2016**, *7*, 79292–79304. [CrossRef]
38. Kiseljak-Vassiliades, K.; Zhang, Y.; Bagby, S.M.; Kar, A.; Pozdeyev, N.; Xu, M.; Gowan, K.; Sharma, V.; Raeburn, C.D.; Albuja-Cruz, M.; et al. Development of new preclinical models to advance adrenocortical carcinoma research. *Endocr. Relat. Cancer* **2018**, *25*, 437–451. [CrossRef] [PubMed]
39. Nicolson, N.G.; Korah, R.; Carling, T. Adrenocortical cancer cell line mutational profile reveals aggressive genetic background. *J. Mol. Endocrinol.* **2019**, *62*, 179–186. [CrossRef]
40. Landwehr, L.S.; Schreiner, J.; Appenzeller, S.; Kircher, S.; Herterich, S.; Sbiera, S.; Fassnacht, M.; Kroiss, M.; Weigand, I. A novel patient-derived cell line of adrenocortical carcinoma shows a pathogenic role of germline MUTYH mutation and high tumour mutational burden. *Eur. J. Endocrinol.* **2021**, *184*, 823–835. [CrossRef] [PubMed]
41. Zsippai, A.; Szabo, D.R.; Tombol, Z.; Szabo, P.M.; Eder, K.; Pallinger, E.; Gaillard, R.C.; Patocs, A.; Toth, S.; Falus, A.; et al. Effects of mitotane on gene expression in the adrenocortical cell line NCI-H295R: A microarray study. *Pharmacogenomics* **2012**, *13*, 1351–1361. [CrossRef] [PubMed]
42. Hermansson, V.; Asp, V.; Bergman, A.; Bergstrom, U.; Brandt, I. Comparative CYP-dependent binding of the adrenocortical toxicants 3-methylsulfonyl-DDE and o,p′-DDD in Y-1 adrenal cells. *Arch. Toxicol.* **2007**, *81*, 793–801. [CrossRef] [PubMed]
43. Martz, F.; Straw, J.A. The in vitro metabolism of 1-(o-chlorophenyl)-1-(p-chlorophenyl)-2,2-dichloroethane (o,p′-DDD) by dog adrenal mitochondria and metabolite covalent binding to mitochondrial macromolecules: A possible mechanism for the adrenocorticolytic effect. *Drug Metab. Dispos.* **1977**, *5*, 482–486.
44. Cai, W.; Benitez, R.; Counsell, R.E.; Djanegara, T.; Schteingart, D.E.; Sinsheimer, J.E.; Wotring, L.L. Bovine adrenal cortex transformations of mitotane [1-(2-chlorophenyl)-1-(4-chlorophenyl)-2,2-dichloroethane; o,p′-DDD] and its p,p′- and m,p′-isomers. *Biochem. Pharmacol.* **1995**, *49*, 1483–1489. [CrossRef]
45. Cohen, S.D.; Pumford, N.R.; Khairallah, E.A.; Boekelheide, K.; Pohl, L.R.; Amouzadeh, H.R.; Hinson, J.A. Selective protein covalent binding and target organ toxicity. *Toxicol. Appl. Pharmacol.* **1997**, *143*, 1–12. [CrossRef] [PubMed]
46. Seidel, E.; Walenda, G.; Messerschmidt, C.; Obermayer, B.; Peitzsch, M.; Wallace, P.; Bahethi, R.; Yoo, T.; Choi, M.; Schrade, P.; et al. Generation and characterization of a mitotane-resistant adrenocortical cell line. *Endocr. Connect.* **2020**, *9*, 122–134. [CrossRef]
47. Hart, M.M.; Straw, J.A. Studies on the site of action of o,p′-DDD in the dog adrenal cortex. 1. Inhibition of ACTH-mediated pregnenolone synthesis. *Steroids* **1971**, *17*, 559–574. [CrossRef]
48. Hart, M.M.; Swackhamer, E.S.; Straw, J.A. Studies on the site of action of o,p′-DDD in the dog adrenal cortex. II. TPNH- and corticosteroid precursor-stimulation of o,p′-DDD inhibited steroidogenesis. *Steroids* **1971**, *17*, 575–586. [CrossRef]
49. Hescot, S.; Amazit, L.; Lhomme, M.; Travers, S.; DuBow, A.; Battini, S.; Boulate, G.; Namer, I.J.; Lombes, A.; Kontush, A.; et al. Identifying mitotane-induced mitochondria-associated membranes dysfunctions: Metabolomic and lipidomic approaches. *Oncotarget* **2017**, *8*, 109924–109940. [CrossRef]
50. Waszut, U.; Szyszka, P.; Dworakowska, D. Understanding mitotane mode of action. *J. Physiol. Pharmacol.* **2017**, *68*, 13–26. [PubMed]
51. Hescot, S.; Slama, A.; Lombes, A.; Paci, A.; Remy, H.; Leboulleux, S.; Chadarevian, R.; Trabado, S.; Amazit, L.; Young, J.; et al. Mitotane alters mitochondrial respiratory chain activity by inducing cytochrome c oxidase defect in human adrenocortical cells. *Endocr. Relat. Cancer* **2013**, *20*, 371–381. [CrossRef] [PubMed]
52. Brown, R.D.; Nicholson, W.E.; Chick, W.T.; Strott, C.A. Effect of o,p′DDD on human adrenal steroid 11 beta-hydroxylation activity. *J. Clin. Endocrinol. Metab.* **1973**, *36*, 730–733. [CrossRef]
53. Hescot, S.; Paci, A.; Seck, A.; Slama, A.; Viengchareun, S.; Trabado, S.; Brailly-Tabard, S.; Al Ghuzlan, A.; Young, J.; Baudin, E.; et al. The lack of antitumor effects of o,p′DDA excludes its role as an active metabolite of mitotane for adrenocortical carcinoma treatment. *Horm. Cancer* **2014**, *5*, 312–323. [CrossRef]
54. Germano, A.; Saba, L.; De Francia, S.; Rapa, I.; Perotti, P.; Berruti, A.; Volante, M.; Terzolo, M. CYP11B1 has no role in mitotane action and metabolism in adrenocortical carcinoma cells. *PLoS ONE* **2018**, *13*, e0196931. [CrossRef] [PubMed]
55. Lala, D.S.; Rice, D.A.; Parker, K.L. Steroidogenic factor I, a key regulator of steroidogenic enzyme expression, is the mouse homolog of fushi tarazu-factor I. *Mol. Endocrinol.* **1992**, *6*, 1249–1258. [CrossRef] [PubMed]
56. Morohashi, K.; Honda, S.; Inomata, Y.; Handa, H.; Omura, T. A common trans-acting factor, Ad4-binding protein, to the promoters of steroidogenic P-450s. *J. Biol. Chem.* **1992**, *267*, 17913–17919. [CrossRef]
57. Poli, G.; Guasti, D.; Rapizzi, E.; Fucci, R.; Canu, L.; Bandini, A.; Cini, N.; Bani, D.; Mannelli, M.; Luconi, M. Morphofunctional effects of mitotane on mitochondria in human adrenocortical cancer cells. *Endocr. Relat. Cancer* **2013**, *20*, 537–550. [CrossRef] [PubMed]
58. Sbiera, S.; Leich, E.; Liebisch, G.; Sbiera, I.; Schirbel, A.; Wiemer, L.; Matysik, S.; Eckhardt, C.; Gardill, F.; Gehl, A.; et al. Mitotane Inhibits Sterol-O-Acyl Transferase 1 Triggering Lipid-Mediated Endoplasmic Reticulum Stress and Apoptosis in Adrenocortical Carcinoma Cells. *Endocrinology* **2015**, *156*, 3895–3908. [CrossRef] [PubMed]
59. Lacombe, A.M.F.; Soares, I.C.; Mariani, B.M.P.; Nishi, M.Y.; Bezerra-Neto, J.E.; Charchar, H.D.S.; Brondani, V.B.; Tanno, F.; Srougi, V.; Chambo, J.L.; et al. Sterol O-Acyl Transferase 1 as a Prognostic Marker of Adrenocortical Carcinoma. *Cancers* **2020**, *12*, 247. [CrossRef]

60. Weigand, I.; Altieri, B.; Lacombe, A.M.F.; Basile, V.; Kircher, S.; Landwehr, L.S.; Schreiner, J.; Zerbini, M.C.N.; Ronchi, C.L.; Megerle, F.; et al. Expression of SOAT1 in Adrenocortical Carcinoma and Response to Mitotane Monotherapy: An ENSAT Multicenter Study. *J. Clin. Endocrinol. Metab.* **2020**, *105*, 2642–2653. [CrossRef]
61. Trotta, F.; Avena, P.; Chimento, A.; Rago, V.; De Luca, A.; Sculco, S.; Nocito, M.C.; Malivindi, R.; Fallo, F.; Pezzani, R.; et al. Statins Reduce Intratumor Cholesterol Affecting Adrenocortical Cancer Growth. *Mol. Cancer Ther.* **2020**, *19*, 1909–1921. [CrossRef] [PubMed]
62. Boulate, G.; Amazit, L.; Naman, A.; Seck, A.; Paci, A.; Lombes, A.; Pussard, E.; Baudin, E.; Lombes, M.; Hescot, S. Potentiation of mitotane action by rosuvastatin: New insights for adrenocortical carcinoma management. *Int. J. Oncol.* **2019**, *54*, 2149–2156. [CrossRef] [PubMed]
63. Linton, M.F.; Tao, H.; Linton, E.F.; Yancey, P.G. SR-BI: A Multifunctional Receptor in Cholesterol Homeostasis and Atherosclerosis. *Trends Endocrinol. Metab.* **2017**, *28*, 461–472. [CrossRef] [PubMed]
64. Weigand, I.; Schreiner, J.; Rohrig, F.; Sun, N.; Landwehr, L.S.; Urlaub, H.; Kendl, S.; Kiseljak-Vassiliades, K.; Wierman, M.E.; Angeli, J.P.F.; et al. Active steroid hormone synthesis renders adrenocortical cells highly susceptible to type II ferroptosis induction. *Cell Death Dis.* **2020**, *11*, 192. [CrossRef] [PubMed]
65. Belavgeni, A.; Bornstein, S.R.; von Massenhausen, A.; Tonnus, W.; Stumpf, J.; Meyer, C.; Othmar, E.; Latk, M.; Kanczkowski, W.; Kroiss, M.; et al. Exquisite sensitivity of adrenocortical carcinomas to induction of ferroptosis. *Proc. Natl. Acad. Sci. USA* **2019**, *116*, 22269–22274. [CrossRef] [PubMed]
66. Warde, K.M.; Schoenmakers, E.; Ribes Martinez, E.; Lim, Y.J.; Leonard, M.; Lawless, S.J.; O'Shea, P.; Chatterjee, K.V.; Gurnell, M.; Hantel, C.; et al. Liver X receptor inhibition potentiates mitotane-induced adrenotoxicity in ACC. *Endocr. Relat. Cancer* **2020**, *27*, 361–373. [CrossRef] [PubMed]
67. Germano, A.; Rapa, I.; Volante, M.; Lo Buono, N.; Carturan, S.; Berruti, A.; Terzolo, M.; Papotti, M. Cytotoxic activity of gemcitabine, alone or in combination with mitotane, in adrenocortical carcinoma cell lines. *Mol. Cell Endocrinol.* **2014**, *382*, 1–7. [CrossRef]
68. Tsakiridou, E.D.; Liberopoulos, E.; Giotaki, Z.; Tigas, S. Proprotein convertase subtilisin-kexin type 9 (PCSK9) inhibitor use in the management of resistant hypercholesterolemia induced by mitotane treatment for adrenocortical cancer. *J. Clin. Lipidol.* **2018**, *12*, 826–829. [CrossRef]
69. Doghman, M.; Lalli, E. Lack of long-lasting effects of mitotane adjuvant therapy in a mouse xenograft model of adrenocortical carcinoma. *Mol. Cell Endocrinol.* **2013**, *381*, 66–69. [CrossRef]
70. Germano, A.; Rapa, I.; Volante, M.; De Francia, S.; Migliore, C.; Berruti, A.; Papotti, M.; Terzolo, M. RRM1 modulates mitotane activity in adrenal cancer cells interfering with its metabolization. *Mol. Cell Endocrinol.* **2015**, *401*, 105–110. [CrossRef]
71. Goyzueta Mamani, L.D.; de Carvalho, J.C.; Bonatto, S.J.R.; Tanobe, V.A.O.; Soccol, C.R. In vitro cytotoxic effect of a chitin-like polysaccharide produced by Mortierella alpina on adrenocortical carcinoma cells H295R, and its use as mitotane adjuvant. *In Vitro Cell Dev. Biol. Anim.* **2021**, *57*, 395–403. [CrossRef] [PubMed]
72. Van der Valk, J.; Bieback, K.; Buta, C.; Cochrane, B.; Dirks, W.G.; Fu, J.; Hickman, J.J.; Hohensee, C.; Kolar, R.; Liebsch, M.; et al. Fetal Bovine Serum (FBS): Past–Present–Future. *ALTEX* **2018**, *35*, 99–118. [CrossRef] [PubMed]

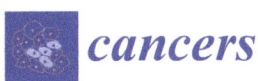

Review

New Insights on the Genetics of Pheochromocytoma and Paraganglioma and Its Clinical Implications

Sakshi Jhawar [1], Yasuhiro Arakawa [2], Suresh Kumar [2], Diana Varghese [2], Yoo Sun Kim [2], Nitin Roper [2], Fathi Elloumi [2], Yves Pommier [2], Karel Pacak [3] and Jaydira Del Rivero [2,*]

1. Life Bridge Health Center, Internal Medicine Program, Sinai Hospital of Baltimore, Baltimore, MD 21215, USA; sakshijhawar24@gmail.com
2. Developmental Therapeutics Branch, National Cancer Institute, National Institutes of Health (NIH), Bethesda, MD 20892, USA; arakawa.yasuhiro@nih.gov (Y.A.); suresh.kumar@nih.gov (S.K.); diana.varghese@nih.gov (D.V.); yoosun.kim@nih.gov (Y.S.K.); nitin.roper@nih.gov (N.R.); fathi.elloumi@nih.gov (F.E.); pommier@nih.gov (Y.P.)
3. Section on Medical Neuroendocrinology, Eunice Kennedy Shriver National Institute of Child Health and Human Development, National Institutes of Health (NIH), Bethesda, MD 20892, USA; karel@mail.nih.gov
* Correspondence: jaydira.delrivero@nih.gov

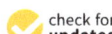

Citation: Jhawar, S.; Arakawa, Y.; Kumar, S.; Varghese, D.; Kim, Y.S.; Roper, N.; Elloumi, F.; Pommier, Y.; Pacak, K.; Del Rivero, J. New Insights on the Genetics of Pheochromocytoma and Paraganglioma and Its Clinical Implications. *Cancers* 2022, 14, 594. https://doi.org/10.3390/cancers14030594

Academic Editor: Peter Igaz

Received: 30 November 2021
Accepted: 20 January 2022
Published: 25 January 2022

Publisher's Note: MDPI stays neutral with regard to jurisdictional claims in published maps and institutional affiliations.

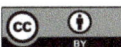

Copyright: © 2022 by the authors. Licensee MDPI, Basel, Switzerland. This article is an open access article distributed under the terms and conditions of the Creative Commons Attribution (CC BY) license (https://creativecommons.org/licenses/by/4.0/).

Simple Summary: Pheochromocytoma and paraganglioma (together PPGL) are rare neuroendocrine tumors that arise from chromaffin tissue and produce catecholamines. Approximately 40% of cases of PPGL carry a germline mutation, suggesting that they have a high degree of heritability. The underlying mutation influences the PPGL clinical presentation such as cell differentiation, specific catecholamine production, tumor location, malignant potential and genetic anticipation, which helps to better understand the clinical course and tailor treatment accordingly. Genetic testing for pheochromocytoma and paraganglioma allows an early detection of hereditary syndromes and facilitates a close follow-up of high-risk patients. In this review article, we present the most recent advances in the field of genetics and we discuss the latest guidelines on the surveillance of asymptomatic *SDHx* mutation carriers.

Abstract: Pheochromocytomas (PHEOs) and paragangliomas (PGLs) are rare neuroendocrine tumors that arise from chromaffin cells. PHEOs arise from the adrenal medulla, whereas PGLs arise from the neural crest localized outside the adrenal gland. Approximately 40% of all cases of PPGLs (pheochromocytomas/paragangliomas) are associated with germline mutations and 30–40% display somatic driver mutations. The mutations associated with PPGLs can be classified into three groups. The pseudohypoxic group or cluster I includes the following genes: *SDHA, SDHB, SDHC, SDHD, SDHAF2, FH, VHL, IDH1/2, MDH2, EGLN1/2* and *HIF2/EPAS*; the kinase group or cluster II includes *RET, NF1, TMEM127, MAX* and *HRAS*; and the Wnt signaling group or cluster III includes *CSDE1* and *MAML3*. Underlying mutations can help understand the clinical presentation, overall prognosis and surveillance follow-up. Here we are discussing the new genetic insights of PPGLs.

Keywords: pheochromocytoma; paraganglioma; genetics; germline; screening

1. Introduction

Pheochromocytomas (PHEOs) and paragangliomas (PGLs) are rare neuroendocrine (NE) tumors arising from chromaffin cells of the adrenal medulla and extra-adrenal ganglia, respectively. The incidence of PHEOs and PGLs (collectively PPGLs) is estimated at approximately 2–8 cases per million per year [1,2]. However, this is likely an underestimate, based upon the finding of up to 0.05–0.1% incidentally detected cases in an autopsy series [3]. PPGLs may occur at any age and they usually peak between the 3rd and 5th decade of life [4]. Patients with PPGL most commonly present with symptoms of excess catecholamine production including headache, diaphoresis, palpitations, tremors, facial pallor and hypertension. These symptoms are often paroxysmal, although persistent hypertension between these episodes is common and occurs in 50–60% patients with PPGL [5].

The field of genomics in PPGL has rapidly evolved over the past two decades. Approximately 40% of all cases of PPGLs are associated with germline mutations, which makes pheochromocytoma and paraganglioma solid tumors with a high heritability rate. A genomic characterization study by The Cancer Genome Atlas (TCGA) group, analyzing a cohort of 173 patients, showed that PPGLs can be driven by either germline, somatic or fusion gene mutations in 27%, 39% and 7% of the cases, respectively [6–8]. It has been proposed that all patients with PPGL should be considered for genetic testing, as the incidence of hereditary syndromes in apparently sporadic cases is as high as 35% [9,10]. Currently, more than 20 susceptibility genes have been identified, including at least 12 distinct genetic syndromes, 15 driver genes and an expanding fraction of potential disease modifying genes [11,12]. Thus, the underlying mutations appear to determine the clinical manifestations, such as tumor location, biochemical profile, malignant potential, imaging signature and overall prognosis, that should help to tailor treatment and guidance for follow-up. Moreover, detection of a mutation in an index case and their family members should also help clinicians to implement a pertinent surveillance program to promptly identify tumors and treat patients accordingly [13,14]. Despite our understanding of PPGL genetics and molecular biology, the treatment options, especially against advanced and metastatic PPGLs, remain limited and require a personalized approach. Surgical resection remains the mainstay of treatment. In cases where surgery is not feasible or if tumor dissemination limits the probability of curative treatment, the options for treatment are localized radiotherapy, radiofrequency or cryoablation and systemic therapy, which includes chemotherapy or targeted molecular therapies.

There has been increasing interest in radionuclide therapy, which includes ^{131}I-MIBG therapy and recently PRRT (peptide receptor radionuclide therapy) ^{177}Lu-DOTATATE [15–17]. In terms of chemotherapy, CVD (cyclophosphamide, vincristine and dacarbazine) is one of the most traditional chemotherapy regimens and has been used to treat PPGLs over the past 30 years [18]. New treatments are emerging for patients with advanced/metastatic PPGL. Understanding the molecular signaling and metabolomics of PPGL has led to the development of therapeutic regimens for cluster-specific targeted molecular therapies. Based on TCGA classification for cluster I, antiangiogenic therapy, HIF inhibitors, PARP (polyADP-ribose polymerase) inhibition and immunotherapy are used. For cluster II, mTOR (mammalian target of rapamycin) inhibitors are used. Currently there are no cluster III Wnt signaling targeted therapies for PPGL patients [19].

At present, clinical genetic testing for patients with a suspected hereditary form of PPGL is carried out using a germline genetic panel rather than using one gene at a time. Based upon its lower financial cost, immunohistochemistry (IHC) can be considered for screening purposes, particularly in patients with suspected succinate dehydrogenase complex (*SDHx*) mutations. However, IHC should be interpreted with caution as there is likelihood of false-positive and false-negative results [20].

In this review, we summarize recent advances in the discovery of new genes during the past five years. Additionally, we summarize the latest guidelines by Amar et al. for the diagnosis and surveillance of asymptomatic *SDHx* mutation carriers [21].

2. Overview of Genetics on What Is Already Known

The identification of the Krebs cycle in the etiology of PPGLs is a milestone in the field of the genetics of PPGLs. The SDH complex plays a pivotal role in energy metabolism in the Krebs cycle, as well as in complex II of the electron transport chain. Mutations in any of the genes encoding the catalytic enzymes of the pathway can lead to an accumulation of their substrates, resulting in hypoxia-inducible factor (HIF) stability and tumorigenesis [22]. These genes include *SDHA, SDHB, SDHC, SDHD, SDHAF2* [23,24], fumarate hydratase (*FH*) [25,26], malate dehydrogenase 2 (*MDH2*) [27,28], hypoxia-inducible factor alpha (*HIF2a*) [29–31], prolyl hydroxylase (*PHD*) [32] and some newly discovered genes that will be discussed further in the review (Figure 1). Mutation of the genes involved in the kinase receptor signaling pathway that are known to cause PPGLs are *RET* (REarranged during Transfection), neurofibromin 1 (*NF1*), Myelocytomatosis-Associated factor X (*MAX*), transmembrane protein 127 (*TMEM127*), and Harvey rat sarcoma viral gene homologue (*HRAS*). Genes such as *ATRX* (Alpha Thalassemia/mental Retardation-X linked) that are involved in chromosomal integrity, are also implicated as drivers in the etiology of PPGLs and are associated with aggressive behavior [33]. To better understand the genetics based on signaling pathways, The Cancer Genome Atlas (TCGA) has classified PPGLs into three clinically useful molecular clusters: (1) Pseudohypoxic PPGLs, (2) Kinase signaling PPGLs and (3) Wnt signaling PPGLs [34] (Figure 1).

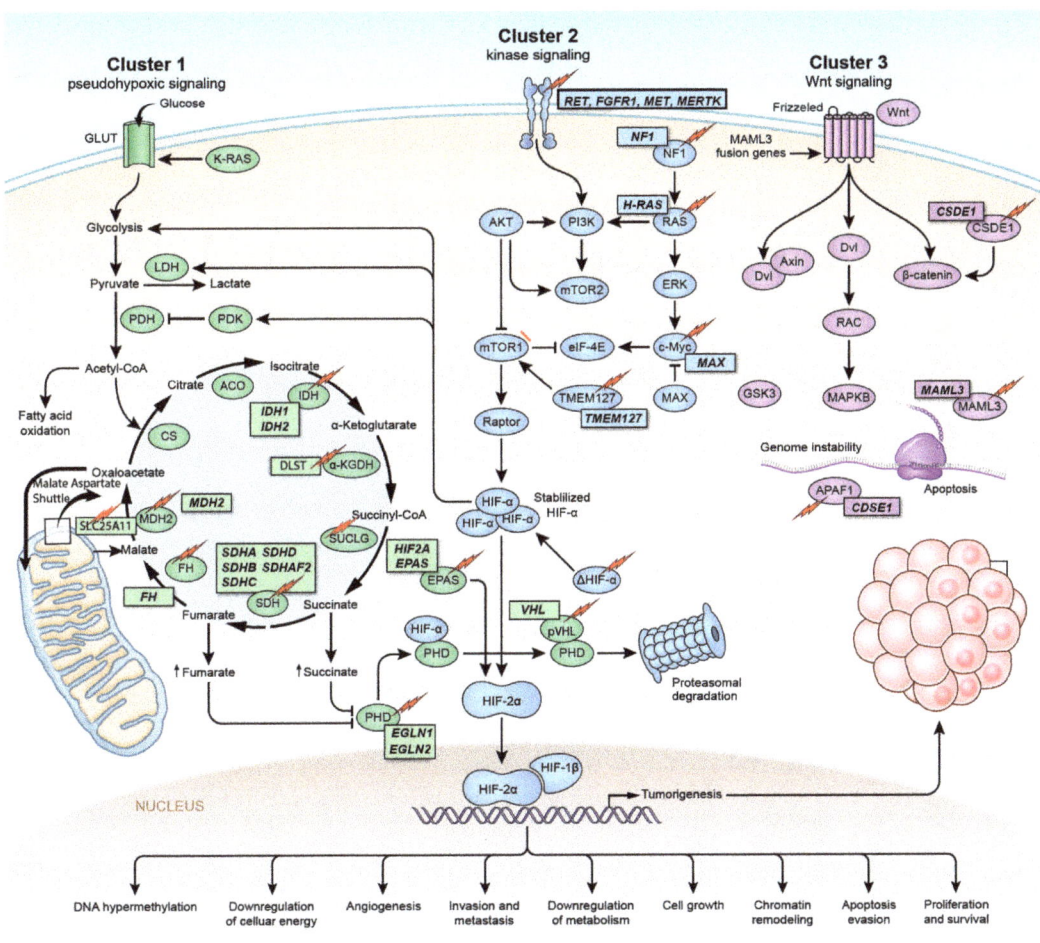

Figure 1. Genetics and molecular pathways for pheochromocytoma and paraganglioma. The genes are classified into three clusters. Cluster I involves mutations in the pseudohypoxic pathway (*SDHx, FH, MDH2, HIF2, PHD, VHL* and *EPAS*). Cluster II involves mutations in the kinase signaling group (*RET, NF1, TMEM127, MAX* and *HRAS*). Lastly, cluster III includes mutations in the Wnt signaling group (*CSDE1* and *UBTF* fusion at *MAML3*). The new genes discovered (SUCLG2, SLC25A11, DLST, MAPK, MET, MERTK, FGFR1) have been depicted as well. ↑ depicts accumulation of substrate. Adapted from ref. [19].

3. Genes Discovered in the Last Five Years

With the expanding genetic landscape of PPGLs, several new genes have been identified recently (Table 1) which can potentially predispose patients to the development of tumors with characteristic biological behaviors.

Table 1. Newly discovered in the pathogenesis of PPGLs.

Gene	Year of Discovery	Pathophysiology	Gene Type	Metabolomics	References
CSDE1	2016	Tumor suppressor gene involved in mRNA stability and cellular apoptosis	Somatic	Adrenergic	[6,7]
H3F3A	2016	Encodes histone H3.3 protein that regulates chromatin formation	Somatic	NA	[35,36]
MET	2016	MAPK signaling pathway	Germline, somatic	NA	[23]
MERTK	2016	Tyrosine kinase receptor	Germline	NA	[11,37,38]
UBTF-MAML3	2017	Unique methylation profile mRNA overexpression involved in Wnt receptor and hedgehog signaling pathways	Fusion	Adrenergic	[6,39]
SLC25A11	2018	Encodes malate-oxalate carrier protein of malate-aspartate shuttle	Germline	Noradrenergic	[40,41]
IRP1	2018	Cellular iron metabolism regulation	Somatic	noradrenergic	[42]
DLST	2019	Encodes E2 subunit of mitochondrial α-KG complex which converts α-KG to succinyl-CoA	Germline	Noradrenergic	[23,43]
SUCLG2	2021	Catalyzes conversion of succinyl-coA and ADP/GTP to succinate and ATP/GTP	Germline	Noradrenergic	[44]

3.1. CSDE1 (Cold Shock Domain Containing E1)

CSDE1 is a tumor suppressor gene located on chromosome 1p13.2 that encodes CSD1 factor, which is involved in messenger RNA (mRNA) stability, internal initiation of translation, apoptosis and neuronal differentiation [7]. Mutation in this gene results in downregulation of the apoptosis protease activator protein 1 (APAF1), which is a critical factor in cellular apoptosis. In the cohort study of 176 patients with PPGL by Feishbein et al. [6], four tumors containing CDSE1 mutations were detected. These mutations were somatic: two frameshift and two splice-site mutations that clustered proximally within the gene. Patients carrying this gene presented with sporadic and aggressive disease with recurrence and metastasis [6].

3.2. H3F3A (Histone Family Member 3A)

The H3F3A gene is located on chromosome 1 and encodes the histone H3.3 protein. Histones are scaffolding proteins and the building blocks of the nucleosome. Mutation of H3F3A affects DNA methylation, chromatin epigenetics and remodeling, and nucleosome positioning. The first case of an association of the H3F3A mutation and PPGL and GCT (giant cell tumor) of the bone was reported in a 2013 case report by Iwata et al. [36]. In 2016, Toledo et al. characterized a new cancer syndrome involving PPGL and GCT of the bone caused by post-zygotic mutation of the H3F3A gene. They analyzed 43 samples from 41 patients by whole exome or transcriptome sequencing and found a post-zygotic H3F3A mutation (c103 G > T, p.Gly34Trp) in three tumors from one patient. That patient had recurrent GCT and bilateral PHEO with no family history and developed bladder and periaortic PGL later. This *H3F3A* mutation was identical to one reported as an oncogenic driver of sporadic GCT (c103 G > T, p.G34W) [35]. With this finding, Toledo et al. obtained and analyzed samples from a patient who had aggressive retroperitoneal PGL with liver metastasis and recurrent GCTs, and identified the same H3F3A mutation.

Other chromatin remodeling genes identified in this study were *SETD2* (sporadic PPGL), *EZH2* (sporadic), *KMT2B, KMT2D* (sporadic, germline), *ATRX, JMJD1C* and *KDM2B* [23].

3.3. UBTF-MAML3 (Upstream Binding Transcription Factor Mastermind-like Transcriptional Coactivator 3)

The Wnt pathway is involved in various developmental processes including cell proliferation, adhesion, motility and differentiation. In 2017, Feishbein et al. first reported the association of *MAML3* fusion genes and *CSDE1* (cold shock domain containing E1) of the Wnt and Hedgehog signaling pathways, with the development of PPGLs [6]. In a cohort of 176 patients with PPGL, 10 were positive for the *UBTF-MAML3* fusion gene. The *UBTF* gene is located on chromosome 17q21.31 and encodes the UBTF protein involved in the expression of ribosomal RNA (rRNA) subunits. Patients carrying this fusion gene show extensive alterations in DNA methylation profiles, predominantly hypomethylation that correlates with mRNA overexpression of target genes. In MAML3 fusion-positive tumors, the Wnt pathway members B-catenin, DVL3 (disheveled segment polarity protein-3) and GSK3 (glycogen synthase kinase-3) are overexpressed; whereas miR-375, which is a negative regulator, is underexpressed [39]. Patients with fusion genes have an increased risk of aggressive and metastatic PPGL [6]. It has been shown that *UBTF-MAML3* fusions are expressed in 7% of human PPGLs and overexpression of MAML3 increases tumorigenicity and invasion. Thus, MAML3 expression can serve as a prognostic marker for aggressive disease [45].

3.4. IRP1 (Iron Regulator Protein 1)

IRP 1 is a regulator of cellular iron metabolism. In iron deficient cells, IRP1 depresses HIF2α mRNA translation, leading to its accumulation and increased EPO expression [46]. In 2018, Pang et al. discovered the association of *IRP1* with PPGL in a patient with concomitant polycythemia and PHEO [42]. An investigational 54-gene panel carried out on this patient's peripheral blood DNA was negative for a genetic mutation. Subsequently, tumor DNA sequencing revealed a somatic loss of function mutation in *IRP1* located on the exon 3 splicing site [42,47].

3.5. SLC25A11 (Solute Carrier Family 25 Member 11)

SLC25A11 is a tumor suppressor gene, whose association with PPGL was first reported in 2018 by Buffet et al., which accounts for approximately 1% of all PPGL cases [40]. *SLC25A11* encodes a carrier protein, malate-oxalate carrier (OGC), mediating malate transport from the cytosol to the mitochondrial matrix in exchange for α-ketoglutarate (αKG), while regenerating NADH in the mitochondrial matrix by the electron transport chain complex I [40,41]. Studies have shown that high levels of aspartate and glutamate due to an *SLC25A11* mutation are potent inhibitors of HIF prolyl hydroxylases, which promote tumorigenesis [48]. Buffet et al. demonstrated that germline mutations in the *SLC25A11* gene are strongly associated with the development of metastatic PPGL as 5% of all metastatic PPGLs in their cohort of 121 patients had underlying germline *SLC25A11* mutations. A malignant phenotype was observed in 5 out of the 7 (71%) cases [40]. Germline *SLC25A11* mutations have been found in 5 out of 30 (17%) patients with single, apparently sporadic, metastatic abdominal PGL. Based upon these data, *SLC25A11* mutations should be considered among the genetic risk factors for metastatic PPGL [49].

3.6. DLST (Dihydrolipoamide S-Succinyltransferase)

Remacha et al. first described the connection between PPGL and *DLST* in 2019 [43]. *DLST* encodes the E2 subunit of the mitochondrial αKG complex, catalyzing the conversion of α-KG to succinyl-CoA and CO_2. Mutation in the *DLST* gene results in depletion of the E2 subunit of the αKGD complex, resulting in impaired enzyme activity. Due to this, αKG accumulates leading to high α-KG/fumarate ratio and dysfunction of the Krebs cycle, thus promoting oncogenesis [43]. Five germline variants have been identified that affected the *DLST* gene in eight unrelated individuals; all except one was diagnosed with multiple PPGLs. The above data, therefore, suggest *DLST* as a susceptibility gene for PPGL [43].

Based on a study by Toledo et al., mutations in chromatin remodeling genes and kinase receptor genes (*MERTK, MET, FGFR1* as described below) are implicated in PPGL pathogenesis [23].

3.7. MERTK (Tyrosine Kinase Protooncogene)

Receptor tyrosine kinase cellular signaling pathways regulate a broad variety of cellular processes driving cell growth, proliferation, differentiation, survival, gene transcription and metabolic regulation. Mutations of genes encoding tyrosine kinase receptors are often associated with cancer development [50]. Toledo et al. detected a germline mutation within the tyrosine kinase domain of the *MERTK* gene (c.2273 G > A, p.Arg758His) in a patient with metastatic PPGL and medullary thyroid carcinoma (MTC) [23]. The association of PPGL and MTC is manifested in multiple endocrine neoplasia type 2 (MEN2), which are usually characterized by mutation in the *RET* gene. However, in this patient, *RET* mutation was not detected. To expand on this finding, sequencing of the *MERTK* kinase domain was carried out in a separate cohort of 136 PPGLs. A germline mutation targeting the same residue, R758C, was identified in a patient with sporadic pheochromocytoma. Moreover, somatic *MERTK* mutations were further reported in two cases of PPGL from TCGA dataset. Thus, these findings are suggestive of the role of *MERTK* mutations in PPGL pathogenesis [11,37,38].

3.8. MET (Mesenchymal to Epithelial Transition)

MET mutations have been reported in multiple cancers [51]. Toledo et al. reported a case of germline mutation of the MET kinase receptor (c.2416 G > A; p.Val806Met) in a patient with a three-generation family history of PPGL [23]. After sequencing 118 unrelated PPGLs, they identified 15 different samples carrying *MET* variants, both germline and somatic, which supports that *MET* mutations are associated with PPGLs [23].

3.9. FGFR1 (Fibroblast Growth Factor Receptor 1)

A somatic mutation in *FGFR1* (c.1638C > A; p.Asn546Lys) was detected in one patient with sporadic PPGL, in a cohort of 130 samples by Toledo et al. [23]. This variant was also detected in samples of PPGL from TCGA dataset [37,38], which suggests the association of *FGFR1* mutations with PPGL.

3.10. SUCLG2 (Succinyl Co-A Ligase G2)

An association of *SUCLG2* gene mutation with PPGL development was first reported by Vanova et al. in 2021 [44]. Succinyl-CoA ligase (SUCL) is an enzyme of the TCA cycle responsible for the conversion of succinyl-CoA and ADP/GDP to succinate and ATP/GTP [52]. Succinate, which is a product of this enzyme, is an oncometabolite that is linked to the pathogenesis of PPGL [53,54]. SUCL has two subunits. The α-subunit is encoded by *SUCLG1* and the β-subunit by *SUCLA2* (ATP-forming) or *SUCLG2* (GTP-forming) [55]. Vanova et al. [44] tested 352 patients with apparently sporadic PPGL, using a 54-gene panel developed at the National Institutes of Health that included *SUCLG2*, and found that 15 patients had eight germline variants located within the GTP-binding domain of SUCGL-2. To confirm the causality of this defect, a progenitor cell line, hPheo1, derived from a human PPGL, was used. *SUCLG2* germline variants showed increased succinate levels and reduced SDH activity leading to TCA cycle disruption. The pattern of malignancy rate and biochemical phenotype was similar to *SDHx*-mutated PPGLs [56]. Moreover, the *SUCLG2* manipulated hPheo1 cell confirmed the link between the *SUCLG2* mutation and *SDHx* complex function. Hence, the association of a *SUCLG2* gene mutation with the development of PPGL is proposed based on this study. Large scale studies are needed to discover more cases of *SUCLG2* mutations that can provide detailed information about prevalence, penetrance, biochemical phenotype and relationship with *SDHx* in disease etiology.

4. New Screening Guidelines for Asymptomatic *SDHx* Carriers

Germline mutations in *SDHx* comprises approximately 20% of cases of PPGL [10,57,58]. When a *SDHx* pathogenic mutation is identified, genetic counselling is proposed for patients' first-degree relatives. However, there are no established guidelines on how to screen and then follow up asymptomatic mutation carriers. A recent consensus algorithm was established for initial screening and follow-up of *SDHx* mutation carriers by an international panel of 29 experts from 12 countries in 2020, using the Delphi method [21] (Table 2).

Table 2. Screening and follow-up guidelines for asymptomatic patients carrying *SDHx* (A, B, C, D-pi) mutations.

Timeline	Children (<18 Years)	Adults (>18 Years)
Initial screening (SDHA, C, D-pi: age 10–15 years, SDHB: age 6–10 years)	• H/P-questionnaire and BP measurement • Biochemical measurements (urinary or plasma M, NM) • Head and neck MRI • Thoracic, abdominal and pelvic MRI	• H/P-questionnaire and BP measurement • Biochemical measurements (plasma M, NM > urinary M, NM) • Head and neck MRI • Abdominal and pelvic MRI • Whole body PET-CT
Follow-up every year	• Symptom questionnaire and BP measurement	• Symptom questionnaire, BP measurement and biochemical measurements
Follow-up every two years	• Biochemical measurements	-
Follow-up every 2–3 years	• Head and neck MRI • Thoracic, abdominal, and pelvic MRI	• Head and neck MRI • Thoracic, abdominal and pelvic MRI
Age 80 years	End of follow-up	

H/P—history and physical, BP—blood pressure, M—metanephrine, NM—normetanephrine. Guidelines published by Amar et al. [21].

The penetrance of *SDHx*-related PPGL is not firmly established. Studies have shown that *SDHB* has a 8–37% penetrance and *SDHD* has a 38–64% penetrance [21,59]. Out of all *SDHx* mutation carriers, patients with an *SDHB* mutation carry the highest risk for metastatic disease [58,60,61]. Patients with *SDHD* mutations have the highest penetrance. Data regarding *SDHC* and *SDHA* mutations are limited but show lower penetrance than *SDHD* mutation carriers [58,62,63]. After analysis of each gene, experts felt that the data are not strong enough to personalize recommendation for each gene separately but concluded that the recommendation for initial screening and follow-up for all *SDHx* genes is the same, with the exception of age of initiation of tumor screening in childhood. Moreover, since *SDHD* has two modes of inheritance—paternal (*SDHD-pi*), which contributes to the majority of transmissions, and maternal (*SDHD-mi*), which is <5% [64], the grade A recommendation is to perform screening for the presence of a tumor once the mutation (*SDHA, SDHB, SDHC* or *SDHD-pi*) is identified in an asymptomatic carrier, and to perform genetic screening only when tumor screening is considered.

The recommendation for the age at which screening should be performed is extrapolated from the age of incidence of a tumor in a particular gene. A small number of *SDHB*-related PPGLs have been reported in 6-year-old children [13,60,62,65], which is associated with a high risk of metastatic diseases compared to other *SDHx* mutation carriers [13,66]. Therefore, it is recommended to start the screening of *SDHB* mutation carriers between the age of 6–10 years. For asymptomatic *SDHA, SDHC, SDHD-pi* mutation carriers, the recommendation is to initiate screening from 10–15 years. Tumor screening of all asymptomatic *SDHx* (*A, B, C, D-pi*) mutation carriers should be started with a history that must include a questionnaire for signs and symptom assessment, followed by clinical examination including blood pressure measurement.

Biochemical testing for tumor screening should include the measurement of either plasma or urine metanephrines and normetanephrines as this seems to be the best diagnostic test with high sensitivity [67,68]. During childhood, the decision of which test to use can be left up to the feasibility and laboratory expertise. On the other hand, for adults, measurement of plasma free metanephrine and normetanephrine should be preferred over urinary tests. It is not recommended to test additionally for catecholamines and vanillylmandelic acid as they are less reliable than metanephrines and normetanephrines [67,68].

Because a significant number of PPGLs are non-functional, especially *SDHx*-related PPGLs, imaging studies must be performed in all asymptomatic *SDHx* mutation carriers. During childhood, a whole-body MRI (head, neck, thoracic, abdomen and pelvic regions) is used as the first-line imaging for initial tumor screening, including patients requiring sedation for MRI. Ultrasound can be used only for children who cannot tolerate MRI [69]. In adults, a combination of head, neck, abdomen and pelvic MRI and PET-CT is recommended for initial tumor screening. Thoracic MRI is not a requirement for initial screening if the PET-CT is normal but it is recommended for subsequent follow-ups. Functional imaging should not be used as first-line screening in children due to radiation exposure. Dedicated cross-sectional imaging should only be carried out if the PET-CT is abnormal. Moreover, use of ^{123}I-MIBG and ^{111}In-pentetreotide is also not recommended for initial tumor screening.

As patients carrying an *SDHx* mutation have an increased risk for tumor development throughout their life, regular interval follow-ups are recommended even if initial screening results are negative [70]. The expert consensus recommends an annual physical in all age groups, including screening for signs and symptoms of PPGL with questionnaires. Biochemical testing (serum or urinary metanephrines and normetanephrines) must be carried out every 2 years in childhood and every year in adulthood. In terms of imaging, MRI should be performed every 2–3 years in all age groups and functional imaging is not recommended for follow-up screening. If *SDHx* (*A, B, C, D-pi*) mutation carriers remain asymptomatic without evidence of a tumor on interval screening, the screening tests should be performed every 5 years after the age of 70, until 80 years of age.

Special consideration should be given to patients who are planning a pregnancy because of complication risks including pre-eclampsia, gestational diabetes and arrhythmias that increase the mortality risk for both the mother and fetus [71]. Therefore, it is recommended to perform complete screening before planning a pregnancy. *SDHx* mutations have been associated with the development of other tumors including renal cell cancer (RCC), gastrointestinal tumors (GIST) and pituitary adenoma [72–75]. However, no additional screening imaging is recommended, although these tumors should be searched for during the screening imaging.

5. Emerging Molecular Genetics and Future Perspectives

The clinical treatment options for patients with PPGL are increasingly based on the underlying molecular biology, genetic and epigenetic analyses of the tumors. In the past two decades, our understanding in the field of genetics, translational research, metabolomics, peptide receptor-based imaging and treatment, as well as immunotherapy, has greatly increased. However, further investigations are needed to deliver precision-based treatment.

Over the last five years, various human- and rodent-derived cell lines and xenografts have been developed. Yet, they do not fully provide subtype classification of tumors and remain challenging for clinical studies. Frankhauser et al. used "immortalized mouse chromaffin cells" (imCCs), MPC/MTT (mouse pheochromocytoma cells/mouse tumor tissue) spheroids, murine pheochromocytoma cell lines and human pheochromocytoma primary cultures, and identified that the PI3Ka inhibitor BYL719 and the MTORC1 inhibitor everolimus are highly effective at tumor shrinkage at clinically relevant doses [76]. To date, there has only been one human cell line progenitor developed successfully: Pheo1 [77]. Moreover, the classic approaches to cell line development, such as SV40-mediated immortalization and newer approaches such as patient-derived tumor xenografts and tumor organoids, have become important preclinical models. Induced pluripotent stem cells (iPSCs) are worth exploring further in this field [78,79]. A recent discovery of the RS0 cell line in 2020 by Powers et al. is a stepping-stone in the field of cell line development and, by far, seems to be the closest model to *SDHB*-mutated human pheochromocytomas [80]. An intrinsic limitation of this model is that it was developed by using irradiation and it is not excluded that the loss of *SDHB* is due to the bystanders effect. Therefore, further characterization by complementation with WT Sdhb must be carried out in the future.

As multiple genetic abnormalities can be associated with a diagnosis of inherited PPGL, next generation sequencing (NGS) is well-suited for carrying out genetic screening. In order to better understand their differences, the classification published by Toledo et al. in 2017 is worth noting as follows: (i) basic panel (including genes mutated at the germline level with the highest evidence for their involvement in the pathogenesis of PPGL), (ii) extended panel (including basic panel genes along with other candidate susceptibility genes that are mutated at the germline level and are found at a low frequency); (iii) comprehensive panel (including extended panel genes along with genes exclusively mutated at the somatic level and those recently found to be mutated at the germline and/or somatic levels, for which the evidence is still limited) [81].

The basic panel encompasses genes involved in germline mutation such as *VHL*, *SDHx*, *FH*, *MAX*, *NF1*, *RET* and *TMEM127* [82]. The extended panel has functionally relevant genes: *EGLN1*, *EPAS1*, *SDHAF2*, *K1F1B* and *MET*. The comprehensive panel includes other recently identified genes [81]. This development has made genetic screening available and affordable in an individual laboratory. However, this comes with the caveat that the analyses become technically challenging with the risk of errors when attempting to add new genes to existing panels [81,83]. The whole exome sequencing (WES) technique is a method of sequencing only the coding regions of DNA and it has led to the identification of several PPGL susceptibility genes such has *MAX*, *FH*, *MDH2*, *HRAS*, *ATRX* and *KMDT2D* [23,81]. Novel NGS techniques, such as RNA sequencing and DNA methylation, can reveal mutational status and can be used as diagnostic or prognostic biomarkers [82].

Several new biomarkers have been discovered that are helpful in differentiating metastatic from non-metastatic tumors and thus prognostication. Major reduction in expression of one putative lncRNA (long non-coding RNA, GenBank: BC063866) has been re-reported in metastatic *SDHx*-related tumors, which itself is an independent risk factor associated with poor clinical outcomes [84,85]. Other metastatic biomarkers identified are hypermethylation of RDBP (negative elongation factor complex member E) promoter and a six-miRNA signature that co-relate time to disease progression [86–88]. Cell-free DNA based methods are becoming more popular for cancer detection, however, no such studies have been performed in PPGL patients.

In terms of immunohistochemical markers, biomarkers such as ATRX, chromogranin B and somatostatin receptor 2A have been reported but need more studies to further characterize their roles for prognostication [33,89,90].

The expanding development in the field of the genetics of PPGL has been translated into clinical practice by the provision of widespread testing for inherited PPGL. Utilization of the knowledge of discovery at a molecular level to enable more personalized strategies for investigation, surveillance and management of affected individuals and their families has not only led to accurate diagnosis and risk prediction but also several challenges. These include improving variant interpretation and reducing the number of variants of uncertain significance (VUS), the need for the development of optimal genotypic-phenotypic protocols that enable both early diagnosis whilst keeping healthcare costs in mind, and lastly, producing targeted therapies for metastatic PPGLs. Comprehensive understanding of molecular biology, genetics and oncogenic pathways will lead to the development of novel targets and therapies, which can potentially help improve the prognosis and survival in patients with PPGL [91].

For metastatic PPGL the treatment options have remained limited. Currently, the practiced standard of therapy includes chemotherapy (CVD scheme or temozolomide monotherapy), radionuclide therapy (^{131}I-MIBG, ^{177}Lu-DOTATATE), tyrosine kinase inhibitors (sunitinib, cabozantinib) and immunotherapy [92–94]. A personalized approach is becoming increasingly popular, in light of a comprehensive understanding of molecular biology. These approaches include ^{177}Lu DOTATATE therapy for patients with the expression of SSTR2 (somatostatin receptor 2), particularly in *SDHx*-mutated PPGL (positive ^{67}Ga-DOTATATE scan); ^{131}I-MIBG therapy for patients who have expression of the norepinephrine transporter system and are less likely positive for *SDHx*-mutated PPGL (positive ^{123}I-MIBG scan); HIF2-α inhibitors for cluster I PPGLs; PARP inhibitors together with temozolomide (especially for *SDHx*-mutated tumors); PDL1 inhibitors (pembrolizumab); and tyrosine kinase inhibitors for cluster II PPGLs [19]. A very recent study by Tabebi et al. showed that downregulation of *SDHB* gene expression in PPGL resulted in increased GLUD1 (glutamate dehydrogenase) expression and can potentially serve as a biomarker and therapeutic target in *SDHB*-mutated PPGLs [95].

Lastly, machine learning algorithms have begun to be used to predict the mutational status in PPGL [96]. Therefore, the combination of artificial intelligence, genetic and immunohistochemical biomarkers, along with metabolomics and clinical features, will be a useful tool for assessing metastatic risk with high accuracy, suggesting long-term prognosis.

6. Conclusions

PPGLs are rare NE tumors with unique molecular landscapes. Cataloging and understanding the germline and somatic mutations associated with PPGLs is a promising approach to understand the clinical behavior and prognosis. Moreover, it can provide guidance on diagnostic strategies and personalized treatments for PPGLs.

Author Contributions: S.J. prepared the initial draft and revised the manuscript. Y.A., S.K., D.V., Y.S.K., N.R. and F.E. reviewed the manuscript. Y.P., K.P. and J.D.R. reviewed and revised the manuscript. All authors have read and agreed to the published version of the manuscript.

Funding: This research received no external funding.

Conflicts of Interest: The authors declare no conflict of interest.

References

1. Beard, C.M.; Sheps, S.G.; Kurland, L.T.; Carney, J.A.; Lie, J.T. Occurrence of pheochromocytoma in Rochester, Minnesota, 1950 through 1979. *Mayo Clin. Proc.* **1983**, *58*, 802–804. [PubMed]
2. Chen, H.; Sippel, R.S.; O'Dorisio, M.S.; Vinik, A.I.; Lloyd, R.V.; Pacak, K. The North American Neuroendocrine Tumor Society consensus guideline for the diagnosis and management of neuroendocrine tumors: Pheochromocytoma, paraganglioma, and medullary thyroid cancer. *Pancreas* **2010**, *39*, 775–783. [CrossRef] [PubMed]
3. Sutton, M.G.; Sheps, S.G.; Lie, J.T. Prevalence of clinically unsuspected pheochromocytoma. Review of a 50-year autopsy series. *Mayo Clin. Proc.* **1981**, *56*, 354–360. [CrossRef]

4. Guerrero, M.A.; Schreinemakers, J.M.; Vriens, M.R.; Suh, I.; Hwang, J.; Shen, W.T.; Gosnell, J.; Clark, O.H.; Duh, Q.-Y. Clinical Spectrum of Pheochromocytoma. *J. Am. Coll. Surg.* **2009**, *209*, 727–732. [CrossRef] [PubMed]
5. Lenders, J.W.; Eisenhofer, G.; Mannelli, M.; Pacak, K. Phaeochromocytoma. *Lancet* **2005**, *366*, 665–675. [CrossRef]
6. Fishbein, L.; Leshchiner, I.; Walter, V.; Danilova, L.; Robertson, A.G.; Johnson, A.R.; Lichtenberg, T.M.; Murray, B.A.; Ghayee, H.K.; Else, T.; et al. Comprehensive Molecular Characterization of Pheochromocytoma and Paraganglioma. *Cancer Cell* **2017**, *31*, 181–193. [CrossRef]
7. Jochmanova, I.; Pacak, K. Genomic Landscape of Pheochromocytoma and Paraganglioma. *Trends Cancer* **2018**, *4*, 6–9. [CrossRef]
8. Burnichon, N.; Vescovo, L.; Amar, L.; Libe, R.; De Reynies, A.; Venisse, A.; Jouanno, E.; Laurendeau, I.; Parfait, B.; Bertherat, J.; et al. Integrative genomic analysis reveals somatic mutations in pheochromocytoma and paraganglioma. *Hum. Mol. Genet.* **2011**, *20*, 3974–3985. [CrossRef]
9. Hampel, H.; Bennett, R.L.; Buchanan, A.; Pearlman, R.; Wiesner, G.L. A practice guideline from the American College of Medical Genetics and Genomics and the National Society of Genetic Counselors: Referral indications for cancer predisposition assessment. *Genet. Med.* **2015**, *17*, 70–87. [CrossRef]
10. Lenders, J.W.M.; Duh, Q.-Y.; Eisenhofer, G.; Gimenez-Roqueplo, A.-P.; Grebe, S.K.G.; Murad, M.H.; Naruse, M.; Pacak, K.; Young, W.F. Pheochromocytoma and Paraganglioma: An Endocrine Society Clinical Practice Guideline. *J. Clin. Endocrinol. Metab.* **2014**, *99*, 1915–1942. [CrossRef]
11. Dahia, P.L.M. Pheochromocytoma and paraganglioma pathogenesis: Learning from genetic heterogeneity. *Nat. Cancer* **2014**, *14*, 108–119. [CrossRef] [PubMed]
12. Favier, J.; Amar, L.; Gimenez-Roqueplo, A.-P. Paraganglioma and phaeochromocytoma: From genetics to personalized medicine. *Nat. Rev. Endocrinol.* **2015**, *11*, 101–111. [CrossRef] [PubMed]
13. King, K.S.; Prodanov, T.; Kantorovich, V.; Fojo, T.; Hewitt, J.; Zacharin, M.; Wesley, R.; Lodish, M.; Raygada, M.; Gimenez-Roqueplo, A.-P.; et al. Metastatic Pheochromocytoma/Paraganglioma Related to Primary Tumor Development in Childhood or Adolescence: Significant Link to SDHB Mutations. *J. Clin. Oncol.* **2011**, *29*, 4137–4142. [CrossRef] [PubMed]
14. Shuch, B.; Ricketts, C.J.; Metwalli, A.R.; Pacak, K.; Linehan, W.M. The Genetic Basis of Pheochromocytoma and Paraganglioma: Implications for Management. *Urology* **2014**, *83*, 1225–1232. [CrossRef]
15. Mak, I.Y.F.; Hayes, A.; Khoo, B.; Grossman, A. Peptide Receptor Radionuclide Therapy as a Novel Treatment for Metastatic and Invasive Phaeochromocytoma and Paraganglioma. *Neuroendocrinology* **2019**, *109*, 287–298. [CrossRef]
16. Kong, G.; Grozinsky-Glasberg, S.; Hofman, M.; Callahan, J.; Meirovitz, A.; Maimon, O.; Pattison, D.; Gross, D.J.; Hicks, R. Efficacy of Peptide Receptor Radionuclide Therapy for Functional Metastatic Paraganglioma and Pheochromocytoma. *J. Clin. Endocrinol. Metab.* **2017**, *102*, 3278–3287. [CrossRef]
17. Yadav, M.P.; Ballal, S.; Bal, C. Concomitant 177Lu-DOTATATE and capecitabine therapy in malignant paragangliomas. *EJNMMI Res.* **2019**, *9*, 13. [CrossRef]
18. Huang, H.; Abraham, J.; Hung, E.; Averbuch, S.; Merino, M.J.; Steinberg, S.M.; Pacak, K.; Fojo, T. Treatment of malignant pheochromocytoma/paraganglioma with cyclophosphamide, vincristine, and dacarbazine. *Cancer* **2008**, *113*, 2020–2028. [CrossRef]
19. Ilanchezhian, M.; Jha, A.; Pacak, K.; Del Rivero, J. Emerging Treatments for Advanced/Metastatic Pheochromocytoma and Paraganglioma. *Curr. Treat. Options Oncol.* **2020**, *21*, 85. [CrossRef]
20. Castelblanco, E.; Santacana, M.; Valls, J.; de Cubas, A.; Cascón, A.; Robledo, M.; Matias-Guiu, X. Usefulness of Negative and Weak-Diffuse Pattern of SDHB Immunostaining in Assessment of SDH Mutations in Paragangliomas and Pheochromocytomas. *Endocr. Pathol.* **2013**, *24*, 199–205. [CrossRef]
21. Amar, L.; Pacak, K.; Steichen, O.; Akker, S.A.; Aylwin, S.J.B.; Baudin, E.; Buffet, A.; Burnichon, N.; Clifton-Bligh, R.J.; Dahia, P.L.M.; et al. International consensus on initial screening and follow-up of asymptomatic SDHx mutation carriers. *Nat. Rev. Endocrinol.* **2021**, *17*, 435–444. [CrossRef] [PubMed]
22. King, A.; Selak, M.A.; Gottlieb, E. Succinate dehydrogenase and fumarate hydratase: Linking mitochondrial dysfunction and cancer. *Oncogene* **2006**, *25*, 4675–4682. [CrossRef] [PubMed]
23. Toledo, R.; Qin, Y.; Cheng, Z.-M.; Gao, Q.; Iwata, S.; Silva, G.M.; Prasad, M.L.; Ocal, I.T.; Rao, S.; Aronin, N.; et al. Recurrent Mutations of Chromatin-Remodeling Genes and Kinase Receptors in Pheochromocytomas and Paragangliomas. *Clin. Cancer Res.* **2016**, *22*, 2301–2310. [CrossRef] [PubMed]
24. Kunst, H.P.; Rutten, M.H.; De Mönnink, J.-P.; Hoefsloot, L.H.; Timmers, H.J.; Marres, H.A.; Jansen, J.; Kremer, H.; Bayley, J.-P.; Cremers, C.W. SDHAF2 (PGL2-SDH5) and Hereditary Head and Neck Paraganglioma. *Clin. Cancer Res.* **2011**, *17*, 247–254. [CrossRef] [PubMed]
25. Castro-Vega, L.J.; Buffet, A.; De Cubas, A.A.; Cascón, A.; Menara, M.; Khalifa, E.; Amar, L.; Azriel, S.; Bourdeau, I.; Chabre, O.; et al. Germline mutations in FH confer predisposition to malignant pheochromocytomas and paragangliomas. *Hum. Mol. Genet.* **2014**, *23*, 2440–2446. [CrossRef]
26. Clark, G.R.; Sciacovelli, M.; Gaude, E.; Walsh, D.M.; Kirby, G.; Simpson, M.; Trembath, R.; Berg, J.N.; Woodward, E.R.; Kinning, E.; et al. Germline FH Mutations Presenting With Pheochromocytoma. *J. Clin. Endocrinol. Metab.* **2014**, *99*, E2046–E2050. [CrossRef]
27. Calsina, B.; Currás-Freixes, M.; Buffet, A.; Pons, T.; Contreras, L.; Letón, R.; Comino-Méndez, I.; Remacha, L.; Calatayud, M.; Obispo, B.; et al. Role of MDH2 pathogenic variant in pheochromocytoma and paraganglioma patients. *Genet. Med.* **2018**, *20*, 1652–1662. [CrossRef]

28. Cascón, A.; Comino-Méndez, I.; Currás-Freixes, M.; de Cubas, A.A.; Contreras, L.; Richter, S.; Peitzsch, M.; Mancikova, V.; Inglada-Pérez, L.; Pérez-Barrios, A.; et al. Whole-Exome Sequencing Identifies MDH2 as a New Familial Paraganglioma Gene. *J. Natl. Cancer Inst.* **2015**, *107*, djv053. [CrossRef]
29. Lorenzo, F.R.; Yang, C.; Ng Tang Fui, M.; Vankayalapati, H.; Zhuang, Z.; Huynh, T.; Grossmann, M.; Pacak, K.; Prchal, J.T. A novel EPAS1/HIF2A germline mutation in a congenital polycythemia with paraganglioma. *J. Mol. Med.* **2013**, *91*, 507–512. [CrossRef]
30. Därr, R.; Nambuba, J.; Del Rivero, J.; Janssen, I.; Merino, M.; Todorovic, M.; Balint, B.; Jochmanova, I.; Prchal, J.T.; Lechan, R.M.; et al. Novel insights into the polycythemia–paraganglioma–somatostatinoma syndrome. *Endocr.-Relat. Cancer* **2016**, *23*, 899–908. [CrossRef]
31. Pacak, K.; Jochmanova, I.; Prodanov, T.; Yang, C.; Merino, M.J.; Fojo, T.; Prchal, J.T.; Tischler, A.S.; Lechan, R.M.; Zhuang, Z. New Syndrome of Paraganglioma and Somatostatinoma Associated With Polycythemia. *J. Clin. Oncol.* **2013**, *31*, 1690–1698. [CrossRef] [PubMed]
32. Yang, C.; Zhuang, Z.; Fliedner, S.; Shankavaram, U.; Sun, M.G.; Bullova, P.; Zhu, R.; Elkahloun, A.G.; Kourlas, P.J.; Merino, M.; et al. Germ-line PHD1 and PHD2 mutations detected in patients with pheochromocytoma/paraganglioma-polycythemia. *Klin. Wochenschr.* **2015**, *93*, 93–104. [CrossRef] [PubMed]
33. Fishbein, L.; Khare, S.; Wubbenhorst, B.; Desloover, D.; D'Andrea, K.; Merrill, S.; Cho, N.W.; Greenberg, R.A.; Else, T.; Montone, K.; et al. Whole-exome sequencing identifies somatic ATRX mutations in pheochromocytomas and paragangliomas. *Nat. Commun.* **2015**, *6*, 6140. [CrossRef] [PubMed]
34. Crona, J.; Taïeb, D.; Pacak, K. New Perspectives on Pheochromocytoma and Paraganglioma: Toward a Molecular Classification. *Endocr. Rev.* **2017**, *38*, 489–515. [CrossRef] [PubMed]
35. Greer, E.L.; Shi, Y. Histone methylation: A dynamic mark in health, disease and inheritance. *Nat. Rev. Genet.* **2012**, *13*, 343–357. [CrossRef] [PubMed]
36. Iwata, S.; Yonemoto, T.; Ishii, T.; Araki, A.; Hagiwara, Y.; Tatezaki, S.I. Multicentric Giant Cell Tumor of Bone and Paraganglioma: A Case Report. *JBJS Case Connect.* **2013**, *3*, e23. [CrossRef]
37. Cerami, E.; Gao, J.; Dogrusoz, U.; Gross, B.E.; Sumer, S.O.; Aksoy, B.A.; Jacobsen, A.; Byrne, C.J.; Heuer, M.L.; Larsson, E.; et al. The cBio Cancer Genomics Portal: An Open Platform for Exploring Multidimensional Cancer Genomics Data: Figure 1. *Cancer Discov.* **2012**, *2*, 401–404. [CrossRef]
38. Gao, J.; Aksoy, B.A.; Dogrusoz, U.; Dresdner, G.; Gross, B.; Sumer, S.O.; Sun, Y.; Jacobsen, A.; Sinha, R.; Larsson, E.; et al. Integrative Analysis of Complex Cancer Genomics and Clinical Profiles Using the cBioPortal. *Sci. Signal.* **2013**, *6*, pl1. [CrossRef]
39. Miao, C.-G.; Shi, W.-J.; Xiong, Y.-Y.; Yu, H.; Zhang, X.-L.; Qin, M.-S.; Du, C.-L.; Song, T.-W.; Li, J. miR-375 regulates the canonical Wnt pathway through FZD8 silencing in arthritis synovial fibroblasts. *Immunol. Lett.* **2015**, *164*, 1–10. [CrossRef]
40. Buffet, A.; Morin, A.; Castro-Vega, L.J.; Habarou, F.; Lussey-Lepoutre, C.; Letouze, E.; Lefebvre, H.; Guilhem, I.; Haissaguerre, M.; Raingeard, I.; et al. Germline Mutations in the Mitochondrial 2-Oxoglutarate/Malate Carrier SLC25A11 Gene Confer a Predisposition to Metastatic Paragangliomas. *Cancer Res.* **2018**, *78*, 1914–1922. [CrossRef]
41. Monné, M.; Palmieri, F. Antiporters of the Mitochondrial Carrier Family. *Chloride Channels* **2014**, *73*, 289–320. [CrossRef]
42. Pang, Y.; Gupta, G.; Yang, C.; Wang, H.; Huynh, T.-T.; Abdullaev, Z.; Pack, S.D.; Percy, M.J.; Lappin, T.R.J.; Zhuang, Z.; et al. A novel splicing site IRP1 somatic mutation in a patient with pheochromocytoma and JAK2V617F positive polycythemia vera: A case report. *BMC Cancer* **2018**, *18*, 286. [CrossRef] [PubMed]
43. Remacha, L.; Pirman, D.; Mahoney, C.E.; Coloma, J.; Calsina, B.; Currás-Freixes, M.; Letón, R.; Torres-Pérez, R.; Richter, S.; Pita, G.; et al. Recurrent Germline DLST Mutations in Individuals with Multiple Pheochromocytomas and Paragangliomas. *Am. J. Hum. Genet.* **2019**, *104*, 1008–1010. [CrossRef] [PubMed]
44. Vanova, K.H.; Pang, Y.; Krobova, L.; Kraus, M.; Nahacka, Z.; Boukalova, S.; Pack, S.D.; Zobalova, R.; Zhu, J.; Huynh, T.-T.; et al. Germline SUCLG2 Variants in Patients With Pheochromocytoma and Paraganglioma. *J. Natl. Cancer Inst.* **2021**, *114*, 130–138. [CrossRef]
45. Alzofon, N.; Koc, K.; Panwell, K.; Pozdeyev, N.; Marshall, C.B.; Albuja-Cruz, M.; Raeburn, C.D.; Nathanson, K.L.; Cohen, D.L.; Wierman, M.E.; et al. Mastermind Like Transcriptional Coactivator 3 (MAML3) Drives Neuroendocrine Tumor Progression. *Mol. Cancer Res.* **2021**, *19*, 1476–1485. [CrossRef]
46. Sanchez, M.; Galy, B.; Muckenthaler, M.; Hentze, M. Iron-regulatory proteins limit hypoxia-inducible factor-2α expression in iron deficiency. *Nat. Struct. Mol. Biol.* **2007**, *14*, 420–426. [CrossRef]
47. Pang, Y.; Lu, Y.; Caisova, V.; Liu, Y.; Bullova, P.; Huynh, T.; Zhou, Y.; Yu, D.; Frysak, Z.; Hartmann, I.; et al. Targeting NAD(+)/PARP DNA Repair Pathway as a Novel Therapeutic Approach to SDHB-Mutated Cluster I Pheochromocytoma and Paraganglioma. *Clin. Cancer Res.* **2018**, *24*, 3423–3432. [CrossRef]
48. Mole, D.R.; Schlemminger, I.; McNeill, L.A.; Hewitson, K.S.; Pugh, C.W.; Ratcliffe, P.J.; Schofield, C.J. 2-Oxoglutarate analogue inhibitors of hif prolyl hydroxylase. *Bioorg. Med. Chem. Lett.* **2003**, *13*, 2677–2680. [CrossRef]
49. Buffet, A.; Burnichon, N.; Favier, J.; Gimenez-Roqueplo, A.-P. An overview of 20 years of genetic studies in pheochromocytoma and paraganglioma. *Best Pract. Res. Clin. Endocrinol. Metab.* **2020**, *34*, 101416. [CrossRef]
50. Greenman, C.; Stephens, P.; Smith, R.; Dalgliesh, G.L.; Hunter, C.; Bignell, G.; Davies, H.; Teague, J.; Butler, A.; Stevens, C.; et al. Patterns of somatic mutation in human cancer genomes. *Nature* **2007**, *446*, 153–158. [CrossRef]

51. Schmidt, L.; Duh, F.-M.; Chen, F.; Kishida, T.; Glenn, G.; Choyke, P.; Scherer, S.; Zhuang, Z.; Lubensky, I.; Dean, M.; et al. Germline and somatic mutations in the tyrosine kinase domain of the MET proto-oncogene in papillary renal carcinomas. *Nat. Genet.* **1997**, *16*, 68–73. [CrossRef] [PubMed]
52. Johnson, J.D.; Mehus, J.G.; Tews, K.; Milavetz, B.I.; Lambeth, D.O. Genetic evidence for the expression of ATP- and GTP-specific succinyl-CoA synthetases in multicellular eucaryotes. *J. Biol. Chem.* **1998**, *273*, 27580–27586. [CrossRef] [PubMed]
53. Selak, M.A.; Armour, S.M.; MacKenzie, E.D.; Boulahbel, H.; Watson, D.G.; Mansfield, K.D.; Pan, Y.; Simon, M.; Thompson, C.B.; Gottlieb, E. Succinate links TCA cycle dysfunction to oncogenesis by inhibiting HIF-α prolyl hydroxylase. *Cancer Cell* **2005**, *7*, 77–85. [CrossRef] [PubMed]
54. Miller, C.; Wang, L.; Ostergaard, E.; Dan, P.; Saada, A. The interplay between SUCLA2, SUCLG2, and mitochondrial DNA depletion. *Biochim. Biophys. Acta-Mol. Basis Dis.* **2011**, *1812*, 625–629. [CrossRef] [PubMed]
55. Kacso, G.; Ravasz, D.; Doczi, J.; Németh, B.; Madgar, O.; Saada, A.; Ilin, P.; Miller, C.; Ostergaard, E.; Iordanov, I.; et al. Two transgenic mouse models for beta-subunit components of succinate-CoA ligase yielding pleiotropic metabolic alterations. *Biochem. J.* **2016**, *473*, 3463–3485. [CrossRef] [PubMed]
56. Amar, L.; Bertherat, J.; Baudin, E.; Ajzenberg, C.; Paillerets, B.B.-D.; Chabre, O.; Chamontin, B.; Delemer, B.; Giraud, S.; Murat, A.; et al. Genetic Testing in Pheochromocytoma or Functional Paraganglioma. *J. Clin. Oncol.* **2005**, *23*, 8812–8818. [CrossRef]
57. Ben Aim, L.; Pigny, P.; Castro-Vega, L.J.; Buffet, A.; Amar, L.; Bertherat, J.; Drui, D.; Guilhem, I.; Baudin, E.; Lussey-Lepoutre, C.; et al. Targeted next-generation sequencing detects rare genetic events in pheochromocytoma and paraganglioma. *J. Med. Genet.* **2019**, *56*, 513–520. [CrossRef]
58. Andrews, K.A.; Ascher, D.B.; Pires, D.E.V.; Barnes, D.R.; Vialard, L.; Casey, R.T.; Bradshaw, N.; Adlard, J.; Aylwin, S.; Brennan, P.; et al. Tumour risks and genotype-phenotype correlations associated with germline variants in succinate dehydrogenase subunit genes SDHB, SDHC and SDHD. *J. Med. Genet.* **2018**, *55*, 384–394. [CrossRef]
59. Marikian, G.G.; Ambartsumian, T.G.; Adamian, S.I. Ouabain-insensitive K+ and Na+ fluxes in frog muscle. *Biofizika* **1983**, *28*, 1019–1021.
60. Benn, D.E.; Gimenez-Roqueplo, A.-P.; Reilly, J.; Bertherat, J.; Burgess, J.; Byth, K.; Croxson, M.; Dahia, P.L.M.; Elston, M.; Gimm, O.; et al. Clinical Presentation and Penetrance of Pheochromocytoma/Paraganglioma Syndromes. *J. Clin. Endocrinol. Metab.* **2006**, *91*, 827–836. [CrossRef]
61. Amar, L.; Baudin, E.; Burnichon, N.; Peyrard, S.; Silvera, S.; Bertherat, J.; Bertagna, X.; Schlumberger, M.; Jeunemaitre, X.; Gimenez-Roqueplo, A.-P.; et al. Succinate Dehydrogenase B Gene Mutations Predict Survival in Patients with Malignant Pheochromocytomas or Paragangliomas. *J. Clin. Endocrinol. Metab.* **2007**, *92*, 3822–3828. [CrossRef] [PubMed]
62. Neumann, H.P.; Pawlu, C.; Peczkowska, M.; Bausch, B.; McWhinney, S.R.; Muresan, M.; Buchta, M.; Franke, G.; Klisch, J.; Bley, T.A.; et al. Distinct clinical features of paraganglioma syndromes associated with SDHB and SDHD gene mutations. *JAMA* **2004**, *292*, 943–951. [CrossRef] [PubMed]
63. Bourdeau, I.; Grunenwald, S.; Burnichon, N.; Khalifa, E.; Dumas, N.; Binet, M.-C.; Nolet, S.; Gimenez-Roqueplo, A.-P. A SDHC Founder Mutation Causes Paragangliomas (PGLs) in the French Canadians: New Insights on the SDHC-Related PGL. *J. Clin. Endocrinol. Metab.* **2016**, *101*, 4710–4718. [CrossRef] [PubMed]
64. Burnichon, N.; Mazzella, J.M.; Drui, D.; Amar, L.; Bertherat, J.; Coupier, I.; Delemer, B.; Guilhem, I.; Herman, P.; Kerlan, V.; et al. Risk assessment of maternally inherited SDHD paraganglioma and phaeochromocytoma. *J. Med. Genet.* **2017**, *54*, 125–133. [CrossRef] [PubMed]
65. Neumann, H.P.H.; Young, W.F., Jr.; Eng, C. Pheochromocytoma and Paraganglioma. *N. Engl. J. Med.* **2019**, *381*, 552–565. [CrossRef] [PubMed]
66. Jochmanova, I.; Abcede, A.M.T.; Guerrero, R.J.S.; Malong, C.L.P.; Wesley, R.; Huynh, T.; Gonzales, M.K.; Wolf, K.I.; Jha, A.; Knue, M.; et al. Clinical characteristics and outcomes of SDHB-related pheochromocytoma and paraganglioma in children and adolescents. *J. Cancer Res. Clin. Oncol.* **2020**, *146*, 1051–1063. [CrossRef]
67. Peaston, R.T.; Lai, L.C. Biochemical detection of phaeochromocytoma: Should we still be measuring urinary HMMA? *J. Clin. Pathol.* **1993**, *46*, 734–737. [CrossRef]
68. Manu, P.; Runge, L.A. Biochemical screening for pheochromocytoma. Superiority of urinary metanephrines measurements. *Am. J. Epidemiol.* **1984**, *120*, 788–790. [CrossRef]
69. Sargar, K.M.; Khanna, G.; Bowling, R.H. Imaging of Nonmalignant Adrenal Lesions in Children. *Radiographics* **2017**, *37*, 1648–1664. [CrossRef]
70. Heesterman, B.L.; de Pont, L.; van der Mey, A.G.; Bayley, J.P.; Corssmit, E.P.; Hes, F.J.; Verbist, B.M.; van Benthem, P.; Jansen, J.C. Clinical progression and metachronous paragangliomas in a large cohort of SDHD germline variant carriers. *Eur. J. Hum. Genet.* **2018**, *26*, 1339–1347. [CrossRef]
71. Lenders, J.W.M.; Langton, K.; Langenhuijsen, J.F.; Eisenhofer, G. Pheochromocytoma and Pregnancy. *Endocrinol. Metab. Clin.* **2019**, *48*, 605–617. [CrossRef] [PubMed]
72. Casey, R.; McLean, M.; Madhu, B.; Challis, B.G.; Hoopen, R.T.; Roberts, T.; Clark, G.; Pittfield, D.; Simpson, H.L.; Bulusu, V.R.; et al. Translating in vivo metabolomic analysis of succinate dehydrogenase deficient tumours into clinical utility. *JCO Precis. Oncol.* **2018**, *2*, 1–12. [CrossRef] [PubMed]

73. Lopez-Jimenez, E.; de Campos, J.M.; Kusak, E.M.; Landa, I.; Leskela, S.; Montero-Conde, C.; Leandro-Garcia, L.J.; Vallejo, L.A.; Madrigal, B.; Rodriguez-Antona, C.; et al. SDHC mutation in an elderly patient without familial antecedents. *Clin. Endocrinol.* **2008**, *69*, 906–910. [CrossRef] [PubMed]
74. Shimizu, T. Stimulation of Oxygen Consumption of Platelets by Solcoseryl and Cardiocrome during In Vitro Aging for 5 Days. *Jpn. J. Pharmacol.* **1990**, *53*, 499–501. [CrossRef]
75. Xekouki, P.; Szarek, E.; Bullova, P.; Giubellino, A.; Quezado, M.; Mastroyannis, S.; Mastorakos, P.; Wassif, C.; Raygada, M.; Rentia, N.; et al. Pituitary Adenoma With Paraganglioma/Pheochromocytoma (3PAs) and Succinate Dehydrogenase Defects in Humans and Mice. *J. Clin. Endocrinol. Metab.* **2015**, *100*, E710–E719. [CrossRef]
76. Fankhauser, M.; Bechmann, N.; Lauseker, M.; Goncalves, J.; Favier, J.; Klink, B.; William, D.; Gieldon, L.; Maurer, J.; Spöttl, G.; et al. Synergistic Highly Potent Targeted Drug Combinations in Different Pheochromocytoma Models Including Human Tumor Cultures. *Endocrinology* **2019**, *160*, 2600–2617. [CrossRef]
77. Ghayee, H.K.; Bhagwandin, V.J.; Stastny, V.; Click, A.; Ding, L.-H.; Mizrachi, D.; Zou, Y.; Chari, R.; Lam, W.L.; Bachoo, R.M.; et al. Progenitor Cell Line (hPheo1) Derived from a Human Pheochromocytoma Tumor. *PLoS ONE* **2013**, *8*, e65624. [CrossRef]
78. Suga, H. Application of pluripotent stem cells for treatment of human neuroendocrine disorders. *Z. Zellforsch. Mikrosk. Anat.* **2018**, *375*, 267–278. [CrossRef]
79. Bleijs, M.; Van De Wetering, M.; Clevers, H.; Drost, J. Xenograft and organoid model systems in cancer research. *EMBO J.* **2019**, *38*, e101654. [CrossRef]
80. Powers, J.F.; Cochran, B.; Baleja, J.D.; Sikes, H.D.; Pattison, A.D.; Zhang, X.; Lomakin, I.; Shepard-Barry, A.; Pacak, K.; Moon, S.J.; et al. A xenograft and cell line model of SDH-deficient pheochromocytoma derived from Sdhb+/− rats. *Endocr. Relat. Cancer* **2020**, *27*, 337–354. [CrossRef]
81. Toledo, R.; The NGS in PPGL (NGSnPPGL) Study Group; Burnichon, N.; Cascon, A.; Benn, D.E.; Bayley, J.-P.; Welander, J.; Tops, C.M.; Firth, H.; Dwight, T.; et al. Consensus Statement on next-generation-sequencing-based diagnostic testing of hereditary phaeochromocytomas and paragangliomas. *Nat. Rev. Endocrinol.* **2017**, *13*, 233–247. [CrossRef] [PubMed]
82. Pillai, S.; Gopalan, V.; Lam, A.K.-Y. Review of sequencing platforms and their applications in phaeochromocytoma and paragangliomas. *Crit. Rev. Oncol.* **2017**, *116*, 58–67. [CrossRef] [PubMed]
83. Liu, P.; Li, M.; Guan, X.; Yu, A.; Xiao, Q.; Wang, C.; Hu, Y.; Zhu, F.; Yin, H.; Yi, X.; et al. Clinical Syndromes and Genetic Screening Strategies of Pheochromocytoma and Paraganglioma. *J. Kidney Cancer VHL* **2018**, *5*, 14–22. [CrossRef] [PubMed]
84. Goncalves, J.; Lussey-Lepoutre, C.; Favier, J.; Gimenez-Roqueplo, A.-P.; Castro-Vega, L.J. Emerging molecular markers of metastatic pheochromocytomas and paragangliomas. *Ann. d'Endocrinol.* **2019**, *80*, 159–162. [CrossRef]
85. Job, S.; Georges, A.; Burnichon, N.; Buffet, A.; Amar, L.; Bertherat, J.; Bouatia-Naji, N.; De Reyniès, A.; Drui, D.; Lussey-Lepoutre, C.; et al. Transcriptome Analysis of lncRNAs in Pheochromocytomas and Paragangliomas. *J. Clin. Endocrinol. Metab.* **2019**, *105*, 898–907. [CrossRef] [PubMed]
86. Calsina, B.; Castro-Vega, L.J.; Torres-Perez, R.; Inglada-Pérez, L.; Currás-Freixes, M.; Roldán-Romero, J.M.; Mancikova, V.; Letón, R.; Remacha, L.; Santos, M.; et al. Integrative multi-omics analysis identifies a prognostic miRNA signature and a targetable miR-21-3p/TSC2/mTOR axis in metastatic pheochromocytoma/paraganglioma. *Theranostics* **2019**, *9*, 4946–4958. [CrossRef]
87. de Cubas, A.A.; Korpershoek, E.; Inglada-Pérez, L.; Letouzé, E.; Currás-Freixes, M.; Fernández, A.F.; Comino-Méndez, I.; Schiavi, F.; Mancikova, V.; Eisenhofer, G.; et al. DNA Methylation Profiling in Pheochromocytoma and Paraganglioma Reveals Diagnostic and Prognostic Markers. *Clin. Cancer Res.* **2015**, *21*, 3020–3030. [CrossRef]
88. Backman, S.; Maharjan, R.; Falk-Delgado, A.; Crona, J.; Cupisti, K.; Stålberg, P.; Hellman, P.; Björklund, P. Global DNA Methylation Analysis Identifies Two Discrete clusters of Pheochromocytoma with Distinct Genomic and Genetic Alterations. *Sci. Rep.* **2017**, *7*, 44943. [CrossRef]
89. Körner, M.; Waser, B.; Schonbrunn, A.; Perren, A.; Reubi, J.C. Somatostatin Receptor Subtype 2A Immunohistochemistry Using a New Monoclonal Antibody Selects Tumors Suitable for In Vivo Somatostatin Receptor Targeting. *Am. J. Surg. Pathol.* **2012**, *36*, 242–252. [CrossRef]
90. Stenman, A.; Svahn, F.; Farsangi, M.H.; Zedenius, J.; Söderkvist, P.; Gimm, O.; Larsson, C.; Juhlin, C.C. Molecular Profiling of Pheochromocytoma and Abdominal Paraganglioma Stratified by the PASS Algorithm Reveals Chromogranin B as Associated With Histologic Prediction of Malignant Behavior. *Am. J. Surg. Pathol.* **2019**, *43*, 409–421. [CrossRef]
91. Casey, R.; Neumann, H.P.; Maher, E. Genetic stratification of inherited and sporadic phaeochromocytoma and paraganglioma: Implications for precision medicine. *Hum. Mol. Genet* **2020**, *29*, R128–R137. [CrossRef] [PubMed]
92. Lenders, J.W.; Kerstens, M.N.; Amar, L.; Prejbisz, A.; Robledo, M.; Taieb, D.; Pacak, K.; Crona, J.; Zelinka, T.; Mannelli, M.; et al. Genetics, diagnosis, management and future directions of research of phaeochromocytoma and paraganglioma: A position statement and consensus of the Working Group on Endocrine Hypertension of the European Society of Hypertension. *J. Hypertens.* **2020**, *38*, 1443–1456. [CrossRef] [PubMed]
93. Nölting, S.; Ullrich, M.; Pietzsch, J.; Ziegler, C.G.; Eisenhofer, G.; Grossman, A.; Pacak, K. Current Management of Pheochromocytoma/Paraganglioma: A Guide for the Practicing Clinician in the Era of Precision Medicine. *Cancers* **2019**, *11*, 1505. [CrossRef] [PubMed]
94. Nölting, S.; Grossman, A.; Pacak, K. Metastatic Phaeochromocytoma: Spinning Towards More Promising Treatment Options. *Exp. Clin. Endocrinol. Diabetes* **2019**, *127*, 117–128. [CrossRef] [PubMed]

95. Tabebi, M.; Dutta, R.K.; Skoglund, C.; Söderkvist, P.; Gimm, O. Loss of SDHB Induces a Metabolic Switch in the hPheo1 Cell Line toward Enhanced OXPHOS. *Int. J. Mol. Sci.* **2022**, *23*, 560. [CrossRef] [PubMed]
96. Wallace, P.W.; Conrad, C.; Brückmann, S.; Pang, Y.; Caleiras, E.; Murakami, M.; Korpershoek, E.; Zhuang, Z.; Rapizzi, E.; Kroiss, M.; et al. Metabolomics, machine learning and immunohistochemistry to predict succinate dehydrogenase mutational status in phaeochromocytomas and paragangliomas. *J. Pathol.* **2020**, *251*, 378–387. [CrossRef]

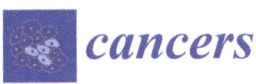

Review

Insights into Mechanisms of Pheochromocytomas and Paragangliomas Driven by Known or New Genetic Drivers

Shahida K. Flores [1], Cynthia M. Estrada-Zuniga [1], Keerthi Thallapureddy [1], Gustavo Armaiz-Peña [1] and Patricia L. M. Dahia [1,2,*]

[1] Department of Medicine, University of Texas Health San Antonio, San Antonio, TX 78229, USA; shahida.flores@gmail.com (S.K.F.); estradazunig@uthscsa.edu (C.M.E.-Z.); thallapuredd@livemail.uthscsa.edu (K.T.); armaizpena@uthscsa.edu (G.A.-P.)
[2] Mays Cancer Center, University of Texas Health San Antonio, San Antonio, TX 78229, USA
* Correspondence: dahia@uthscsa.edu

Simple Summary: Pheochromocytomas and paragangliomas are rare neuroendocrine tumors that are often hereditary. Although research has advanced considerably, significant gaps still persist in understanding risk factors, predicting metastatic potential and treating aggressive tumors. The study of rare mutations can provide new insights into how pheochromocytomas and paragangliomas develop. In this review, we provide examples of such rare events and how they can inform our understanding of the spectrum of mutations that can lead to these tumors and improve our ability to provide a genetic diagnosis.

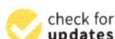

Citation: Flores, S.K.; Estrada-Zuniga, C.M.; Thallapureddy, K.; Armaiz-Peña, G.; Dahia, P.L.M. Insights into Mechanisms of Pheochromocytomas and Paragangliomas Driven by Known or New Genetic Drivers. *Cancers* **2021**, *13*, 4602. https://doi.org/10.3390/cancers13184602

Academic Editor: Peter Igaz

Received: 30 August 2021
Accepted: 12 September 2021
Published: 14 September 2021

Publisher's Note: MDPI stays neutral with regard to jurisdictional claims in published maps and institutional affiliations.

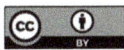

Copyright: © 2021 by the authors. Licensee MDPI, Basel, Switzerland. This article is an open access article distributed under the terms and conditions of the Creative Commons Attribution (CC BY) license (https://creativecommons.org/licenses/by/4.0/).

Abstract: Pheochromocytomas and paragangliomas are rare tumors of neural crest origin. Their remarkable genetic diversity and high heritability have enabled discoveries of bona fide cancer driver genes with an impact on diagnosis and clinical management and have consistently shed light on new paradigms in cancer. In this review, we explore unique mechanisms of pheochromocytoma and paraganglioma initiation and management by drawing from recent examples involving rare mutations of hypoxia-related genes *VHL*, *EPAS1* and *SDHB*, and of a poorly known susceptibility gene, *TMEM127*. These models expand our ability to predict variant pathogenicity, inform new functional domains, recognize environmental-gene connections, and highlight persistent therapeutic challenges for tumors with aggressive behavior.

Keywords: pheochromocytomas; paragangliomas; mutations; susceptibility genes; driver mutations; hereditary; germline; somatic; environment; variants; tumor suppressor genes; metastatic; treatment; RNAseq; next generation sequencing

1. Overview and Current Status of Genetic Drivers

Pheochromocytomas and paragangliomas (PPGLs) are rare neural crest derived tumors with an incidence of 500 to 1600 cases per year [1,2]. Pheochromocytomas arise from adrenomedullary chromaffin cells and paragangliomas arise from extra-adrenal chromaffin cells of the sympathetic paravertebral ganglia of thorax, abdomen, and pelvis or chief cells that form the paraganglia of glossopharyngeal and vagal nerves in the neck and base of the skull [3]. While pheochromocytomas and thoracic-abdominal paragangliomas often produce catecholamines, head and neck paragangliomas are almost invariably non-secreting [4]. PPGLs are predominantly benign, and malignancy is only established by the detection of metastasis, which occurs in approximately 30% of paragangliomas and 10–15% of pheochromocytomas. Currently there are limited options for treatment of metastatic PPGLs [5,6].

PPGLs are remarkable for their high heritability rate and genetic diversity. More than 20 genes have been implicated in PPGL [7–9]. Mutations of these genes occur in a mutually exclusive manner through germline (~30–40%) or somatic (30%) transmission

(Figure 1A) [10,11]. Within the domain of hereditary mutations, genes that predispose to genetic syndromes include *RET* (multiple endocrine neoplasia type 2A and 2B), *VHL* (von Hippel Lindau disease), *NF1* (neurofibromatosis type 1) and *SDH* subunit genes (hereditary paraganglioma syndromes types 1–5) [12]. *TMEM127, MAX, FH* and *MDH2* genes have also been linked to germline mutations [13]. However, *NF1, VHL, RET,* and *MAX* can also be somatically mutated. Genes exclusively associated with somatic mutations include *EPAS1, ATRX,* and *HRAS*. [10,14–17]. Besides germline and somatic mutations, mosaicism (post-zygotic mutation) has been reported in *EPAS1, H3F3A, VHL* and *SDHB*, and has been historically associated with *NF1*, although not specifically in the context of PPGLs [16,18]. Recently, gene fusions have been recognized in PPGLs, especially those involving the MAML3 transcription factor, including the *UBTF-MAML3* fusion [14]. Other genes (listed in Figure 1A) have only been reported in a few cases, and the evidence supporting their direct role in PPGLs still remains limited [19].

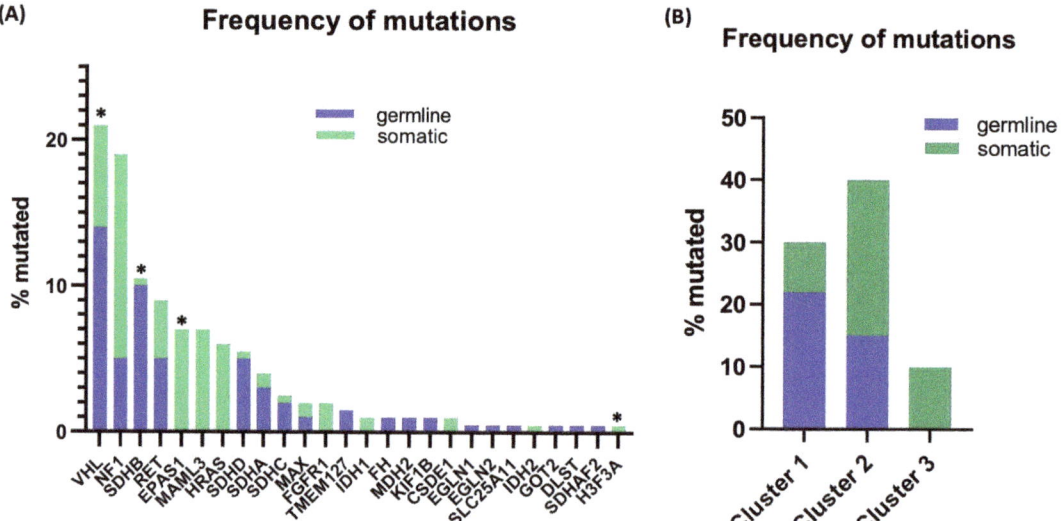

Figure 1. Approximate mutation frequency of genes implicated in PPGLs with a known genetic driver. Data were compiled from published series [10,14,16–18] and our own cohort regardless of age groups and may reflect referral bias. (**A**) Mutation distribution based on individual genes and (**B**) cluster type. Tumors with unknown genetic drivers are not shown. For the purpose of this representation, mutation frequencies of uncommon genes have been depicted as 0.5%. * genes that can be post-zygotically mutated. The genes implicated in PPGLs, with various degrees of supporting evidence are: *NF1, VHL, RET, SDHA, SDHB, SDHC, SDHD, SDHAF2, TMEM127, MAX, EPAS1, HRAS, FH, EGLN1, EGLN2, MDH2, FGFR1, CSDE1, MAML3, GOT2, SLC25A11, H3F3A, DLST, IDH1, IDH2, KIF1B, MET*.

PPGLs have been classified into three clusters according to the molecular pathways involved in their pathogenesis [14]. Cluster 1 consists of the pseudohypoxia pathway and includes tumors with either germline or somatic mutations in *VHL, SDHA/B/C/D/AF2, EPAS1, EGLN1, EGLN2, FH, SLC25A11,* and *MDH2* (Figure 1B). This cluster is also subdivided into genes associated with the tricarboxylic acid (TCA) or mitochondrial function (*SDH, FH, MDH2, SLC25A11, IDH1/2*), also referred to as C1A group, and other hypoxia pathway-related genes, or C1B (*VHL, EPAS1, EGLN1/2* genes) [20]. Cluster 2 is characterized by kinase signaling and protein translation pathways and includes PPGLs with germline or somatic mutations of *RET, NF1, TMEM127, HRAS, FGFR1,* and *MAX*. Cluster 3 has been recognized more recently, is related to activation of targets of the *WNT1* transcription factor and includes *MAML3* fusion genes and truncating mutations in *CSDE1* [14,21]. This classification underlies the diverse mechanisms and signals that can initiate PPGLs, although it remains challenging to predict the disease course [22]. Although the biological behavior of PPGLs cannot be anticipated, specific genotypes have been associated with an increased risk of metastasis. For example, *SDHB* mutations confer a higher risk of metastatic progression. Similarly, somatic *MAML3* fusions, often accompanied by disruption of *TERT* and/or *ATRX* mutations are enriched in aggressive and/or metastatic tumors [5,23,24].

2. Leveraging Clinical and Genetic Data for Classification and Patient Management

Current evidence supports genetic testing as a key component of the management of patients with PPGL to guide treatment selection and follow-up surveillance [1,25]. Disease presentation and the likelihood of identifying a causative germline mutation will vary depending on the molecular class of the PPGL [26]. For example, tumors belonging to Cluster 1 (pseudohypoxia) may present as either pheochromocytoma or paraganglioma, often occur at a younger age (especially those with germline *VHL* mutation) and frequently manifest as multiple and/or recurrent. Metastatic disease, especially if *SDHB* related, is enriched in this group [27]. These tumors are characteristically deficient for the enzyme which converts norepinephrine (NE) to epinephrine (Epi), phenyl-ethanolamine N-methyltransferase (PMNT). For these reasons these PPGLs are strictly noradrenergic and can be diagnosed preferentially by elevated NE levels [26,28]. A germline mutation can be detected in most cases of C1A-related PPGLs, while the rate of germline mutation is lower in C1B cases [26]. In contrast, around 20% of Cluster 2 cases (kinase signaling group) are associated with a germline mutation. These patients have a broad age of presentation that can be modulated by the specific gene mutated, usually peaks between 40–50 years of age and present as benign pheochromocytomas [26,29]. Not infrequently these tumors are multiple, especially related to MEN 2A/2B, but to a lesser extent *TMEM127*- and *MAX*-mutant cases. Cluster 3 (Wnt-altered) presents as pheochromocytomas that are often metastatic or recurrent, although studies are still limited to few cases. There have not been germline variants associated with this cluster to date. Both Cluster 2 and 3 express PMNT and are associated with elevated Epi/NE levels [14,30].

PPGL localization and possible metastasis identification usually involve computed tomography (CT) or magnetic resonance imaging (MRI) as the initial step, regardless of genotype. However, in suspected metastatic cases, recurrent disease, or if radionuclide-based therapy is being considered, distinct functional imaging studies can be utilized, such as ^{123}I-metaiodobenzylguanidine (MIBG), 6-^{18}F-fluoro-L-dopa (^{18}F-FDOPA), ^{18}F-fluorodeoxyglucose (^{18}F-FDG), and gallium-68 DOTATATE (^{68}Ga-DOTATATE). Once again, molecular knowledge can influence the functional imaging choice. For example, Cluster 2-type PPGLs have high avidity for ^{18}F-FDOPA but a low-to-moderate ^{18}F-FDG uptake [26]. In contrast, cluster 1-related PPGLs with *VHL* or *EPAS1* mutations display high uptake of ^{18}F-FDOPA and ^{18}F-FDG [26,31]. Genotype-functional imaging associations are more complex in *SDH*-related PPGLs. In these tumors, nuclear imaging studies will depend mainly on the tissue of origin, with ^{18}F-FDOPA being characteristically positive for head and neck PGLs but not for sympathetic PPGLs [31]. Also, *SDH*-related tumors, particularly *SDHB* mutants, are known to show poor sensitivity to $^{123/131}$I-MIBG compared to other radiopharmaceuticals, like ^{18}F-FDG PET/CT and ^{68}Ga-DOTATATE [32,33]. Furthermore, ^{68}Ga-DOTATATE demonstrates superiority to other available functional studies regardless of location, if *SDH*-related parasympathetic PGL or metastatic PPGL is identified [34].

The first line of treatment for all PPGLs should be tumor resection with pre-operative management of catecholamine-related symptoms that are usually achieved by alpha-blockade, regardless of mutation status [1,35]. However, knowledge of the genotype impacts on surgical planning, as patients diagnosed with, or at risk of, bilateral pheochromocytomas are recommended to undergo cortical-sparing surgery [36]. However, not all PPGLs are amenable for surgery due to metastatic disease, surgically challenging tumor location, or extensive recurrence. In cases where surgery is not feasible, tumor burden, disease progression, or symptomatic status should guide treatment options that include local therapies (radiotherapy, radiofrequency ablation, embolization, among others), radionucleotide therapy and chemotherapy [5]. Radionucleotide therapy with ^{131}MIBG can be considered when ^{123}MIBG diagnostic scans demonstrate avid uptake. A recently FDA-approved, high-specific activity version of ^{131}MIBG showed a response in more than 90% of patients, with tumor reduction in 25% of cases [37], although long-term follow-up of this drug is still lacking. Cytotoxic radionuclide therapy with ^{177}Lu-DOTATATE shows promise as a therapeutic option that provides less toxicity than ^{131}MIBG; however, although studies are still limited [38]. Systemic chemotherapy with cyclophosphamide, vincristine, doxorubicin (CVD) can reduce tumor burden, decrease catecholamines, and improve blood pressure in only 30–40% of patients, and data with other agents, such as temozolomide are limited to small cohorts [5]. Given this limited effectiveness of systemic therapies, targeted therapies have been tested, though usually outside of clinical trials [5,39]. The highly vascular nature of PPGLs, and increased VEGF expression and activity especially notable in cluster 1 tumors justifies the use of tyrosine kinase inhibitors (TKI) with antiangiogenic properties, such as sunitinib, pazopanib, axitinib, cabozantinib, lenvantinib, and dovitinib [40,41]. Another potential and even more promising therapy targeting molecular disruption of PPGLs involve HIF inhibitors, in particular HIF-2α, which has been identified as one of the main oncogenic drivers in PPGL development and is overexpressed in *VHL*, *SDH*, and *EPAS1*-mutant PPGLs [42,43]. A novel class of HIF-2α-specific inhibitors showed promising results in advanced clear cell-renal cell carcinoma (cc-RCC) [44]. This drug, belzutifan (previously known as PT2977), received FDA approval in August 2021 for the treatment of VHL-related cc-RCC, hemangioblastomas and pancreatic neuroendocrine tumors (https://www.fda.gov/drugs/resources-information-approved-drugs/fda-approves-belzutifan-cancers-associated-von-hippel-lindau-disease, accessed on 27 August 2021). This is an important milestone that will accelerate the development of new trials [42,43], including advanced and/or metastatic PPGLs (NCT04924075). Immunotherapy is another area of interest in the treatment of cluster 1 related PPGLs, as pseudohypoxia may prevent immune recognition of the tumors via mechanisms involving increased expression of the immune checkpoint protein programmed death-ligand 1 (PD-L1) and inactivating cytotoxic T cell lymphocytes. Pembrolizumab, nivolumab and ipilimumab are being studied as possible therapeutic options [45]. Figure 2 illustrates the challenges of treating patients with metastatic PPGL and the need for additional research to better understand the events underlying rapid disease progression after months or years of indolent metastatic growth, and molecular determinants of acquired resistance to targeted therapy. Advances on these fronts will be critical to refine treatment strategies and improve patient outcomes.

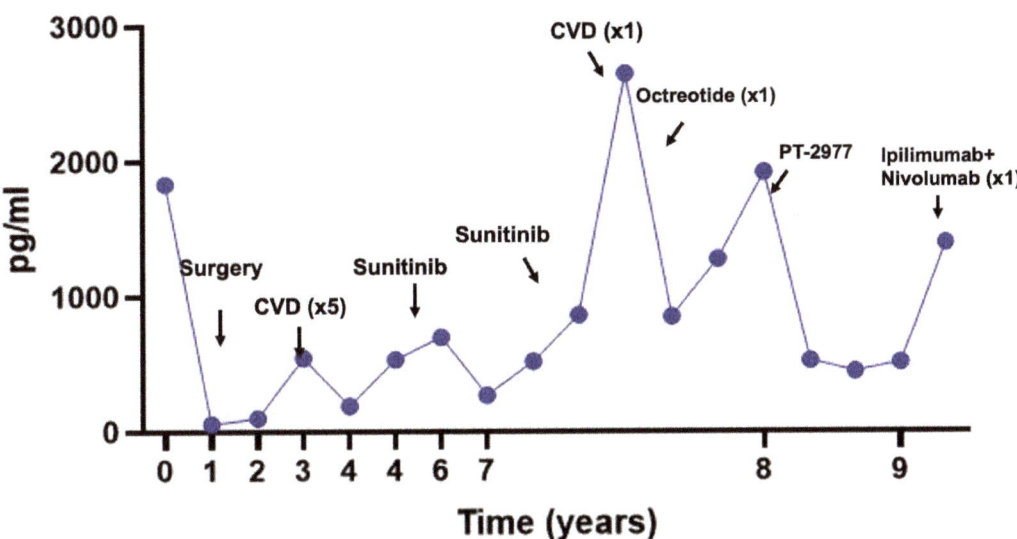

Figure 2. Plasma norepinephrine (NE) levels of a patient with a pathogenic germline *SDHB* mutation diagnosed with a retroperitoneal paraganglioma, who progressed with metastases and underwent multiple lines of treatment over the course of her disease. NE levels are tracked closely with the tumor burden and symptoms. Bone metastases were detected two years post-surgery. The patient received CVD followed by sunitinib, with the initial control of disease, however, both therapies were eventually discontinued (DC) due to adverse side effects. After disease progression, new attempts were made with sunitinib and CVD, although once again drugs were poorly tolerated. One dose of octreotide depot was given to attempt symptomatic control of the disease. Next, the patient was enrolled in the Phase 1 clinical trial for a HIF2α inhibitor (PT-2977/ MK6484, NCT02974738). The patient had clinical, biochemical, cellular, and molecular responses mainly demonstrated by a decrease in NE, development of anemia, a common on-target effect of HIF2 inhibition, and reduced expression of HIF2α target genes (not shown) and remained stable for 8 months. Despite this improvement, the disease progressed, and the HIF2α inhibitor was discontinued. The patient initiated a trial with CTLA-4 and PD-1 inhibitors (NCT02834013) but only tolerated one cycle. Disease progressed rapidly and the patient died a few months later. This case illustrates two critical timepoints during disease evolution that remain gaps in the field: determining the basis for the rapid increase in disease burden and emergence of resistance to targeted therapy could inform treatment choices in patients with metastatic pheochromocytoma and/or paraganglioma.

3. Detecting and Interpreting Variants: Protocols and Challenges

Patients with PPGLs should be engaged in genetic testing [1,35]. The relevance of genetic diagnosis is demonstrated by its positive impact on patient outcomes [46]. Next-generation sequencing (NGS) technology has emerged as a valuable tool capable of simultaneously evaluating multiple susceptibility genes in the same assay [47]. This methodology significantly improves the performance of PPGLs genetic testing compared with conventional methods, increasing the rate of variant identification [10,16]. At the same time, this approach leads to the detection of rare and novel variants, and the task of defining their pathogenicity becomes a relevant challenge [47].

According to the ACMG Standards and Guidelines [48], several lines of evidence are needed to support the classification of a variant as pathogenic or likely pathogenic. Variant classification requires careful interpretation of a combination of information including (a) the type of variant, (b) the frequency of the variant, (c) the occurrence of the variant in clinically-related databases, (d) literature citations of the variant, (e) functional evaluation of the variant, (f) in silico predictions of variant effect, (g) analysis of co-segregation of disease in the family, (h) concordance with phenotype, and (i) co-occurrence of pathogenic variants [47]. The latter is an increasingly likely scenario observed in NGS-based studies, which adds to the complexity of interpreting variant relevance [49]; however, this subject will not be discussed in this brief review. Not uncommonly, very strong evidence (a null variant in a gene where the loss of function is an established disease mechanism) and strong evidence (functional studies support a damaging effect; higher prevalence of variant in affected individuals vs. controls, etc.) that would support pathogenicity is not available. This is especially true for rare, genetically heterogeneous diseases, such as PPGLs which can arise due to a germline, somatic or mosaic variant in one of many susceptibility genes. As a result, a substantial number of variants, especially missense substitutions, identified in PPGL susceptibility genes are currently classified as variants of uncertain significance (VUS) pending additional support for pathogenicity [10,16]. Functional studies are recommended to assess the pathogenicity of variants, which may be resource-intensive [18,22,47].

4. A Workflow to Identify a Driver Mutation in PPGLs

Multiple strategies have been employed for the genetic diagnosis of PPGLs. Our group adopted a flexible workflow (NCT03160274) depicted in Figure 3A. This process involves parallel testing of blood and tumor tissue, either fresh frozen or as formalin-fixed, paraffin-embedded material (Figure 3B). While this protocol includes both germline and tumor samples for DNA-based screening whenever possible, it prioritizes tumor tissue processing. This approach allows for improved data interpretation [50], by enabling the detection of somatic events or suspected areas of copy number variation, including loss of heterozygosity.

For clearly syndromic cases, the first step of this workflow may include targeted testing. For non-syndromic PPGLs, a next-generation sequencing (NGS)-based custom panel of 28 genes is used (Figure 3A). Libraries are processed and sequenced at high depth (>500× average) in an Illumina MiSeq instrument, easily scalable to higher capacity instruments for higher throughput, as needed (e.g., Illumina NextSeq). Data are analyzed for sequence variants of interest and copy number changes, or, if tumor tissue is available, suggestive systematic gain/loss patterns of known fusion partner genes. If high-quality tumor RNA is available, sequencing is followed by a focused transcription profiling step based on real-time PCR of tumor cDNA. This step has two purposes: (i) to determine whether the expression pattern of tumors with a detected candidate driver mutation matches the expected cluster group, and (ii) to guide the subsequent investigation of mechanisms that drive pathogenicity in tumors with suspected VUS or those with an unknown driver event based on cluster membership. The genes included in this focused classification were modeled on top classifiers of the three main expression clusters previously reported [14,21,51,52] and other curated expression data.

Tumor samples without an identifiable variant are subjected to whole transcriptome sequencing (RNAseq). This approach can provide multiple levels of information to improve driver gene detection [53–55]. Although comprehensive analysis of whole transcriptome data requires bioinformatics expertise, the broad use of RNAseq-based algorithms has simplified this process [53,56]. First, it provides sequence data of the whole transcriptome, beyond the known PPGL genes, enabling the identification of potentially novel candidate driver genes. Although the depth of coverage of conventional RNAseq data tends to be generally lower than that provided by typical custom DNA panels, and can be subject to variability dependent on transcription instability of certain mutants, high-depth RNAseq can improve detectability [57]. Secondly, the data can also reveal genes targeted by aberrant splicing that may explain atypical and/or suspect variants. Thirdly, RNAseq data also generates expression classifications that can help support putative candidate variants (e.g., pseudohypoxia expression signature of a sample with a *SDHB* VUS). A fourth advantage of RNAseq is its ability to predict putative in-frame gene fusions that may have an oncogenic role in PPGLs. Putative fusions can be orthogonally verified by designing specific breakpoint spanning primers and by sequencing independent tumor samples with a shared expression profile. Thus, the incorporation of tumor RNAseq for fusion and splicing aberration detection can expand the characterization of novel structural variants. When integrated with expression profiles, these data can also provide insights into the potential dominant signaling disruption (e.g., pseudohypoxia).

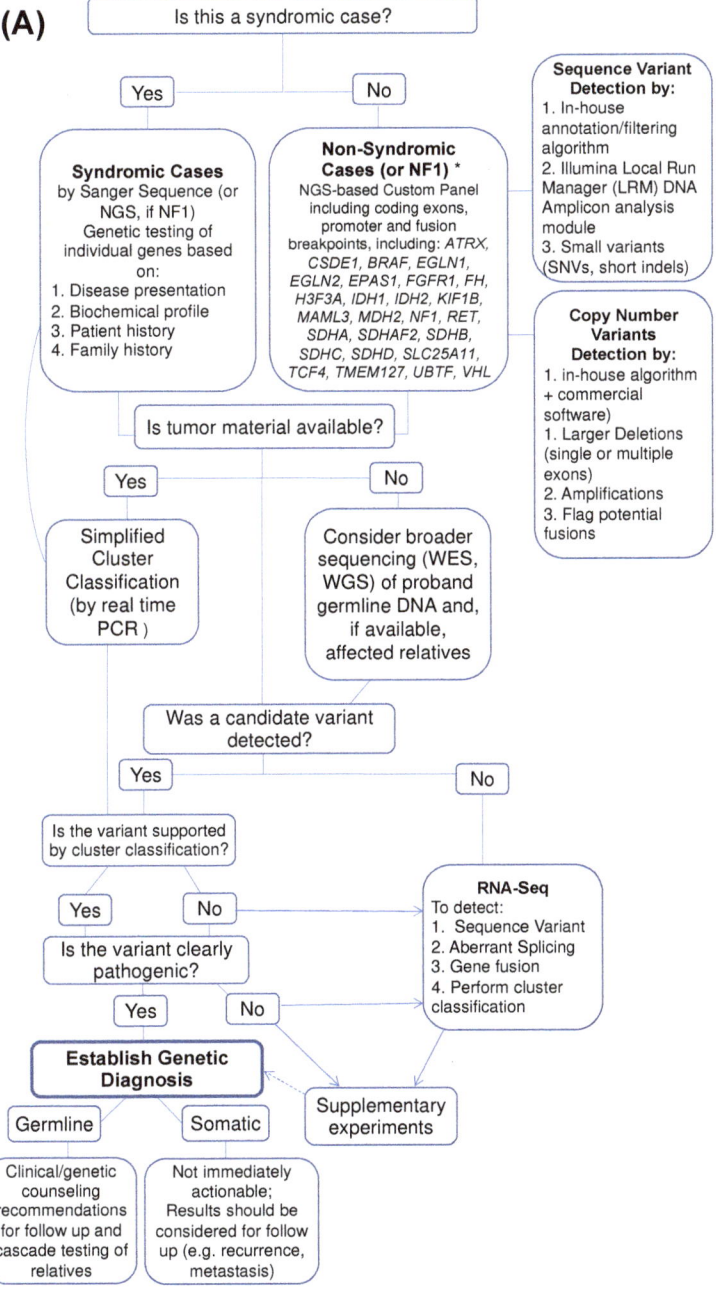

Figure 3. *Cont.*

(B)

Source of sample	Cell type	Mode of collection
Germline/ Mosaic	Blood	Fresh blood
		Filter paper
	Saliva	Fresh
	Normal (non-tumoral) tissue	Fresh*
		Frozen
		FFPE
Somatic	Tumor	Frozen
		FFPE

Figure 3. (**A**) A proposed workflow to identify driver mutations in pheochromocytoma and/or paragangliomas (PPGLs). The process is modified based on the type of sample available for analysis and initial clinical information. The ultimate goal is to establish a germline or somatic genetic diagnosis. In some cases, extensive experimentation may be necessary, as shown by directional lines. A definitive, unambiguous diagnosis may not be achieved in all cases (dashed line), and additional research is required. Limitations may include samples with only germline material available, without family history/or samples from informative relatives, and no clear candidate variant. * areas with lower coverage are supplemented by Sanger sequencing; NGS = next-generation sequencing; WES = whole exome sequencing; WGS = whole genome sequencing (**B**) Materials used for analysis; FFPE = formalin-fixed, paraffin-embedded; * cell culture compatible media.

Additional steps of the workflow are guided by individual findings [47]. For example, these analyses can be complemented by immunohistochemical staining of selected, well-established targets [58], or novel targets, to help support cluster membership and the functional impact of candidate variants. Additional functional experiments are usually tailored to the candidate gene and variant type, as exemplified in the next section. Other analytical platforms also contribute to improved diagnosis and classification, when integrated with sequencing, transcription and immunohistochemical analyses. Epigenetic (especially DNA methylation profiling, but also analysis of posttranslational modifications) and metabolite profiling can help to narrow down the classes of possible susceptibility gene mutations, as well as potential consequences of candidate variants [19,50,59,60].

5. Lessons Learned from Atypical/Novel/Unsuspected Genetic Disruptions

This session addresses the relevance of exploring rarer or atypical variants and how these investigations can reveal driver mutations and mechanisms of PPGL tumorigenesis, illustrated with examples from our cohort. Some PPGL susceptibility genes, like the transmembrane protein encoding gene *TMEM127*, are poorly known upon their identification [61]. TMEM127 has been previously described as a tumor suppressor, an endomembrane protein, and a negative regulator of mTOR signaling [61,62]. Tumor suppressor genes are often inactivated by frameshift and nonsense/truncating variants, but the effects of missense variants are more difficult to characterize. Individually, missense variants observed in PPGL patients and families may not reveal much information, but collectively, they can highlight specific functional protein hotspots. Recently we used in vitro transient expression of cDNA constructs to investigate a cluster of missense *TMEM127* variants that suggested the presence of a putative functional domain not previously described in the N-terminal region [63]. We had reported earlier that membrane binding ability appears to be required for TMEM127 function [64,65], therefore analysis of variant subcellular localization patterns served as an efficient first-pass approach in evaluating loss of structure/function. All missense variants in the N-terminal cluster had a diffuse/cytoplasmic pattern, in contrast with the punctate, endomembrane pattern of wild-type (WT) TMEM127 indicating that these variants lost their membrane binding ability. Moreover, these variants were rapidly degraded, in favor of a loss of function defect. Through this process and additional topology studies, a fourth TMEM127 transmembrane domain was identified [63]. These findings were recently supported by highly accurate deep learning protein structure predictions [66]. At the same time, distinctive variants can also reveal key protein features. A C-terminal, frameshift variant, disrupting the region downstream of the last transmembrane domain of *TMEM127*, was found to display a unique, plasma membrane bound pattern. This observation suggested that the variant lost its internalization capability. Further analysis revealed that an atypical endocytic signaling motif resided in the C-terminal tail and was necessary for effective localization of TMEM127 [63].

Another example of atypical variants with unsuspected functional consequences is illustrated by synonymous variants. Unless they are located close to exon-intron boundaries, where they could disrupt donor and acceptor splice sites, synonymous variants are often filtered out during screening because they are not predicted to result in a change to the protein sequence. However, considerations need to be made that synonymous variants occurring in the middle of an exon may also have an effect on splicing, as demonstrated recently with *VHL* [67,68]. Although the mechanism is not understood, a synonymous variant in the middle of exon 2 of *VHL* at proline 138 (c.414A > G, p.138=) results in a splicing effect that omits exon 2 from the transcript, resulting in an in-frame transcript consisting of exon 1 and exon 3 [67,68]. Importantly, exon 2 encodes most of the oxygen-dependent degradation domain (ODD) of VHL, the HIF binding site, and its absence leads to reduced HIF2α degradation, similar to other loss-of-function *VHL* mutations. Several families carrying this variant have now been reported, enabling reclassification of this variant as pathogenic [67,68].

The reports above demonstrate the utility of functional studies in expanding and redefining our knowledge of existing genes as well as supporting variant classification. Over time and with long-term follow up these observations may be updated to uncover new genotype-phenotype associations of value in implementing clinical surveillance practices. Despite these efforts, there remain tumors with undefined driver events. These tumors may carry disruptions of the noncoding genome, epigenetic events, or involvement of multiple genes, and their study will require additional approaches [69].

6. Epistatic Interactions between Genetics and the Environment

Establishing causality of gene-environment interactions in cancer, defined by co-participation in the same causal mechanism, is challenging [70]. Several disease models have emerged in which cancer development has been traced to specific types of environmental stress [70]. However, the ability to precisely measure the impact of exposure to environmental stressors, such as radiation, toxins, or oxygen variability, and define their direct role in the acquisition of genetic mutations which can influence disease risk and severity is limited.

An intriguing natural model of environmental risk is represented by patients with cyanotic congenital heart disease (CCHD), a group of diseases caused by complex heart defects present at birth that result in low blood oxygen levels (hypoxemia) [71]. Even after corrective surgeries, some degree of hypoxemia may remain, which creates a state of chronic systemic hypoxia in these patients [72]. It has long been recognized that CCHD patients have a higher incidence (~5-fold) and earlier occurrence of PPGLs compared to the general population [72–74]. Although a molecular basis had not been previously established, it was considered that these two diseases might share an inherited genetic susceptibility. However, recent studies support that the development of PPGLs in CCHD patients is linked to a somatic event in one of the PPGL susceptibility genes. Specifically, the *EPAS1* gene, which codes for the hypoxia inducible factor HIF2α, which plays a significant role in the hypoxia-response pathway, was found to be susceptible to somatic mutations at critical residues [75]. In a study of six tumor samples from five CCHD patients, including five sympathetic PPGLs and one carotid body paraganglioma (CB-PGL), we found that four out of five sympathetic PPGLs displayed a somatic *EPAS1* mutation affecting either alanine 530 or proline 531 [75]. As these residues play a key role in regulating HIF2α stability, the resulting amino acid changes prevent degradation and, hence, confer a constitutively active status for HIF2α [76]. Notably, these patients had no germline mutations of known PPGL susceptibility genes, supporting a driver role for the somatic *EPAS1* mutations [75]. Interestingly, the PGL of the single patient without a somatic *EPAS1* mutation showed an SDHA/SDHB immunohistochemistry pattern compatible with deficient SDH function, suggesting a qualitatively distinct mechanism of tumorigenesis in this case. The single carotid body PGL in this series, which arose in the same patient with an *EPAS1* mutant pheochromocytoma, also did not carry a somatic *EPAS1* mutation.

In the sections above, we emphasized the overrepresentation of hypoxia-related genes in mutated PPGLs (*VHL, SDH* subunits, *EGLN1/2, FH, IDH, EPAS1*), highlighting the relevance of this pathway for tumor development [42]. While most PPGLs within the pseudohypoxia cluster result from germline variants, suggesting an early event, the *EPAS1* gene is targeted instead by somatic mutations [14,77]. These somatic *EPAS1* mutations are detected at a frequency no higher than 7% in cohorts of generic PPGLs [14,77]. In contrast, in PPGLs arising in patients with CCHD the frequency of *EPAS1* mutations is markedly elevated, at 80% [75]. The timing of the emergence of the *EPAS1* mutation within the PPGL tumorigenesis process in CCHD patients remains unknown. However, the specific conditions experienced by these patients, which include prolonged tissue exposure to low circulating oxygen levels, may act as an environmental cue that favors PPGL development through somatic mutations that selectively target a key component of the hypoxia response. These observations suggest that sympathetic cells of the adrenal and paraganglia are uniquely sensitive to the CCHD environment, similar to other cell types that experience specific genetic vulnerabilities in the presence of particular external factors, much like targeted therapy-induced resistant mutations in cancer [78].

At the same time, CB-PGLs differ from other PPGLs in the cell of origin (chief cells instead of chromaffin cells), and, hence, may have genetic vulnerabilities distinct from chromaffin-derived PPGLs [79]. Of note, individuals living in certain high-altitude areas, such as the Andes, who are exposed to low relative ambient oxygen pressure have a higher incidence of CB-PGLs [73,74]. In some cases, CB-PGL development has been attributed to germline variants in *SDHB* [80] or *SDHD* [81]. However, not all tumors have detectable variants in SDH genes [82]. Future studies will be needed to determine whether chief cells have a distinct vulnerability to mutations and whether other genes related to the hypoxia response can also be implicated in these tumors. Regardless, the remarkable association between CCHD and *EPAS1* mutated-PPGLs should spur studies to further investigate and model the impact of environmental influences in PPGL tumorigenesis that may also illuminate our knowledge of other cancers.

7. Conclusions

Great advances have been achieved in the knowledge of the genetic basis of PPGLs. However, the driver event remains unidentified in at least one-third of the cases. Importantly, the ability to recognize molecular identifiers of metastatic risk persists as an unattained goal. Bridging these gaps will require optimization of workflows for genetic diagnosis, improvement of variant annotation and the recognition of atypical genetic disruptions that shed light on novel disease mechanisms. Overcoming these challenges will require unified efforts of researchers in this field.

Author Contributions: All authors: S.K.F., C.M.E.-Z., K.T., G.A.-P. and P.L.M.D. were responsible for writing the original draft and editing the manuscript. Figure 2 was designed by G.A.-P., Figure 3A was designed by C.M.E.-Z. Figure 1A,B was designed by P.L.M.D. and revised by all authors. P.L.M.D. conceptualized and supervised the manuscript. All authors have read and agreed to the published version of the manuscript.

Funding: P.L.M.D. is a recipient of funds from the NIH (GM114102), Neuroendocrine Tumor Research Foundation and the University of Texas System STARS award which supported the work reported in this review. P.L.M.D. is a Robert Tucker Hayes Distinguished Chair in Oncology.

Acknowledgments: The authors are grateful to patients who participated in our studies, our multiple collaborators and regret not citing many important references due to space constraints.

Conflicts of Interest: The authors declare no conflict of interest.

References

1. Lenders, J.W.; Duh, Q.Y.; Eisenhofer, G.; Gimenez-Roqueplo, A.P.; Grebe, S.K.; Murad, M.H.; Naruse, M.; Pacak, K.; Young, W.F., Jr.; Endocrine, S. Pheochromocytoma and paraganglioma: An endocrine society clinical practice guideline. *J. Clin. Endocrinol. Metab.* **2014**, *99*, 1915–1942. [CrossRef] [PubMed]
2. Neumann, H.P.H.; Young, W.F., Jr.; Eng, C. Pheochromocytoma and Paraganglioma. *N. Engl. J. Med.* **2019**, *381*, 552–565. [CrossRef]
3. Thompson, L.D.R.; Gill, A.J.; Asa, S.L.; Clifton-Bligh, R.J.; de Krijger, R.R.; Kimura, N.; Komminoth, P.; Lack, E.E.; Lenders, J.W.M.; Lloyd, R.V.; et al. Data set for the reporting of pheochromocytoma and paraganglioma: Explanations and recommendations of the guidelines from the International Collaboration on Cancer Reporting. *Hum. Pathol.* **2021**, *110*, 83–97. [CrossRef] [PubMed]
4. Fishbein, L. Pheochromocytoma and Paraganglioma: Genetics, Diagnosis, and Treatment. *Hematol. Oncol. Clin. N. Am.* **2016**, *30*, 135–150. [CrossRef] [PubMed]
5. Fishbein, L.; Del Rivero, J.; Else, T.; Howe, J.R.; Asa, S.L.; Cohen, D.L.; Dahia, P.L.M.; Fraker, D.L.; Goodman, K.A.; Hope, T.A.; et al. The North American Neuroendocrine Tumor Society Consensus Guidelines for Surveillance and Management of Metastatic and/or Unresectable Pheochromocytoma and Paraganglioma. *Pancreas* **2021**, *50*, 469–493. [CrossRef] [PubMed]
6. Ayala-Ramirez, M.; Feng, L.; Johnson, M.M.; Ejaz, S.; Habra, M.A.; Rich, T.; Busaidy, N.; Cote, G.J.; Perrier, N.; Phan, A.; et al. Clinical risk factors for malignancy and overall survival in patients with pheochromocytoma and sympathetic paragangliomas: Primary tumor size and primary tumor location as prognostic indicators. *J. Clin. Endocrinol. Metab.* **2011**, *96*, 717–725. [CrossRef]
7. Dahia, P.L. Pheochromocytoma and paraganglioma pathogenesis: Learning from genetic heterogeneity. *Nat. Rev. Cancer* **2014**, *14*, 108–119. [CrossRef] [PubMed]
8. Remacha, L.; Currás-Freixes, M.; Torres-Ruiz, R.; Schiavi, F.; Torres-Pérez, R.; Calsina, B.; Letón, R.; Comino-Méndez, I.; Roldán-Romero, J.M.; Montero-Conde, C.; et al. Gain-of-function mutations in DNMT3A in patients with paraganglioma. *Genet. Med.* **2018**, *20*, 1644–1651. [CrossRef]
9. Remacha, L.; Pirman, D.; Mahoney, C.E.; Coloma, J.; Calsina, B.; Currás-Freixes, M.; Letón, R.; Torres-Pérez, R.; Richter, S.; Pita, G.; et al. Recurrent Germline DLST Mutations in Individuals with Multiple Pheochromocytomas and Paragangliomas. *Am. J. Hum. Genet.* **2019**, *104*, 651–664. [CrossRef]
10. Curras-Freixes, M.; Pineiro-Yanez, E.; Montero-Conde, C.; Apellaniz-Ruiz, M.; Calsina, B.; Mancikova, V.; Remacha, L.; Richter, S.; Ercolino, T.; Rogowski-Lehmann, N.; et al. PheoSeq: A Targeted Next-Generation Sequencing Assay for Pheochromocytoma and Paraganglioma Diagnostics. *J. Mol. Diagn.* **2017**, *19*, 575–588. [CrossRef]
11. Buffet, A.; Burnichon, N.; Favier, J.; Gimenez-Roqueplo, A.P. An overview of 20 years of genetic studies in pheochromocytoma and paraganglioma. *Best Pract. Res. Clin. Endocrinol. Metab.* **2020**, *34*, 101416. [CrossRef]
12. Castro-Vega, L.J.; Lepoutre-Lussey, C.; Gimenez-Roqueplo, A.P.; Favier, J. Rethinking pheochromocytomas and paragangliomas from a genomic perspective. *Oncogene* **2016**, *35*, 1080–1089. [CrossRef]
13. Favier, J.; Amar, L.; Gimenez-Roqueplo, A.P. Paraganglioma and phaeochromocytoma: From genetics to personalized medicine. *Nat. Rev. Endocrinol.* **2015**, *11*, 101–111. [CrossRef] [PubMed]
14. Fishbein, L.; Leshchiner, I.; Walter, V.; Danilova, L.; Robertson, A.G.; Johnson, A.R.; Lichtenberg, T.M.; Murray, B.A.; Ghayee, H.K.; Else, T.; et al. Comprehensive Molecular Characterization of Pheochromocytoma and Paraganglioma. *Cancer Cell* **2017**, *31*, 181–193. [CrossRef] [PubMed]
15. Dahia, P.L. The genetic landscape of pheochromocytomas and paragangliomas: Somatic mutations take center stage. *J. Clin. Endocrinol. Metab.* **2013**, *98*, 2679–2681. [CrossRef] [PubMed]
16. Ben Aim, L.; Pigny, P.; Castro-Vega, L.J.; Buffet, A.; Amar, L.; Bertherat, J.; Drui, D.; Guilhem, I.; Baudin, E.; Lussey-Lepoutre, C.; et al. Targeted next-generation sequencing detects rare genetic events in pheochromocytoma and paraganglioma. *J. Med. Genet.* **2019**, *56*, 513–520. [CrossRef]
17. Welander, J.; Larsson, C.; Backdahl, M.; Hareni, N.; Sivler, T.; Brauckhoff, M.; Soderkvist, P.; Gimm, O. Integrative genomics reveals frequent somatic NF1 mutations in sporadic pheochromocytomas. *Hum. Mol. Genet.* **2012**, *21*, 5406–5416. [CrossRef]
18. Toledo, R.A.; Qin, Y.; Cheng, Z.M.; Gao, Q.; Iwata, S.; Silva, G.M.; Prasad, M.L.; Ocal, I.T.; Rao, S.; Aronin, N.; et al. Recurrent Mutations of Chromatin-Remodeling Genes and Kinase Receptors in Pheochromocytomas and Paragangliomas. *Clin. Cancer Res.* **2016**, *22*, 2301–2310. [CrossRef] [PubMed]
19. Cascón, A.; Remacha, L.; Calsina, B.; Robledo, M. Pheochromocytomas and Paragangliomas: Bypassing Cellular Respiration. *Cancers* **2019**, *11*, 683. [CrossRef]
20. Castro-Vega, L.J.; Buffet, A.; de Cubas, A.A.; Cascon, A.; Menara, M.; Khalifa, E.; Amar, L.; Azriel, S.; Bourdeau, I.; Chabre, O.; et al. Germline mutations in FH confer predisposition to malignant pheochromocytomas and paragangliomas. *Hum. Mol. Genet.* **2014**, *23*, 2440–2446. [CrossRef]

21. Dahia, P.L.; Ross, K.N.; Wright, M.E.; Hayashida, C.Y.; Santagata, S.; Barontini, M.; Kung, A.L.; Sanso, G.; Powers, J.F.; Tischler, A.S.; et al. A HIF1alpha regulatory loop links hypoxia and mitochondrial signals in pheochromocytomas. *PLoS Genet.* 2005, *1*, e8. [CrossRef] [PubMed]
22. Koopman, K.; Gaal, J.; de Krijger, R.R. Pheochromocytomas and Paragangliomas: New Developments with Regard to Classification, Genetics, and Cell of Origin. *Cancers* 2019, *11*, 1070. [CrossRef]
23. Job, S.; Draskovic, I.; Burnichon, N.; Buffet, A.; Cros, J.; Lepine, C.; Venisse, A.; Robidel, E.; Verkarre, V.; Meatchi, T.; et al. Telomerase Activation and ATRX Mutations Are Independent Risk Factors for Metastatic Pheochromocytoma and Paraganglioma. *Clin. Cancer Res.* 2019, *25*, 760–770. [CrossRef]
24. Fishbein, L.; Khare, S.; Wubbenhorst, B.; De Sloover, D.; D'Andrea, K.; Merrill, S.; Cho, N.W.; Greenberg, R.A.; Else, T.; Montone, K.; et al. Whole-exome sequencing identifies somatic ATRX mutations in pheochromocytomas and paragangliomas. *Nat. Commun.* 2015, *6*, 6140. [CrossRef]
25. Lenders, J.W.M.; Kerstens, M.N.; Amar, L.; Prejbisz, A.; Robledo, M.; Taieb, D.; Pacak, K.; Crona, J.; Zelinka, T.; Mannelli, M.; et al. Genetics, diagnosis, management and future directions of research of phaeochromocytoma and paraganglioma: A position statement and consensus of the Working Group on Endocrine Hypertension of the European Society of Hypertension. *J. Hypertens.* 2020, *38*, 1443–1456. [CrossRef]
26. Crona, J.; Taieb, D.; Pacak, K. New Perspectives on Pheochromocytoma and Paraganglioma: Toward a Molecular Classification. *Endocr. Rev.* 2017, *38*, 489–515. [CrossRef]
27. Nolting, S.; Grossman, A.; Pacak, K. Metastatic Phaeochromocytoma: Spinning Towards More Promising Treatment Options. *Exp. Clin. Endocrinol. Diabetes* 2019, *127*, 117–128. [CrossRef]
28. Eisenhofer, G.; Huynh, T.-T.; Hiroi, M.; Pacak, K. Understanding Catecholamine Metabolism as a Guide to the Biochemical Diagnosis of Pheochromocytoma. *Rev. Endocr. Metab. Disord.* 2001, *2*, 297–311. [CrossRef] [PubMed]
29. Nolting, S.; Bechmann, N.; Taieb, D.; Beuschlein, F.; Fassnacht, M.; Kroiss, M.; Eisenhofer, G.; Grossman, A.; Pacak, K. Personalized management of pheochromocytoma and paraganglioma. *Endocr. Rev.* 2021, bnab019. [CrossRef] [PubMed]
30. Wachtel, H.; Fishbein, L. Genetics of pheochromocytoma and paraganglioma. *Curr. Opin. Endocrinol. Diabetes Obes.* 2021, *28*, 283–290. [CrossRef] [PubMed]
31. Taieb, D.; Pacak, K. New Insights into the Nuclear Imaging Phenotypes of Cluster 1 Pheochromocytoma and Paraganglioma. *Trends Endocrinol. Metab.* 2017, *28*, 807–817. [CrossRef] [PubMed]
32. Timmers, H.J.; Chen, C.C.; Carrasquillo, J.A.; Whatley, M.; Ling, A.; Havekes, B.; Eisenhofer, G.; Martiniova, L.; Adams, K.T.; Pacak, K. Comparison of 18F-fluoro-L-DOPA, 18F-fluoro-deoxyglucose, and 18F-fluorodopamine PET and 123I-MIBG scintigraphy in the localization of pheochromocytoma and paraganglioma. *J. Clin. Endocrinol. Metab.* 2009, *94*, 4757–4767. [CrossRef] [PubMed]
33. Han, S.; Suh, C.H.; Woo, S.; Kim, Y.J.; Lee, J.J. Performance of (68)Ga-DOTA-Conjugated Somatostatin Receptor-Targeting Peptide PET in Detection of Pheochromocytoma and Paraganglioma: A Systematic Review and Metaanalysis. *J. Nucl. Med.* 2019, *60*, 369–376. [CrossRef]
34. Janssen, I.; Blanchet, E.M.; Adams, K.; Chen, C.C.; Millo, C.M.; Herscovitch, P.; Taieb, D.; Kebebew, E.; Lehnert, H.; Fojo, A.T.; et al. Superiority of [68Ga]-DOTATATE PET/CT to Other Functional Imaging Modalities in the Localization of SDHB-Associated Metastatic Pheochromocytoma and Paraganglioma. *Clin. Cancer Res.* 2015, *21*, 3888–3895. [CrossRef] [PubMed]
35. Fassnacht, M.; Assie, G.; Baudin, E.; Eisenhofer, G.; de la Fouchardiere, C.; Haak, H.R.; de Krijger, R.; Porpiglia, F.; Terzolo, M.; Berruti, A.; et al. Adrenocortical carcinomas and malignant phaeochromocytomas: ESMO-EURACAN Clinical Practice Guidelines for diagnosis, treatment and follow-up. *Ann. Oncol.* 2020, *31*, 1476–1490. [CrossRef] [PubMed]
36. Neumann, H.P.H.; Tsoy, U.; Bancos, I.; Amodru, V.; Walz, M.K.; Tirosh, A.; Kaur, R.J.; McKenzie, T.; Qi, X.; Bandgar, T.; et al. Comparison of Pheochromocytoma-Specific Morbidity and Mortality Among Adults With Bilateral Pheochromocytomas Undergoing Total Adrenalectomy vs Cortical-Sparing Adrenalectomy. *JAMA Netw. Open* 2019, *2*, e198898. [CrossRef]
37. Pryma, D.A.; Chin, B.B.; Noto, R.B.; Dillon, J.S.; Perkins, S.; Solnes, L.; Kostakoglu, L.; Serafini, A.N.; Pampaloni, M.H.; Jensen, J.; et al. Efficacy and Safety of High-Specific-Activity (131)I-MIBG Therapy in Patients with Advanced Pheochromocytoma or Paraganglioma. *J. Nucl. Med.* 2019, *60*, 623–630. [CrossRef] [PubMed]
38. Kong, G.; Grozinsky-Glasberg, S.; Hofman, M.S.; Callahan, J.; Meirovitz, A.; Maimon, O.; Pattison, D.A.; Gross, D.J.; Hicks, R.J. Efficacy of Peptide Receptor Radionuclide Therapy for Functional Metastatic Paraganglioma and Pheochromocytoma. *J. Clin. Endocrinol. Metab.* 2017, *102*, 3278–3287. [CrossRef]
39. Ayala-Ramirez, M.; Feng, L.; Habra, M.A.; Rich, T.; Dickson, P.V.; Perrier, N.; Phan, A.; Waguespack, S.; Patel, S.; Jimenez, C. Clinical benefits of systemic chemotherapy for patients with metastatic pheochromocytomas or sympathetic extra-adrenal paragangliomas: Insights from the largest single-institutional experience. *Cancer* 2012, *118*, 2804–2812. [CrossRef]
40. Druce, M.R.; Kaltsas, G.A.; Fraenkel, M.; Gross, D.J.; Grossman, A.B. Novel and evolving therapies in the treatment of malignant phaeochromocytoma: Experience with the mTOR inhibitor everolimus (RAD001). *Horm. Metab. Res.* 2009, *41*, 697–702. [CrossRef]
41. Jimenez, C.; Fazeli, S.; Roman-Gonzalez, A. Antiangiogenic therapies for pheochromocytoma and paraganglioma. *Endocr. Relat. Cancer* 2020, *27*, R239–R254. [CrossRef]
42. Dahia, P.L.M.; Toledo, R.A. Recognizing hypoxia in phaeochromocytomas and paragangliomas. *Nat. Rev. Endocrinol.* 2020, *16*, 191–192. [CrossRef]

43. Toledo, R.A. New HIF2alpha inhibitors: Potential implications as therapeutics for advanced pheochromocytomas and paragangliomas. *Endocr. Relat. Cancer* **2017**, *24*, C9–C19. [CrossRef]
44. Choueiri, T.K.; Bauer, T.M.; Papadopoulos, K.P.; Plimack, E.R.; Merchan, J.R.; McDermott, D.F.; Michaelson, M.D.; Appleman, L.J.; Thamake, S.; Perini, R.F.; et al. Inhibition of hypoxia-inducible factor-2alpha in renal cell carcinoma with belzutifan: A phase 1 trial and biomarker analysis. *Nat. Med.* **2021**, *27*, 802–805. [CrossRef] [PubMed]
45. Jimenez, C.; Subbiah, V.; Stephen, B.; Ma, J.; Milton, D.; Xu, M.; Zarifa, A.; Akhmedzhanov, F.O.; Tsimberidou, A.; Habra, M.A.; et al. Phase II Clinical Trial of Pembrolizumab in Patients with Progressive Metastatic Pheochromocytomas and Paragangliomas. *Cancers* **2020**, *12*, 2307. [CrossRef] [PubMed]
46. Buffet, A.; Ben Aim, L.; Leboulleux, S.; Drui, D.; Vezzosi, D.; Libe, R.; Ajzenberg, C.; Bernardeschi, D.; Cariou, B.; Chabolle, F.; et al. Positive Impact of Genetic Test on the Management and Outcome of Patients With Paraganglioma and/or Pheochromocytoma. *J. Clin. Endocrinol. Metab.* **2019**, *104*, 1109–1118. [CrossRef] [PubMed]
47. Group, N.G.S.i.P.S.; Toledo, R.A.; Burnichon, N.; Cascon, A.; Benn, D.E.; Bayley, J.P.; Welander, J.; Tops, C.M.; Firth, H.; Dwight, T.; et al. Consensus Statement on next-generation-sequencing-based diagnostic testing of hereditary phaeochromocytomas and paragangliomas. *Nat. Rev. Endocrinol.* **2017**, *13*, 233–247. [CrossRef]
48. Richards, S.; Aziz, N.; Bale, S.; Bick, D.; Das, S.; Gastier-Foster, J.; Grody, W.W.; Hegde, M.; Lyon, E.; Spector, E.; et al. Standards and guidelines for the interpretation of sequence variants: A joint consensus recommendation of the American College of Medical Genetics and Genomics and the Association for Molecular Pathology. *Genet. Med.* **2015**, *17*, 405–424. [CrossRef]
49. Holcomb, D.; Hamasaki-Katagiri, N.; Laurie, K.; Katneni, U.; Kames, J.; Alexaki, A.; Bar, H.; Kimchi-Sarfaty, C. New approaches to predict the effect of co-occurring variants on protein characteristics. *Am. J. Hum. Genet.* **2021**, *108*, 1502–1511. [CrossRef]
50. Gieldon, L.; William, D.; Hackmann, K.; Jahn, W.; Jahn, A.; Wagner, J.; Rump, A.; Bechmann, N.; Nölting, S.; Knösel, T.; et al. Optimizing Genetic Workup in Pheochromocytoma and Paraganglioma by Integrating Diagnostic and Research Approaches. *Cancers* **2019**, *11*, 809. [CrossRef]
51. Flynn, A.; Dwight, T.; Harris, J.; Benn, D.; Zhou, L.; Hogg, A.; Catchpoole, D.; James, P.; Duncan, E.L.; Trainer, A.; et al. Pheo-Type: A Diagnostic Gene-expression Assay for the Classification of Pheochromocytoma and Paraganglioma. *J. Clin. Endocrinol. Metab.* **2016**, *101*, 1034–1043. [CrossRef] [PubMed]
52. Castro-Vega, L.J.; Letouze, E.; Burnichon, N.; Buffet, A.; Disderot, P.H.; Khalifa, E.; Loriot, C.; Elarouci, N.; Morin, A.; Menara, M.; et al. Multi-omics analysis defines core genomic alterations in pheochromocytomas and paragangliomas. *Nat. Commun.* **2015**, *6*, 6044. [CrossRef]
53. Creason, A.; Haan, D.; Dang, K.; Chiotti, K.E.; Inkman, M.; Lamb, J.; Yu, T.; Hu, Y.; Norman, T.C.; Buchanan, A.; et al. A community challenge to evaluate RNA-seq, fusion detection, and isoform quantification methods for cancer discovery. *Cell Syst.* **2021**, *12*, 827–838.e5. [CrossRef]
54. Maher, C.A.; Kumar-Sinha, C.; Cao, X.; Kalyana-Sundaram, S.; Han, B.; Jing, X.; Sam, L.; Barrette, T.; Palanisamy, N.; Chinnaiyan, A.M. Transcriptome sequencing to detect gene fusions in cancer. *Nature* **2009**, *458*, 97–101. [CrossRef] [PubMed]
55. Kahles, A.; Lehmann, K.V.; Toussaint, N.C.; Hüser, M.; Stark, S.G.; Sachsenberg, T.; Stegle, O.; Kohlbacher, O.; Sander, C.; Rätsch, G. Comprehensive Analysis of Alternative Splicing Across Tumors from 8705 Patients. *Cancer Cell* **2018**, *34*, 211–224.e6. [CrossRef]
56. Beaubier, N.; Bontrager, M.; Huether, R.; Igartua, C.; Lau, D.; Tell, R.; Bobe, A.M.; Bush, S.; Chang, A.L.; Hoskinson, D.C.; et al. Integrated genomic profiling expands clinical options for patients with cancer. *Nat. Biotechnol.* **2019**, *37*, 1351–1360. [CrossRef] [PubMed]
57. Levin, J.Z.; Berger, M.F.; Adiconis, X.; Rogov, P.; Melnikov, A.; Fennell, T.; Nusbaum, C.; Garraway, L.A.; Gnirke, A. Targeted next-generation sequencing of a cancer transcriptome enhances detection of sequence variants and novel fusion transcripts. *Genome Biol.* **2009**, *10*, R115. [CrossRef] [PubMed]
58. Papathomas, T.G.; Oudijk, L.; Persu, A.; Gill, A.J.; van Nederveen, F.; Tischler, A.S.; Tissier, F.; Volante, M.; Matias-Guiu, X.; Smid, M.; et al. SDHB/SDHA immunohistochemistry in pheochromocytomas and paragangliomas: A multicenter interobserver variation analysis using virtual microscopy: A Multinational Study of the European Network for the Study of Adrenal Tumors (ENS@T). *Mod. Pathol.* **2015**, *28*, 807–821. [CrossRef]
59. Richter, S.; Gieldon, L.; Pang, Y.; Peitzsch, M.; Huynh, T.; Leton, R.; Viana, B.; Ercolino, T.; Mangelis, A.; Rapizzi, E.; et al. Metabolome-guided genomics to identify pathogenic variants in isocitrate dehydrogenase, fumarate hydratase, and succinate dehydrogenase genes in pheochromocytoma and paraganglioma. *Genet. Med.* **2019**, *21*, 705–717. [CrossRef]
60. Qiu, Z.; Lin, A.P.; Jiang, S.; Elkashef, S.M.; Myers, J.; Srikantan, S.; Sasi, B.; Cao, J.Z.; Godley, L.A.; Rakheja, D.; et al. MYC Regulation of D2HGDH and L2HGDH Influences the Epigenome and Epitranscriptome. *Cell Chem. Biol.* **2020**, *27*, 538–550.e7. [CrossRef] [PubMed]
61. Qin, Y.; Yao, L.; King, E.E.; Buddavarapu, K.; Lenci, R.E.; Chocron, E.S.; Lechleiter, J.D.; Sass, M.; Aronin, N.; Schiavi, F.; et al. Germline mutations in TMEM127 confer susceptibility to pheochromocytoma. *Nat. Genet.* **2010**, *42*, 229–233. [CrossRef]
62. Deng, Y.; Qin, Y.; Srikantan, S.; Luo, A.; Cheng, Z.M.; Flores, S.K.; Vogel, K.S.; Wang, E.; Dahia, P.L.M. The TMEM127 human tumor suppressor is a component of the mTORC1 lysosomal nutrient-sensing complex. *Hum. Mol. Genet.* **2018**, *27*, 1794–1808. [CrossRef] [PubMed]
63. Flores, S.K.; Deng, Y.; Cheng, Z.; Zhang, X.; Tao, S.; Saliba, A.; Chu, I.; Burnichon, N.; Gimenez-Roqueplo, A.P.; Wang, E.; et al. Functional Characterization of TMEM127 Variants Reveals Novel Insights into Its Membrane Topology and Trafficking. *J. Clin. Endocrinol. Metab.* **2020**, *105*, e3142–e3156. [CrossRef] [PubMed]

64. Qin, Y.; Deng, Y.; Ricketts, C.J.; Srikantan, S.; Wang, E.; Maher, E.R.; Dahia, P.L. The tumor susceptibility gene TMEM127 is mutated in renal cell carcinomas and modulates endolysosomal function. *Hum. Mol. Genet.* **2014**, *23*, 2428–2439. [CrossRef] [PubMed]
65. Yao, L.; Schiavi, F.; Cascon, A.; Qin, Y.; Inglada-Perez, L.; King, E.E.; Toledo, R.A.; Ercolino, T.; Rapizzi, E.; Ricketts, C.J.; et al. Spectrum and prevalence of FP/TMEM127 gene mutations in pheochromocytomas and paragangliomas. *JAMA* **2010**, *304*, 2611–2619. [CrossRef]
66. Jumper, J.; Evans, R.; Pritzel, A.; Green, T.; Figurnov, M.; Ronneberger, O.; Tunyasuvunakool, K.; Bates, R.; Žídek, A.; Potapenko, A.; et al. Highly accurate protein structure prediction with AlphaFold. *Nature* **2021**, *596*, 583–589. [CrossRef]
67. Flores, S.K.; Cheng, Z.; Jasper, A.M.; Natori, K.; Okamoto, T.; Tanabe, A.; Gotoh, K.; Shibata, H.; Sakurai, A.; Nakai, T.; et al. A synonymous VHL variant in exon 2 confers susceptibility to familial pheochromocytoma and von Hippel-Lindau disease. *J. Clin. Endocrinol. Metab.* **2019**, *104*, 3826–3834. [CrossRef] [PubMed]
68. Lenglet, M.; Robriquet, F.; Schwarz, K.; Camps, C.; Couturier, A.; Hoogewijs, D.; Buffet, A.; Knight, S.J.L.; Gad, S.; Couve, S.; et al. Identification of a new VHL exon and complex splicing alterations in familial erythrocytosis or von Hippel-Lindau disease. *Blood* **2018**, *132*, 469–483. [CrossRef]
69. Dahia, P.L. Pheochromocytomas and Paragangliomas, Genetically Diverse and Minimalist, All at Once! *Cancer Cell* **2017**, *31*, 159–161. [CrossRef]
70. Mucci, L.A.; Wedren, S.; Tamimi, R.M.; Trichopoulos, D.; Adami, H.O. The role of gene-environment interaction in the aetiology of human cancer: Examples from cancers of the large bowel, lung and breast. *J. Intern. Med.* **2001**, *249*, 477–493. [CrossRef]
71. Hoffman, J.I.; Kaplan, S. The incidence of congenital heart disease. *J. Am. Coll. Cardiol.* **2002**, *39*, 1890–1900. [CrossRef]
72. Opotowsky, A.R.; Moko, L.E.; Ginns, J.; Rosenbaum, M.; Greutmann, M.; Aboulhosn, J.; Hageman, A.; Kim, Y.; Deng, L.X.; Grewal, J.; et al. Pheochromocytoma and paraganglioma in cyanotic congenital heart disease. *J. Clin. Endocrinol. Metab.* **2015**, *100*, 1325–1334. [CrossRef]
73. Saldana, M.J.; Salem, L.E.; Travezan, R. High altitude hypoxia and chemodectomas. *Hum. Pathol.* **1973**, *4*, 251–263. [CrossRef]
74. Rodriguez-Cuevas, H.; Lau, I.; Rodriguez, H.P. High-altitude paragangliomas diagnostic and therapeutic considerations. *Cancer* **1986**, *57*, 672–676. [CrossRef]
75. Vaidya, A.; Flores, S.K.; Cheng, Z.M.; Nicolas, M.; Deng, Y.; Opotowsky, A.R.; Lourenco, D.M., Jr.; Barletta, J.A.; Rana, H.Q.; Pereira, M.A.; et al. EPAS1 Mutations and Paragangliomas in Cyanotic Congenital Heart Disease. *N. Engl. J. Med.* **2018**, *378*, 1259–1261. [CrossRef] [PubMed]
76. Kaelin, W.G., Jr. The VHL Tumor Suppressor Gene: Insights into Oxygen Sensing and Cancer. *Trans. Am. Clin. Climatol. Assoc.* **2017**, *128*, 298–307. [PubMed]
77. Toledo, R.A.; Qin, Y.; Srikantan, S.; Morales, N.P.; Li, Q.; Deng, Y.; Kim, S.W.; Pereira, M.A.; Toledo, S.P.; Su, X.; et al. In vivo and in vitro oncogenic effects of HIF2A mutations in pheochromocytomas and paragangliomas. *Endocr. Relat. Cancer* **2013**, *20*, 349–359. [CrossRef] [PubMed]
78. Dagogo-Jack, I.; Shaw, A.T. Tumour heterogeneity and resistance to cancer therapies. *Nat. Rev. Clin. Oncol.* **2018**, *15*, 81–94. [CrossRef] [PubMed]
79. Lotti, L.V.; Vespa, S.; Pantalone, M.R.; Perconti, S.; Esposito, D.L.; Visone, R.; Veronese, A.; Paties, C.T.; Sanna, M.; Verginelli, F.; et al. A Developmental Perspective on Paragangliar Tumorigenesis. *Cancers* **2019**, *11*, 273. [CrossRef] [PubMed]
80. Cerecer-Gil, N.Y.; Figuera, L.E.; Llamas, F.J.; Lara, M.; Escamilla, J.G.; Ramos, R.; Estrada, G.; Hussain, A.K.; Gaal, J.; Korpershoek, E.; et al. Mutation of SDHB is a Cause of Hypoxia-Related High-Altitude Paraganglioma. *Clin. Cancer Res.* **2010**, *16*, 4148. [CrossRef] [PubMed]
81. Astrom, K.; Cohen, J.E.; Willett-Brozick, J.E.; Aston, C.E.; Baysal, B.E. Altitude is a phenotypic modifier in hereditary paraganglioma type 1: Evidence for an oxygen-sensing defect. *Hum. Genet.* **2003**, *113*, 228–237. [CrossRef] [PubMed]
82. Jech, M.; Alvarado-Cabrero, I.; Albores-Saavedra, J.; Dahia, P.L.; Tischler, A.S. Genetic analysis of high altitude paragangliomas. *Endocr. Pathol.* **2006**, *17*, 201–202. [CrossRef] [PubMed]

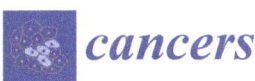

Article

Analytical Performance of NGS-Based Molecular Genetic Tests Used in the Diagnostic Workflow of Pheochromocytoma/Paraganglioma

Balazs Sarkadi [1], Istvan Liko [1,2], Gabor Nyiro [2,3], Peter Igaz [3,4], Henriett Butz [1,5,6] and Attila Patocs [1,2,5,6,*]

1. MTA-SE Hereditary Tumors Research Group, Eotvos Lorand Research Network, H-1089 Budapest, Hungary; sharkadi@gmail.com (B.S.); istvanliko@gmail.com (I.L.); butz.henriett@med.semmelweis-univ.hu (H.B.)
2. Bionics Innovation Center, H-1089 Budapest, Hungary; nyirogabor1@gmail.com
3. MTA-SE Molecular Medicine Research Group, Eotvos Lorand Research Network, H-1083 Budapest, Hungary; igaz.peter@med.semmelweis-univ.hu
4. Department of Endocrinology, Department of Internal Medicine and Oncology, Semmelweis University, H-1083 Budapest, Hungary
5. Department of Laboratory Medicine, Semmelweis University, H-1089 Budapest, Hungary
6. Department of Molecular Genetics, National Institute of Oncology, H-1122 Budapest, Hungary
* Correspondence: patocs.attila@med.semmelweis-univ.hu

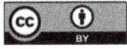

Citation: Sarkadi, B.; Liko, I.; Nyiro, G.; Igaz, P.; Butz, H.; Patocs, A. Analytical Performance of NGS-Based Molecular Genetic Tests Used in the Diagnostic Workflow of Pheochromocytoma/Paraganglioma. *Cancers* **2021**, *13*, 4219. https://doi.org/10.3390/cancers13164219

Academic Editor: Karel Pacak

Received: 6 August 2021
Accepted: 18 August 2021
Published: 22 August 2021

Publisher's Note: MDPI stays neutral with regard to jurisdictional claims in published maps and institutional affiliations.

Copyright: © 2021 by the authors. Licensee MDPI, Basel, Switzerland. This article is an open access article distributed under the terms and conditions of the Creative Commons Attribution (CC BY) license (https://creativecommons.org/licenses/by/4.0/).

Simple Summary: The escalating use of next generation sequencing in the routine clinical setting greatly facilitates the genetic diagnosis of hereditary cancer syndromes. However, these novel methods pose new and unique challenges. In our study we sought to demonstrate the evolution of these techniques, especially whole exome sequencing and targeted panel sequencing. This study highlights the multi-layered workflow and how each step affects the diagnostic outcome and demonstrates the effectiveness of an in-house developed targeted panel sequencing for hereditary endocrine tumor syndromes.

Abstract: Next Generation Sequencing (NGS)-based methods are high-throughput and cost-effective molecular genetic diagnostic tools. Targeted gene panel and whole exome sequencing (WES) are applied in clinical practice for assessing mutations of pheochromocytoma/paraganglioma (PPGL) associated genes, but the best strategy is debated. Germline mutations of the at least 18 PPGL genes are present in approximately 20–40% of patients, thus molecular genetic testing is recommended in all cases. We aimed to evaluate the analytical and clinical performances of NGS methods for mutation detection of PPGL-associated genes. WES (three different library preparation and bioinformatics workflows) and an in-house, hybridization based gene panel (**en**docrine-**o**nco-**gen**e-panel- ENDOGENE) was evaluated on 37 (20 WES and 17 ENDOGENE) samples with known variants. After optimization of the bioinformatic workflow, 61 additional samples were tested prospectively. All clinically relevant variants were validated with Sanger sequencing. Target capture of PPGL genes differed markedly between WES platforms and genes tested. All known variants were correctly identified by all methods, but methods of library preparations, sequencing platforms and bioinformatical settings significantly affected the diagnostic accuracy. The ENDOGENE panel identified several pathogenic mutations and unusual genotype–phenotype associations suggesting that the whole panel should be used for identification of genetic susceptibility of PPGL.

Keywords: next-generation sequencing; pheochromocytoma; paraganglioma; hereditary cancer; endocrine tumor syndrome

1. Introduction

Pheochromocytomas and paragangliomas (PPGL) are rare chromaffin cell tumors arising from the adrenal medulla or the sympathetic or parasympathetic paraganglia.

PPGL have strong genetic determinism, overall approximately 40% of patients carry a germline mutation that predispose to the disease. The majority of these germline mutations occur in *SDHB, SDHD, VHL, NF1, RET* and *KIF1B* genes, but in rare or extremely rare cases, germline mutations of *SDHA, SDHAF2, EGLN1,* DLST, *FH, MAX, MDH2, KMT2D, TMEM127, MERTK, MET* and *SLC25A11* genes [1–23]. Moreover, several somatic driver mutations of *EPAS1, ATRX, IDH1,* MET, *BRAF, HRAS,* and *FGFR1* genes have also been identified which may serve as target for specific therapeutical approaches as causative factors of the tumor [24,25].

It is recommended to perform genetic testing for certain groups at high risk for hereditary PPGL syndromes, which consists of positive family history, coexistence of multiple syndromic features, early onset, multiple primary PPGL, malignancy, extra-adrenal location, or combination of these features [26]. According to the actual guideline, phenotype-related genetic screening is suggested [26]. However, not all mutations manifest with specific phenotype, and in some cases, due to the low number of documented patients, genotype–phenotype correlations are not yet established [1].

Next generation sequencing (NGS) methods are categorized as high-throughput techniques that allow the parallel sequencing of multiple (even million) samples covering numerous genes or even the whole exome/genome. The appropriate informatics background is obligatory for the operation of these systems. The spreading of these techniques revolutionized the genetic and the hereditary disease diagnostics and reformed the everyday clinical practice. Beside their advantages, these methods yielded novel obstacles to overcome: the distribution of NGS techniques required technological upgrades, new expertise and workflow to be developed. Alongside the clinical practitioner, laboratory staff, bioinformatics specialists and molecular biologists synchronized work is mandatory for the correct assessment of the results. The appropriate choice for use is of utmost important due to the sheer amount of data generated by the process [27]. The indication varies between different tumors, but the American Society of Oncology recommends that if the chance of carrying an oncogene germline mutation exceeds 10% the patient should undergo genetic testing of the predisposing cancer genes [28] and patients affected with PPGL with the overall ~40% heterogeneity certainly exceed this criterion. This recommendation is supported by the fact that at least 10% of patients with "low risk" cases may carry predisposing mutation [4]. Due to the high number of various genomic aberrations that could lead to developing PPGL, the molecular genetic diagnosis easily becomes costly and burdensome [29–33]. WES started to emerge as both a research and a diagnostic tool for PPGL in the recent past [2,34,35]. Exome sequencing identified novel PPGL susceptibility genes and novel genes are predicted to be identified in the future [16–21,36]. NGS technologies are capable of screening familial [37–41] and sporadic cases [20,34]. With these technologies, novel somatic mutations can be identified [20,42–45] and screening large cohorts of PPGL patients became available [20,37,39]. Moreover, WES contributed to the complex profiling of these tumors [22,46].

However, despite the gradual decrease of experimental costs, whole-exome sequencing is still only sporadically used in routine diagnostics as the costs remain relatively high. Due to the various designs available, it is urgent to make a consensus to determine the indispensable quality standards for both technical processing and the interpretation of the results [2]. Various guidelines have set the standards and goals of genomic screening with NGS [47–56].

As a national reference center for Hereditary Endocrine Tumor syndromes in Hungary and part of European Reference Network for Endocrine Diseases (ENDO-ERN) our laboratory performs the molecular genetic analysis of patients with hereditary endocrine tumors. The incidence of these syndromes is low, but in order to provide the genetic test result within an acceptable time, we decided to use next generation sequencing in the routine molecular genetic diagnostic workflow. In this recent work, we summarize our experience with NGS based methods in molecular testing of PPGL. WES along with an in-house targeted gene sequencing panel (ENDOGENE) was tested on 82 patients and the analytical performance was evaluated.

2. Materials and Methods

2.1. Patients and the Genetic Testing of the RET, VHL, SDHB, SDHC, SDHD and TMEM127 Genes Using Sanger Sequencing

A retrospective medical and laboratory record review was performed on all patients diagnosed with hereditary endocrine tumor syndrome including suspicion of hereditary pheochromocytoma and paraganglioma during the period 1998–2020 under care at Semmelweis University, Budapest, Hungary. Our center is a national reference and part of European Reference Network (ERN) expertise center for hereditary endocrine tumors. After genetic counseling and having obtained informed consent, all patients with PPGL underwent genetic testing for the *RET, VHL, SDHB, SDHC, SDHD, MAX* and *TMEM127* genes using conventional methods including PCR amplification followed by Sanger sequencing as previously reported [57]. Blood DNA was extracted using commercially available DNA extraction kits (DNA isolation from mammalian blood, Roche, or DNA isolation kit from blood, Qiagen LTD). Bidirectional DNA sequencing of all these genes and large deletion analysis of the *VHL, SDHB, SDHC* and *SDHD* and *TMEM127* genes were performed using multiplex ligation probe amplification [58]. Of these samples 20 were used for determination of analytical sensitivity of whole exome sequencing (WES) performed between 2015–2019. In 2015, an in-house NGS based gene panel (ENDOGENE panel) was developed and introduced into clinical practice. Fifteen samples were used for the validation of ENDOGENE panel and additional 61 patients were tested prospectively. The study was approved by the Hungarian National Public Health Center (NPHC: 41189-7/2018/EÜIG, 13 December 2018) and the Scientific and Research Committee of the Medical Research Council of Ministry of Health, Hungary (ETT-TUKEB 4457/2012/EKU).

2.2. Whole Exome Sequencing

Seven members of two families presenting PPGL and 13 unrelated patients affected with PPGL were selected from our database containing the clinical and laboratory data of 241 patients and relatives diagnosed and treated at the 2nd Department of Internal Medicine, Semmelweis University with clinical diagnosis of PPGL between 1998–2019. Twelve patients carried *SDHB* mutations, two *SDHD* mutations and one *SDHC* mutation (Table 1). Six patients had no mutation in *SDHB, SDHC, SDHD, VHL, RET, TMEM127* and *MAX* genes. A total number of 29 missense/nonsense variants were identified with Sanger sequencing in this cohort. These variants were used as positive references, while wild type sequences were considered as negative references during evaluation of analytical performances of WES.

WES was performed in all 20 samples; four samples from a family presenting *SDHB* mutation were prepared using Agilent 51 M SureSelect Biotinylated RNA Library kit, 12 unrelated samples, were prepared using BGI 59 Mb exome kit and four samples were prepared using Illumina's Rapid Capture Exome library preparation kit. WES was performed at NGS certified provider BGI Hong Kong (for libraries prepared with Agilent and BGI kits) [59,60] and by Omega Biotech, USA (samples prepared by Rapid Capture Exome). Library preparation and sequencing strategies are summarized in Supplementary Table S1.

For Illumina workflow, the bioinformatics analysis followed the routine Illumina pipeline. The adapter sequence was removed, and low-quality reads which had too many Ns and low base quality bases were discarded. Burrows–Wheeler Aligner (BWA) [61] was used for the alignment. Single Nucleotide Polymorphisms (SNPs) were determined by SOAPsnp, Small Insertion/Deletion (InDels) were detected by Samtools/Genome Analysis ToolKit (GATK) [62], Single Nucleotide Variants (SNVs) were analyzed by Varscan, CNVs were detected by ExomeCNV/Varscan [63,64]. ANNOVAR and GATK FUNCOTATOR was used for annotation [62,65].

Table 1. Genetic alterations of samples used for analytical testing of WES.

Patient ID	Known Mutation Detected by Sanger Sequencing	Characteristics of Mutation Identified by Exome Sequencing				
		NGS Platform Used	Library Preparation Kit Used	Mutation Confirmed	ACMG Category	Coverage, Read Number (Ratio and Read Numbers for Wild Type and Mutant Alleles)
1/F1	SDHB(NM_003000.3):c.586T>G (p.Cys196Gly)	Illumina Hiseq 2000	Agilent 51 M SureSelect	Yes	Pathogenic	50 (0.46: 27/23)
2/F1	SDHB(NM_003000.3):c.586T>G (p.Cys196Gly)			Yes	Pathogenic	58 (0.55: 26/32)
3/F1	No mutation detected				No mutation detected	
4/F1	No mutation detected				No mutation detected	
5	SDHB(NM_003000.2):c.649C>T (p.Arg217Cys)	Complete Genomics	BGI 59Mb Exome kit	Yes	Pathogenic	59 (0.38: 36/23)
6	SDHB(NM_003000.2):c.758G>A (p.Cys253Tyr)			Yes	Pathogenic	56 (0.59: 23/33)
7	SDHB(NM_003000.3):c.728G>A (p.Cy243Tyr)			Yes	Pathogenic	37 (0.62: 14/23)
8	SDHB (NM_003000.2):c.286+1G>A			Yes	Pathogenic	34 (0.5: 17/17)
9	SDHB(NM_003000.2): c.607G>T (p.Gly203 *)			Yes	Pathogenic	33 (0.36: 21/12)
10	SDHC(NM_003001.3):c.405+1G>T			Yes	Pathogenic	50 (0.42:29/21)
11	SDHD(NM_003002.4): c.147_148dupA (p.His50fs)			Yes	Pathogenic	33 (0.27: 24/9)
12	SDHD(NM_003002.4):c.149A>G (p.His50Arg)			Yes	VUS	36 (0.47: 19/17)
13	No mutation detected				No mutation detected	
14	No mutation detected				No mutation detected	
15	No mutation detected				No mutation detected	
16	No mutation detected				No mutation detected	
17	No mutation detected				No mutation detected	
18/F2	SDHB(NM_003000.3):c.586T>C (p.Cys196Arg)	Illumina Hiseq 2000	Rapid Capture Exome Library Preparation Kit	Yes	Pathogenic	185 (0.55:84/101)
19/F2	SDHB(NM_003000.3):c.586T>C (p.Cys196Arg)			Yes	Pathogenic	102 (0.48:53/49)
20/F2	SDHB(NM_003000.3):c.586T>C (p.Cys196Arg)			Yes	Pathogenic	170 (0.45:93/77)

* nomenclature.

For *Complete genomics workflow* the VCF files were received from the sequencing provider. The minimum sequencing depth for Illumina workflow was 10 reads/allele (20x) while for Complete Genomics data this threshold was set to 5 reads/allele (10x). Using in-house scripts written in phyton, the outputs of VCF files obtained either by Illumina or Complete Genomics platforms were merged into a single database file. Mean depth of coverage of PPGL genes were calculated using samtools bedcov utility on the CDS regions of genes obtained from gencode.hg19_v29 annotation.

2.3. Developing the ENDOGENE Panel

In the first version of ENDOGENE Panel (version 1.0), the covered genes included the *EGLN1, EPAS1, FH, KIF1B, MAX, MEN1, NF1, RET, SDHA, SDHAF2, SDHB, SDHC, SDHD, TMEM127* and *VHL* genes. During the development of the panel novel PPGL susceptibility genes were identified, therefore, the second version (version 2.0) included the *GOT2, MDH2* and *SLC25A11* genes as well. For targeted library preparation, a hybridization-based Roche NimbleGene SeqCap technology was used. Probes were designed for every exon and ±30 bp intronic sites. The micro format of the MiSeq Reagent kit was used for ENDOGEN Panel v1.0, whereas the nano format was used for ENDOGEN Panel v2.0 (Illumina Inc., Foster City, CA, USA). The sequencing was carried out in our laboratory on Illumina MiSeq sequencing device (Illumina Inc., Foster City CA, USA).

The sequencing data was assessed with GATK (Genome Analysis Toolkit) following Best Practice guides [66]. The adapter sequences were removed with Cutadapt software [67]. The raw FASTQ format data was aligned to the UCSC hg19 human reference genome with BWA [61]. The reads below quality score 30 were removed GATK HaplotypeCaller [68]. PCR duplicates were removed with Picard MarkDuplicates (http://broadinstitute.github.io/picard; 6 August 2021) software. The indel realignment and the recalibration of the quality score was carried out with GATK v2.5-2 [62,66,69]. High quality InDels were filtered by criteria: "QD < 2.0, ReadPosRankSum < −20.0. The minimum sequencing depth was 20 reads/allele (40x)

Variant annotation was carried out with FUNCOTATOR, SNPEFFECT, SIFT, ClinVar, Varsome and PolyPhen applications [62,70–72]. The prevalence and the clinical impact of the variants were assessed using data from dbSNP [73], the American Exome Project Variants Server (National Heart, Lung, and Blood Institute Exome Sequencing Project Exome Variant Server (http://evs.gs.washington.edu/EVS; 15 March 2021)), Hapmap [74], ClinVar, Varsome 1000Genomes [75], gnomad [76] and LOVD [77] databases.

Variant calls were subject to the same filtering parameters, eliminating non-exonic (untranslated region: UTR), synonymous and common (>1% MAF from the 1000 genome project, the exome sequencing project, and the Exome Aggregation Consortium) variants, as well as variants categorized as benign using ACMG criteria (ACMG criteria and PolyPhen-2 score = benign and SIFT < 0.05). All variants were categorized by recommendation of the NGS study group in PPGL, too [25].

All pathogenic, likely-pathogenic or variants with unknown significance were validated by Sanger sequencing.

3. Results

3.1. Whole Exome Sequencing

WES was performed on a set of 20 germline DNA samples obtained from patients with PPGL. Of these patients, seven belonged to two kindreds (F1 and F2) with already known *SDHB* p.Cys196Gly and *SDHB* p.Cys196Arg mutations.

3.2. Depth of coverage

For WES, the offered minimum mean depth of coverage per sample by the manufacturers was 100 reads. This coverage was achieved with all three library preparations and sequencing platforms. No significant differences were found in the number of unique reads, bases corresponding to targeted sequences and bases with no coverage (Supplementary Table S2).

However, analyzing the depth of coverage of PPGL-associated genes, significant differences were observed between genes and platforms. The most under covered regions belonged to *SDHA*, *SDHC* and *SDHD* genes in Agilent library preparation (Figure 1, Supplementary Table S3).

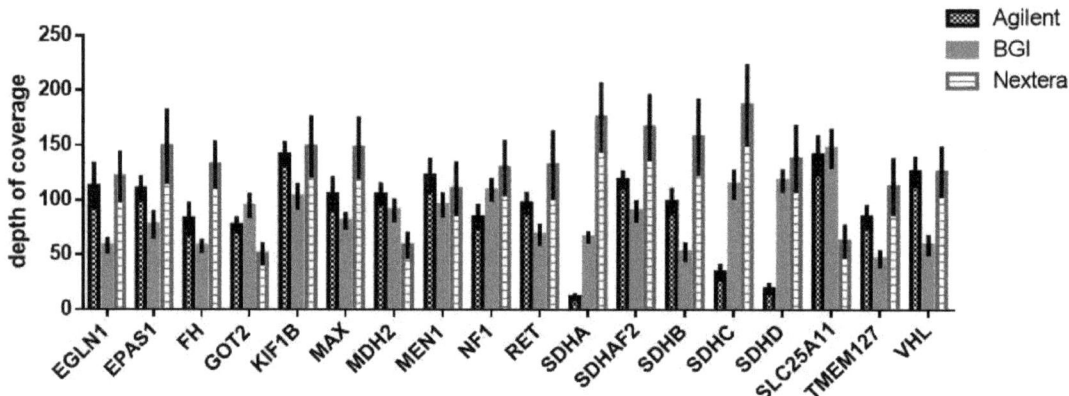

Figure 1. Coverage of PPGL associated genes by whole exome sequencing. Data is represented as mean ± SD.

3.3. Analytical Validation

For analytical validation, Sanger sequencing was performed of all exons of *SDHB*, *SDHC*, *SDHD*, *TMEM127* and *VHL* genes and exons 10,11,14–16 of *RET* gene in all samples sequenced by WES. The number of nucleotides covered by Sanger sequencing was 3569.

The total number of heterozygous, non-synonymous variants in these genes in these 20 samples were 29 variants. WES correctly detected all of them using an optimization of filtering strategy. The genetic alterations of samples used for analytical testing of WES are summarized in Table 1.

3.4. Optimization of Bioinformatical Workflow, Role of Allelic Ratio

As PPGL-associated pathogenic variants are heterozygous in germline DNA, we used this criterion for optimization of our bioinformatical workflow. In our study, the term of deviation (expressed in %) stands for the difference in modulus from the ideal allele fraction range (AFR) for heterozygote calls. For a heterozygote call the ratio of wild type and mutated allele is 1. The AFR shows the deviation of certain heterozygote variant from this number expressed in percentage (i.e., for a heterozygote call with 15/20 reads/alleles the AFR would be 75%). During WES data filtering we observed that some heterozygote variants showed larger allelic ratio. Based on the AFR the sensitivity of workflows was evaluated. Samples sequenced with BGI library preparation an AFR between 27–73% was needed for the correct identification of all true non-synonymous variants. For Agilent workflow, an AFR between 44.8–55.2% whereas for Nextera kit a ratio between 45.4–54.6% was necessary in order to achieve 100% sensitivity (Table 2).

Table 2. Analytical performances of WES for genes associated with PPGL using different cut-off values of allelic ratio for heterozygote calls.

	Agilent 51M SureSelect (n = 4)		Complete Genomics (n = 12)		Illumina Rapid Capture (n = 4)	
Allelic Ratio (%, Range)	30–70	41.1–58.8	30–70	41.1–58.8	30–70	41.1–58.8
True variants (mutations and polymorphisms) detected by Sanger sequencing	9		29		14	
Variants detected by WES	9	8	28	16	14	14
False positive variants	0	0	4	2	0	0
False negative variants	0	1	1	13	0	0
Sensitivity	100	88.9	96.5	55	100	100

3.5. Design of the ENDOGENE Panel v1.0

Due to the need of an in-house validated assay, we developed a hybridization-based library preparation method. ENDOGENE Panel v1.0 was capable of the simultaneous sequencing of *EGLN1, EPAS1, FH, KIF1B, MAX, MEN1, NF1, RET, SDHA, SDHB, SDHC, SDHD, SDHAF2, TMEM127* and *VHL* genes. A total number of 509 fragments covered the genes listed above. The complete sequence spanned 126,116 nucleotides.

For analytical validation of the ENDOGENE Panel v1.0, 15 patients with 10 verified pathogenic mutations (2 *RET*, 5 *SDHB*, 2 *TMEM127* and 1 *VHL*) were included. The coverage of the analyzed genomic regions was above 20 reads per allele (total 40x). Variants of 3′ and 5′ UTRs, of intron regions, synonymous variants and variants with coverage <10 reads were excluded from further analysis. In total 155 variants mapped to the coding regions. Of these variants, 41 were true positive while 114 were false positive. No false negative variants were detected. Fifteen of the false positive calls were due to a single *MEN1* variant. The *MEN1* p.T546A (rs2959656) was labeled as normal in the reference sequence used. The reference genome of the *MEN1* gene differs in the databases, therefore a special caution is needed during annotation of the *MEN1* variants.

In order to decrease the number of false positives, we applied a filter based on the allelic fraction range (AFR%) described above. Variants with a ratio less than 0.3 or higher than 0.7 were excluded. All the previously verified 12 pathogenic variants were correctly identified. Two variants of unknown significance (VUS) and 25 benign polymorphisms were found. Using this additional filter, the sensitivity of the ENDOGEN Panel v1.0 was 100%, accompanied with 99.1% specificity.

3.6. The Prospective Group of ENDOGENE Panel v1.0

The diagnostic use of the ENDOGENE Panel v1.0 was tested in the clinical setting on 24 samples which had no previous genetic diagnosis. Using the criteria detailed above, 62 variants were identified. In all cases, the already mentioned *MEN1* variant was called and categorized as false positive. Out of the 24 patients, 9 (37.5%) carried pathogenic variants (2 *SDHB*, 7 *NF1*) and in one patient a novel *VHL* variant, classified as VUS was detected (*VHL*: p.36_37insSGPEE) in a young patient presenting with carotid body paraganglioma. The remaining 28 variants were variants categorized as benign polymorphisms. It is worth noting that in a patient the panel sequencing identified two different *SDHB* mutations which were verified with Sanger sequencing: beside a p.R90 frameshift mutation, an *SDHB* p.T88I variant was found too.

3.7. Upgrading the ENDOGENE Panel v1.0 to v2.0

During the last three years novel genetic susceptibility loci have been identified for PPGL. Therefore, we had to upgrade our panel by including 3 additional (*GOT2*, *MDH2* and *SLC25A11*) genes. The same bioinformatical pipeline was used. The effectiveness of the ENDOGENE Panel v2.0 was tested on 37 patients with no previous genetic diagnosis. Pathogenic variants were identified in 10 patients (27%). Mutations in *SDHB* (three patients), *FH* (two patients), *NF1* (four patients), and *VHL* (one patient) genes were detected and confirmed with Sanger sequencing. Four variants were categorized as VUS; the *SDHC*: c.94A > G (p.Thr32Ala) was found alongside one pathogenic variant suggesting that this variant might be a benign or a likely-benign variant. The pathogenic role of the *MDH2*: c.365G>A (p.Arg122Gln) and the *SDHA*: c.837G>T (p.Met279Ile) should be further tested following recommendation provided by the NGS in PPGL consensus statement [25]. Confronting data about the pathogenicity of the *RET* c.2372A>T (p.Tyr791Phe) have been presented, the detailed phenotype of our case is presented in Discussion section.

In summary, of 61 prospectively tested cases 19 (31.1%) harbored pathogenic/likely pathogenic variants (all variants detected in our cohort are summarized in Table 3). Of these variants, eight could be considered as novel as they have not been reported in any database to the best of our knowledge (Table 4). All these variants were confirmed by Sanger sequencing. Five of these is classified as pathogenic or likely pathogenic (all of these variants are truncating variants). Three variants are classified as VUS. Two *SDHB* variants: SDHB(NM_003000.3):c.263C>T (p.Thr88Ile); SDHB(NM_003000.3):c.268C>G (p.Arg90Gly) occurred in a patient where another pathogenic or likely pathogenic variant was identified (Figure 2, Panel A). The distribution of sequencing reads containing these variants show that these variants occurred at the same chromosome, therefore they are all in cis. The third VUS was detected in a patient with NF1 syndrome (Case 24). This is a complex alteration which has been annotated differently by various tools. However, looking at the sequence, this variant would is named NF1(NM_001042492.2):c.5047_5053delinsGGAG (p.Asn1683_Ser1684_Trp1685delinsGlyGly) (Figure 2, Panel B).

Table 3. Variants identified with ENDOGEN panels v1.0, and v2.0 and the associated phenotypes.

ID	Panel	Phenotype	ACMG Classification Pathogenic/Likely Pathogenic Variants	VUS	Clinical Classification Based on PPGL Consensus Guideline [25]
1	EP 1.0V	malignant PGL	SDHB(NM_003000.3):c.728G>A (p.Cys243Tyr)	-	pathogenic
2	EP 1.0V	Pheo	-	-	
3	EP 1.0V	malignant PGL	SDHB(NM_003000.3):c.586T>G (p.Cys196Gly)	-	pathogenic
4	EP 1.0V	malignant PGL	-	-	
5	EP 1.0V	Pheo	-	-	
6	EP 1.0V	MEN2	RET(NM_020975.6):c.1832G>A (p.Cys611Tyr)	-	pathogenic
7	EP 1.0V	Pheo	TMEM127(NM_001193304.3):c.419G>A (p.Cys140Tyr)	-	likely pathogenic
8	EP 1.0V	Pheo	-	-	
9	EP 1.0V	malignant PGL	SDHB(NM_003000.3):c.745T>C (p.Cys249Arg)	-	likely pathogenic
10	EP 1.0V	malignant PGL	SDHB(NM_003000.3):c.649C>T (p.Arg217Cys)	-	likely pathogenic
11	EP 1.0V	malignant PGL	SDHB(NM_003000.3):c.758G>A (p.Cys253Tyr)	-	pathogenic
12	EP 1.0V	MEN2B	RET(NM_020975.6):c.2753T>C (p.Met918Thr)	-	pathogenic
13	EP 1.0V	Pheo	TMEM127(NM_001193304.3):c.320delG (p.Ser107Ilefs*17)	-	likely pathogenic
14	EP 1.0V	VHL	VHL(NM_000551.4):c.407T>G (p. Phe136Cys)	-	likely pathogenic
15	EP 1.0V	Pheo	-	-	
16	EP 1.0P	Pheo	-	-	
17	EP 1.0P	Pheo	-	-	
18	EP 1.0P	Pheo	-	-	
19	EP 1.0P	malignant PGL	SDHB(NM_003000.3):c.286+2T>A	-	likely pathogenic
20	EP 1.0P	PGL	-	-	
21	EP 1.0P	NF1	NF1(NM_001042492.3):c.1756_1759delACTA (p.Thr586ValfsTer18)	-	pathogenic

Table 3. Cont.

ID	Panel	Phenotype	ACMG Classification Pathogenic/Likely Pathogenic Variants	VUS	Clinical Classification Based on PPGL Consensus Guideline [25]
22	EP 1.0P	NF1	NF1(NM_001042492.2):c.5047_5053delinsGGAG (p.Asn1683_Ser1684_Trp1685delinsGlyGly)	-	VUS
23	EP 1.0P	NF1	NF1(NM_001042492.2):c.4230_4231delCC (p.Leu1411GlnfsTer12)	-	likely pathogenic
24	EP 1.0P	NF1	NF1(NM_001042492.2):c.1466A>G (p.Tyr489Cys)	-	pathogenic
25	EP 1.0P	NF1	NF1(NM_001042492.2):c.2251+1G>A	-	likely pathogenic
26	EP 1.0P	NF1	NF1(NM_001042492.2):c.7465_7466insG (p.Lys2489ArgfsTer13)	-	likely pathogenic
27	EP 1.0P	Pheo	-	-	
28	EP 1.0P	NF1	NF1(NM_001042492.2):c.4175dupT (p.Val1393GlyfsTer2)	-	likely pathogenic
29	EP 1.0P	Pheo	-	-	
30	EP 1.0P	Pheo	-	-	
31	EP 1.0P	Pheo	-	-	
32	EP 1.0P	Pheo	-	-	
33	EP 1.0P	Pheo	-	-	
34	EP 1.0P	PGL-glomus caroticum	-	VHL(NM_000551.4):c.123_137dupAGAGTCCGGCCCGGA (p.Ser43_Glu47dup) = NM_000551.3(VHL):c.123_137dup (p.38_42SGPEE [3])	VUS
35	EP 1.0P	Pheo	-	-	VUS
36	EP 1.0P	malignant PGL	SDHB(NM_003000.3):c.263C>T (p.Thr88Ile) SDHB(NM_003000.3):c.268C>G (p.Arg90Gly) SDHB(NM_003000.3):c.271_273del (p.Arg91del)	-	VUS likely pathogenic

Table 3. Cont.

ID	Panel	Phenotype	ACMG Classification Pathogenic/Likely Pathogenic Variants	VUS	Clinical Classification Based on PPGL Consensus Guideline [25]
37	EP 1.0P	Pheo	-	-	
38	EP 1.0P	Pheo	-	-	
39	EP 1.0P	Pheo	-	-	
40	EP 2.0	Pheo	-	-	
41	EP 2.0	Pheo	SDHB(NM_003000.3):c.193C>T (p.Leu65Phe)	-	likely pathogenic
42	EP 2.0	Pheo	-	-	
43	EP 2.0	Pheo	-	-	
44	EP 2.0	Pheo	-	-	
45	EP 2.0	Pheo	-	-	
46	EP 2.0	Pheo	-	-	
47	EP 2.0	Pheo	-	-	
48	EP 2.0	Pheo	VHL(NM_000551.4):c.576delA (p.Asn193MetfsTer9)	-	likely pathogenic
49	EP 2.0	Pheo	-	-	
50	EP 2.0	Pheo&PGL	SDHB(NM_003000.3):c.286+2T>A	-	likely pathogenic
51	EP 2.0	Pheo	FH(NM_000143.4):c.1127A>C (p.Gln376Pro)	-	likely pathogenic
52	EP 2.0	Pheo	-	-	
53	EP 2.0	Pheo	-	-	
54	EP 2.0	abdominal PGL	SDHB(NM_003000.3):c.689G>A(p.Arg230His)	-	pathogenic
55	EP 2.0	Pheo	-	-	
56	EP 2.0	Pheo	-	-	
57	EP 2.0	malignant PGL	-	-	

Table 3. *Cont.*

ID	Panel	Phenotype	ACMG Classification		Clinical Classification Based on PPGL Consensus Guideline [25]
			Pathogenic/Likely Pathogenic Variants	VUS	
58	EP 2.0	Pheo	-	-	
59	EP 2.0	Pheo	-	-	
60	EP 2.0	cervical PGL	-	-	
61	EP 2.0	NF1	NF1(NM_001042492.2):c.3456dupA (p.Leu1153ThrfsTer42)	-	pathogenic
62	EP 2.0	Pheo	-	-	
63	EP 2.0	NF1	NF1(NM_001042492.2):c.888+2T>G	-	pathogenic
64	EP 2.0	Pheo	-	-	
65	EP 2.0	Fumarase deficient leiomyoma	FH(NM_000143.4):c.1256C>T (p.Ser419Leu)	-	likely pathogenic
66	EP 2.0	Pheo	-	-	
67	EP 2.0	Pheo	-	MDH2(NM_005918.4):c.686G>A (p.Arg229Gln)	VUS
68	EP 2.0	Pheo	-	SDHA(NM_004168.4):c.837G>T (p.Met279Ile)	VUS
69	EP 2.0	Pheo	-	-	
70	EP 2.0	Pheo	-	-	
71	EP 2.0	Pheo	-	RET(NM_020975.6):c.2372A>T (p.Tyr791Phe)-	VUS
72	EP 2.0	NF1	NF1(NM_001042492.2):c.6850_6853delACTT (p.Tyr2285fs)	SDHC(NM_003001.5):c.94A>G (p.Thr32Ala)	The *NF1* variant pathogenic The *SDHC* variant VUS
73	EP 2.0	Pheo	-	-	
74	EP 2.0	Pheo	-	-	
75	EP 2.0	Pheo	-	-	
76	EP 2.0	NF1	NF1(NM_001042492.3):c.2991-1G>C	-	pathogenic

EP1.0V: ENDOGENE Panel version 1-validation group; EP1.0P: ENDOGENE Panel version 1-prospective group; Pheo: pheochromocytoma; PGL: paraganglioma; MEN: multiple endocrine neoplasia; NF1: Neurofibromatosis type 1; VUS: variant of uncertain significance. Patients tested by EP 1.0V had genetic diagnosis before panel sequencing. Patients tested by EP 1.0P and EP2.0 did not have a genetic diagnosis before testing.

Table 4. Novel genetic variants and associated clinical phenotypes identified in our recent cohort.

Sample ID	Manifestations	Age (Years)	Benign/ Malignant	Genetic Variant	Clinical Significance
22	Neurofibromatosis Type 1: multiple neurofibromas	30	B	NF1(NM_001042492.2):c.5047 _5053delinsGGAG(p.Asn1683_Ser1684 _Trp1685delinsGlyGly)	VUS
	Adrenal pheochromocytoma	30	B		
23	Neurofibromatosis Type 1: multiple neurofibromas	32	B	NF1(NM_001042492.2):c.4230 _4231delCC (p.Leu1411GlnfsTer12)	likely pathogenic
26	Neurofibromatosis Type 1: Adrenal pheochromocytoma	15	B	NF1(NM_001042492.2):c.7465 _7466insG (p.Lys2489ArgfsTer13)	likely pathogenic
28	Neurofibromatosis Type 1	26	B	NF1(NM_001042492.2):c.4175dupT (p.Val1393GlyfsTer2)	likely pathogenic
36	Extra-adrenal PGL	14	M	SDHB(NM_003000.3):c.263C>T (p.Thr88Ile)	VUS
				SDHB(NM_003000.3):c.268C>G (p.Arg90Gly)	VUS
				SDHB(NM_003000.3):c.271_273del (p.Arg91del)	likely pathogenic
48	Adrenal pheochromocytoma	15	B	VHL(NM_000551.4):c.576delA (p.Asn193MetfsTer9)	likely pathogenic

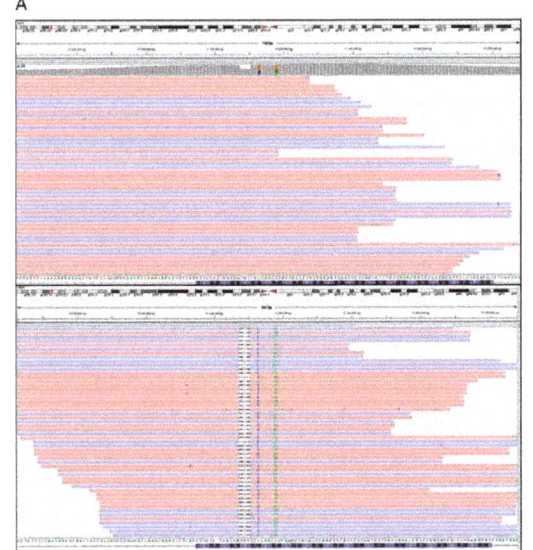 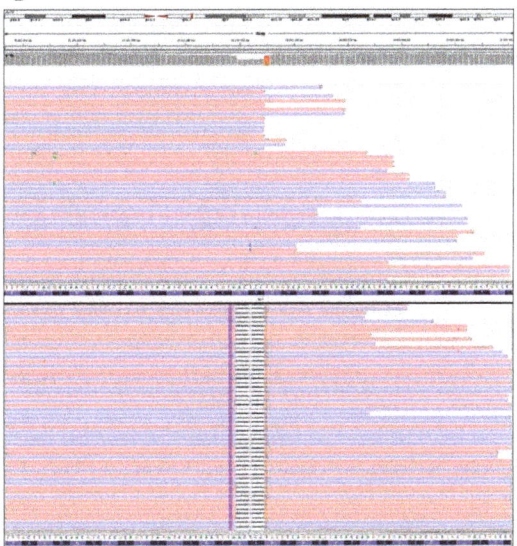

Figure 2. Schematic presentation of sequencing reads containing the variants SDHB(NM_003000.3):c.263C>T (p.Thr88Ile), SDHB(NM_003000.3):c.268C>G (p.Arg90Gly), SDHB(NM_003000.3):c.271_273del(p.Arg91del) (Case 38, (**A**)) and NF1(NM_001042492.2):c.5047_5053delinsGGAG(p.Asn1683_Ser1684_Trp1685delinsGlyGly) (Case 24, (**B**)). Each line represents one read. Half of the reads shows normal sequence (**upper part**) and half of the reads (**lower part**) show the mutated sequences.

No large deletions or copy number alterations were detected in our cases. Multiplex ligation-dependent probe amplification assays were used for analysis of *VHL* (probemix P016), *SDHB*, *SDHC*, *SDHD*, *SDHAF1* and *SDHAF2* (probemix P226).

4. Discussion

Next generation sequencing and especially the targeted sequencing of certain chromosome regions and genes became the prime focus in the clinical management and the research of PPGL [36,78–81]. Even though methods covering the whole exome or even the whole genome are available, the targeted sequencing of certain genes is preferred in the clinical setting due to their cost-effectiveness [82–84].

PPGLs accompany various hereditary tumor syndromes. The genetic counseling and screening of these patients and their family are essential. Life-long monitoring is also compulsory for asymptomatic individuals carrying a pathogenic variant in PPGL-related gene. Depending on the affected gene, the childhood or even the prenatal genetic screening could be recommended, especially in case of *FH* and *SDHB* mutations due to their often aggressive, malignant phenotype [17,85]. This recommendation for early screening is further supported by the fact that there is no reliable marker for the malignant potential [86]. Tumor metabolomics and detailed immunohistochemistry of SDHB, FH and GLS1 enzymes may provide help in the future [87].

Molecular genetic tests for PPGL are recommended by recent guidelines [25,26,88]. Based on clinic-pathological conditions, a successive testing of genes associating with PPGL is recommended [24], but currently the availability and cost effectiveness of NGS methods are attractive options. However, the analytical and the clinical validation of these methods is mandatory before applying them in the clinical setting. During a test development of an in-house sequencing method, both gene panel and WES should follow the recommendation of The European Society of Human Genetics and only genes with known genotype–phenotype correlations can be investigated for diagnostic purposes [52]. Following this recommendation, we tested three independent library preparations and two sequencing strategies for their performances in testing of PPGL associated genes. First, a critical parameter was the coverage of our target genes with WES methods. The minimal coverage is highly depends on library preparation and sequencing devices, so universal recommendation for the minimal coverage cannot be made. The differences in them are represented in the pipeline of the sequencing method. Low coverage could indicate false negative variants, therefore the declaration of the minimal coverage of certain laboratories is mandatory [48]. However, high coverage is neither optimal due to the increasing sequencing costs and it yields more false positive calls. In germline testing, a min. 30x coverage is recommended, and in our study the 40-reads (20 per allele) coverage was enough for the identification of all pathogenic variants after an optimization of bioinformatical analysis. The sequencing depth of all the three tested library preparation provided sufficient coverage of all PPGL associated genes, but for the Agilent 51M exome kit the coverage of *SDHA*, *SDHC* and *SDHD* genes was the lowest. This observation is in line with previously reported data showing an inadequate coverage for the majority of variants in seven genes including *SDHC* and *SDHD* [89]. Despite this disadvantage, our data confirmed that WES can be a suitable tool for molecular genetic testing of inherited diseases. Position-specific comparative analysis of disease-causing variants of PPGL genes identified through NGS panels demonstrated that exome sequencing with a validated bioinformatical pipeline can be used for clinical testing [90]. Therefore, targeted analysis of PPGL genes from WES data may be suitable for clinical diagnostic purposes.

Parallel with WES, we developed an in-house gene panel sequencing (ENDOGENE Panel) for cost effect analysis of PPGL-associated genes together with *MEN1* gene. As a reference center for Hereditary Endocrine Tumors our laboratory routinely tests patients with PPGL and hereditary endocrine cancer syndromes. The first version of ENDOGENE was designed in 2015 and it was capable for sequencing of 15 hereditary endocrine tumor syndrome candidate genes. In order to assess the analytical performance, we first tested the effectiveness of the panel on samples with known pathogenic mutations and genetic diagnosis. The ENDOGENE panel successfully identified all known pathogenic mutations. In case of genetically negative cases, the panel sequencing did not identify a pathogenic mutation either. The sensitivity of our test was 100% with a specificity of 99.1%. These parameters are in line with those requirements established for germline testing by the Food and Drug Administration [91].

After validation, we used the ENDOGENE panel for prospective analysis of all patients referred for genetic analysis. In total, we identified pathogenic mutations in 19 of 61 (31.1%) of patients tested prospectively, which is in line with data previously reported [22,92]. It is important to note that mutations detected in Hungarian population were unique, no "founder" mutations have been detected. Therefore, only the specific phenotypes may guide the clinician in choosing the most accurate genetic test, but the successive testing of genes related to the well-known hereditary tumor syndromes (MEN2, VHL, NF1 and paraganglioma syndromes) would lead to a long and burdensome process. Our data confirms that both NGS approaches (gene panel and WES) have similar diagnostic yield in PPGL. The diagnostic yield, however, varies by diseases [93,94], but in apparently sporadic PPGL patients the prevalence of germline mutations is around 20–40%. Currently there is no recommendation for using NGS in molecular genetic testing of PPGL. However, for rare diseases the gene panel testing is preferred over WES. Based on our experience for non-syndromic PPGL the choice between panel and exome sequencing can be traced back to the availability of NGS platforms and cost. The major advantages of exome sequencing over targeted NGS panel testing is the evaluation of all coding regions in the genome. As shown in our study, even within this short period we had to upgrade our panel sequencing strategy because of the newly discovered genes. Based on our study, WES coverage depth was adequate for detection for close to all pathogenic variants identified on targeted NGS panel testing, along with newly-discovered PPGL genes. In addition, the repeated analysis of WES data may further increase the diagnostic yield of exome sequencing. The turn around time (TAT) for providing the genetic test report is 4–5 weeks, which includes Sanger validation from a separate DNA sample isolated from the same patient and pre- and posttest genetic counselling. Our panel sequencing is performed usually 1–2 times/month, depending on the requested number of tests. Generally, batches of eight to 24 samples are sequenced. With this strategy the cost of sequencing per sample is approx. 250 EUR. Contrarily, with Sanger sequencing the cost of sequencing only the most recommended PPGL genes (basic set: *SDHB*, *SDHD*, *SDHC*, *VHL*, *TMEM127*, *RET* and *MAX*), the TAT would take 3 months and the cost would be more than the 1000 EUR/sample.

Our study resulted in discoveries of unusual genotype–phenotype associations (Table 3). A VUS *VHL* variant (NM_000551.4): c.123_137dupAGAGTCCGGCCCGGA (p.Ser43_Glu47dup) was identified in a patient with carotid body paraganglioma, which would have been missed or delayed significantly if the routine protocol had been applied. In this case, testing of *SDHx* genes is recommended as a first test, while testing of the *VHL* gene is recommended only in case of other specific manifestations of the disease or the presence of von Hippel–Lindau syndrome in the family [95]. Since neither criterion was present in our patient, the genetic diagnosis with Sanger sequencing would have been a long and burdensome process. Genetic testing of the index patient's parents showed the absence of this variant suggesting that it occurred de novo in our case.

The ENDOGENE Panel was capable of identifying a complex genetic variation in the *SDHB* gene in one patient. The SDHB(NM_003000.3):c.263C>T (p.Thr88Ile), SDHB(NM_003000.3):c.268C>G (p.Arg90Gly), SDHB(NM_003000.3):c.271_273del (p.Arg91del) variants was detected in a 14-year-old patient presenting with a large (14 × 8 × 17.5 cm) intraabdominal mass at the right side spanning the midline. Multiple bone metastases were also detected. The patient underwent a surgical intervention but, due to bleeding and the localization of the tumor, complete surgical removal was not possible. The histological examination showed pheochromocytoma. Chemotherapy with cyclophosphamide, vincristine and dacarbazine (CVD) and after 10 month of radiotherapy with administration of ^{131}I-MIBG. After three years, the patient is in remission. The bone lesions are without any change. The family history was negative for any malignant disorder. DNA sample was available only from the index patient's mother, but none of the identified variants were present. The pathogenic role, based on multiple predictions is attributed to the SDHB(NM_003000.3):c.271_273del (p.Arg91del) variant whereas the two other variants are classified as VUSs. These alterations located close to the pathogenic variant. Looking at the mapped sequencing reads it is evident that all these variants are present in the same reads, while other reads are normal. These distributions suggest that this complex rearrangment affects one chromosome and all these variants are in cis.

Mutations of *FH* gene are associated with hereditary leiomyomatosis, "fumarate hydratase deficient renal cell cancer (RCC)" ("FH-deficient RCC") [96] and in a very few cases with PPGL [17]. We identified a novel variant (c.1256C>T (p.S419L)) in a patient with this phenotype and the pathogenicity of this variant was supported by the lack of staining of the tumor sample with FH antibody on immunohistochemistry [97].

The ENDOGENE Panel v1.0 identified the *RET* p.M918T (rs74799832) mutation in a 33-year-old male patient in whom the referring clinical diagnosis was a unilateral pheochromocytoma. This mutation associates with a severe MEN2B phenotype, usually causing medullary thyroid cancer (MTC) at a very young age [98]. Eight years earlier the patient had a total thyroidectomy and lymph node dissection due to MTC. At that time the most common *RET* mutations (exon 10 and exon 11) were tested in another laboratory and no *RET* mutation was identified. After our genetic test result clinical, biochemical and imaging studies revealed that his serum calcitonin level was still elevated and a mediastinal lymph node metatasis was detected with Positron Emission Tomography and Computed Tomography (PET-CT) Scans. Although the patient received chemotherapy and recently tyrosine kinase inhibitor therapy, further progression of the disease was observed. Other MEN2B related manifestations were not documented. This patient carries the *SDHD* p.H50R variant as well. Currently this variant is categorized as benign, but there are confronting results about its association with PPGL. Our data may support its benign role.

Beside pathogenic or likely pathogenic variants, numerous variants classified as with uncertain significance were identified. These VUSs present major challenges in clinical practice. Following the recommendations of The American College of Medical Genetics and Genomics and the European Society of Human Genetics, these variants should be reported and interpreted on the molecular genetic test report but taking a clinical action is not recommended [48,51,52]. During their interpretation, various factors such as their minor allelic frequency, in silico predictions for the protein function and other supplementary evaluations must be carried out. The *SDHD* p.G12S variant's phenotype altering effect was previously studied by our working group [99]. Our results implied that this variant is significantly more frequent in MEN2 patients than in the healthy population. This variant occurred in a *NF1* and a *VHL* mutation carrier patients suggesting that this variant has a minor role in disease development.

The classification of the *RET* c.2372A>T (p.Y791F) variant is also debated (note 1 January 2021 in ClinVar). This variant was identified in a 59-year-old patient presenting with unilateral adrenal pheochromocytoma. After genetic test result, routine clinical, biochemical and imaging studies were performed for MEN2 related manifestations. His serum calcitonin, serum calcium and parathormone levels were within the reference range and no thyroid abnormalities were observed on thyroid ultrasonography. There are data showing that this variant does not increase the susceptibility for MTC [100] and recently a functional study proved that this variant exerted no pathogenetic effect in vivo in mice [101]. Taken together these data we suggest that this variant can be considered as a variant with unknown significance.

The *MDH2* c.686G>A (p.Arg229Gln) and the *SDHA* c.837G>T (p.Met279Ile) variants are classified as VUS. Both were identified in patients presenting with unilateral, adrenal pheochromocytomas. In these cases, no other clinical manifestations were detected. The pathogenicity of these variants should be considered given their MAFs and the lack of other pathogen variants in these patients. In these cases, evaluation of the metabolic features together with expression of enzymes on protein level could clarify their pathogenic role. For interpretation of the clinical relevance of a rare VUS additional studies (somatic mutation analysis, functional assays) are needed. These VUS should be reported on molecular genetic test reports, but no clinical action can be made until their pathogenic role has been confirmed [25]. Therefore, in our cases, yearly medical examinations were carried out.

The VHL(NM_000551.4):c.576delA (p.Asn193MetfsTer9) variant was identified in young male patient (15 years old) presenting with hormonally active adrenal pheochromocytoma. After genetic test, his regular (yearly performed) clinical, biochemical, imaging and ophthalmological studies revealed no sign of other VHL-related manifestations. Genetic screening was performed in his parents and the same variant was detected in her clinically healthy mother (45 years old). Her screening for VHL-associated manifestation showed no VHL-related manifestations.

Several novel variants were identified in patients presenting with typical signs of Neurofibromatosis type 1. Earlier, due to the size of the gene and the obvious clinical symptoms (skin alterations: café au lait spot, neurofibromas, Lisch nodules) the genetic analysis was not performed in these cases. However, as NF1 is an autosomal dominant disorder with significant alterations which associate with decreased life expectancy [102], early diagnosis and adequate interventions are indicated. Patient No. 28 represents a 33-year-old female patient presented 6 years ago with multiple neurofibromas. Clinical, hormone laboratory and imaging studies detected no other manifestations. After 7 years no progression and no new manifestation occurred

5. Conclusions

In summary, our research group developed a hybridization based targeted sequencing panel for hereditary endocrine syndromes. The ENDOGENE Panel effectively verified the previously known mutations and uncovered novel variants in patients without genetic diagnosis in a cost-effective way. Respecting the limitations of our panel, it can be simply expanded by novel genes in the future. In the case of targeted sequencing the most important value to reach is 100% sensitivity. As false positive variants can be excluded via Sanger sequencing, the false negative results pose the greatest threat to the patients and their families.

Supplementary Materials: The following are available online at https://www.mdpi.com/article/10.3390/cancers13164219/s1, Table S1: Sequencing platforms of WES, Table S2: Table Distribution of sequencing reads obtained by different WES platforms, Table S3: Mean depth of coverage of PPGL genes obtained during WES.

Author Contributions: Conceptualization, A.P.; formal analysis, B.S., G.N., H.B. and A.P.; funding acquisition: A.P.; bioinformatical investigation: I.L.; methodology: B.S., G.N. and H.B.; project administration B.S. and A.P.; resources, A.P. and H.B.; supervision, A.P. and H.B.; writing—original draft: B.S. and A.P.; review and editing: B.S., I.L., G.N., P.I., H.B. and A.P. All authors have read and agreed to the published version of the manuscript.

Funding: The research was financed by the Higher Education Institutional Excellence Programme of the Ministry of Human Capacities in Hungary, within the framework of the Molecular Biology thematic program of the Semmelweis University to Attila Patócs and by Hungarian Scientific Research Grant of National Research, Development and Innovation Office (K125231 to Attila Patócs). The authors would like to acknowledge the National Program of Bionics (subtheme medical bionics lead by Attila Patócs). Henriett Butz is a recipient of Bolyai Research Fellowship of Hungarian Academy of Sciences and her work is supported by the ÚNKP-19-4 New National Excellence Program of the Ministry for Innovation and Technology.

Institutional Review Board Statement: The study was approved by the Hungarian National Public Health Center (NPHC: 41189-7/2018/EÜIG, 13 December 2018) and the Scientific and Research Committee of the Medical Research Council of Ministry of Health, Hungary (ETT-TUKEB 4457/2012/EKU).

Informed Consent Statement: Informed consent was obtained from all subjects involved in the study.

Data Availability Statement: The data presented in this study are available on request from the corresponding author.

Acknowledgments: The authors are grateful to clinicians all over Hungary sending patients for genetic counseling and genetic testing for hereditary endocrine tumor syndromes.

Conflicts of Interest: The authors declare no conflict of interest.

References

1. Toledo, R.A. Genetics of Pheochromocytomas and Paragangliomas: An Overview on the Recently Implicated Genes MERTK, MET, Fibroblast Growth Factor Receptor 1, and H3F3A. *Endocrinol. Metab. Clin. North. Am.* **2017**, *46*, 459–489. [CrossRef] [PubMed]
2. Toledo, R.A.; Dahia, P.L. Next-generation sequencing for the diagnosis of hereditary pheochromocytoma and paraganglioma syndromes. *Curr. Opin. Endocrinol. Diabetes Obes.* **2015**, *22*, 169–179. [CrossRef] [PubMed]
3. Neumann, H.P.; Bausch, B.; McWhinney, S.R.; Bender, B.U.; Gimm, O.; Franke, G.; Schipper, J.; Klisch, J.; Altehoefer, C.; Zerres, K.; et al. Germ-line mutations in nonsyndromic pheochromocytoma. *N. Engl. J. Med.* **2002**, *346*, 1459–1466. [CrossRef]
4. Gimenez-Roqueplo, A.P.; Dahia, P.L.; Robledo, M. An update on the genetics of paraganglioma, pheochromocytoma, and associated hereditary syndromes. *Horm. Metab. Res. = Horm. Stoffwechs. = Horm. Metab.* **2012**, *44*, 328–333. [CrossRef] [PubMed]
5. Dahia, P.L.M. Pheochromocytoma and paraganglioma pathogenesis: Learning from genetic heterogeneity. *Nat. Rev. Cancer* **2014**, *14*, 108–119. [CrossRef] [PubMed]
6. Favier, J.; Amar, L.; Gimenez-Roqueplo, A.P. Paraganglioma and phaeochromocytoma: From genetics to personalized medicine. *Nat. Rev. Endocrinol.* **2015**, *11*, 101–111. [CrossRef] [PubMed]
7. Baysal, B.E.; Ferrell, R.E.; Willett-Brozick, J.E.; Lawrence, E.C.; Myssiorek, D.; Bosch, A.; van der Mey, A.; Taschner, P.E.; Rubinstein, W.S.; Myers, E.N.; et al. Mutations in SDHD, a mitochondrial complex II gene, in hereditary paraganglioma. *Science* **2000**, *287*, 848–851. [CrossRef]
8. Niemann, S.; Muller, U. Mutations in SDHC cause autosomal dominant paraganglioma, type 3. *Nat. Genet.* **2000**, *26*, 268–270. [CrossRef]
9. Astuti, D.; Latif, F.; Dallol, A.; Dahia, P.L.; Douglas, F.; George, E.; Skoldberg, F.; Husebye, E.S.; Eng, C.; Maher, E.R. Gene mutations in the succinate dehydrogenase subunit SDHB cause susceptibility to familial pheochromocytoma and to familial paraganglioma. *Am. J. Hum. Genet.* **2001**, *69*, 49–54. [CrossRef]
10. Hao, H.X.; Khalimonchuk, O.; Schraders, M.; Dephoure, N.; Bayley, J.P.; Kunst, H.; Devilee, P.; Cremers, C.W.; Schiffman, J.D.; Bentz, B.G.; et al. SDH5, a gene required for flavination of succinate dehydrogenase, is mutated in paraganglioma. *Science* **2009**, *325*, 1139–1142. [CrossRef]
11. Burnichon, N.; Briere, J.J.; Libe, R.; Vescovo, L.; Riviere, J.; Tissier, F.; Jouanno, E.; Jeunemaitre, X.; Benit, P.; Tzagoloff, A.; et al. SDHA is a tumor suppressor gene causing paraganglioma. *Hum. Mol. Genet.* **2010**, *19*, 3011–3020. [CrossRef] [PubMed]
12. Yeh, I.T.; Lenci, R.E.; Qin, Y.; Buddavarapu, K.; Ligon, A.H.; Leteurtre, E.; Do Cao, C.; Cardot-Bauters, C.; Pigny, P.; Dahia, P.L. A germline mutation of the KIF1B beta gene on 1p36 in a family with neural and nonneural tumors. *Hum. Genet.* **2008**, *124*, 279–285. [CrossRef]
13. Ladroue, C.; Carcenac, R.; Leporrier, M.; Gad, S.; Le Hello, C.; Galateau-Salle, F.; Feunteun, J.; Pouyssegur, J.; Richard, S.; Gardie, B. PHD2 mutation and congenital erythrocytosis with paraganglioma. *N. Engl. J. Med.* **2008**, *359*, 2685–2692. [CrossRef] [PubMed]
14. Qin, Y.; Yao, L.; King, E.E.; Buddavarapu, K.; Lenci, R.E.; Chocron, E.S.; Lechleiter, J.D.; Sass, M.; Aronin, N.; Schiavi, F.; et al. Germline mutations in TMEM127 confer susceptibility to pheochromocytoma. *Nat. Genet.* **2010**, *42*, 229–233. [CrossRef] [PubMed]
15. Yao, L.; Schiavi, F.; Cascon, A.; Qin, Y.; Inglada-Perez, L.; King, E.E.; Toledo, R.A.; Ercolino, T.; Rapizzi, E.; Ricketts, C.J.; et al. Spectrum and prevalence of FP/TMEM127 gene mutations in pheochromocytomas and paragangliomas. *JAMA* **2010**, *304*, 2611–2619. [CrossRef] [PubMed]
16. Comino-Mendez, I.; Gracia-Aznarez, F.J.; Schiavi, F.; Landa, I.; Leandro-Garcia, L.J.; Leton, R.; Honrado, E.; Ramos-Medina, R.; Caronia, D.; Pita, G.; et al. Exome sequencing identifies MAX mutations as a cause of hereditary pheochromocytoma. *Nat. Genet.* **2011**, *43*, 663–667. [CrossRef] [PubMed]
17. Castro-Vega, L.J.; Buffet, A.; De Cubas, A.A.; Cascon, A.; Menara, M.; Khalifa, E.; Amar, L.; Azriel, S.; Bourdeau, I.; Chabre, O.; et al. Germline mutations in FH confer predisposition to malignant pheochromocytomas and paragangliomas. *Hum. Mol. Genet.* **2014**, *23*, 2440–2446. [CrossRef]
18. Cascon, A.; Comino-Mendez, I.; Curras-Freixes, M.; de Cubas, A.A.; Contreras, L.; Richter, S.; Peitzsch, M.; Mancikova, V.; Inglada-Perez, L.; Perez-Barrios, A.; et al. Whole-exome sequencing identifies MDH2 as a new familial paraganglioma gene. *J. Natl. Cancer Inst.* **2015**, *107*, 1915–1942. [CrossRef]
19. Juhlin, C.C.; Stenman, A.; Haglund, F.; Clark, V.E.; Brown, T.C.; Baranoski, J.; Bilguvar, K.; Goh, G.; Welander, J.; Svahn, F.; et al. Whole-exome sequencing defines the mutational landscape of pheochromocytoma and identifies KMT2D as a recurrently mutated gene. *Genes Chromosomes Cancer* **2015**, *54*, 542–554. [CrossRef]

20. Toledo, R.A.; Qin, Y.; Srikantan, S.; Morales, N.P.; Li, Q.; Deng, Y.; Kim, S.W.; Pereira, M.A.; Toledo, S.P.; Su, X.; et al. In vivo and in vitro oncogenic effects of HIF2A mutations in pheochromocytomas and paragangliomas. *Endocr. Relat. Cancer* **2013**, *20*, 349–359. [CrossRef] [PubMed]
21. Castro-Vega, L.J.; Lepoutre-Lussey, C.; Gimenez-Roqueplo, A.P.; Favier, J. Rethinking pheochromocytomas and paragangliomas from a genomic perspective. *Oncogene* **2016**, *35*, 1080–1089. [CrossRef]
22. Fishbein, L.; Leshchiner, I.; Walter, V.; Danilova, L.; Robertson, A.G.; Johnson, A.R.; Lichtenberg, T.M.; Murray, B.A.; Ghayee, H.K.; Else, T.; et al. Comprehensive Molecular Characterization of Pheochromocytoma and Paraganglioma. *Cancer Cell* **2017**, *31*, 181–193. [CrossRef]
23. Buffet, A.; Morin, A.; Castro-Vega, L.J.; Habarou, F.; Lussey-Lepoutre, C.; Letouze, E.; Lefebvre, H.; Guilhem, I.; Haissaguerre, M.; Raingeard, I.; et al. Germline Mutations in the Mitochondrial 2-Oxoglutarate/Malate Carrier SLC25A11 Gene Confer a Predisposition to Metastatic Paragangliomas. *Cancer Res.* **2018**, *78*, 1914–1922. [CrossRef] [PubMed]
24. Nölting, S.; Bechmann, N.; Taieb, D.; Beuschlein, F.; Fassnacht, M.; Kroiss, M.; Eisenhofer, G.; Grossman, A.; Pacak, K. Personalized management of pheochromocytoma and paraganglioma. *Endocr. Rev.* **2021**. [CrossRef]
25. Toledo, R.A.; Burnichon, N.; Cascon, A.; Benn, D.E.; Bayley, J.P.; Welander, J.; Tops, C.M.; Firth, H.; Dwight, T.; Ercolino, T.; et al. Consensus Statement on next-generation-sequencing-based diagnostic testing of hereditary phaeochromocytomas and paragangliomas. *Nat. Rev. Endocrinol.* **2017**, *13*, 233–247. [CrossRef] [PubMed]
26. Lenders, J.W.; Duh, Q.Y.; Eisenhofer, G.; Gimenez-Roqueplo, A.P.; Grebe, S.K.; Murad, M.H.; Naruse, M.; Pacak, K.; Young, W.F., Jr. Pheochromocytoma and paraganglioma: An endocrine society clinical practice guideline. *J. Clin. Endocrinol. Metab.* **2014**, *99*, 1915–1942. [CrossRef] [PubMed]
27. Patócs, A.; Likó, I.; Butz, H.; Baghy, K.; Rácz, K. Novel methods and their applicability in the evaluation of the genetic background of endocrine system tumours. Új módszertani lehetőségek és ezek alkalmazása a hormonális rendszer daganatainak genetikai kivizsgálásában. *Orv. Hetil.* **2015**, *156*, 2063–2069. [CrossRef]
28. Robson, M.E.; Storm, C.D.; Weitzel, J.; Wollins, D.S.; Offit, K. American Society of Clinical Oncology policy statement update: Genetic and genomic testing for cancer susceptibility. *J. Clin. Oncol. Off. J. Am. Soc. Clin. Oncol.* **2010**, *28*, 893–901. [CrossRef]
29. Jafri, M.; Maher, E.R. The genetics of phaeochromocytoma: Using clinical features to guide genetic testing. *Eur. J. Endocrinol.* **2012**, *166*, 151–158. [CrossRef]
30. Amar, L.; Bertherat, J.; Baudin, E.; Ajzenberg, C.; Bressac-de Paillerets, B.; Chabre, O.; Chamontin, B.; Delemer, B.; Giraud, S.; Murat, A.; et al. Genetic testing in pheochromocytoma or functional paraganglioma. *J. Clin. Oncol. Off. J. Am. Soc. Clin. Oncol.* **2005**, *23*, 8812–8818. [CrossRef]
31. Erlic, Z.; Rybicki, L.; Peczkowska, M.; Golcher, H.; Kann, P.H.; Brauckhoff, M.; Mussig, K.; Muresan, M.; Schaffler, A.; Reisch, N.; et al. Clinical predictors and algorithm for the genetic diagnosis of pheochromocytoma patients. *Clin. Cancer Res. Off. J. Am. Assoc. Cancer Res.* **2009**, *15*, 6378–6385. [CrossRef] [PubMed]
32. Cascon, A.; Lopez-Jimenez, E.; Landa, I.; Leskela, S.; Leandro-Garcia, L.J.; Maliszewska, A.; Leton, R.; de la Vega, L.; Garcia-Barcina, M.J.; Sanabria, C.; et al. Rationalization of genetic testing in patients with apparently sporadic pheochromocytoma/paraganglioma. *Horm. Metab. Res. = Horm. Stoffwechs. = Horm. Metab.* **2009**, *41*, 672–675. [CrossRef]
33. Mannelli, M.; Castellano, M.; Schiavi, F.; Filetti, S.; Giacche, M.; Mori, L.; Pignataro, V.; Bernini, G.; Giache, V.; Bacca, A.; et al. Clinically guided genetic screening in a large cohort of italian patients with pheochromocytomas and/or functional or nonfunctional paragangliomas. *J. Clin. Endocrinol. Metab.* **2009**, *94*, 1541–1547. [CrossRef]
34. Crona, J.; Verdugo, A.D.; Granberg, D.; Welin, S.; Stalberg, P.; Hellman, P.; Bjorklund, P. Next-generation sequencing in the clinical genetic screening of patients with pheochromocytoma and paraganglioma. *Endocr. Connect.* **2013**, *2*, 104–111. [CrossRef]
35. McInerney-Leo, A.M.; Marshall, M.S.; Gardiner, B.; Benn, D.E.; McFarlane, J.; Robinson, B.G.; Brown, M.A.; Leo, P.J.; Clifton-Bligh, R.J.; Duncan, E.L. Whole exome sequencing is an efficient and sensitive method for detection of germline mutations in patients with phaeochromcytomas and paragangliomas. *Clin. Endocrinol.* **2014**, *80*, 25–33. [CrossRef]
36. Remacha, L.; Comino-Mendez, I.; Richter, S.; Contreras, L.; Curras-Freixes, M.; Pita, G.; Leton, R.; Galarreta, A.; Torres-Perez, R.; Honrado, E.; et al. Targeted Exome Sequencing of Krebs Cycle Genes Reveals Candidate Cancer-Predisposing Mutations in Pheochromocytomas and Paragangliomas. *Clin. Cancer Res. Off. J. Am. Assoc. Cancer Res.* **2017**, *23*, 6315–6324. [CrossRef] [PubMed]
37. Bennedbaek, M.; Rossing, M.; Rasmussen, A.K.; Gerdes, A.M.; Skytte, A.B.; Jensen, U.B.; Nielsen, F.C.; Hansen, T.V. Identification of eight novel SDHB, SDHC, SDHD germline variants in Danish pheochromocytoma/paraganglioma patients. *Hered Cancer Clin. Pract.* **2016**, *14*, 13. [CrossRef] [PubMed]
38. Qi, X.-P.; Ma, J.-M.; Du, Z.-F.; Ying, R.-B.; Fei, J.; Jin, H.-Y.; Han, J.-S.; Wang, J.-Q.; Chen, X.-L.; Chen, C.-Y.; et al. RET Germline Mutations Identified by Exome Sequencing in a Chinese Multiple Endocrine Neoplasia Type 2A/Familial Medullary Thyroid Carcinoma Family. *PLoS ONE* **2011**, *6*, e20353. [CrossRef]
39. Rattenberry, E.; Vialard, L.; Yeung, A.; Bair, H.; McKay, K.; Jafri, M.; Canham, N.; Cole, T.R.; Denes, J.; Hodgson, S.V.; et al. A comprehensive next generation sequencing-based genetic testing strategy to improve diagnosis of inherited pheochromocytoma and paraganglioma. *J. Clin. Endocrinol. Metab.* **2013**, *98*, E1248–E1256. [CrossRef]
40. Latteyer, S.; Klein-Hitpass, L.; Khandanpour, C.; Zwanziger, D.; Poeppel, T.D.; Schmid, K.W.; Fuhrer, D.; Moeller, L.C. A 6-Base Pair in Frame Germline Deletion in Exon 7 Of RET Leads to Increased RET Phosphorylation, ERK Activation, and MEN2A. *J. Clin. Endocrinol. Metab.* **2016**, *101*, 1016–1022. [CrossRef] [PubMed]

41. Clark, G.R.; Sciacovelli, M.; Gaude, E.; Walsh, D.M.; Kirby, G.; Simpson, M.A.; Trembath, R.C.; Berg, J.N.; Woodward, E.R.; Kinning, E.; et al. Germline FH mutations presenting with pheochromocytoma. *J. Clin. Endocrinol. Metab.* **2014**, *99*, E2046–E2050. [CrossRef] [PubMed]
42. Flynn, A.; Benn, D.; Clifton-Bligh, R.; Robinson, B.; Trainer, A.H.; James, P.; Hogg, A.; Waldeck, K.; George, J.; Li, J.; et al. The genomic landscape of phaeochromocytoma. *J. Pathol.* **2015**, *236*, 78–89. [CrossRef] [PubMed]
43. Fishbein, L.; Khare, S.; Wubbenhorst, B.; DeSloover, D.; D'Andrea, K.; Merrill, S.; Cho, N.W.; Greenberg, R.A.; Else, T.; Montone, K.; et al. Whole-exome sequencing identifies somatic ATRX mutations in pheochromocytomas and paragangliomas. *Nat. Commun.* **2015**, *6*, 6140. [CrossRef]
44. Wilzen, A.; Rehammar, A.; Muth, A.; Nilsson, O.; Tesan Tomic, T.; Wangberg, B.; Kristiansson, E.; Abel, F. Malignant pheochromocytomas/paragangliomas harbor mutations in transport and cell adhesion genes. *Int. J. Cancer* **2016**, *138*, 2201–2211. [CrossRef] [PubMed]
45. Crona, J.; Delgado Verdugo, A.; Maharjan, R.; Stalberg, P.; Granberg, D.; Hellman, P.; Bjorklund, P. Somatic mutations in H-RAS in sporadic pheochromocytoma and paraganglioma identified by exome sequencing. *J. Clin. Endocrinol. Metab.* **2013**, *98*, E1266–E1271. [CrossRef] [PubMed]
46. Castro-Vega, L.J.; Letouzé, E.; Burnichon, N.; Buffet, A.; Disderot, P.-H.; Khalifa, E.; Loriot, C.; Elarouci, N.; Morin, A.; Menara, M.; et al. Multi-omics analysis defines core genomic alterations in pheochromocytomas and paragangliomas. *Nat. Commun.* **2015**, *6*, 6044. [CrossRef] [PubMed]
47. Green, R.C.; Berg, J.S.; Grody, W.W.; Kalia, S.S.; Korf, B.R.; Martin, C.L.; McGuire, A.L.; Nussbaum, R.L.; O'Daniel, J.M.; Ormond, K.E.; et al. ACMG recommendations for reporting of incidental findings in clinical exome and genome sequencing. *Genet. Med. Off. J. Am. Coll. Med. Genet.* **2013**, *15*, 565–574. [CrossRef]
48. Rehm, H.L.; Bale, S.J.; Bayrak-Toydemir, P.; Berg, J.S.; Brown, K.K.; Deignan, J.L.; Friez, M.J.; Funke, B.H.; Hegde, M.R.; Lyon, E. ACMG clinical laboratory standards for next-generation sequencing. *Genet. Med. Off. J. Am. Coll. Med. Genet.* **2013**, *15*, 733–747. [CrossRef]
49. Weiss, M.M.; Van der Zwaag, B.; Jongbloed, J.D.; Vogel, M.J.; Bruggenwirth, H.T.; Lekanne Deprez, R.H.; Mook, O.; Ruivenkamp, C.A.; van Slegtenhorst, M.A.; van den Wijngaard, A.; et al. Best practice guidelines for the use of next-generation sequencing applications in genome diagnostics: A national collaborative study of Dutch genome diagnostic laboratories. *Hum. Mutat.* **2013**, *34*, 1313–1321. [CrossRef]
50. Aziz, N.; Zhao, Q.; Bry, L.; Driscoll, D.K.; Funke, B.; Gibson, J.S.; Grody, W.W.; Hegde, M.R.; Hoeltge, G.A.; Leonard, D.G.; et al. College of American Pathologists' laboratory standards for next-generation sequencing clinical tests. *Arch. Pathol. Lab. Med.* **2015**, *139*, 481–493. [CrossRef]
51. Richards, S.; Aziz, N.; Bale, S.; Bick, D.; Das, S.; Gastier-Foster, J.; Grody, W.W.; Hegde, M.; Lyon, E.; Spector, E.; et al. Standards and guidelines for the interpretation of sequence variants: A joint consensus recommendation of the American College of Medical Genetics and Genomics and the Association for Molecular Pathology. *Genet. Med. Off. J. Am. Coll. Med. Genet.* **2015**, *17*, 405–424. [CrossRef] [PubMed]
52. Matthijs, G.; Souche, E.; Alders, M.; Corveleyn, A.; Eck, S.; Feenstra, I.; Race, V.; Sistermans, E.; Sturm, M.; Weiss, M.; et al. Guidelines for diagnostic next-generation sequencing. *Eur. J. Hum. Genet.* **2016**, *24*, 2–5. [CrossRef] [PubMed]
53. Asan; Xu, Y.; Jiang, H.; Tyler-Smith, C.; Xue, Y.; Jiang, T.; Wang, J.; Wu, M.; Liu, X.; Tian, G.; et al. Comprehensive comparison of three commercial human whole-exome capture platforms. *Genome. Biol.* **2011**, *12*, R95. [CrossRef] [PubMed]
54. Clark, M.J.; Chen, R.; Lam, H.Y.K.; Karczewski, K.J.; Chen, R.; Euskirchen, G.; Butte, A.J.; Snyder, M. Performance comparison of exome DNA sequencing technologies. *Nat. Biotechnol.* **2011**, *29*, 908–914. [CrossRef] [PubMed]
55. Chilamakuri, C.S.; Lorenz, S.; Madoui, M.A.; Vodák, D.; Sun, J.; Hovig, E.; Myklebost, O.; Meza-Zepeda, L.A. Performance comparison of four exome capture systems for deep sequencing. *BMC Genom.* **2014**, *15*, 449. [CrossRef]
56. Biesecker, L.G.; Green, R.C. Diagnostic clinical genome and exome sequencing. *N. Engl. J. Med.* **2014**, *371*, 1170. [CrossRef]
57. Patocs, A.; Lendvai, N.K.; Butz, H.; Liko, I.; Sapi, Z.; Szucs, N.; Toth, G.; Grolmusz, V.K.; Igaz, P.; Toth, M.; et al. Novel SDHB and TMEM127 Mutations in Patients with Pheochromocytoma/Paraganglioma Syndrome. *Pathol. Oncol. Res. POR* **2016**, *22*, 673–679. [CrossRef]
58. Gergics, P.; Toke, J.; Szilagyi, A.; Szappanos, A.; Kender, Z.; Barta, G.; Toth, M.; Igaz, P.; Racz, K.; Patocs, A. Methods for the analysis of large gene deletions and their application in some hereditary diseases. *Orv. Hetil.* **2009**, *150*, 2258–2264. [CrossRef]
59. Shen, R.; Fan, J.B.; Campbell, D.; Chang, W.; Chen, J.; Doucet, D.; Yeakley, J.; Bibikova, M.; Wickham Garcia, E.; McBride, C.; et al. High-throughput SNP genotyping on universal bead arrays. *Mutat. Res.* **2005**, *573*, 70–82. [CrossRef]
60. Bentley, D.R.; Balasubramanian, S.; Swerdlow, H.P.; Smith, G.P.; Milton, J.; Brown, C.G.; Hall, K.P.; Evers, D.J.; Barnes, C.L.; Bignell, H.R.; et al. Accurate whole human genome sequencing using reversible terminator chemistry. *Nature* **2008**, *456*, 53–59. [CrossRef]
61. Li, H.; Durbin, R. Fast and accurate long-read alignment with Burrows–Wheeler transform. *Bioinformatics* **2010**, *26*, 589–595. [CrossRef]
62. DePristo, M.A.; Banks, E.; Poplin, R.E.; Garimella, K.V.; Maguire, J.R.; Hartl, C.; Philippakis, A.A.; del Angel, G.; Rivas, M.A.; Hanna, M.; et al. A framework for variation discovery and genotyping using next-generation DNA sequencing data. *Nat. Genet.* **2011**, *43*, 491–498. [CrossRef]
63. Koboldt, D.C.; Chen, K.; Wylie, T.; Larson, D.E.; McLellan, M.D.; Mardis, E.R.; Weinstock, G.M.; Wilson, R.K.; Ding, L. VarScan: Variant detection in massively parallel sequencing of individual and pooled samples. *Bioinformatics* **2009**, *25*, 2283–2285. [CrossRef]

64. Koboldt, D.C.; Zhang, Q.; Larson, D.E.; Shen, D.; McLellan, M.D.; Lin, L.; Miller, C.A.; Mardis, E.R.; Ding, L.; Wilson, R.K. VarScan 2: Somatic mutation and copy number alteration discovery in cancer by exome sequencing. *Genome. Res.* **2012**, *22*, 568–576. [CrossRef] [PubMed]
65. Wang, K.; Li, M.; Hakonarson, H. ANNOVAR: Functional annotation of genetic variants from high-throughput sequencing data. *Nucleic Acids Res.* **2010**, *38*, e164. [CrossRef] [PubMed]
66. McKenna, A.; Hanna, M.; Banks, E.; Sivachenko, A.; Cibulskis, K.; Kernytsky, A.; Garimella, K.; Altshuler, D.; Gabriel, S.; Daly, M.; et al. The Genome Analysis Toolkit: A MapReduce framework for analyzing next-generation DNA sequencing data. *Genome Res.* **2010**, *20*, 1297–1303. [CrossRef] [PubMed]
67. Martin, M. Cutadapt removes adapter sequences from high-throughput sequencing reads. *Bioinformatics* **2011**, *27*, 2957–2963. [CrossRef]
68. Li, H.; Handsaker, B.; Wysoker, A.; Fennell, T.; Ruan, J.; Homer, N.; Marth, G.; Abecasis, G.; Durbin, R. The Sequence Alignment/Map format and SAMtools. *Bioinformatics* **2009**, *25*, 2078–2079. [CrossRef]
69. Van der Auwera, G.A.; Carneiro, M.O.; Hartl, C.; Poplin, R.; Del Angel, G.; Levy-Moonshine, A.; Jordan, T.; Shakir, K.; Roazen, D.; Thibault, J.; et al. From FastQ data to high confidence variant calls: The Genome Analysis Toolkit best practices pipeline. *Curr. Protoc. Bioinform.* **2013**, *43*, 10–11. [CrossRef]
70. Cingolani, P.; Platts, A.; Wang le, L.; Coon, M.; Nguyen, T.; Wang, L.; Land, S.J.; Lu, X.; Ruden, D.M. A program for annotating and predicting the effects of single nucleotide polymorphisms, SnpEff: SNPs in the genome of Drosophila melanogaster strain w1118; iso-2; iso-3. *Fly* **2012**, *6*, 80–92. [CrossRef]
71. Cingolani, P.; Patel, V.M.; Coon, M.; Nguyen, T.; Land, S.J.; Ruden, D.M.; Lu, X. Using Drosophila melanogaster as a Model for Genotoxic Chemical Mutational Studies with a New Program, SnpSift. *Front. Genet.* **2012**, *3*, 35. [CrossRef]
72. Adzhubei, I.A.; Schmidt, S.; Peshkin, L.; Ramensky, V.E.; Gerasimova, A.; Bork, P.; Kondrashov, A.S.; Sunyaev, S.R. A method and server for predicting damaging missense mutations. *Nat. Methods* **2010**, *7*, 248–249. [CrossRef]
73. Sherry, S.T.; Ward, M.H.; Kholodov, M.; Baker, J.; Phan, L.; Smigielski, E.M.; Sirotkin, K. dbSNP: The NCBI database of genetic variation. *Nucleic Acids Res.* **2001**, *29*, 308–311. [CrossRef] [PubMed]
74. Gibbs, R.A.; Belmont, J.W.; Hardenbol, P.; Willis, T.D.; Yu, F.; Yang, H.; Ch'ang, L.-Y.; Huang, W.; Liu, B.; Shen, Y.; et al. The International HapMap Project. *Nature* **2003**, *426*, 789–796. [CrossRef]
75. Auton, A.; Brooks, L.D.; Durbin, R.M.; Garrison, E.P.; Kang, H.M.; Korbel, J.O.; Marchini, J.L.; McCarthy, S.; McVean, G.A.; Abecasis, G.R. A global reference for human genetic variation. *Nature* **2015**, *526*, 68–74. [CrossRef] [PubMed]
76. Karczewski, K.J.; Francioli, L.C.; Tiao, G.; Cummings, B.B.; Alföldi, J.; Wang, Q.; Collins, R.L.; Laricchia, K.M.; Ganna, A.; Birnbaum, D.P.; et al. The mutational constraint spectrum quantified from variation in 141,456 humans. *Nature* **2020**, *581*, 434–443. [CrossRef] [PubMed]
77. Fokkema, I.F.; Taschner, P.E.; Schaafsma, G.C.; Celli, J.; Laros, J.F.; den Dunnen, J.T. LOVD v.2.0: The next generation in gene variant databases. *Hum. Mutat.* **2011**, *32*, 557–563. [CrossRef]
78. Gieldon, L.; William, D.; Hackmann, K.; Jahn, W.; Jahn, A.; Wagner, J.; Rump, A.; Bechmann, N.; Nolting, S.; Knosel, T.; et al. Optimizing Genetic Workup in Pheochromocytoma and Paraganglioma by Integrating Diagnostic and Research Approaches. *Cancers* **2019**, *11*, 809. [CrossRef]
79. Ben Aim, L.; Pigny, P.; Castro-Vega, L.J.; Buffet, A.; Amar, L.; Bertherat, J.; Drui, D.; Guilhem, I.; Baudin, E.; Lussey-Lepoutre, C.; et al. Targeted next-generation sequencing detects rare genetic events in pheochromocytoma and paraganglioma. *J. Med. Genet.* **2019**, *56*, 513–520. [CrossRef]
80. Richter, S.; Gieldon, L.; Pang, Y.; Peitzsch, M.; Huynh, T.; Leton, R.; Viana, B.; Ercolino, T.; Mangelis, A.; Rapizzi, E.; et al. Metabolome-guided genomics to identify pathogenic variants in isocitrate dehydrogenase, fumarate hydratase, and succinate dehydrogenase genes in pheochromocytoma and paraganglioma. *Genet. Med. Off. J. Am. Coll. Med. Genet.* **2019**, *21*, 705–717. [CrossRef]
81. Pillai, S.; Gopalan, V.; Lo, C.Y.; Liew, V.; Smith, R.A.; Lam, A.K. Silent genetic alterations identified by targeted next-generation sequencing in pheochromocytoma/paraganglioma: A clinicopathological correlations. *Exp. Mol. Pathol.* **2017**, *102*, 41–46. [CrossRef]
82. Di Resta, C.; Galbiati, S.; Carrera, P.; Ferrari, M. Next-generation sequencing approach for the diagnosis of human diseases: Open challenges and new opportunities. *EJIFCC* **2018**, *29*, 4–14.
83. Wang, L.; Zhang, J.; Chen, N.; Wang, L.; Zhang, F.; Ma, Z.; Li, G.; Yang, L. Application of Whole Exome and Targeted Panel Sequencing in the Clinical Molecular Diagnosis of 319 Chinese Families with Inherited Retinal Dystrophy and Comparison Study. *Genes* **2018**, *9*, 360. [CrossRef]
84. Graziola, F.; Garone, G.; Stregapede, F.; Bosco, L.; Vigevano, F.; Curatolo, P.; Bertini, E.; Travaglini, L.; Capuano, A. Diagnostic Yield of a Targeted Next-Generation Sequencing Gene Panel for Pediatric-Onset Movement Disorders: A 3-Year Cohort Study. *Front. Genet.* **2019**, *10*, 1026. [CrossRef]
85. Gimenez-Roqueplo, A.P.; Favier, J.; Rustin, P.; Rieubland, C.; Crespin, M.; Nau, V.; Khau Van Kien, P.; Corvol, P.; Plouin, P.F.; Jeunemaitre, X. Mutations in the SDHB gene are associated with extra-adrenal and/or malignant phaeochromocytomas. *Cancer Res.* **2003**, *63*, 5615–5621.

86. Ayala-Ramirez, M.; Feng, L.; Johnson, M.M.; Ejaz, S.; Habra, M.A.; Rich, T.; Busaidy, N.; Cote, G.J.; Perrier, N.; Phan, A.; et al. Clinical risk factors for malignancy and overall survival in patients with pheochromocytomas and sympathetic paragangliomas: Primary tumor size and primary tumor location as prognostic indicators. *J. Clin. Endocrinol. Metab.* **2011**, *96*, 717–725. [CrossRef]
87. Sarkadi, B.; Meszaros, K.; Krencz, I.; Canu, L.; Krokker, L.; Zakarias, S.; Barna, G.; Sebestyen, A.; Papay, J.; Hujber, Z.; et al. Glutaminases as a Novel Target for SDHB-Associated Pheochromocytomas/Paragangliomas. *Cancers* **2020**, *12*, 599. [CrossRef] [PubMed]
88. Plouin, P.F.; Amar, L.; Dekkers, O.M.; Fassnacht, M.; Gimenez-Roqueplo, A.P.; Lenders, J.W.M.; Lussey-Lepoutre, C.; Steichen, O. European Society of Endocrinology Clinical Practice Guideline for long-term follow-up of patients operated on for a phaeochromocytoma or a paraganglioma. *Eur. J. Endocrinol.* **2016**, *174*, G1–G10. [CrossRef] [PubMed]
89. Park, J.Y.; Clark, P.; Londin, E.; Sponziello, M.; Kricka, L.J.; Fortina, P. Clinical exome performance for reporting secondary genetic findings. *Clin. Chem.* **2015**, *61*, 213–220. [CrossRef] [PubMed]
90. LaDuca, H.; Farwell, K.D.; Vuong, H.; Lu, H.M.; Mu, W.; Shahmirzadi, L.; Tang, S.; Chen, J.; Bhide, S.; Chao, E.C. Exome sequencing covers >98% of mutations identified on targeted next generation sequencing panels. *PLoS ONE* **2017**, *12*, e0170843. [CrossRef]
91. Considerations for Design, Development, and Analytical Validation of Next Generation Sequencing (NGS)—Based In Vitro Diagnostics (IVDs) Intended to Aid in the Diagnosis of Suspected Germline Diseases. Available online: https://www.fda.gov/regulatory-information/search-fda-guidance-documents/considerations-design-development-and-analytical-validation-next-generation-sequencing-ngs-based (accessed on 22 May 2021).
92. Welander, J.; Andreasson, A.; Juhlin, C.C.; Wiseman, R.W.; Bäckdahl, M.; Höög, A.; Larsson, C.; Gimm, O.; Söderkvist, P. Rare germline mutations identified by targeted next-generation sequencing of susceptibility genes in pheochromocytoma and paraganglioma. *J. Clin. Endocrinol. Metab.* **2014**, *99*, E1352–E1360. [CrossRef] [PubMed]
93. Wooderchak-Donahue, W.L.; O'Fallon, B.; Furtado, L.V.; Durtschi, J.D.; Plant, P.; Ridge, P.G.; Rope, A.F.; Yetman, A.T.; Bayrak-Toydemir, P. A direct comparison of next generation sequencing enrichment methods using an aortopathy gene panel- clinical diagnostics perspective. *BMC Med. Genom.* **2012**, *5*, 50. [CrossRef] [PubMed]
94. Lee, H.; Deignan, J.L.; Dorrani, N.; Strom, S.P.; Kantarci, S.; Quintero-Rivera, F.; Das, K.; Toy, T.; Harry, B.; Yourshaw, M.; et al. Clinical exome sequencing for genetic identification of rare Mendelian disorders. *JAMA* **2014**, *312*, 1880–1887. [CrossRef]
95. Boedeker, C.C.; Erlic, Z.; Richard, S.; Kontny, U.; Gimenez-Roqueplo, A.-P.; Cascon, A.; Robledo, M.; de Campos, J.M.; van Nederveen, F.H.; de Krijger, R.R.; et al. Head and Neck Paragangliomas in Von Hippel-Lindau Disease and Multiple Endocrine Neoplasia Type 2. *J. Clin. Endocrinol. Metab.* **2009**, *94*, 1938–1944. [CrossRef]
96. Trpkov, K.; Hes, O.; Williamson, S.R.; Adeniran, A.J.; Agaimy, A.; Alaghehbandan, R.; Amin, M.B.; Argani, P.; Chen, Y.B.; Cheng, L.; et al. New developments in existing WHO entities and evolving molecular concepts: The Genitourinary Pathology Society (GUPS) update on renal neoplasia. *Mod. Pathol.* **2021**, *34*, 1392–1424. [CrossRef] [PubMed]
97. Patel, V.M.; Handler, M.Z.; Schwartz, R.A.; Lambert, W.C. Hereditary leiomyomatosis and renal cell cancer syndrome: An update and review. *J. Am. Acad.Dermatol.* **2017**, *77*, 149–158. [CrossRef]
98. Wells, S.A., Jr.; Asa, S.L.; Dralle, H.; Elisei, R.; Evans, D.B.; Gagel, R.F.; Lee, N.; Machens, A.; Moley, J.F.; Pacini, F.; et al. Revised American Thyroid Association guidelines for the management of medullary thyroid carcinoma. *Thyroid* **2015**, *25*, 567–610. [CrossRef]
99. Lendvai, N.; Tóth, M.; Valkusz, Z.; Bekő, G.; Szücs, N.; Csajbók, E.; Igaz, P.; Kriszt, B.; Kovács, B.; Rácz, K.; et al. Overrepresentation of the G12S polymorphism of the SDHD gene in patients with MEN2A syndrome. *Clinics* **2012**, *67* (Suppl. 1), 85–89. [CrossRef]
100. Toledo, R.A.; Hatakana, R.; Lourenço, D.M., Jr.; Lindsey, S.C.; Camacho, C.P.; Almeida, M.; Lima, J.V., Jr.; Sekiya, T.; Garralda, E.; Naslavsky, M.S.; et al. Comprehensive assessment of the disputed RET Y791F variant shows no association with medullary thyroid carcinoma susceptibility. *Endocr. Relat. Cancer* **2015**, *22*, 65–76. [CrossRef] [PubMed]
101. Nakatani, T.; Iwasaki, M.; Yamamichi, A.; Yoshioka, Y.; Uesaka, T.; Bitoh, Y.; Maeda, K.; Fukumoto, T.; Takemoto, T.; Enomoto, H. Point mutagenesis in mouse reveals contrasting pathogenetic effects between MEN2B- and Hirschsprung disease-associated missense mutations of the RET gene. *Dev. Growth Differ.* **2020**, *62*, 214–222. [CrossRef] [PubMed]
102. Rasmussen, S.A.; Yang, Q.; Friedman, J.M. Mortality in neurofibromatosis 1: An analysis using U.S. death certificates. *Am. J. Hum. Genet.* **2001**, *68*, 1110–1118. [CrossRef] [PubMed]

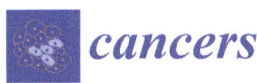

Article

Analysis of Telomere Maintenance Related Genes Reveals *NOP10* as a New Metastatic-Risk Marker in Pheochromocytoma/Paraganglioma

María Monteagudo [1,2,†], Paula Martínez [3,†], Luis J. Leandro-García [1], Ángel M. Martínez-Montes [1], Bruna Calsina [1], Marta Pulgarín-Alfaro [1], Alberto Díaz-Talavera [1,4], Sara Mellid [1], Rocío Letón [1], Eduardo Gil [1], Manuel Pérez-Martínez [5], Diego Megías [5], Raúl Torres-Ruiz [6], Sandra Rodriguez-Perales [6], Patricia González [7], Eduardo Caleiras [7], Scherezade Jiménez-Villa [8], Giovanna Roncador [8], Cristina Álvarez-Escolá [9], Rita M. Regojo [10], María Calatayud [11], Sonsoles Guadalix [11], Maria Currás-Freixes [12], Elena Rapizzi [13], Letizia Canu [13], Svenja Nölting [14], Hanna Remde [15], Martin Fassnacht [15,16], Nicole Bechmann [17,18], Graeme Eisenhofer [17,18], Massimo Mannelli [13], Felix Beuschlein [14,19], Marcus Quinkler [20], Cristina Rodríguez-Antona [1,4], Alberto Cascón [1,4], María A. Blasco [3], Cristina Montero-Conde [1,4] and Mercedes Robledo [1,4,*]

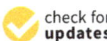

Citation: Monteagudo, M.; Martínez, P.; Leandro-García, L.J.; Martínez-Montes, Á.M.; Calsina, B.; Pulgarín-Alfaro, M.; Díaz-Talavera, A.; Mellid, S.; Letón, R.; Gil, E.; et al. Analysis of Telomere Maintenance Related Genes Reveals *NOP10* as a New Metastatic-Risk Marker in Pheochromocytoma/Paraganglioma. *Cancers* **2021**, *13*, 4758. https://doi.org/10.3390/cancers13194758

Academic Editor: Peter Igaz

Received: 26 August 2021
Accepted: 19 September 2021
Published: 23 September 2021

Publisher's Note: MDPI stays neutral with regard to jurisdictional claims in published maps and institutional affiliations.

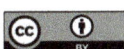

Copyright: © 2021 by the authors. Licensee MDPI, Basel, Switzerland. This article is an open access article distributed under the terms and conditions of the Creative Commons Attribution (CC BY) license (https://creativecommons.org/licenses/by/4.0/).

1. Hereditary Endocrine Cancer Group, Human Cancer Genetics Program, Spanish National Cancer Research Centre (CNIO), 28029 Madrid, Spain; mmonteagudo@cnio.es (M.M.); ljleandro@cnio.es (L.J.L.-G.); ammontes@cnio.es (Á.M.M.-M.); bcalsina@cnio.es (B.C.); mpulgarin@cnic.es (M.P.-A.); adiazt@ext.cnio.es (A.D.-T.); smellid@cnio.es (S.M.); rleton@cnio.es (R.L.); edgilv@cnio.es (E.G.); crodriguez@cnio.es (C.R.-A.); acascon@cnio.es (A.C.); cmontero@cnio.es (C.M.-C.)
2. PhD Program in Neuroscience, Autonoma de Madrid University, 28029 Madrid, Spain
3. Telomeres and telomerase Group, Molecular Oncology Program, Spanish National Cancer Research Centre (CNIO), 28029 Madrid, Spain; pmartinez@cnio.es (P.M.); mblasco@cnio.es (M.A.B.)
4. Centro de Investigación Biomédica en Red de Enfermedades Raras (CIBERER), 28029 Madrid, Spain
5. Confocal Microscopy Core Unit, Biotechnology Program, Spanish National Cancer Research Centre (CNIO), 28029 Madrid, Spain; mperez@cnio.es (M.P.-M.); dmegias@cnio.es (D.M.)
6. Molecular Citogenetic, Unit Human Cancer Genetics Program, Spanish National Cancer Research Centre (CNIO), 28029 Madrid, Spain; rtorresr@cnio.es (R.T.-R.); srodriguezp@cnio.es (S.R.-P.)
7. Histopathology Core Unit, Biotechnology Program, Spanish National Cancer Research Centre (CNIO), 28029 Madrid, Spain; pgonzalez@cnio.es (P.G.); ejcaleiras@cnio.es (E.C.)
8. Monoclonal Antibodies Core Unit, Biotechnology Program, Spanish National Cancer Research Centre (CNIO), 28029 Madrid, Spain; sjimenez@cnio.es (S.J.-V.); groncador@cnio.es (G.R.)
9. Department of Endocrinology, La Paz University Hospital, 28046 Madrid, Spain; calvareze@salud.madrid.org
10. Department of Pathology La Paz University Hospital, 28046 Madrid, Spain; ritamaria.regojo@salud.madrid.org
11. Department of Endocrinology, 12 de Octubre University Hospital, 28041 Madrid, Spain; maria.calatayud@salud.madrid.org (M.C.); sonsoguadalix@gmail.com (S.G.)
12. Department of Endocrinology, Clínica Universidad de Navarra, 28027 Madrid, Spain; mcurras@unav.es
13. Department of Experimental and Clinical Medicine, University of Florence, 50121 Florence, Italy; elena.rapizzi@unifi.it (E.R.); letizia.canu@unifi.it (L.C.); massimo.mannelli@unifi.it (M.M.)
14. Medizinische Klinik und Poliklinik IV, Klinikum der Universität München, 80336 Munich, Germany; Svenja.Noelting@usz.ch (S.N.); Felix.Beuschlein@usz.ch (F.B.)
15. Department of Internal Medicine I, Division of Endocrinology and Diabetes, University Hospital Würzburg, University of Würzburg, 97070 Würzburg, Germany; remde_h@ukw.de (H.R.); fassnacht_m@ukw.de (M.F.)
16. Comprehensive Cancer Center, Mainfranken University of Würzburg, 97070 Würzburg, Germany
17. Institute of Clinical Chemistry and Laboratory Medicine, University Hospital Carl Gustav Carus, Technische Universität Dresden, 01069 Dresden, Germany; nicole.bechmann@uniklinikum-dresden.de (N.B.); graeme.eisenhofer@uniklinikum-dresden.de (G.E.)
18. Department of Medicine III, University Hospital Carl Gustav Carus, Technische Universität Dresden, 01069 Dresden, Germany
19. Klinik für Endokrinologie Diabetologie und Klinische Ernährung, Universitätsspital Zürich, 8091 Zürich, Switzerland
20. Endocrinology in Charlottenburg Stuttgarter Platz 1, 10627 Berlin, Germany; marcusquinkler@t-online.de
* Correspondence: mrobledo@cnio.es
† These authors contributed equally to this work.

Simple Summary: Telomere maintenance involving *TERT* and *ATRX* genes has been recently described in metastatic pheochromocytoma and paraganglioma, reinforcing the importance of immortalization mechanisms in the progression of these tumors. Thus, the aim of this study was to analyze additional telomere-related genes to uncover potential new markers capable of identifying metastatic-risk patients more accurately. After analyzing 29 telomere-related genes, we were able to validate the predictive value of *TERT* and *ATRX* in mPPGL progression. In addition, we were able to identify *NOP10* as a novel prognostic risk marker of mPPGLs, which also facilitates telomerase-dependent telomere length maintenance in these tumors. Interestingly, NOP10 overexpression assessment by IHC could be easily included within the current battery of markers for stratifying PPGL patients to fine-tune their clinical diagnoses.

Abstract: One of the main problems we face with PPGL is the lack of molecular markers capable of predicting the development of metastases in patients. Telomere-related genes, such as *TERT* and *ATRX*, have been recently described in PPGL, supporting the association between the activation of immortalization mechanisms and disease progression. However, the contribution of other genes involving telomere preservation machinery has not been previously investigated. In this work, we aimed to analyze the prognostic value of a comprehensive set of genes involved in telomere maintenance. For this study, we collected 165 PPGL samples (97 non-metastatic/63 metastatic), genetically characterized, in which the expression of 29 genes of interest was studied by NGS. Three of the 29 genes studied, *TERT*, *ATRX* and *NOP10*, showed differential expression between metastatic and non-metastatic cases, and alterations in these genes were associated with a shorter time to progression, independent of *SDHB*-status. We studied telomere length by Q-FISH in patient samples and in an *in vitro* model. *NOP10* overexpressing tumors displayed an intermediate-length telomere phenotype without ALT, and in vitro results suggest that *NOP10* has a role in telomerase-dependent telomere maintenance. We also propose the implementation of NOP10 IHC to better stratify PPGL patients.

Keywords: pheochromocytoma; paraganglioma; PPGL; telomeres; *TERT*; *ATRX*; *NOP10*; prognostic biomarker; ALT

1. Introduction

Pheochromocytomas (PCC) and paragangliomas (PGL), all together called PPGLs, are rare neuroendocrine tumors derived from the adrenal medulla or extra-adrenal paraganglia [1]. PPGLs are known as the most hereditary neoplasms, since at least 40% are caused by germline mutations in one of the 23 genes associated so far with the susceptibility to develop this kind of tumor [2]. In addition, 30–40% of PPGLs are due to somatic mutations in these same genes, other cancer-related genes or chromosomal translocations involving the *MAML3* gene [3].

Approximately 15–20% of the patients develop metastatic disease (mPPGL) in the first two-three years after diagnosis [4,5]. In this regard, it is important to note that although synchronous metastases occur in 35–50% of cases, metachronous lesions can be developed during the decade following the initial diagnosis [4]. Prognosis of mPPGL is poor and heterogeneous, showing a 5-year overall survival of 40–77% from diagnosis of the first metastasis [6].

Risk factors associated with metastatic disease in PPGLs are scarce, inaccurate and remain poorly defined, mainly due to the low prevalence of the disease, which makes it difficult to recruit large series of patients to reach robust conclusions. Therefore, the early detection of mPPGLs becomes highly relevant for early detection of metastatic disease for which treatment options and therapies remain limited for these patients beyond surgery [7–11].

Even so, there are some clinical features that provide useful information about the potential for developing metastases, such as transcriptional clusters, tumor size and location or plasma metabolites concentration [3,7–11]. Among molecular metastatic risk markers, it is accepted that *SDHB* mutations are associated with poor prognosis [12]. Although, it has been suggested that additional factors must be involved in disease progression [13]. Recent studies reported that immortalization mechanisms common in other types of carcinomas, which involve telomere deregulation, also play a role in PPGL progression. In fact, the activation of the telomerase gene, *TERT*, and *ATRX* loss of function mutations have been reported to be associated with poor prognosis in PPGL [3,14,15].

Telomeres are DNA regions associated with the shelterin protein complex located at the end of chromosomes. The function of these structures is to protect the DNA *termini* from degradation and from being recognized as DNA double-strand breaks (DSB), to prevent end-to-end interchromosomal fusions [16–20]. Telomeric regions shorten with each cell division [21,22], due to the "end replication" problem and other processes, such as DNA processing and oxidative damage [16,17]. When they reach a critical short length, cells become senescent/quiescent, affecting the generative capacity of tissues [23]. Telomere shortening can be compensated through the *de novo* addition of telomeric repeats by telomerase, a reverse transcriptase composed of a catalytic subunit (TERT) and an RNA component (TERC), used as a template for telomere elongation [24]. *TERT* is downregulated in the majority of tissues post-natally, with the exception of adult stem cells [25]. Noteworthy, human tumors reach an indefinite proliferative capacity by either upregulating telomerase or activating the alternative lengthening of the telomeres mechanism [15,26–28].

The enzyme telomerase (TERT/TERC) is associated with additional factors that are required for telomerase biogenesis, localization and activity in vivo. Among other factors, telomerase forms a complex with the H/ACA-motif RNA-binding proteins, i.e., DKC1, NOP10, GAR1 and NHP2, that are involved in the proper stability, regulation and intracellular trafficking of telomerase and therefore are key for telomerase-dependent telomere lengthening [29,30].

Since telomere regulation is an important event in the metastatic progression of PPGLs, the aim of this study was to analyze other genes directly or indirectly related to telomere maintenance, in order to uncover potential new markers capable of identifying PPGL patients at risk of developing metastatic disease more accurately. For this purpose, we performed an exhaustive analysis of the expression of 29 genes related to telomere maintenance in a series of 165 metastatic and non-metastatic PPGL tumor samples with clinical and genetic information. The 29 telomere-related genes, henceforth called *telomerome*, are grouped into different categories: telomerase holoenzyme complex, shelterin complex, ALT (alternative lengthening of telomeres) phenotype and genes indirectly related to telomere maintenance. We were able to validate the predictive value of *TERT* and *ATRX* for mPPGL. Furthermore, our findings from patient samples showed that *NOP10* is a novel prognostic risk marker of developing mPPGLs. On the other hand, *in vitro* experiments supported a mechanism in which *NOP10* overexpression facilitates telomerase-dependent telomere length maintenance in these tumors.

2. Materials and Methods

2.1. PPGL Cohort and Genetic Characterization

The CNIO study cohort included 149 patients: 81 women, 64 men and 4 of unknown gender, with a mean age at diagnosis of 45 years and a mean follow-up time of 6 years. Among patients, 47 were classified as metastatic (from which 54 primary tumors and 9 metastases were available), diagnosed either with synchronous or metachronous metastasis. This series also included 5 patients with tumors classified as clinically aggressive, characterized by detection of capsular, vascular or adipose tissue infiltration in the pathology report, and/or multiple local recurrences, but without confirmed metastases. The 97 remaining tumors corresponded to non-metastatic PPGL patients with a mean follow-up of 7.67 years (2800 days; min: 0-max: 5895). The series included 96 formalin-fixed paraffin embedded tissues (FFPE) and 69 frozen samples. Clinical data are summarized in Table 1.

Table 1. Summary of PPGL series clinical data.

Characteristics	Patients
CNIO series (*n* = 149)	
Gender	
Female	54.4% (81)
Male	43% (64)
Unknown	2.7% (4)
Age at initial diagnosis of PCC/PGL; (range) in years	
	45 (9–82)
Cluster	
C1A	40.3% (55)
C1B	9.4% (14)
C2	36.9% (54)
C3	4.7% (7)
WT	13.4% (19)
Clinical behavior	
Metastatic	34.6% (47)
Synchronous	19.9% (28)
Metachronous	14.7% (19)
Clinically aggressive	3.2% (5)
Non-metastatic	62.2% (97)
Driver	
SDHB	21.2% (30)
Tumor type	
PCC	54.4% (81)
PGL	29.5% (44)
Bilateral PCC	3.4% (5)
Multiple PGL	3.4% (5)
PCC+PGL	7.4% (11)
Unknown	2% (3)

Germline and somatic mutational status characterization were performed using a customized NGS panel. The targeted gene panel was designed using the AmpliSeq Custom DNA Panel (Illumina, San Diego, CA, USA), and included the main susceptibility PPGL genes (*VHL, RET, SDHA, SDHB, SDHC, SDHD, SDHAF2, SDHAF1, MAX, HIF1A (exon 12), HIF2A (exon 12), TMEM127, HRAS, KRAS, NF1, GOT2, FH, MDH2, SLC25A11, DNMT3A (exon 8), DLST (exon 14), MERTK (exon 17), IDH1, IDH2, CSDE1, EGLN1, EGLN2, BRAF (exon 15), MET (exons 14–21), FGFR1 (exons 12 and 14), KIF1B, CDKN1B, MEN1, PTEN, H3F3a*) and *ATRX*. The panel was used according to the manufacturer's instructions, starting with 200ng of DNA. Interpretation of variants was performed following the recommendations of the NGS in PPGL Study Group and the American College of Medical Genetics and Genomics-Association for Molecular Pathology (ACMG-AMP) [31,32], and mutations detected were confirmed by Sanger sequencing (Figure 1).

Written informed consent for the use of specimens and clinical data were obtained from all patients, according to the institutional ethics committee guidelines. All subjects gave their informed consent for inclusion before they participated in the study. The study was conducted in accordance with the Declaration of Helsinki, and the protocol was approved by the following ethics committees: Hospital Universitario 12 de Octubre (15/024), Madrid, Spain; Universität Spital (2017-00771), Zurich, Germany; Klinikum der Universität (379-10), Munich, Germany; University Hospital Würzburg (ENS@T Ethics Committee 88/11), Würzburg, Germany; Azienda Ospedaliera Universitaria Careggi (Prot. N. 2011/0020149) Florence, Italy; Berlin Chamber of Physicians (Eth-S-R/14), Berlin, Germany.

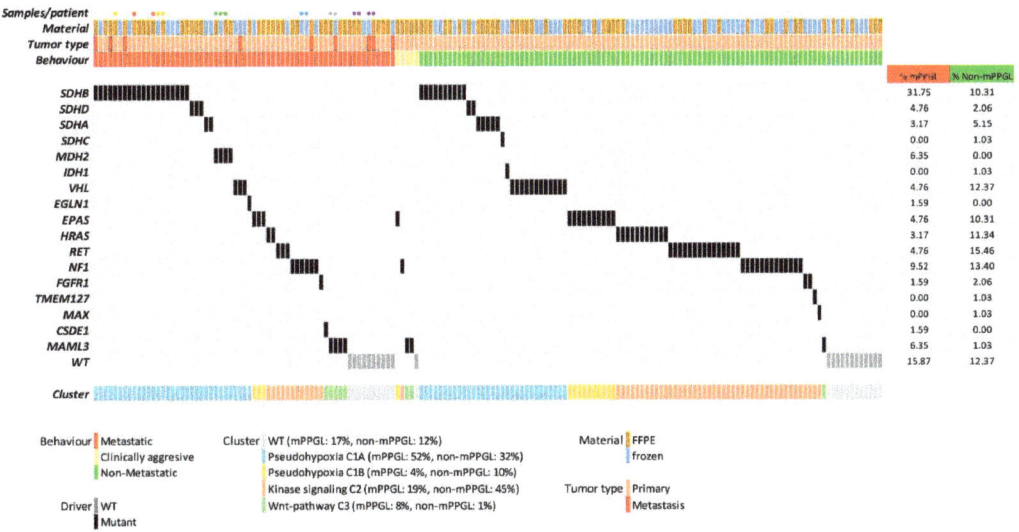

Figure 1. CNIO discovery series: genetic characterization of PPGL series: tumor driver gene and cluster classification. The frequency of each driver gene (percentage) per group, material for each sample and tumor tissue type (primary/metastasis) are shown in the figure. The colored dots represent tumors from the same patient; each color corresponds to a different patient.

2.2. Tumor DNA Extraction

Total DNA was isolated from FFPE samples using the Maxwell® RSC DNA Formalin-fixed paraffin embedded Kit (Promega, Madison, WI, USA) and a Maxwell® RSC Instrument (Promega). DNA from frozen tissue was extracted with DNeasy® Blood and Tissue Kit (Qiagen, Hilden, Germany), following the manufacturer's protocols. In FFPE, at least 2 cores were obtained from selected tumor areas. DNA was quantified using QuantiFluor® ONE dsDNA System kit (Promega) or Quant-iT™ PicoGreen™ dsDNA protocol (Invitrogen, Carlsbad, CA, USA).

2.3. Tumor RNA Extraction and Quality Test

Three or four 5 µm sections, or at least 2 cores from tumor enriched areas, were used for total RNA extraction from FFPE specimens using Maxwell® RSC RNA FFPE Kit (Promega). Frozen sample RNA extraction was performed using TRIzol™ reagent (Invitrogen) following manufacturers' protocol. After extraction, RNA was quantified by Nanodrop (NanoDrop™, Waltham, MA, USA). RNA integrity was assessed using Agilent Bioanalyzer 2100 (Agilent Technologies, Santa Clara, CA, USA) and the percentage of RNA fragments over 200 nt (DV200) was determined. RNA input was adjusted to DV_{200} values according to the following criteria: $DV_{200} > 70\%$, 200 ng; $DV_{200} = 50–70\%$, 400 ng; $DV_{200} = 30–50\%$, 600 ng, and poor integrity RNAs ($DV_{200} < 30\%$) were discarded. High quality commercial RNA from human placenta tissue and RNAs from human cancer cell lines were included in all runs as inter-assay controls. Three frozen/FFPE pairs of tumors, for which both types of preservation were available, were included to evaluate technique reliability for samples with different RNA integrity.

2.4. TREx RNA Sequencing

A customized TruSeq Targeted RNA expression (TREx) panel (Illumina, San Diego, CA, USA), capable of analyzing paraffin-embedded and frozen tissues, was designed to assess telomere-related gene expressions. A total of 29 telomere maintenance genes were included in the assay, belonging directly and indirectly to telomere maintenance pathways: telomerase complex (*TERT, TERC, DKC1, GAR1, NOP10, NHP2*); shelterin–

telosome protein complex (*POT1, TERF1, TERF2, TERF2IP, TINF2, TPP1*); histone binding and alternative telomere lengthening mechanism (*ATRX, DAXX, TNKS*); *non*-canonical telomere maintenance (*ACD, FBXO4, GPX2, MCRS1, MKRN1, NAT10, NFX1, RLIM, SMG5, SMG6, SOX7, TEP1, WRAP53, YLPM1*).

Sequencing runs of 150bp single-end reads were successfully performed in an Illumina MiSeq system. The output data were mapped to the reference genome version GRCh37, adapted for the TREx custom panel, using TopHat [33] included in the Nextpresso suite [34]. Random down-sampling of each sample was performed to obtain a final number of ≈170,000 mapped reads. Samples with less than 170,000 aligned reads were discarded due to low read depth (<700 reads/amplicon). A total of 165 samples (96 FFPE and 69 frozen) passed this cut-off and were used for the analysis: 143 samples had >1000 reads/amplicon, 23 samples had between 1000–750 reads/amplicon and 4 were excluded with <750 reads/amplicon. New mapping process and different quality steps were performed with the down-sampled FASTQ files. Briefly, to decrease the bias effect between FFPE and frozen samples, we used limma package [35], which allowed obtaining unbiased log2CPMs (counts per million) for all the selected samples.

TERT expression was detected using 3 specific probes, and only samples with at least 3 raw counts in each one of the probes and average raw counts ≥ 4 were considered as positive for expression, in order to minimize false positive identification due to *TERT* low-expressor condition.

2.5. ATRX Mutations

Mutations in *ATRX* were detected by the customized NGS panel in a set of 120 tumors. Exome data were available for 45 additional PPGLs (unpublished data). WES (whole exome sequencing) was performed using two different Illumina sequencing platforms, HiSeq and NovaSeq, generating 100bp paired-end reads. RubioSeq suite was used for the exome analysis [36], and data were processed and aligned to the human reference genome GRCh37 using Burrows–Wheeler Aligner (BWA). Germline and somatic variants were detected with Haplotype Caller [37] and MuTect [38] (Table S1).

2.6. Identification of TERT PROMOTER Mutations (TPMs)

Mutations causing altered *TERT* expression were studied using NGS, following the 16S Metagenomic Sequencing Library Preparation (Illumina, San Diego, CA, USA) protocol. To identify TPMs (chr5:1,295,228 C > T and chr5: 1,295,250 C > T), amplicons of 151bp were amplified from 50 ng of tumor DNA (primer sequences provided in Table S2). Amplicon PCR was performed using Multiplex QIAGEN 2X Master Mix following manufacturer's instructions. Index PCR was later executed with the EasyTaq DNA polymerase (TransGen Biotech, Beijing, China) using synthetic indices from the Nextera XT Index Kit (Illumina, San Diego, CA, USA). Both PCR products were purified using AMPure XP beads (Beckman Coulter, Pasadena, IN, USA) and quantified by PicoGreen (Thermo Fisher Scientific, Waltham, MA, USA). Amplicon concentration was normalized and pooled up to 96 samples for a single run.

Libraries were sequenced according to manufacturer's instructions in a MiSeq sequencer (Illumina). The sequencing module used was the "PCR Amplicon" protocol with a paired-end design with 150 base pairs reads. Illumina software was used to perform the variant calling, and Illumina VariantStudio software (Illumina) was used to obtain the sequencing results. *TERT* promoter mutations detected by NGS were confirmed by PCR and Sanger sequencing (primers are provided in Table S2).

2.7. Analysis of TERT Promoter Methylation Levels

To analyze THOR (*TERT* hypermethylated oncological region) methylation levels, bisulfite-modified DNA was used to amplify four THOR sections: A1, A2, A3 and A4, as described in Lee et al., 2019. Within the fourth THOR amplicon is located the UTSS region (upstream of the transcription start site), which contains a subset of five CpG sites (CpG

1295586, 1295590, 1295593, 1295605 & 1295618) whose average methylation level accurately correlates with the average methylation level of the whole THOR.

An amount of 100 ng of tumor DNA was bisulfite-modified using the EZ-96 DNA MethylationTM Kit (ZYMO RESEARCH, Irvine, CA, USA) research for the analysis of promoter hypermethylation. Bisulfite-modified DNA results in the conversion of unmethylated cytosine to uracil, which will be copied as thymine upon PCR, thus distinguishing methylated (thymine) from unmethylated (cytosine) DNA bases. Preparation and sequencing of the four THOR PCR amplicons were performed following the protocol "16S Metagenomic Sequencing Library Preparation" for the Illumina MiSeq platform with a paired-end design of 150 base pairs reads. Primers were chosen according to Lee et al., 2019 (Table S2).

Paired-end FASTQ files of each sample were generated. Only forward reads were used in the analysis. Trimming was performed with cut-adapt software to eliminate the sequences corresponding to the Illumina adapters incorporated during the sequencing process. The first step was to generate a reference genome adapted to bisulfite modification from the human genome assembly hg19. Reads were aligned to this modified reference genome using BS-Seeker2 software (2), taking into account changes introduced by bisulfite modification and favoring correct alignment. Secondly, we obtained the coverage at the positions of interest (UTSS region) using bam-readcount software (https://github.com/genome/bam-readcount, accessed on 16 January 2019). Finally, we calculated for each CpG site of interest the percentage of methylation observed as a function of the number of reads showing "C" or "T" at that position. Only samples with a mean UTSS-region value $\geq 16.1\%$ were considered as hypermethylated, as previously established by Lee et al., 2019.

2.8. TERT Copy Number Alterations (CNAs)

TERT CNAs analysis was performed in those samples from which WES data were available (unpublished data). Anaconda pipeline was used to detect somatic copy number alterations [39]. CNA profiles at gene level were identified using GISTIC 2.tool [40]. Data from frozen and FFPE samples were analyzed separately to minimize the preservation type bias in the analysis. Thresholds for gain detection were set to 4 and 8 for frozen and FFPE samples, respectively.

2.9. Telomerome Significant Genes and Metastasis Prediction Risk Model

To determine tumors with altered expression of telomere maintenance genes, we estimated the interquartile range (IQR) of the expression values of the non-metastatic samples with long follow-up (≥ 8 years) from diagnosis ($n = 45$). We considered deregulated gene expression tumors those with values below or above the threshold set using lower/upper whiskers (Q1 − (1.5 × IQR) or Q3 + (1.5 × IQR), respectively) of the gene expression dispersion. Candidate genes were chosen according to Fisher exact test after Bonferroni correction. Expression outlier data of candidate genes were transformed into dichotomous variables. For this analysis, tumors with clinically aggressive phenotype ($n = 5$) and non-metastatic samples with <8 years or unknown follow-up ($n = 52$) were excluded, leaving a total of 108 samples (63 metastatic and 45 non-metastatic).

A logistic regression analysis to assess the odds of metastatic risk was executed including as variables SDHB, TERT/ATRX, NOP10 and FBXO4. Selection of the best gene classifier was evaluated using a stepwise conditional logistic regression model. Non-metastatic patients with unknown follow-up, and those with clinically aggressive tumors, were excluded from the analysis.

The classification power of *telomerome* genes selected in the previous step was evaluated by computing receiver operating characteristic (ROC) curves and area under the curve analysis (AUC). A total number of 45 non-metastatic (≥ 8 years of follow-up) and 54 primary-metastatic samples were included. This analysis was applied considering 3 scenarios: 1) tumors with any event in TERT (expression outliers, TPMs, promoter hypermethylation or gains in 5p region) and/or ATRX (expression outliers and loss of function mutations), 2) tumors with only outlier expression of *NOP10* but excluding events in *TERT* and *ATRX*, and 3) considering any event in any of the 3 aforementioned *telomerome* genes. Data were analyzed using IBM-SPSS Version 19 (Armonk, NY, USA) and GraphPad Prism Version 5 (San Diego, CA, USA).

2.10. Time to Progression and Validated Telomerome Genes

Time to progression was evaluated using the Kaplan–Meier analysis for the whole series with follow-up data, testing differences using the log-rank test (IBM-SPSS Version 19) Metastasis ($n = 9$), clinically aggressive ($n = 5$) and non-metastatic cases with unknown follow-up ($n = 6$) were excluded from the analysis. *TERT+ATRX* (considering *TERT* expression outliers, TPMs, *TERT* promoter hypermethylation, gains and *ATRX* down expression outliers and loss of function mutations) and *TERT+ATRX+NOP10* (considering *NOP10* overexpression outliers) were studied for association with time to progression. The latter was defined as the number of days between surgery of the primary PPGL and the appearance of the first confirmed metastasis. The inclusion criteria were the presence of either synchronous or metachronous metastases (those that appeared before and after one year since surgery of the primary tumor, respectively) or at least 2 years' follow-up in the case of non-metastatic patients. Patients with non-metastatic tumors were censored at the date of last follow-up available.

2.11. Telomere Length Q-FISH, High-Throughput Quantification

Telomere length was studied by Q-FISH in selected representative FFPE samples. Hematoxylin and eosin-stained tumor sections were evaluated by a pathologist in order to select the areas of interest. Samples with a high tumor content were cut into complete sections (4 µm), and for those samples with a low tumor content, representative cores (1 mm) were selected for study in a tissue micro array (TMA). After deparaffinization and rehydration, tissues were washed in PBS 1X and fixed in 4% formaldehyde for 5 min. After washing, slides were dehydrated in a 70–90%–100% ethanol series (5 min each).

Slides were air dried and 30 µL of the telomere probe mix (10 mM TrisHCl, pH 7.2, 25 mM $MgCl_2$, 9 mM citric acid, 82 mM Na_2HPO_4, 50% deionized formamide (Sigma-Aldrich, Darmstadt, Germany), 0.25% blocking reagent (Roche, Basel, Switzerland), and 0.5 µg/mL Telomeric PNA probe (Panagene, Daejeon, Korea) was added. Slides were incubated for 3 min at 85 °C and then 2 h at room temperature in a wet chamber in the dark. Slides were washed twice for 15 min each in 10 mM TrisCl (pH 7.2) and 0.1% BSA in 50% formamide and then three times for 5 min each in TBS 0.08% Tween 20. After washing, slides were stained with DAPI (0.2 µg/mL) and dehydrated in a 70–90%–100% ethanol series. Dried samples were finally mounted with VECTASHIELD mounting media (Vector Laboratories, Burlingame, CA, USA).

Telomere length analysis is based on the specific and stable hybridization of the PNA with the telomeric region; the intensity of this PNA is directly related to telomere length allowing the measurement of telomeres at each individual chromosome end. Samples were imaged and quantified by confocal microscopy. For each sample evaluation, five representative areas from each tumor were imaged for an unbiased study of telomere length. Q-FISH images were acquired in a confocal microscope equipped with a 63×/NA 1.4 oil immersion objective and LAS AF v2.6 software (Leica-Microsystems, Wetzlar, Germany), and maximum projection images were created with the LAS AF 2.7.3.9723 software. Telomere signal intensity from Z-stacks was quantified using Definiens Developer Cell software version XD 64 2.5. Telomere length was estimated as the mean telomere intensity value per nucleus.

2.12. Promelocytic Leukaemia (PML) Bodies and Telomere Co-Localization by Immuno-Q-FISH

FFPE tissue samples were fixed in 10% buffered formalin, dehydrated, embedded in paraffin wax and sectioned at 4 µm. Tissue sections were deparaffinized in xylene and re-hydrated through a series of decreasing ethanol concentrations up to water. Immunofluorescence (IF) was performed on deparaffined tissue sections processed with 10 mM sodium citrate (pH 6.5) cooked under pressure for 2 min. Tissue sections were permeabilized with 0.5% Triton in PBS and blocked with 5% BSA in PBS. Samples were incubated overnight at 4 °C with rabbit polyclonal anti-PML (1:100; Santa Cruz Biotechnology, Santa Cruz, CA, USA, H-238). Q-FISH was performed on IF-stained slides fixed with 4% formaldehyde for 20 min. The DAPI images were used to detect telomeric signals inside each nucleus. Immunofluorescence images were obtained with a TCS-SP8 STED 3X confocal microscope equipped with a 63×/NA 1.4 oil immersion objective, a white light laser and LAS X v3.5 software (Leica-Microsystems). Z-stacks of the samples were acquired and then analyzed with Definiens Developer XD 64 v2.5 software (Definiens Inc., Munich, Bayern, Germany).

2.13. Characterization of NOP10 Expression Mechanisms

The coding regions (exons 1 and 2) of *NOP10* gene were analyzed by Sanger sequencing in order to detect activating mutations (primers in Table S2). Additionally, *NOP10* promoter region (200 bp upstream of the transcription start site or TSS) was checked for activating mutations using the previously mentioned WES data. Epigenetic mechanisms were also studied, including methylation 450K array data from PPGL TCGA project ([3], https://xenabrowser.net/datapages/, accessed on 19 February 2021) and PPGL CNIO series previously published data [41–44] as well as miRNA expression data from PPGL TCGA project (https://xenabrowser.net/datapages/, accessed on 19 February 2021) and from the PPGL CNIO series [45].

NOP10 protein expression was assessed by immunohistochemistry (IHC) in metastatic and non-metastatic PPGLs, previously selected according to *NOP10* overexpression. Sections of 2 μm thick were prepared from FFPE tissue and were dried in a 60 °C oven overnight. The sections were placed in a BOND-MAX Automated Immunohistochemistry Vision Biosystem (Leica Microsystems GmbH, Wetzlar, Germany) using standard protocol. First, tissues were deparaffinized and pre-treated with the Epitope Retrieval Solution 2 (EDTA-buffer pH8.8) at 98 °C for 20 min. After washing steps, peroxidase blocking was carried out for 10 min using the Bond Polymer Refine Detection Kit DC9800 (Leica Microsystems GmbH). Tissues were again washed and then incubated with the primary antibody anti-NOP10 (rabbit monoclonal antibody (EPR8857) (ab134902, Abcam)) diluted 1:1000 for 30 min. Subsequently, tissues were incubated with polymer for 10 min and developed with DAB-chromogen for 10 min. Human kidney slides were used as positive staining control following manufacturer's recommendations. Additionally, patients with long-term follow-up (>8 years), *TERT* over-expressing samples and *ATRX* down-expressing samples and normal adrenal medulla FFPE slides were included as controls.

Images of whole sections were taken with a slide scanner (AxioScan Z1, Zeiss, Jena, Germany). For analysis, an appropriate script was created using QuPath software (Belfast, UK) [46]. Representative areas from each slide were chosen for quantification program training, creating an appropriate script for *NOP10* antibody according to the intensity method: positivity was evaluated in three stages from high to low (3+, 2+, 1+) and negative. After training and script optimization, the quantification step was run, and results were exported as excel files with scoring data for each file.

Staining was classified as: low staining (negative and 1+) and high staining (2+ and 3+). Tumor staining was compared with negative staining from normal adrenal medulla. The percentage of high positivity staining was compared between samples (Neuwman–Keuls multiple comparison test, p-value < 0.05).

2.14. Cell Culture and Generation of TERT and NOP10 Overexpression Models

Human mesenchymal cells [47] were cultured in MesenPRO RS™ (Gibco) medium with L-Glutamin (5%; Gibco) and penicillin/streptomycin (1%; Gibco). Cells were maintained in monolayer in an incubator at 37 °C and 5% CO_2. For the experiments performed *in vitro*, two different plasmids were used:

1. *pLV-TERT-IRES-puro*: to generate TERT *overexpressing cells, lentiviral plasmid pLV-TERT-IRES-hygro was acquired from Addgene repository (Addgene Plasmid #85140 [48])*. Selection antibiotic was changed from hygromycin to puromycin.
2. *pLV-NOP10-IRES-hygro*: NOP10 expression plasmid (NM_018648) was acquired from OriGene (CAT#: RC209038). Using pLV-TERT-IRES-hygro backbone, *TERT* gene was replaced by *NOP10* ORF sequence from the aforementioned plasmid, generating a new pLV-*NOP10*-IRES-hygro vector.

Lentiviral plasmids were introduced in HEK293T cells (CRL-1573, ATCC) [47] using lipofectamine (Thermo Fisher). After cell culture, supernatant-carrying lentiviral particles were collected and used for mesenchymal cell infection. The infection was performed by using a small volume from the viral supernatant, allowing viral particles to physically contact mesenchymal cells. Once cells were selected with their respective antibiotics (Puromycin 0.35 µg/mL, Gibco; Hygromicin: 20 µg/mL; Invitrogen), overexpression of both *TERT* and *NOP10* was confirmed by RT-PCR. Briefly, each cell line was seeded in 60 mm plates. After expansion (3×10^6 cells), RNA was isolated using TRIzol Reagent® (Ambion-Life Technologies, Waltham, MA, USA) following the manufacturer's instructions. cDNAs were prepared from 500 ng of RNA using the qScriptTM cDNA Synthesis Kit (Quanta Biosciences, Gaithersburg, MD, USA) and mRNA levels were quantified by real-time PCR using the Universal ProbeLibrary set (Roche), as described by the vendor, on a QuantStudio 6 Flex Real-Time PCR System (Applied Biosystems, Waltham, MA, USA) using TaqMan® Universal PCR Master Mix No AmpErase® UNG (Applied Biosystems). Normalization was carried out with the *β-ACTIN* housekeeping gene and relative mRNA levels were estimated by the ΔΔCt method [49]. Primers and probes used for RT-PCR shown in Table S2.

2.15. Telomere Length Q-FISH on Cell Spreads

For telomere length analysis, non-confluent hMSC were harvested. Cells were collected by centrifugation and after hypotonic swelling in 0.03 M sodium citrate for 30 min at 37 °C, hMSC were fixed in methanol–acetic acid (3:1). Cell suspension was dropped onto wet microscope slides and dried overnight. After drying, we proceeded to carry out quantitative telomere fluorescence in situ hybridization (Q-FISH), as previously described [50].

3. Results

3.1. Description of the PPGL-Telomerome Series

The series comprises a collection of 165 tumors, representative of the genetic landscape of the different susceptibility genes in PPGLs. After genetic characterization, 38.78% of tumors (64/165) belonged to cluster C1A, 8.48% (14/165) to cluster C1B, 33.93% (56/165) to C2 and 4.84% (8/165) to C3. Among the 63 mPPGLs, 52.38% (33/63) belong to the C1A cluster, associated with a high risk of progression. The other ones belong to clusters C1B (3/63), C2 (12/63) and C3 (5/63). This series also included 23 WT samples (23/165) (Figure 1, Table 1).

3.2. Study of the Telomerome Expression Profile and Outlier Selection

After assessing the telomerome expression data, interquartile range analysis was applied for detecting expression outliers of candidate genes, and the number of outliers was compared between metastatic and long follow-up non-metastatic samples (more than 8 years). A total of 3 out of 29 genes, *TERT*, *NOP10* and *FBXO4*, showed differences between metastatic and non-metastatic PPGLs by Fisher´s exact test after Bonferroni correction. Although not significant, we added *ATRX* as a prognostic marker because it had already been associated with mPPGLs [14], selecting a final number of four candidate genes for further analyses (Figure S1).

3.3. Mechanisms That Trigger Aberrant Expression of Telomerome Genes in mPPGL

Six tumors carried loss of function mutations in *ATRX* that correlated with a decreased *ATRX* expression, three of them being outliers (Table S1). Five of them corresponded to the pseudohypoxia cluster and the remaining one to the Wnt-pathway cluster (Figure 2).

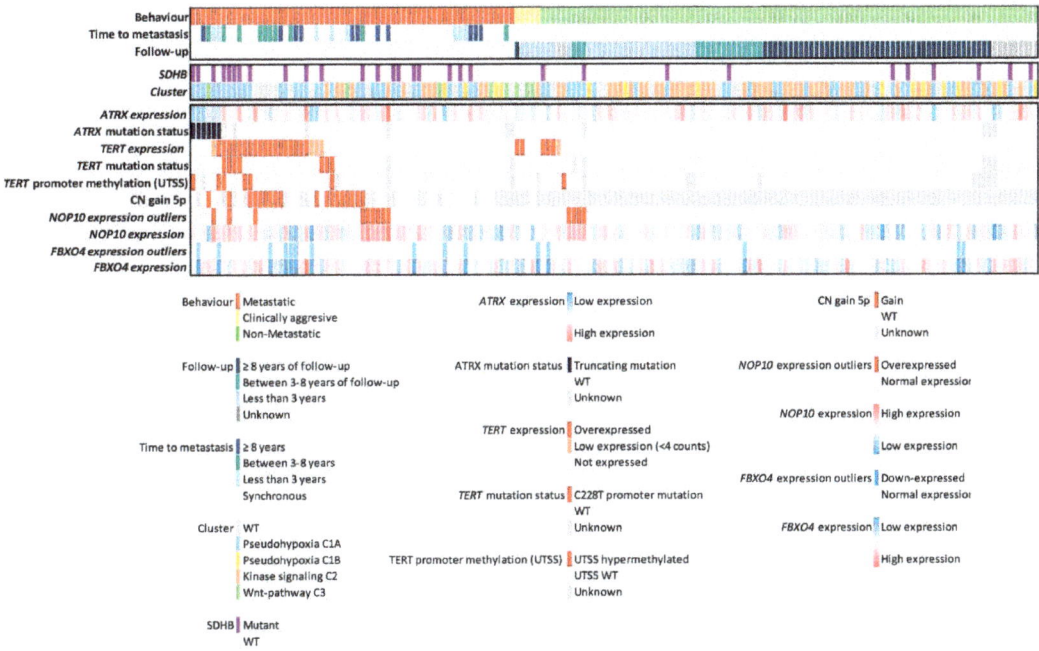

Figure 2. Summary of genomic alterations in PPGL series linked to *telomerome* events. Tumor behavior and patient follow-up are shown, non-metastatic patients mean follow-up = 7.67 years (min: 9 days, max: 36 years). Patients classification was made according to driver mutations. Events in *ATRX* include *ATRX* low expression and *ATRX* loss of function mutations. *TERT* events include: *TERT* overexpression, *TERT* promoter mutation, *TERT* promoter hypermethylation (UTSS median value > 16.1%) and CN gain 5p. *NOP10* and *FBXO4* expression outliers and continuous expression data are shown.

TERT reactivated expression was detected in 23/63 (36.5%) mPPGLs, as well as in two clinically aggressive tumor samples and four non-mPPGLs with short/unknown follow-up (Figure 2). Aberrantly high *TERT* expression could arise through four major mechanisms: enhancing promoter mutations, promoter hypermethylation in the THOR-UTSS (*TERT* hypermethylated oncological region untranscribed site), *TERT* locus amplification and rearrangements involving the super enhancer region located upstream *TERT* TSS and up to 5.4 Mb [51].

The sequencing of the *TERT* promoter from 158 PPGLs with available material revealed seven mPPGLs carrying the C228T mutation, from which five showed reactivation of *TERT* expression. These five mutants with *TERT* overexpression were also carrying *SDHB* driver mutations (5/7, 71.4%) (Figure 2).

TERT promoter methylation analysis was performed in 147 tumors with good quality DNA available (Figure S2A). The median hypermethylation value was significantly higher in metastatic samples when compared with non-mPPGLs (mPPGL median 8.34%, SD: 12.7; non-mPPGL median: 3.57%, SD: 3.4; unpaired *t*-test) (Figure S2B). Seven tumors were considered hypermethylated as they showed median UTSS-THOR methylation value over 16.1%, as previously established [51] (Figure S2A,B). Among them, six were mPPGLs, and the remaining case corresponded to a non-metastatic PPGL without follow-up data. Notably, 6/7 (86%) *TERT* promoter hypermethylated cases belong to the C1A cluster.

Simultaneous events in the *TERT* promoter (mutation and hypermethylation) were present in one sample (Figure 2).

Among the 44 samples with the copy number data available, we found that gains in the *TERT* locus (5p15.33) were present in 8 out of 18 *TERT* expressing samples (40%) and 10/26 non-expressing samples (38%). *TERT* locus gain overlapped with promoter mutation and/or methylation in 2/18 (11.1%) specimens. Among metastatic samples with *TERT* locus gains, two of them were *SDHB*-mutated (2/18, 11.1%), and 5/18 (27.7%) belonged to the C1A cluster. Among the 50 PPGLs showing any type of *TERT* event, 25 (50%) belonged to the C1A cluster, 1 (0.2%) to cluster C1B, 7 (14%) to C2, 3 (6%) to C3 and 14 (28%) were classified as wild type samples with an unknown driver mutation (Figure 2). Finally, we analyzed the association between events in the *TERT* locus and its expression. CNAs were the event associated with the highest median *TERT* expression (Figure S2C).

Regarding *NOP10*, no pathogenic mutations were found that could explain its upregulation, neither in the exons nor in the studied part of the gene promoter (200 bp upstream the TSS). Furthermore, no significant correlation was found between *NOP10* expression and the methylation status of any of the nine CpG sites studied at the gene locus (2 CpG) or promoter region (7 CpG) (up to 230 bp from TSS), according to TCGA and CNIO data sets. Similarly, the expression of miRNAs with conserved binding sites at the *NOP10* locus, according to TargetScan tool (http://www.targetscan.org/vert_72/, accessed on 17 February 2021), miRNAs -204, -211, -194, -27, -128 and -135 did not inversely correlate with *NOP10* expression. Additionally, no alterations in the number of copies for the *NOP10* locus were detected in our sample set. Therefore, none of the canonical mechanisms associated with an altered gene expression underlay the significantly higher *NOP10* expression levels found in mPPGLs (Figure 2). Nevertheless, a selection of samples with high *NOP10* expression showed a significantly higher NOP10 staining at the nuclear and nucleolar levels by immunohistochemistry (Figure 3A,B). Moreover, NOP10 IHC staining and gene expression were highly correlated (Pearson r = 0.784; *p*-value: 0.012) (Figure 3C).

3.4. Telomerome Significant Genes Identification and Predictive Value

The risk given by the two candidate genes (*NOP10* and *FBXO4*) was evaluated using a univariate logistic regression model, as well as *TERT+ATRX* as a single variable (bona fide markers of immortalization) and *SDHB* as a genetic variable associated with worse prognosis. The univariate regression model revealed that each of them were associated with a higher risk to develop metastatic disease. Finally, a step-wise model selected *TERT+ATRX* and *NOP10* as the best classifier of metastasis (Table S3). *FBXO4* and *SDHB* were excluded from the model, suggesting that they did not confer malignancy by themselves.

We applied the AUC analysis to determine the metastatic risk predictive value of the selected genes. Although events in *TERT/ATRX* explained a significant number of metastatic cases (AUC = 0.767, 95%CI = 0.678–0.856, *p*-value = $2.46 \times E^{-6}$), the *TERT/ATRX/NOP10* combination was a better predictor (AUC = 0.798, 95%CI = 0.714–0.882, *p*-value = $1.35 \times E^{-7}$), suggesting that *NOP10* aberrant expression contributes to the PPGL progression (Figure 4A). In addition, patients carrying alterations in *TERT/ATRX/NOP10* showed a significant shorter time to progression than those without events (*p*-value: $4.73 \times E^{-10}$, HR: 5.05, 95%CI: 2.76–9.23) (Figure 4B).

3.5. TERT, ATRX and NOP10 Events Affect Telomere Length

We measured telomere length in samples with *TERT*, *ATRX* and *NOP10*-altered profiles by Q-FISH technique. Additionally, three non-metastatic samples without any alterations in any of these genes and three normal adrenal medullae were included as controls.

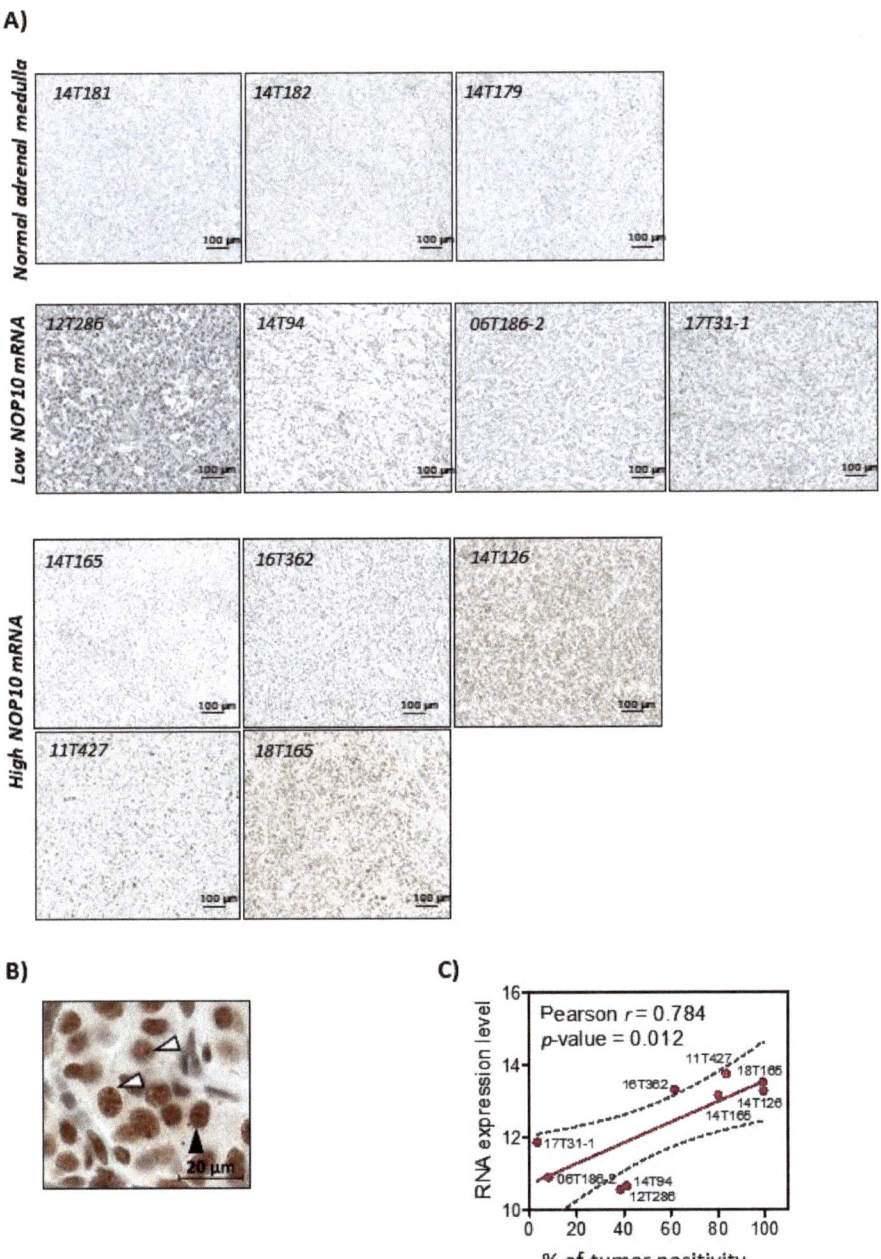

Figure 3. NOP10 immunohistochemistry. (**A**) Representative staining images of normal adrenal medulla ($n = 3$), tumors with low *NOP10* expression ($n = 4$) and *NOP10* overexpressing tumors ($n = 5$). (**B**) Magnified image from an NOP10-positive staining (14T126). Black arrow: representative nuclear staining. White arrows: representative nucleolar staining. (**C**) Linear regression plot of *NOP10* RNA expression and percentage of tumor positivity. Pearson correlation r and *p*-value are shown.

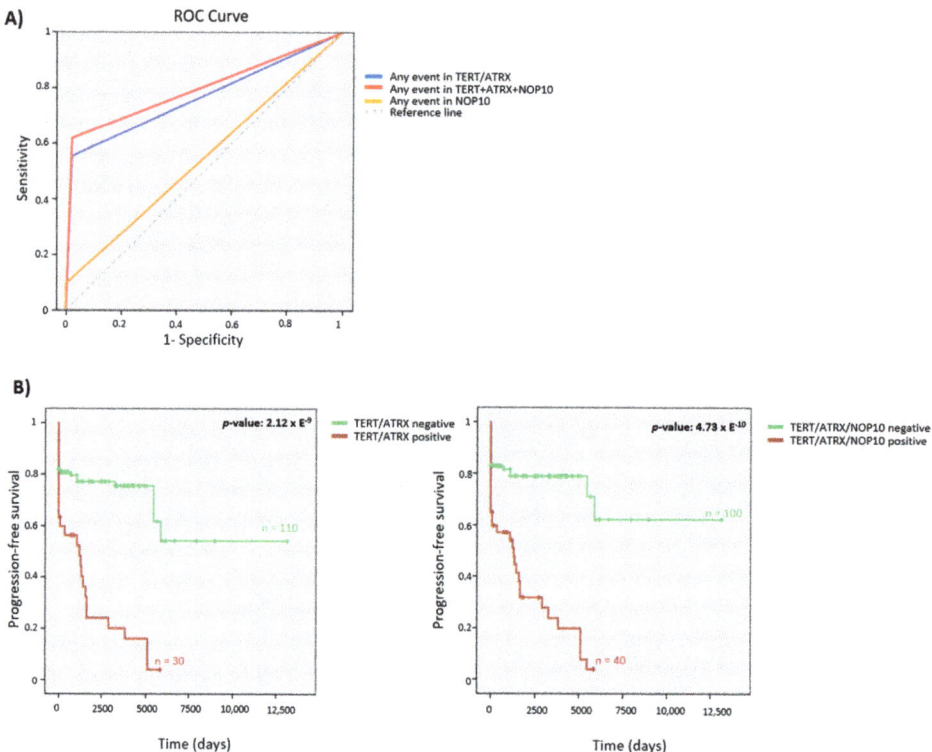

Figure 4. (**A**) Receiver operating characteristic curve (ROC) analysis showing the accuracy of telomerome events to distinguish between metastatic and non-metastatic samples. This data corresponds to all metastatic ($n = 54$) and non-metastatic cases with ≥ 8 years of follow-up ($n = 45$). Metastases ($n = 9$), clinically aggressive samples ($n = 5$) and non-metastatic cases with <8 years' follow-up ($n = 52$) were excluded. Genes were introduced as a dichotomous variable based on outlier expressors. *TERT* events: overexpression, promoter mutation, promoter hypermethylation or gains; *ATRX* events: low expression outliers and mutations; *NOP10* events: overexpression outliers. Any event in *TERT+ATRX*: p-value: $2.46 \times E^{-6}$, AUC: 0.767; 95%CI: 0.678–0.856; any event in *TERT+ATRX+NOP10*: p-value: $1.35 \times E^{-7}$, AUC: 0.798; 95%CI: 0.714–0.882; any event in *NOP10*: p-value: 0.439, AUC: 0.548; 95%CI: 0.439–0.656. (**B**) Kaplan–Meier plots of time to progression of patients, according to the events in *TERT/ATRX* (left) and to the events in the three telomerome significant genes (*TERT/ATRX/NOP10*) (right). n = number of samples. Log-rank test p-value is shown. Non-metastatic patients with unknown follow-up and those with clinically aggressive tumors were excluded from the analysis.

Confocal microscopy analysis revealed that tumors harboring *TERT* alterations had shorter telomeres than the controls. Those with *ATRX* mutations presented higher heterogeneity in the telomere length, as observed by the wider telomere distribution shown and the high number of extremely long telomeres. Tumors overexpressing *NOP10* showed an intermediate phenotype between short and long telomeres (Figure 5A,B). Differences in the distribution of telomere average intensity between groups were statistically significant, showing a higher frequency of long telomeres in *ATRX* mutants and *NOP10*-altered samples compared with the normal and non-metastatic ones, and a higher frequency of short telomeres in *TERT*-altered samples (Figure 5C). Differences in the mean of telomere spot size were also observed, confirming the results obtained with the mean telomere intensity analysis (Figure 5D).

The alternative telomere lengthening (ALT) phenotype is characterized by the high heterogeneity of telomere length and the presence of extremely long telomeres. ALT has unequivocally been associated with *ATRX* alterations [52,53]. We analyzed the colocalization of PML nuclear bodies with telomeres (ALT-associated PML nuclear bodies or

APBs), a phenomenon previously described in ALT-positive cells with increased telomere recombination [54]. Representative samples were selected for APB assays (Figure S3A). The percentage of PML-positive cells was significantly higher in *ATRX* mutated samples as compared to *ATRX* WT ones (Figure S3B). In addition, a larger number of APBs was observed in the *ATRX* mutants (Figure S3C). Samples without *ATRX* mutations did not show APBs, whereas three out of four *ATRX* mutant samples presented a high number of APBs and were therefore classified as ALT⁺. Interestingly, samples with *NOP10* alteration presenting intermediate/long telomeres, though showing PML-positive cells (5%) did not present APBs (Figure S3A–C), ruling out ALT mechanism in *NOP10* overexpressing samples.

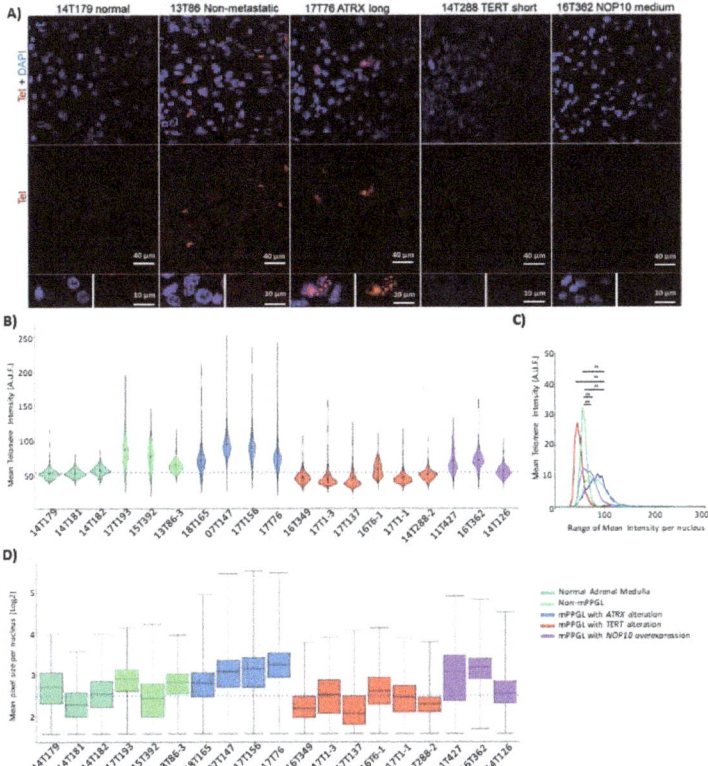

Figure 5. (**A**) Representative Q-FISH images from different tumors. 14T179: normal adrenal medulla with short telomeres. 13T86: non-metastatic PPGL with short telomeres. 17T76: mPPGL with *ATRX* mutation (c.3622dup, p.Ile1208AsnfsTer4) and long telomeres. 14T288: mPPGL with extremely short telomeres, this patient has *TERT* overexpression, promoter hypermethylation and 5p amplification. 16T362: mPPGL with medium-long telomeres and *NOP10* overexpression. (**B**) Violin plot of telomere mean intensity per nucleus. Highest values (upper end) represent long telomeric regions. Black dots inside each violin box represent median intensity value. Dashed line represents the median value of normal samples intensity (normal adrenal medulla, $n = 3$). Non-mPPGL: 17T193 (*FGFR1*-mutated); 15T392 (WT); 13T86-3 (*SDHB*-mutated). (**C**) Mean telomere intensity distribution for each group of samples (Wilcoxon matched-pairs signed rank test, Gaussian Approximation). (**D**) Box plot representing the mean telomere size (mean pixel size per nucleus) for each tumor: *ATRX* mutants have extremely long telomeres, *NOP10*-altered samples show intermediate-long telomeres, *TERT*-altered present extremely short telomeres. Normal and non-metastatic samples have medium-short telomeres. Dashed line represents the median value of normal samples' telomere size. The color code chart applies to panels **B**, **C** and **D** (one-way ANOVA Tukey's multiple comparison test: **: p-value < 0.01).

3.6. NOP10 and TERT Expression in Primary Cultures Affect Telomere Length Maintenance

To determine the role of *NOP10* overexpression in cell immortalization and telomere lengthening, primary cultures from human umbilical cord mesenchymal stem cells (hUCMSC) were modeled to overexpress either *NOP10*, *TERT* or both genes simultaneously (Figure S4A,B). An unmodified primary culture (parental) of hUCMSC was used as the control condition.

Cell growth curve analysis of the isogenic primary cultures showed that both the parental control and *NOP10* cells became quiescent/non-replicative after three passages, acquiring an expanded/quiescent morphology. *TERT* expression alone or in combination with *NOP10* delayed the non-replicative status until passage 8 and 10, respectively, in accordance with a higher number of fibroblastic/dividing cell morphology in both conditions (Figure 6A and Figure S4A–C).

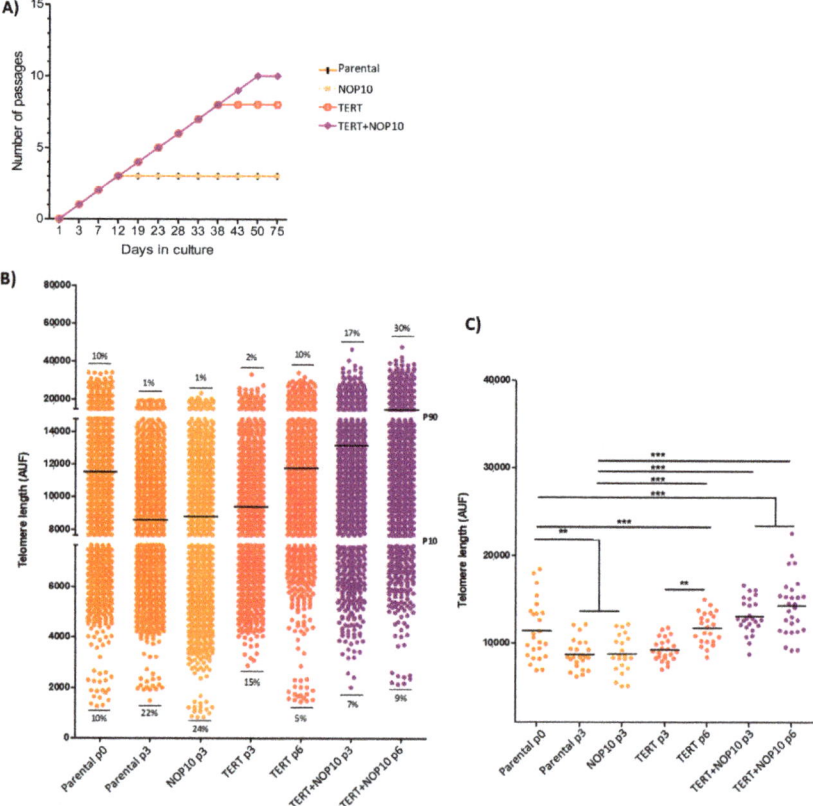

Figure 6. *In vitro* telomere length analysis. (**A**) Cell proliferation per condition. X axis: number of days in culture since antibiotic selection; Y axis: accumulative number of passages. Parental and *NOP10* become quiescent after 3 passages. *TERT* cells become quiescent after 8 passages and *TERT+NOP10* after 10 passages. (**B**) Scatter dot plot showing telomere length. Percentages of short and long telomeres for each isogenic primary culture are shown. Graph separations were made according to percentile 10 and 90 (P10 and P90) based on "Parental p0". Median telomere length value graphed in black. (**C**) Median telomere length value per cell (one-way ANOVA Tukey's multiple comparison test: **: *p*-value < 0.01; ***: *p*-value < 0.001).

Analysis of telomere length by Q-FISH of all isogenic primary cultures at passage three, when parental and *NOP10* conditions reached the replicative quiescent state (Figure 6A), showed that both cultures presented equally short telomeres and a similar percentage of critically short telomeric signals (>20% below 10th percentile of parental cells) (Figure 6B, Figure S4A,C). In contrast, *TERT* overexpressing cells presented a progressive reduction in the percentage of short telomeres and an increase in median telomere length from passage three to passage six (p-value < 0.001), indicating a *TERT*-dependent telomere lengthening (Figure 6A,B). Notably, *TERT+NOP10* overexpressing primary cultures had the longest median telomeric lengths of all the tested conditions (p-values < 0.001), suggesting an enhanced effect of *TERT* and *NOP10* on telomere length maintenance (Figure 6B,C). Indeed, the proportion of long telomeres (>90th percentile) was 3-fold higher in *TERT+NOP10* cells as compared to *TERT* cells at passage six (Figure 6B,C).

4. Discussion

To date, some PPGL-specific markers have been described [8,10–12,41–43,45]. However, the problem still facing PPGL patients is the lack of molecular markers capable of predicting the development of metastases at an earlier stage. PPGL patients can develop metastases up to 10 years after the diagnosis of the first tumor, and any PPGL should be considered as potentially metastatic, as the most recent WHO classification states [34,55].

Additionally, mechanisms that appear widely de-regulated in cancer, such as cell immortality, have also been described in PPGL [56]. In this regard, there is sufficient evidence to support the association of *TERT* and *ATRX* alterations with disease progression [14]. In this work, we aimed to analyze the prognostic value of these and other additional genes involved in this biological process.

Our results are in consonance with previous studies: *TERT* expression is commonly mediated by genetic and epigenetic mechanisms [3,14,15,57,58] and only detectable in metastatic PPGL but not in non-metastatic cases [59]. In addition, among all the mechanisms associated with *TERT* expression, we found that copy number gains of *TERT* locus showed the highest levels of *TERT* transcriptional activation [14,15,60,61]. Similarly, rearrangements in the *TERT* promoter have been reported to be associated with high levels of *TERT* expression [60]. This mechanism could explain the data observed in three *TERT*-WT samples of our series, which showed equally high levels as samples with *TERT* locus gains. Additionally, some samples that harbor events involving *TERT* have not shown significant changes in *TERT* expression levels. However, the prognostic value of these alterations remains significant, as they are almost exclusive of mPPGLs. We found that mutations in *ATRX* were also exclusive of mPPGLs and associated with a decreased expression [14,62,63].

We validated the distribution of *TERT* and *ATRX* events among PPGL genetic classes [14,64–66]. Most of these samples belong to C1A, although they are not exclusive of this cluster nor *SDHB*-mutant tumors, as previously reported [14,15]. These data reinforce previous evidence of the role of *TERT* and *ATRX* as prognostic markers in PPGL [13,67–70].

Additionally, our study identified *NOP10* overexpression as a novel prognostic marker in PPGL. Probably both the size of the series of available metastatic cases, the extensive follow-up time for a considerable number of patients and the comprehensive analysis of genes related to telomere maintenance have allowed the identification of *NOP10* as a new risk marker, which until now had gone unnoticed in other previous studies. In this regard, a pan-cancer study based on the systematic analysis of immortalization mechanisms identified the TCGA-PPGL series as a tumor type with limited occurrence of immortalization hallmarks [56]. This is probably due to the reduced number of metastatic cases of this latter series in comparison to ours. Our prognostic model prioritized alterations in telomere maintenance genes (*TERT+ATRX+NOP10*) over *SDHB*-mutation status. The *SDHB* prognostic role has already been questioned when a comprehensive set of clinico-pathological features was considered [13]. Notably, the *TERT+ATRX+NOP10* combination identified the group of patients with the shortest time to progression in our series.

NOP10 belongs to the family of H/ACA small nucleolar ribonucleoproteins (snoRNPs), which is also comprised by DKC1, NHP2 and GAR1. These snoRNPs have a constitutive expression at the nuclear and nucleolar level and have two functions: as part of the telomerase complex, they are involved in its stabilization [71,72], and they also participate in rRNA post-transcriptional modifications through pseudourydilation [73,74].

Highly positive NOP10 IHC staining has been already associated with shorter time to progression and aggressiveness in lung and breast cancer [75–78]. Our IHC results have demonstrated that *NOP10* expression outliers have a highly positive staining. The good correlation between expression and IHC supports the implementation of NOP10 immunohistochemistry as an additional prognostic tool. Additionally, NOP10 protein is located both at the nuclear and nucleolar level, suggesting the dual role of NOP10 in our mPGGL.

Regarding the role of *NOP10* in telomere maintenance, our *in vitro* results showed that *NOP10* on its own has not had a direct effect on the telomere length. However, when *NOP10* overexpression coexists with *TERT*, telomeres lengthen and cells delay the entrance on a quiescent state. In agreement with this finding, Q-FISH analysis of telomeric lengths on tumors showed that the mPPGL 16T362, with a *TERT* copy gain and *NOP10* overexpression, had a significantly higher median telomeric length as compared to that of mPPGLs bearing only *TERT* alterations. In addition, *NOP10* overexpressing mPPGLs displayed a higher mean telomere length and a lower percentage of short telomeres compared with *TERT*-only mPPGLs. None of these samples were classified as ALT(+), strongly supporting a *NOP10* role in facilitating telomerase-dependent telomere lengthening in these tumors.

Given the fact that *NOP10* is involved in the anchorage of the telomerase complex to the Cajal bodies [79,80], we speculate that the overexpression of this protein could help to generate a more durable interaction favoring telomere lengthening. However, based on our *NOP10* nucleolar staining, we cannot rule out additional indirect effects in telomere lengthening through RNA stabilization.

One of the limitations of this study, as occurs in many other tumors, is that we cannot rule out that intratumoral heterogeneity is limiting the discriminatory ability of our analysis. Therefore, it is plausible that we are not detecting the immortalization markers reported in this study in some of the PPGLs.

5. Conclusions

In summary, we showed that *NOP10* is a novel metastatic risk marker in PPGLs, which in combination with alterations in *TERT* and *ATRX*, provided the strongest means of stratification in our series, independently of *SDHB*-mutation status. In *NOP10* overexpressing tumors, we observed an intermediate-length telomere phenotype without ALT, which together with *in vitro* results, suggest that *NOP10* has a role in telomerase-dependent telomere maintenance.

We propose to include NOP10 immunostaining within the current battery of markers for stratifying PPGL patients to fine-tune their prognosis, thereby providing early detection of metastatic disease and ultimately bettering the planning of treatment options.

Supplementary Materials: The following are available online at https://www.mdpi.com/article/10.3390/cancers13194758/s1, Figure S1: Print of telomerome expression outliers, Figure S2: Mechanisms altering TERT expression, Figure S3: APBs detection, Figure S4: Summary of in-vitro experiment. Table S1: Summary of the mutations found in *ATRX* by NGS (exome sequencing and customized panel). Table S2: Summary of the primers used for NGS in blue, Sanger sequencing in green and RT-PCR in purple, Table S3: Univariate logistic regression analysis and stepwise conditional logistic regression model to assess the odds of metastasis risk.

Author Contributions: Conceptualization, M.R. and C.M.-C.; methodology, M.M. (María Monteagudo), L.J.L.-G., P.M., B.C., M.P.-A., R.L., E.G., A.D.-T. and S.M.; software Á.M.M.-M., M.P.-M. and D.M.; validation, C.M.-C., Á.M.M.-M., L.J.L.-G., B.C., E.C., P.G. and M.M. (María Monteagudo); formal analysis, M.M. (María Monteagudo), L.J.L.-G., P.M. and C.M.-C.; investigation, M.M. (María Monteagudo), L.J.L.-G., P.M., M.P.-A., R.T.-R., S.R.-P., G.R., S.J.-V., B.C., E.C. and M.A.B.; resources, M.R., C.Á.-E., R.M.R., M.C., S.G., M.C.-F., E.R., L.C., S.N., H.R., M.F., N.B., G.E., M.M. (Massimo Mannelli), F.B. and M.Q.; data curation, M.M. (María Monteagudo), P.M., Á.M.M.-M. and C.M.-C.;

writing—original draft preparation, M.M. (María Monteagudo); writing—review and editing, M.M., L.J.L.-G., C.M.-C., C.R.-A., A.C., M.R., Á.M.M.-M. and A.D.-T.; visualization, M.M. (María Monteagudo); supervision, L.J.L.-G., C.M.-C. and M.R.; project administration, M.R.; funding acquisition, M.R. All authors have read and agreed to the published version of the manuscript.

Funding: This work was supported by Project PI17/01796 and PI20/01169 to M.R. [Instituto de Salud Carlos III (ISCIII), Acción Estratégica en Salud, cofinanciado a través del Fondo Europeo de Desarrollo Regional (FEDER)], Paradifference Foundation [no grant number applicable to M.R.] and Pheipas Association [no grant number applicable to M.R.]. Research in the M.A.B. lab was funded by the Spanish State Research Agency (AEI), Ministry of Science and Innovation, cofounded by the European Regional Development Fund (ERDF) (SAF2017-82623-R and SAF2015-72455-EXP), the Comunidad de Madrid Project (S2017/BMD-3770), the World Cancer Research (WCR) Project (16-1177), the European Research Council (ERC-AvG Shelterines GA882385) and the Fundación Botín (Spain). International collaborators research has been supported by the Deutsche Forschungsgemeinschaft (DFG) within the CRC/Transregio 205/1 "The Adrenal: Central Relay in Health and Disease" to F.B., S.N., M.F.-C., N.B. and G.E. and by the Immuno-TargET project under the umbrella of the University Medicine Zurich to F.B. and S.N. M.M. was supported by the Spanish Ministry of Science, Innovation and Universities "Formación del Profesorado Universitario—FPU" fellowship with ID number FPU18/00064. L.J.L.-G. was supported both by the Banco Santander Foundation and La Caixa Postdoctoral Junior Leader Fellowship (LCF/BQ/PI20/11760011). C.M.-C. was supported by a grant from the AECC Foundation (AIO15152858 MONT). A.M.M.-M. was supported by CAM (S2017/BMD-3724; TIRONET2-CM). B.C. was supported by the Rafael del Pino Foundation (Becas de Excelencia Rafael del Pino 2017) and currently by the ISCIII project PI17/01796. A.D.-T. is supported by the Centro de Investigacion Biomédica en Red de Enfermedades Raras (CIBERER). We thank the Spanish National Tumor Bank Network (RD09/0076/00047) for the support in obtaining tumor samples and all patients, physicians and tumor biobanks involved in the study.

Institutional Review Board Statement: The study was conducted according to the guidelines of the Declaration of Helsinki and approved by the following ethics committees: Hospital Universitario 12 de Octubre (15/024), Madrid, Spain; Universität Spital (2017-00771) Zurich, Germany; Klinikum der Universität (379-10), Munich, Germany; University Hospital Würzburg (ENS@T Ethics Committee 88/11); Azienda Ospedaliera Universitaria Careggi (Prot. N. 2011/0020149) Florence, Italy; Berlin Chamber of Physicians (Eth-S-R/14) Berlin, Germany.

Informed Consent Statement: Informed consent was obtained from all subjects involved in the study.

Data Availability Statement: Data will be available upon reasonable request.

Conflicts of Interest: The authors declare no conflict of interest. The funders had no role in the design of the study; in the collection, analyses or interpretation of data; in the writing of the manuscript or in the decision to publish the results.

References

1. Favier, J.; Amar, L.; Gimenez-Roqueplo, A.P. Paraganglioma and phaeochromocytoma: From genetics to personalized medicine. *Nat. Rev. Endocrinol.* **2015**, *11*, 101–111. [CrossRef]
2. Cascón, A.; Remacha, L.; Calsina, B.; Robledo, M. Pheochromocytomas and paragangliomas: Bypassing cellular respiration. *Cancers* **2019**, *11*, 683. [CrossRef] [PubMed]
3. Fishbein, L.; Leshchiner, I.; Walter, V.; Danilova, L.; Robertson, A.G.; Johnson, A.R.; Lichtenberg, T.M.; Murray, B.A.; Ghayee, H.K.; Else, T.; et al. Comprehensive molecular characterization of pheochromocytoma and paraganglioma. *Cancer Cell* **2017**, *31*, 181–193. [CrossRef]
4. Baudin, E.; Habra, M.A.; Deschamps, F.; Cote, G.; Dumont, F.; Cabanillas, M.; Arfi-Roufe, J.; Berdelou, A.; Moon, B.; Ghuzlan, A.A.; et al. Therapy of endocrine disease: Treatment of malignant pheochromocytoma and paraganglioma. *Eur. J. Endocrinol.* **2014**, *171*, R111–R122. [CrossRef] [PubMed]
5. Jimenez, C. Treatment for patients with malignant pheochromocytomas and paragangliomas: A perspective from the hallmarks of cancer. *Front. Endocrinol.* **2018**, *9*, 277. [CrossRef] [PubMed]
6. De Filpo, G.; Maggi, M.; Mannelli, M.; Canu, L. Management and outcome of metastatic pheochromocytomas/paragangliomas: An overview. *J. Endocrinol. Investig.* **2021**, *44*, 15–25. [CrossRef]
7. Jochmanova, I.; Pacak, K. Pheochromocytoma: The first metabolic endocrine cancer. *Clin. Cancer Res.* **2016**, *22*, 5001–5011. [CrossRef] [PubMed]

8. Plouin, P.F.; Amar, L.; Dekkers, O.M.; Fassnach, M.; Gimenez-Roqueplo, A.P.; Lenders, J.W.M.; Lussey-Lepoutre, C.; Steichen, O. European society of endocrinology clinical practice guideline for long-term follow-up of patients operated on for a phaeochromocytoma or a paraganglioma. *Eur. J. Endocrinol.* **2016**, *174*, G1–G10. [CrossRef]
9. Plouin, P.F.; Fitzgerald, P.; Rich, T.; Ayala-Ramirez, M.; Perrier, N.D.; Baudin, E.; Jimenez, C. Metastatic pheochromocytoma and paraganglioma: Focus on therapeutics. *Horm. Metab. Res.* **2012**, *44*, 390–399. [CrossRef]
10. John, H.; Ziegler, W.H.; Hauri, D.; Jaeger, P. Pheochromocytomas: Can malignant potential be predicted? *Urology* **1999**, *53*, 679–683. [CrossRef]
11. Eisenhofer, G.; Lenders, J.W.M.; Siegert, G.; Bornstein, S.R.; Friberg, P.; Milosevic, D.; Mannelli, M.; Linehan, W.M.; Adams, K.; Timmers, H.J.; et al. Plasma methoxytyramine: A novel biomarker of metastatic pheochromocytoma and paraganglioma in relation to established risk factors of tumour size, location and SDHB mutation status. *Eur. J. Cancer* **2012**, *48*, 1739–1749. [CrossRef] [PubMed]
12. Gimenez-Roqueplo, A.P.; Favier, J.; Rustin, P.; Rieubland, C.; Crespin, M.; Nau, V.; van Kien, P.K.; Corvol, P.; Plouin, P.F.; Jeunemaitre, X. Mutations in the SDHB gene are associated with extra-adrenal and/or malignant phaeochromocytomas. *Cancer Res.* **2003**, *63*, 5615–5621. [PubMed]
13. Hescot, S.; Curras-Freixes, M.; Deutschbein, T.; van Berkel, A.; Vezzosi, D.; Amar, L.; de La Fouchardiere, C.; Valdes, N.; Riccardi, F.; Do Cao, C.; et al. Prognosis of malignant pheochromocytoma and paraganglioma (MAPP-PronO Study): A European network for the study of adrenal tumors retrospective study. *J. Clin. Endocrinol. Metab.* **2019**, *104*, 2367–2374. [CrossRef] [PubMed]
14. Job, S.; Draskovic, I.; Burnichon, N.; Buffet, A.; Cros, J.; Lepine, C.; Venisse, A.; Robidel, E.; Verkarre, V.; Meatchi, T.; et al. Telomerase Activation and ATRX Mutations Are Independent Risk Factors for Metastatic Pheochromocytoma and Paraganglioma. *Clin. Cancer Res.* **2019**, *25*, 760–770. [CrossRef]
15. Dwight, T.; Flynn, A.; Amarasinghe, K.; Benn, D.E.; Lupat, R.; Li, J.; Cameron, D.L.; Hogg, A.; Balachander, S.; Candiloro, I.L.M.; et al. TERT Structural Rearrangements in Metastatic Pheochromocytomas. *Endocr. Relat. Cancer* **2018**, *25*, 1–9. [CrossRef]
16. De Lange, T. Shelterin: The protein complex that shapes and safeguards human telomeres. *Genes Dev.* **2005**, *19*, 2100–2110. [CrossRef]
17. Chan, S.W.-L.; Blackburn, E.H. New ways not to make ends meet: Telomerase, DNA damage proteins and heterochromatin. *Oncogene* **2002**, *21*, 553–563. [CrossRef]
18. Funk, W.D.; Wang, C.K.; Shelton, D.N.; Harley, C.B.; Pagon, G.D.; Hoeffler, W.K. Telomerase expression restores dermal integrity to in vitro-aged fibroblasts in a reconstituted skin model. *Exp. Cell Res.* **2000**, *258*, 270–278. [CrossRef] [PubMed]
19. Blasco, M.A.; Funk, W.; Villeponteau, B.; Greider, C.W. Functional characterization and developmental regulation of mouse telomerase RNA. *Science* **1995**, *269*, 1267–1270. [CrossRef]
20. Shay, J.W.; Wright, W.E. Role of telomeres and telomerase in cancer. *Semin. Cancer Biol.* **2011**, *21*, 349–353. [CrossRef]
21. Maciejowski, J.; de Lange, T. Telomeres in cancer: Tumour suppression and genome instability. *Nat. Rev. Mol. Cell Biol.* **2017**, *18*, 175–186. [CrossRef] [PubMed]
22. Wright, W.E.; Piatyszek, M.A.; Rainey, W.E.; Shgy, J.W.; Byrd, W. Telomerase activity in human germline embryonic tissues and cells. *Dev. Genet.* **1996**, *18*, 18173–18179. [CrossRef]
23. Martínez, P.; Blasco, M.A. Telomeric and extra-telomeric roles for telomerase and the telomere-binding proteins. *Nat. Rev. Cancer* **2011**, *11*, 161–176. [CrossRef] [PubMed]
24. Greider, C.W.; Blackburn, E.H. Identification of a specific telomere terminal transferase activity in tetrahymena extracts. *Cell* **1985**, *43*, 405–413. [CrossRef]
25. Ulaner, G.A.; Hu, J.-F.; Vu, T.H.; Giudice, L.C.; Hoffman2, A.R. Telomerase activity in human development is regulated by human telomerase reverse transcriptase (HTERT) transcription and by alternate splicing of HTERT Transcripts1. *CANCER Res.* **1998**, *58*, 4168–4172. [PubMed]
26. Dunham, M.A.; Neumann, A.A.; Fasching, C.L.; Reddel, R.R. Telomere maintenance by recombination in human cells. *Nat. Genet.* **2000**, *26*, 447–450. [CrossRef]
27. Shay, J.W.; Bacchetti, S. A survey of telomerase activity in human cancer. *Eur. J. Cancer Part A* **1997**, *33*, 787–791. [CrossRef]
28. Dilley, R.L.; Greenberg, R.A. Alternative telomere maintenance and cancer. *Trends Cancer* **2015**, *1*, 145–156. [CrossRef]
29. Schmidt, J.C.; Cech, T.R. Human telomerase: Biogenesis, trafficking, recruitment, and activation. *Genes Dev.* **2015**, *29*, 1095–1105. [CrossRef]
30. Venteicher, A.S.; Abreu, E.B.; Meng, Z.; McCann, K.E.; Terns, R.M.; Veenstra, T.D.; Terns, M.P.; Artandi, S.E. A human telomerase holoenzyme protein required for cajal body localization and telomere synthesis. *Science* **2009**, *323*, 644–648. [CrossRef]
31. Nykamp, K.; Anderson, M.; Powers, M.; Garcia, J.; Herrera, B.; Ho, Y.-Y.; Kobayashi, Y.; Patil, N.; Thusberg, J.; Westbrook, M.; et al. Sherloc: A comprehensive refinement of the ACMG–AMP variant classification criteria. *Genet. Med.* **2017**, *19*, 1105–1117. [CrossRef] [PubMed]
32. Toledo, R.A.; Burnichon, N.; Cascon, A.; Benn, D.E.; Bayley, J.P.; Welander, J.; Tops, C.M.; Firth, H.; Dwight, T.; Ercolino, T.; et al. Consensus statement on next-generation-sequencing-based diagnostic testing of hereditary phaeochromocytomas and paragangliomas. *Nat. Rev. Endocrinol.* **2017**, *13*, 233–247. [CrossRef]
33. Trapnell, C.; Pachter, L.; Salzberg, S.L. TopHat: Discovering splice junctions with RNA-Seq. *Bioinformatics* **2009**, *25*, 1105–1111. [CrossRef] [PubMed]

34. Graña, O.; Rubio-Camarillo, M.; Fdez-Riverola, F.; Pisano, D.G.; Glez-Peña, D. Nextpresso: Next generation sequencing expression analysis pipeline. *Curr. Bioinform.* **2017**, *13*, 583–591. [CrossRef]
35. Ritchie, M.E.; Phipson, B.; Wu, D.; Hu, Y.; Law, C.W.; Shi, W.; Smyth, G.K. Limma powers differential expression analyses for RNA-sequencing and microarray studies. *Nucleic Acids Res.* **2015**, *43*, e47. [CrossRef]
36. Rubio-Camarillo, M.; López, G.G.; Fernández, J.M.; Valencia, A.; Pisano, D. RUbioSeq: A suite of parallelized pipelines to automate exome variation and bisulfite-seq analyses. *Bioinformatics* **2013**, *29*, 1687–1689. [CrossRef]
37. Poplin, R.; Ruano-Rubio, V.; DePristo, M.; Fennell, T.; Carneiro, M.; van der Auwera, G.; Kling, D.; Gauthier, L.; Levy-Moonshine, A.; Roazen, D.; et al. Scaling accurate genetic variant discovery to tens of thousands of samples. *bioRxiv* **2017**. [CrossRef]
38. Cibulskis, K.; Lawrence, M.S.; Carter, S.L.; Sivachenko, A.; Jaffe, D.; Sougnez, C.; Gabriel, S.; Meyerson, M.; Lander, E.S.; Getz, G. Sensitive detection of somatic point mutations in impure and heterogeneous cancer samples. *Nat. Biotechnol.* **2013**, *31*, 213–219. [CrossRef]
39. Gao, J.; Wan, C.; Zhang, H.; Li, A.; Zang, Q.; Ban, R.; Ali, A.; Yu, Z.; Shi, Q.; Jiang, X.; et al. Anaconda: An automated pipeline for somatic copy number variation detection and annotation from tumor exome sequencing data. *BMC Bioinform.* **2017**, *18*, 1–6. [CrossRef]
40. Mermel, C.H.; Schumacher, S.E.; Hill, B.; Meyerson, M.L.; Beroukhim, R.; Getz, G. GISTIC2.0 facilitates sensitive and confident localization of the targets of focal somatic copy-number alteration in human cancers. *Genome Biol.* **2011**, *12*, 1–14. [CrossRef]
41. Cascón, A.; Comino-Méndez, I.; Currás-Freixes, M.; de Cubas, A.A.; Contreras, L.; Richter, S.; Peitzsch, M.; Mancikova, V.; Inglada-Pérez, L.; Pérez-Barrios, A.; et al. Whole-exome sequencing identifies MDH2 as a new familial paraganglioma gene. *J. Natl. Cancer Inst.* **2015**. [CrossRef] [PubMed]
42. De Cubas, A.A.; Korpershoek, E.; Inglada-Pérez, L.; Letouzé, E.; Currás-Freixes, M.; Fernández, A.F.; Comino-Méndez, I.; Schiavi, F.; Mancikova, V.; Eisenhofer, G.; et al. DNA methylation profiling in pheochromocytoma and paraganglioma reveals diagnostic and prognostic markers. *Clin. Cancer Res.* **2015**, *21*, 3020–3030. [CrossRef] [PubMed]
43. Remacha, L.; Currás-Freixes, M.; Torres-Ruiz, R.; Schiavi, F.; Torres-Pérez, R.; Calsina, B.; Letón, R.; Comino-Méndez, I.; Roldán-Romero, J.M.; Montero-Conde, C.; et al. Gain-of-function mutations in DNMT3A in patients with paraganglioma. *Genet. Med.* **2018**, *20*, 1644–1651. [CrossRef] [PubMed]
44. Remacha, L.; Pirman, D.; Mahoney, C.E.; Coloma, J.; Calsina, B.; Currás-Freixes, M.; Letón, R.; Torres-Pérez, R.; Richter, S.; Pita, G.; et al. Recurrent germline DLST mutations in individuals with multiple pheochromocytomas and paragangliomas. *Am. J. Hum. Genet.* **2019**, *104*, 651–664. [CrossRef]
45. Calsina, B.; Castro-Vega, L.J.; Torres-Pérez, R.; Inglada-Pérez, L.; Currás-Freixes, M.; Roldán-Romero, J.M.; Mancikova, V.; Letón, R.; Remacha, L.; Santos, M.; et al. Integrative multi-omics analysis identifies a prognostic MiRNA signature and a targetable MiR-21-3p/TSC2/MTOR axis in metastatic pheochromocytoma/paraganglioma. *Theranostics* **2019**, *9*, 4946–4958. [CrossRef]
46. Bankhead, P.; Loughrey, M.B.; Fernández, J.A.; Dombrowski, Y.; McArt, D.G.; Dunne, P.D.; McQuaid, S.; Gray, R.T.; Murray, L.J.; Coleman, H.G.; et al. QuPath: Open source software for digital pathology image analysis. *Sci. Rep.* **2017**, *7*, 1–7. [CrossRef]
47. Torres-Ruiz, R.; Martinez-Lage, M.; Martin, M.C.; Garcia, A.; Bueno, C.; Castaño, J.; Ramirez, J.C.; Menendez, P.; Cigudosa, J.C.; Rodriguez-Perales, S. Efficient recreation of t(11;22) EWSR1-FLI1+ in human stem cells using CRISPR/Cas9. *Stem Cell Rep.* **2017**, *8*, 1408–1420. [CrossRef]
48. Hayer, A.; Shao, L.; Chung, M.; Joubert, L.M.; Yang, H.W.; Tsai, F.C.; Bisaria, A.; Betzig, E.; Meyer, T. Engulfed cadherin fingers are polarized junctional structures between collectively migrating endothelial cells. *Nat. Cell Biol.* **2016**, *18*, 1311–1323. [CrossRef]
49. Livak, K.J.; Schmittgen, T.D. Analysis of relative gene expression data using real-time quantitative PCR and the 2-ΔΔCT method. *Methods* **2001**, *25*, 402–408. [CrossRef]
50. Samper, E.; Flores, J.M.; Blasco, M.A. Restoration of telomerase activity rescues chromosomal instability and premature aging in Terc$^{-/-}$ mice with short telomeres. *EMBO Rep.* **2001**, *2*, 800–807. [CrossRef]
51. Lee, D.D.; Leão, R.; Komosa, M.; Gallo, M.; Zhang, C.H.; Lipman, T.; Remke, M.; Heidari, A.; Nunes, N.M.; Apolónio, J.D.; et al. DNA hypermethylation within TERT promoter upregulates TERT expression in cancer. *J. Clin. Investig.* **2019**, *129*, 223–229. [CrossRef]
52. de Nonneville, A.; Reddel, R.R. Alternative lengthening of telomeres is not synonymous with mutations in ATRX/DAXX. *Nat. Commun.* **2021**, *12*, 1–4. [CrossRef] [PubMed]
53. Amorim, J.P.; Santos, G.; Vinagre, J.; Soares, P. The role of ATRX in the alternative lengthening of telomeres (ALT) phenotype. *Genes* **2016**, *7*, 66. [CrossRef] [PubMed]
54. Cesare, A.J.; Reddel, R.R. Alternative lengthening of telomeres: Models, mechanisms and implications. *Nat. Rev. Genet.* **2010**, *11*, 319–330. [CrossRef]
55. Klöppel, G.; Couvelard, A.; Hruban, R.H.; Klimstra, D.S.; Komminoth, P.; Osamura, R.Y.; Perren, A.; Rindi, G. Neoplasms of the neuroendocrine pancreas. In *WHO Classification of Tumours of the Endocrine Organs; WHO/IARC Classification of Tumours*; Lioyd, R.V., Osamura, R.Y., Kloppel, G., Eds.; IARC Press: Lyon, France, 2017; Volume 10, pp. 210–239. ISBN 978-92-832-4493-6.
56. Barthel, F.P.; Wei, W.; Tang, M.; Martinez-Ledesma, E.; Hu, X.; Amin, S.B.; Akdemir, K.C.; Seth, S.; Song, X.; Wang, Q.; et al. Systematic analysis of telomere length and somatic alterations in 31 cancer types. *Nat. Genet.* **2017**, *49*, 349–357. [CrossRef] [PubMed]
57. Stern, J.L.; Theodorescu, D.; Vogelstein, B.; Papadopoulos, N.; Cech, T.R. Mutation of the TERT promoter, switch to active chromatin, and monoallelic TERT expression in multiple cancers. *Genes Dev.* **2015**, *29*, 2219. [CrossRef]

58. Bell, R.J.A.; Rube, H.T.; Xavier-Magalhães, A.; Costa, B.M.; Mancini, A.; Song, J.S.; Costello, J.F. Understanding TERT promoter mutations: A common path to immortality. *Mol. Cancer Res.* **2016**, *14*, 315–323. [CrossRef] [PubMed]
59. Liu, T.; Brown, T.C.; Juhlin, C.C.; Andreasson, A.; Wang, N.; Bäckdahl, M.; Healy, J.M.; Prasad, M.L.; Korah, R.; Carling, T.; et al. The activating TERT promoter mutation C228T is recurrent in subsets of adrenal tumors. *Endocr. Relat. Cancer* **2014**, *21*, 427–434. [CrossRef]
60. Gupta, S.; Vanderbilt, C.M.; Lin, Y.-T.; Benhamida, J.K.; Jungbluth, A.A.; Rana, S.; Momeni-Boroujeni, A.; Chang, J.C.; Mcfarlane, T.; Salazar, P.; et al. A pan-cancer study of somatic TERT promoter mutations and amplification in 30,773 tumors profiled by clinical genomic sequencing. *J. Mol. Diagnostics* **2021**, *23*, 253–263. [CrossRef]
61. Zhang, A.; Zheng, C.; Hou, M.; Lindvall, C.; Wallin, K.-L.; Ångström, T.; Yang, X.; Hellström, A.-C.; Blennow, E.; Björkholm, M.; et al. Amplification of the telomerase reverse transcriptase (HTERT) gene in cervical carcinomas. *Genes Chromosom. Cancer* **2002**, *34*, 269–275. [CrossRef]
62. Dagg, R.A.; Pickett, H.A.; Neumann, A.A.; Napier, C.E.; Henson, J.D.; Teber, E.T.; Arthur, J.W.; Reynolds, C.P.; Murray, J.; Haber, M.; et al. Extensive proliferation of human cancer cells with ever-shorter telomeres. *Cell Rep.* **2017**, *19*, 2544–2556. [CrossRef] [PubMed]
63. Viceconte, N.; Dheur, M.S.; Majerova, E.; Pierreux, C.E.; Baurain, J.F.; van Baren, N.; Decottignies, A. Highly aggressive metastatic melanoma cells unable to maintain telomere length. *Cell Rep.* **2017**, *19*, 2529–2543. [CrossRef]
64. Papathomas, T.G.; Oudijk, L.; Zwarthoff, E.C.; Post, E.; Duijkers, F.A.; van Noesel, M.M.; Hofland, L.J.; Pollard, P.J.; Maher, E.R.; Restuccia, D.F.; et al. Telomerase reverse transcriptase promoter mutations in tumors originating from the adrenal gland and extra-adrenal paraganglia. *Endocr. Relat. Cancer* **2014**, *21*, 653–661. [CrossRef] [PubMed]
65. Vinagre, J.; Almeida, A.; Pópulo, H.; Batista, R.; Lyra, J.; Pinto, V.; Coelho, R.; Celestino, R.; Prazeres, H.; Lima, L.; et al. Frequency of TERT promoter mutations in human cancers. *Nat. Commun.* **2013**, *4*, 1–6. [CrossRef] [PubMed]
66. Letouzé, E.; Martinelli, C.; Loriot, C.; Burnichon, N.; Abermil, N.; Ottolenghi, C.; Janin, M.; Menara, M.; Nguyen, A.T.; Benit, P.; et al. SDH mutations establish a hypermethylator phenotype in paraganglioma. *Cancer Cell* **2013**, *23*, 739–752. [CrossRef]
67. Xu, Y.; Goldkorn, A. Telomere and telomerase therapeutics in cancer. *Genes* **2016**, *7*, 22. [CrossRef] [PubMed]
68. Reddel, R. Telomere maintenance mechanisms in cancer: Clinical implications. *Curr. Pharm. Des.* **2014**, *20*, 6361–6374. [CrossRef]
69. Benn, D.E.; Robinson, B.G.; Clifton-Bligh, R.J. 15 years of paraganglioma: Clinical manifestations of paraganglioma syndromes types 1–5. *Endocr. Relat. Cancer* **2015**, *22*, T91–T103. [CrossRef]
70. Heaphy, C.M.; Subhawong, A.P.; Hong, S.M.; Goggins, M.G.; Montgomery, E.A.; Gabrielson, E.; Netto, G.J.; Epstein, J.I.; Lotan, T.L.; Westra, W.H.; et al. Prevalence of the alternative lengthening of telomeres telomere maintenance mechanism in human cancer subtypes. *Am. J. Pathol.* **2011**, *179*, 1608–1615. [CrossRef]
71. Qin, J.; Autexier, C. Regulation of human telomerase RNA biogenesis and localization. *RNA Biol.* **2021**, *18*, 305–315. [CrossRef]
72. Grozdanov, P.N.; Roy, S.; Kittur, N.; Meier, U.T. SHQ1 is required prior to NAF1 for assembly of H/ACA small nucleolar and telomerase RNPs. *RNA* **2009**, *15*, 1188–1197. [CrossRef]
73. Kiss, T. Small nucleolar RNA-guided post-transcriptional modification of cellular RNAs. *EMBO J.* **2001**, *20*, 3617–3622. [CrossRef]
74. Kiss, A.M.; Jády, B.E.; Darzacq, X.; Verheggen, C.; Bertrand, E.; Kiss, T. A cajal body-specific pseudouridylation guide RNA is composed of two box H/ACA SnoRNA-like domains. *Nucleic Acids Res.* **2002**, *30*, 4643–4649. [CrossRef]
75. Mcmahon, M.; Contreras, A.; Ruggero, D. Small RNAs with big implications: New insights into H/ACA SnoRNA function and their role in human disease. *Wiley Interdiscip. Rev. RNA* **2015**, *6*, 173–189. [CrossRef] [PubMed]
76. von Stedingk, K.; Koster, J.; Piqueras, M.; Noguera, R.; Navarro, S.; Påhlman, S.; Versteeg, R.; Øra, I.; Gisselsson, D.; Lindgren, D.; et al. SnoRNPs regulate telomerase activity in neuroblastoma and are associated with poor prognosis. *Transl. Oncol.* **2013**, *6*, 447–IN6. [CrossRef]
77. Elsharawy, K.A.; Althobiti, M.; Mohammed, O.J.; Aljohani, A.I.; Toss, M.S.; Green, A.R.; Rakha, E.A. Nucleolar protein 10 (NOP10) predicts poor prognosis in invasive breast cancer. *Breast Cancer Res. Treat.* **2021**, *185*, 615–627. [CrossRef]
78. Cui, C.; Liu, Y.; Gerloff, D.; Rohde, C.; Pauli, C.; Köhn, M.; Misiak, D.; Oellerich, T.; Schwartz, S.; Schmidt, L.H.; et al. NOP10 predicts lung cancer prognosis and its associated small nucleolar RNAs drive proliferation and migration. *Oncogene* **2020**, *40*, 909–921. [CrossRef]
79. Cristofari, G.; Adolf, E.; Reichenbach, P.; Sikora, K.; Terns, R.M.; Terns, M.P.; Lingner, J. Human telomerase RNA accumulation in cajal bodies facilitates telomerase recruitment to telomeres and telomere elongation. *Mol. Cell* **2007**, *27*, 882–889. [CrossRef]
80. Ghanim, G.E.; Fountain, A.J.; van Roon, A.-M.M.; Rangan, R.; Das, R.; Collins, K.; Nguyen, T.H.D. Structure of human telomerase holoenzyme with bound telomeric DNA. *Nature* **2021**, *593*, 449–453. [CrossRef]

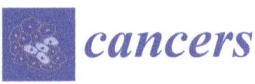

Review

MicroRNAs, Long Non-Coding RNAs, and Circular RNAs: Potential Biomarkers and Therapeutic Targets in Pheochromocytoma/Paraganglioma

Peter Istvan Turai [1], Gábor Nyírő [2], Henriett Butz [3,4,5], Attila Patócs [3,4,5] and Peter Igaz [1,2,*]

1. Department of Endocrinology, Department of Internal Medicine and Oncology, Faculty of Medicine, Semmelweis University, Korányi str. 2/a, H-1083 Budapest, Hungary; peteturai@gmail.com
2. MTA-SE Molecular Medicine Research Group, H-1083 Budapest, Hungary; nyirogabor1@gmail.com
3. Department of Laboratory Medicine, Faculty of Medicine, Semmelweis University, H-1089 Budapest, Hungary; butz.henriett@med.semmelweis-univ.hu (H.B.); patocs.attila@med.semmelweis-univ.hu (A.P.)
4. Department of Molecular Genetics, National Institute of Oncology, H-1122 Budapest, Hungary
5. MTA-SE Hereditary Endocrine Tumors Research Group, H-1089 Budapest, Hungary
* Correspondence: igaz.peter@med.semmelweis-univ.hu; Tel.: +36-1-266-0816

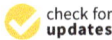

Citation: Turai, P.I.; Nyírő, G.; Butz, H.; Patócs, A.; Igaz, P. MicroRNAs, Long Non-Coding RNAs, and Circular RNAs: Potential Biomarkers and Therapeutic Targets in Pheochromocytoma/Paraganglioma. *Cancers* **2021**, *13*, 1522. https://doi.org/10.3390/cancers13071522

Academic Editor: Alberto Cascón

Received: 7 March 2021
Accepted: 22 March 2021
Published: 26 March 2021

Publisher's Note: MDPI stays neutral with regard to jurisdictional claims in published maps and institutional affiliations.

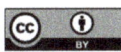

Copyright: © 2021 by the authors. Licensee MDPI, Basel, Switzerland. This article is an open access article distributed under the terms and conditions of the Creative Commons Attribution (CC BY) license (https://creativecommons.org/licenses/by/4.0/).

Simple Summary: Pheochromocytomas/paragangliomas (PPGL) are rare tumors originating from chromaffin tissues. Around 40% of pheochromocytomas/paragangliomas (PPGL) harbor germline mutations, representing the highest heritability among human tumors. Unfortunately, there are no available molecular markers for the metastatic potential of these tumors, and the prognosis of metastatic forms is rather dismal. In this review, we present the potential relevance of non-coding RNA molecules including microRNAs, long non-coding RNAs and circular RNAs in PPGL pathogenesis and diagnosis. The pathomechanisms presented might also represent potential novel therapeutic targets.

Abstract: Around 40% of pheochromocytomas/paragangliomas (PPGL) harbor germline mutations, representing the highest heritability among human tumors. All PPGL have metastatic potential, but metastatic PPGL is overall rare. There is no available molecular marker for the metastatic potential of these tumors, and the diagnosis of metastatic PPGL can only be established if metastases are found at "extra-chromaffin" sites. In the era of precision medicine with individually targeted therapies and advanced care of patients, the treatment options for metastatic pheochromocytoma/paraganglioma are still limited. With this review we would like to nurture the idea of the quest for non-coding ribonucleic acids as an area to be further investigated in tumor biology. Non-coding RNA molecules encompassing microRNAs, long non-coding RNAs, and circular RNAs have been implicated in the pathogenesis of various tumors, and were also proposed as valuable diagnostic, prognostic factors, and even potential treatment targets. Given the fact that the pathogenesis of tumors including pheochromocytomas/paragangliomas is linked to epigenetic dysregulation, it is reasonable to conduct studies related to their epigenetic expression profiles and in this brief review we present a synopsis of currently available findings on the relevance of these molecules in these tumors highlighting their diagnostic potential.

Keywords: pheochromocytoma; paraganglioma; genetics; non-coding RNA; malignancy; biomarker; treatment

1. Introduction

Non-coding RNA molecules encompassing microRNAs, long non-coding RNAs, and circular RNAs have been implicated in the pathogenesis of various tumors, and were also proposed as valuable diagnostic and prognostic factors, and even potential therapeutic targets. Given the fact that the pathogenesis of tumors including pheochromocytomas/paragangliomas (PPGL) is partly linked to epigenetic dysregulation [1], it is reasonable to investigate their epigenetic expression profiles.

Pheochromocytomas are rare (incidence is approximately 0.8 per 100,000 people per year) catecholamine-producing endocrine tumors, arising from neural-crest-derived chromaffin cells. They have a strong genetic background and originate either in the adrenal medulla (80%) or in the sympathetic or parasympathetic paraganglia (20%), "extra-adrenal pheochromocytomas" (paraganglioma) as formerly referred to in [2]. A considerable proportion (40%) of pheocromocytoma/paraganglioma (PPGL) is diagnosed as manifestations of hereditary tumor syndromes, including familial paraganglioma syndrome types 1–5 (mutations in genes coding for subunits and associated factors of succinate dehydrogenase (SDH), e.g., *SDHB*, *SDHC*, *SDHD*, *SDHA* and *SDHAF2* (collectively called *SDHx*), von Hippel-Lindau syndrome (mutations of *VHL* tumor suppressor), multiple endocrine neoplasia type 2 (mutations of the *RET* protooncogene), neurofibromatosis type 1 (mutations of *NF1* tumor suppressor) and other germline mutations of various genes linked to major pathogenic processes in PPGL pathogenesis (e.g., *HIF2A*, *MAX*, *MDH2*, *FH*, *TMEM127*, *KIF1B*, *PHD/EGLN1*) [3–5]. At present, there are more than 12 genetic syndromes and 22 PPGL driver genes that contribute to PPGL formation [6,7]. This proportion of germline mutations has the highest degree of heritability among human tumors [8]. Moreover, sporadic PPGL were found to harbor somatic mutations in genes corresponding to their germline counterparts [9].

The molecular etiology of PPGL is especially important to explore as PPGL display various driver mutations with serious impact on diagnosis, prognosis and therapy as well. As a familial disease, early genetic diagnosis can not only facilitate the treatment of the proband, but is also an important step to detect potentially mutation carriers in the family [10]. Another reason for genetic testing is the well-known causative link between some driver mutations and their metastatic potential [8]. The rate of metastatic forms of catecholamine-secreting tumors is rather variable in different studies ranging between 5–26%. On the other side up to 50% of patients with metastatic PPGL have specific germline mutations [11–13]. The risk of metastasis is particularly high in individuals harboring germline *SDHB* mutations [12]. PPGL susceptibility can be associated with mutations either in tumor suppressor genes (e.g., *VHL*, *NF1*, *SDHB*) or in proto-oncogenes (e.g., *RET*, *HRAS*) [7].

In order to further specify PPGL types and their tumor behavior, according to another recent paper, PPGL can further be classified into four molecular subtypes [14] (Figure 1). These groups include Wnt-altered, kinase signaling, pseudohypoxia, and cortical admixture subtypes with different molecular features and also clinical behavior. For example, the Wnt-altered subtype seems to be specific for sporadic PPGL as no germline mutations were observed within these tumors. The pseudohypoxia type generally had no epinephrine or metanephrine secretion, and also showed overexpression of the previously described tumor hypoxia marker microRNA-210 (*miR-210*) [15]. The cortical admixture type was found to be correlated with *MAX* (*MYC* associated factor X) mutations, which is also included as one of the susceptibility genes for hereditary PPGL [16]. Finally, kinase signaling exhibited the highest expression of *PNMT* (phenylethanolamine N-methyltransferase), an enzyme known to convert norepinephrine to epinephrine and according to that, was found mainly in pheochromocytomas.

From the clinical point of view, primary symptoms of excessive catecholamine secretion are episodic headache, sweating, and tachycardia (palpitations), also called the "classic triad" [17,18]. Either sustained or paroxysmal hypertension and even unexplained orthostatic hypotension are also characteristic features of PPGL. Other non-specific signs related to catecholamine-excess are anxiety, panic attacks, tremor, pallor, frequent urination, constipation, vision disturbances, hyperglycemia, and severe cardiovascular complications including stroke, aortic dissection, and stress-induced (takotsubo) cardiomyopathy [19]. In the so-called "pheochromocytoma crisis" patients suffer from hyperthermia, mental status change, and multisystem dysfunction, hence they require immediate medical attention [20]. Signs related to the general properties of a tumor are pain—depending on tumor location—weight loss, hematuria, and rarely erythrocytosis due to overproduction of erythropoietin [21]. Ever-increasingly, PPGL often appear with no associated symptoms as an incidental finding on imaging performed for other purposes (approximately 5–8% of adrenal incidentalomas), and also due to genetic screening in the context of familial disease [5].

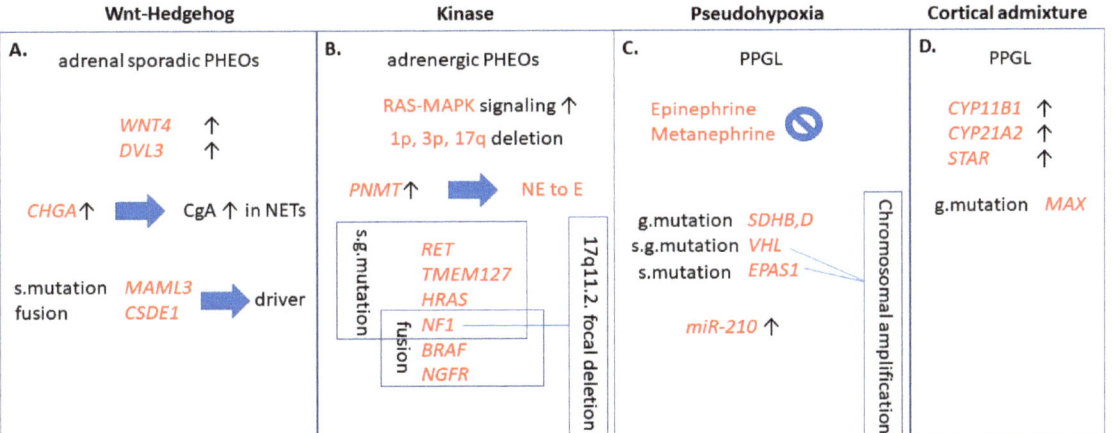

Figure 1. Clinically relevant functions of the four molecular pathways contributing to pheochromocytomas/paragangliomas (PPGL). (A) Wnt-Hedgehog overexpressed subtype included mainly adrenal sporadic pheochromocytomas and high chromogranin A levels. *MAML3* and *CSDE1* are independently important driver mutations leading to Wnt-Hedgehog activation. (B) Kinase signaling pathway is correlated to pheochromocytomas of adrenergic phenotype due to overexpression of *PNMT*, comprising somatic- and germline mutations and chromosomal deletions, as well. (C): Pseudohypoxia subtype, in addition to somatic- and germline mutations and chromosomal amplification, also exhibited overexpression of *miR-210*. (D) Overexpression of *CYP11B1*, *CYP21A2*, and *STAR* adrenal cortex markers was characteristic to cortical admixture subtype, along with *MAX* mutation in PPGL. g. mutation: germline mutation; s. mutation: somatic mutation; s.g. mutation: somatic and germline mutation; *WNT4*: wingless-related integration site 4; *DVL3*: dishevelled 3; *CHGA*: encodes chromogranin A (CgA); NET: neuroendocrine tumor; *MAML3*: mastermind-like transcriptional coactivator 3; *CSDE1*: cold shock domain containing E1; *RAS*: rat entry sarcoma; *MAPK*: mitogen-activated protein kinase; *PNMT*: phenylethanolamine N-methyltransferase; NE: norepineprhrine; E: epinephrine; *RET*: rearranged during transfection; *TMEM127*: transmembrane protein 127; *HRAS*: Harvey rat sarcoma viral oncogene homolog; *NF1*: neurofibromatosis 1; *BRAF*: v-raf murine sarcoma viral oncogene homolog B1; *NGFR*: nerve growth factor receptor; *SDH*: succinate dehydrogenase; *VHL*: Von-Hippel Lindau; *EPAS1*: endothelial PAS domain 1; *CYP11B1*: cytochrome P450 family 11 subfamily B member 1; *CYP21A2*: cytochrome P450 family 21 subfamily A member 2; *STAR*: steroid acute regulatory protein; *MAX*: myc associated factor X.

Diagnosis of PPGL is based on a thorough clinical examination and medical history followed by biochemical tests, diagnostic imaging, and genetic testing. Biochemical tests include measuring 24 h urinary fractionated metanephrines and catecholamines or plasma metanephrine [22–24]. The general neuroendocrine tumor marker chromogranin A (CgA) is also useful. However, CgA is not specific for PPGL, but as its serum levels correlate with tumor burden, it is applicable for monitoring PPGL patients [25]. Patients with positive biochemical test results need to proceed on radiological evaluation, such as ^{123}I-MIBG scan (meta-iodobenzylguanidine), MRI (magnetic resonance imaging), CT (computed tomography), ^{18}FDG PET-CT (fluorodeoxyglucose positron emission tomography), or ^{68}Ga-DOTATATE-PET (dodecanetetraacetic tyrosine-3-octreotate) [26].

Beside the clinical evaluation, at present, there are no reliable histomorphological features to distinguish between benign and metastatic PPGL, however Pheochromocytoma of the Adrenal Gland Scaled Score (PASS) and the Grading System for Adrenal Pheochromocytoma and Paraganglioma (GAPP) have been evaluated in a recent meta-analysis as promising tools with a good negative predictive value [27]. The recent WHO classification omitted the terms benign and malignant pheochromocytoma, and defined metastatic

PPGL as a tumor with metastases at "extra-chromaffin" sites [28]. Patients with metastatic PPGL have poor prognosis with an estimated 44% overall survival (OS) at 5 years due to limited treatment options [29]. Whereas some patients present with synchronous metastases, metastases occur in several patients after the removal of the primary tumor, i.e., in a metachronous fashion. Long-term monitoring in all patients is warranted, even in those patients seemingly cured from the disease, which is obviously a life-long burden for such patients [30]. Metastasis in PPGL can occur as long as 53 years after surgery [31]. Unfortunately, despite intensive efforts, there are no reliable molecular markers of the metastatic potential of PPGL either. Altogether, according to the current WHO classification, all PPGL should be regarded as potentially malignant/metastatic, and followed up, but only a minority of PPGL will actually metastasize [32,33].

Currently, the primary treatment of PPGL is surgical resection, although removal of the tumor does not always lead to the cure of PPGL or to normotension [30]. However, it is possible that successful surgical treatment can not only be curative, but can also lead to normotension, normalization of blood pressure variability, and even normalization of urinary metanephrines [34]. Undiagnosed or not properly treated PPGL has high morbidity and mortality rate mainly due to cardiovascular complications. Other complications can also be life-threatening, such as drug interactions, hypertensive crises due to diagnostic- or therapeutic manipulations—owing to the sympathetic activation, and also malignancy or associated neoplasms [35]. For metastatic PPGL, there is no curative treatment, and currently available systemic chemotherapeutic approaches (e.g., CVD—cyclophosphamide-vincristin-dacarbazin chemotherapy) have limited efficacy [36]. Novel treatment options including *VEGF* (vascular endothelial growth factor) and tyrosine kinase inhibitors (e.g., axitinib, dovitinib, lenvatinib, sunitinib) exist for patients with *SDHA*, *SDHB*, *SDHD*, *RET*, *VHL*, and *FH* mutations in renal cell carcinoma and PPGL; furthermore, immunotherapies targeting PD-L1 (programmed death-ligand 1) checkpoint protein (e.g., pembrolizumab, ipilimumab, nivolumab) are currently under clinical investigation [37–41]. Poly ADP-ribose polymerase (PARP) inhibitors (e.g., olaparib) represent another perspective in patients harboring *SDHx* mutations due to elevated levels of succinate and NAD$^+$ inhibiting homologous recombination-based DNA repair mechanism which is known to be corrected by PARP, thus keeping aberrant cells alive [42]. Furthermore, there are two kinase signaling pathways (PI3K-Akt-mTOR and Ras-Raf-Erk) affected by mutations of *RET*, *MAX*, *NF1*, and *TMEM127*, which can be inhibited by kinase signaling inhibitors (e.g., the mTOR inhibitor everolimus) [43]. Isotope therapies such as ^{131}I-MIBG or somatostatin-analogue-based radiotherapies are also effective [32]. For more details on the current trials in PPGL, the reader is referred to the article by Ilanchezian et al., 2020 [44].

Given the difficulties in PPGL diagnosis, especially the lack of markers of malignancy, non-coding RNA (ncRNA) molecules are gaining increasing attention, as they have been proven to be useful in other neoplasms, as well [45].

2. Classification of ncRNA

Recent progress in the field of molecular biology has revealed that only 1–2% of the transcripts encode for protein (mRNA: messenger RNA), while 90% of the genomic DNA is transcribed. Most of these are transcribed as non-coding RNA; nevertheless, ncRNAs still bear major biological functions [46]. They are epigenetic modulators of gene expression by chromatin remodeling, transcriptional regulation, and posttranscriptional modification. ncRNAs can further be classified as structural ncRNAs, like ribosomal RNAs (rRNAs), transfer RNAs (tRNAs), small nuclear RNAs (snRNAs), small nucleolar RNAs (snoRNAs), and as regulatory ncRNAs, including microRNAs (miRNAs, miRs), PiWi-interacting RNAs (piRNAs), small interfering RNAs (siRNAs), long non-coding RNAs (lncRNA), enhancer RNAs (eRNAs), and circular RNAs (circRNAs) [47,48]. These molecules span across the landscape of cancer biology. Tumors are inherently genetic diseases that derange cellular homeostasis and work towards cellular growth. Non-coding RNA molecules have been shown to be implicated in the pathogenesis of tumors [49,50].

Long non-coding RNAs (usually from 200 to thousands of nucleotides long) are evolutionarily conserved and highly specific to cell/tissue types [51]. lncRNAs have been recently shown to be implicated in important regulatory mechanisms, as it was a long standing view not only about lncRNAs, but also about circRNAs to add no further values than being byproducts of their cognate mRNAs [52]. Surprisingly, the number of lncRNA coding genes even exceeds the number of protein coding genes, but the function of the bulk of them remains to be identified. Cellular mechanisms of lncRNAs relate to their localization within the cell. For example, nuclear transcripts control chromatin functions, transcription, and RNA processing; on the other hand, cytoplasmic lncRNAs have an effect on mRNA stability, translation, and cellular signaling (Figure 2). In different circumstances, functions of lncRNAs not only involve intracellular mechanisms, but may also act on an intercellular level, e.g., contribute to development of the tumor microenvironment and other hallmarks of cancer [53].

Overview of functions and localization of non-coding RNAs

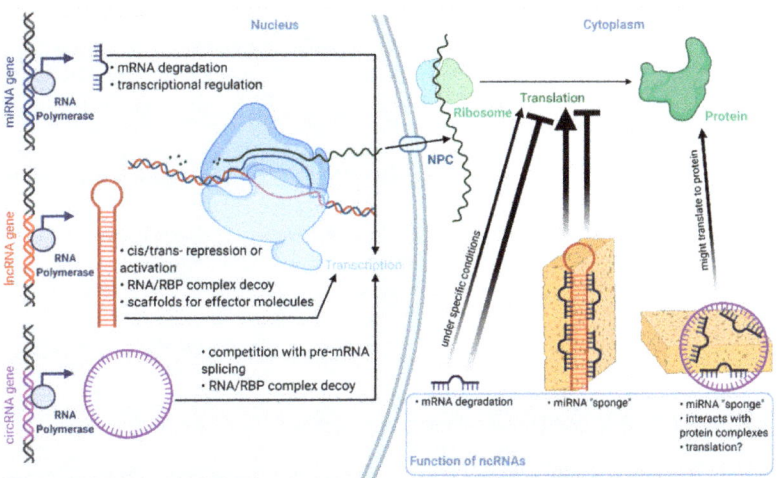

Figure 2. Overview of functions and localization of non-coding RNAs. RBP: RNA binding protein; NPC: nuclear pore complex. Faded arrowhead lines indicate activation; faded blunt-head lines indicate inhibition.

The relevance of circular RNAs (covalently bonded 3′ and 5′ ends) in biological and pathological processes has been shown only recently [54]. These peculiarly stable, evolutionarily conserved molecules play major roles mainly in the post-transcriptional regulation of gene expression e.g., by acting upon transcriptional, translational machinery or by sponging microRNAs (Figure 2). Furthermore, altered expression of circRNAs has been described in various tumors; for example, *circHIPK* functions as a miRNA sponge in colorectal, hepatocellular, kidney, prostate, breast, gastric, and bladder cancer, while *hsa_circ_0004277* seems to be a potential biomarker and therapeutic target in acute myelogenous leukemia [55,56]. CircRNAs are formed from the intron-containing pre-mRNA in a process called "backsplicing", but they are expressed in a different manner to their linear counterparts. Differential expression of circRNAs is explicable via, e.g., different structures of introns (reverse complementary repeat sequences) [57]. Furthermore, one of the most interesting aspect of circRNAs is their potential as biomarkers, as they exhibit high stability compared to other linear RNAs and they show cell-type-specific expression profiles [58,59]. There are four different types of circular RNAs: i. 2′-5′ intronic circRNA (ciRNA) localized in the nucleus, ii. 3′-5′ exon-intron circRNA (EIciRNA) also with nuclear localization, iii. intergenic circRNA located in the cytoplasm, and the most abundant, iv. exonic circRNA (ecircRNA), also localized in the cytoplasm [60,61]. Circular RNAs exert their biological potential via two mechanisms: via backsplicing and subsequent competition with their linear counterpart from the host gene and via trans-regulatory effect of the circRNA end product. Their effect on gene expression can further be divided into six mechanisms: i. sequestration of miRNA, so-called miRNA "sponges"; ii. stimulation of initiation and elongation of transcription by acting upon RNA polymerase II; iii. down-regulation of cognate mRNAs by attenuation of linear splicing; iv. through protein binding they are able to inhibit translational activity; v. a portion of them is protein coding circRNA; vi. circRNAs can alter enzymatic reactions by forming ternary complexes [62,63].

MicroRNAs (miR, miRNA) have been proposed to have a major impact on biological function of tumors and are of great interest as candidates of liquid biopsy. Mature miRs are single-stranded, short RNA molecules comprising 19–25 nucleotides, that are also evolutionarily conserved and encoded by proper miRNA genes [64]. They have a role in the regulation of 30–60% of human genes in epigenetic, posttranscriptional modification, without altering the very sequence of DNA. MicroRNAs are shown to behave similarly to transcription factors (TF). While TFs exert their activating or silencing effect by binding to a specific region of the promoter in the nucleus, miRNAs bind to the 3' UTR (*untranslated region*) of their mRNA target, hence degrading them or blocking their translation in the cytoplasm; however, they can also act in the nucleus (Figure 2) [65,66]. Today, we see an abundance of the biological functions of miRs. Their pleiotropic effects include the regulation of cell cycle and differentiation, cell proliferation, hormone secretion, apoptosis and are also implicated in the regulation of hemopoiesis, immune functioning, and ontogenesis. Several pathogenic processes including tumorigenesis, autoimmune disorders, and vascular diseases among others can be found to be associated with altered miRNA expression [67]. Another important aspect of miRs is their cell- and tissue-specific expression. Cell-specificity means that the expression of miR is different in various tissues, moreover a certain miR can act differently, either as a silencer or rarely an activator in different tissues [65]. In line with this, a miR can be a tumor suppressor in one tissue and an oncogene in another making regulation via miR rather complex and local. Thanks to their abundance and exceptionally high stability, miR expression profiles can be studied in easily accessible archived formalin-fixed paraffin-embedded tissue samples and—being secreted—even in bodily fluids [68,69]. These aforementioned features make microRNAs some of the most studied molecules in the field of minimally invasive diagnostics of neoplastic and non-neoplastic diseases—especially true with "hard-to-diagnose" entities like adrenal tumors or thyroid tumors [70].

3. Non-Coding RNAs in PPGL

3.1. CircRNAs in PPGL

To date, only one study has investigated the expression pattern of circular RNAs in PPGL, suggesting its role in histone methylation [71]. The authors performed RNA sequencing on circRNA transcripts of tumor tissue compared to adjacent normal tissue from PPGL patients. In the discovery cohort, seven patients were randomly assigned in order to perform transcriptome analysis, which revealed 3927 mRNAs, 283 miRNAs, and 367 circRNAs to be differentially expressed. The top 11 differentially expressed circRNAs have been validated by real-time quantitative PCR (RT-qPCR) on 33 pairs of PPGL tumor tissues and adjacent normal tissues from snap-frozen samples. Out of 367 differentially expressed circRNAs 112 were shown to be down-regulated and 255 were up-regulated. The top three overexpressed histone methylation-related circRNAs (*hsa_circ_0000567*, *hsa_circ_0002897*, and *hsa_circ_0004473*) related to histone methylation were identified and validated as well as their miRNA targets (Table 1). These three circRNAs were also found to be differentially expressed in the peripheral blood from 16 PPGL patients and 16 healthy individuals. By bioinformatical analysis, *hsa_circ_0000567* was predicted to bind *hsa-miR-96-3p*, which is involved in the regulation of histone methylation [71]. Furthermore, a coding-non-coding gene co-expression network (CNC) was established by mapping of circRNA-miRNA-mRNA transcripts involving known PPGL susceptibility genes. It has been proposed that these circRNAs related to histone methylation function as miRNA sponges.

Table 1. Functions of ncRNAs with altered expression in PPGL.

ncRNA	Method and Sample (Number of Patients)	Expression Alteration and Suggested Role	Ref.
hsa-circ-0000567	RNA-seq (M = 7, N = 7)/ RT-qPCR (M = 33, N = 33)	related to histone methylation; predicted to bind hsa-miR-96-3p	[71]
hsa-circ-0002897	RNA-seq (M = 7, N = 7)/ RT-qPCR (M = 33, N = 33)	related to histone methylation	[71]
hsa-circ-0004473	RNA-seq (M = 7, N = 7)/ RT-qPCR (M = 33, N = 33)	related to histone methylation	[71]
hsa-miR-15a	Microarray (M = 12, B = 12, N = 5)/ RT-qPCR (B = 10, M = 10)	tumor suppressor; promotes cell death via downregulation of CCND1; underexpressed in metastatic pheochromocytoma	[72]
hsa-miR-16	Microarray (M = 12, B = 12, N = 5)/ RT-qPCR (B = 10, M = 10)	tumor suppressor; promotes cell death via downregulation of CCND1; underexpressed in metastatic pheochromocytoma	[72]
hsa-miR-21-3p	Discovery cohort: 443 metastatic vs. non-metastatic samples; Validation cohort: 49 non-metastatic and 8 non-metastatic vs. metastatic	regulates TSC2/mTOR axis; association in expression with sensitivity to rapamycin	[73]
hsa-miR-96-3p	RNA-seq (M = 7, N = 7)/ RT-qPCR (M = 33, N = 33)	regulates histone methylation; predicted to bind hsa-circ-0000567	[64]
hsa-miR-101	Microarray (M = 8, B = 42, N = 21)/ RT-qPCR (M = 25, B = 36, N = 21)	overexpression in SDHB mutant; overexpression in metastatic pheochromocytoma	[74]
hsa-miR-133b	Microarray (M = 5, B = 58, N = 6)/ RT-qPCR (M/B = 28, N = 2)	overexpression in VHL type PPGLs	[75]
hsa-miR-137	Microarray (M = 5, B = 58, N = 6)/ RT-qPCR (M/B = 28, N = 2)	overexpression in PPGL; downregulates RUNX2, KDM5B, IDH1	[75]
hsa-miR-139-3p	Microarray (M/B = 24)/ RT-qPCR (M/B = 33)	overexpression in VHL pheochromocytoma	[68]
hsa-miR-183	Microarray (M = 8, B = 42, N = 21)/ RT-qPCR (M = 25, B = 36, N = 21)	overexpression in SDHB mutant; overexpression in metastatic pheochromocytoma	[74]
hsa-miR-193b	RNA-seq (B/M = 183, N = 3)	underexpression in PPGL; mediates TGFBR3 expression through BSN-AS2 competition	[76]
hsa-miR-195	RNA-seq (B/M = 183, N = 3)	underexpression in PPGL; mediates TGFBR3 expression through BSN-AS2 competition	[76]
hsa-miR-210	RT-qPCR (B/M = 39)	overexpression in pseudohypoxia subtype; tumor hypoxia marker; associated with SDHx or VHL mutations	[15,77,78]

Table 1. Cont.

ncRNA	Method and Sample (Number of Patients)	Expression Alteration and Suggested Role	Ref.
hsa-miR-375	RNA-seq (B/M = 183, N = 3)	overexpression is PPGL	[76]
hsa-miR-382	Microarray (M = 5, B = 58, N = 6)/ RT-qPCR (M/B = 28, N = 2)	overexpression in tumors with VHL, SDHB, SDHD, RET mutations; targeting SOD2, C-MYC	[75]
hsa-miR-483-5p	Microarray (M = 12, B = 12, N = 5)/ RT-qPCR (B = 10, M = 10)	overexpression in metastatic PPGL; underexpression in SDHB among metastatic PPGL; worse disease-free survival in metastatic PPGL; co-amplification with IGF2 in metastatic adrenal tumors	[72,74,79]
hsa-miR-488	Microarray (M = 5, B = 58, N = 6)/ RT-qPCR (M/B = 28, N = 2)	overexpression in RET PPGL	[75]
hsa-miR-497	RNA-seq (B/M = 183, N = 3)	underexpression in PPGL; mediates TGFBR3 expression through BSN-AS2 competition	[76]
hsa-miR-508	RNA-seq (B/M = 183, N = 3)	underexpression in PPGL	[76]
hsa-miR-541	Microarray (M/B = 24)/ RT-qPCR (M/B = 33)	overexpression in VHL pheochromocytoma	[68]
hsa-miR-765	Microarray (M/B = 24)/ RT-qPCR (M/B = 33)	overexpression in VHL pheochromocytoma	[68]
hsa-miR-885-5p	Microarray (M/B = 24)/ RT-qPCR (M/B = 33)	overexpression in MEN2 PPGL	[68]
hsa-miR-1225-3p	Microarray (M/B = 24)/ RT-qPCR (M/B = 33)	overexpression in sporadic recurrent PPGL	[68]
lncRNA BSN-AS2	RNA-seq (B/M = 183, N = 3)	negative association with OS; mediate TGFBR3 expression through miR-193b, miR-195, miR-497 competition	[76]
lncRNA C9orf147	RNA-seq (B/M = 183, N = 3)	positive association with OS	[76]

B—benign; M—metastatic; N—normal/control; OS—overall survival.

Limitations of this study include the small number of patients included and that the control samples were derived from normal tissues adjacent to the tumor, instead of from individuals adrenalectomized for other (non-PPGL-related) causes. Epigenetic alterations can precede tumor formation (hence the prognostic value) and play major role in cell-to-cell communication (hence the therapeutic value) and by analyzing differential expression profiles, protein-protein interactions, gene set enrichment, dimensionality reduction, and tissue composition, it was elucidated that normal tissues adjacent to the tumor represent a unique in-between state concerning the molecular landscape [80]. Pan-cancer proinflammatory reaction in the adjacent endothelium was also suggested to bias the outcome of the normal tissue adjacent to the tumor as control tissue. Moreover, in this study, pathway analyses were also restricted only to bioinformatical predictions and the physical interaction between hsa_circ_0000567 and hsa-miR-96-3p has not been confirmed, either.

3.2. Long Non-Coding RNAs in PPGL

It is important not only to detect the expression profiles of non-coding RNAs, but also to have an understanding of their mechanistic interaction with other regulatory molecules.

For example, some lncRNAs have binding sites with microRNAs, thus sequestering them, thereby increasing the expression of their target genes.

In a competing endogenous RNAs (ceRNA) bioinformatics study, the expression of mRNAs, miRNAs, and lncRNAs in PPGL related to non-tumorous tissues were analyzed in datasets downloaded from the Cancer Genome Atlas (TCGA) [76]. To design a ceRNA study, it is a basic principle that the more binding sites the lncRNA have, the stronger they can down-regulate miRNA, thus inhibiting mRNA degradation. The authors observed 554 lncRNAs, 1775 mRNAs, and 40 miRNAs to be differentially expressed, from which 23 lncRNAs, 22 mRNAs, and 6 miRNAs were selected to build the ceRNA network. Twenty-three lncRNAs were identified to be differentially expressed in PPGL, and among them two were related to overall survival, i.e., lncRNA *BSN-AS2* and *C9orf147*, without having been described previously as related to other diseases. LncRNA *BSN-AS2* and *C9orf147* are future candidates to investigate their roles in tumorigenesis as their overexpression was associated with poor prognosis; moreover, the underexpression of *C9orf147* was associated with good prognosis (Table 1). Up-regulation of *BSN-AS2* has been observed in 183 pheochromocytoma patients related to a very low number (3) of control samples. As reported by the study, *BSN-AS2* might exert its impact on prognosis through altering receptor-type tyrosine-protein phosphatase eta (*PTPRJ*) mRNA expression by interacting with *miR-195* based on bioinformatical predictions. *PTPRJ* underexpression was found to be correlated with good prognosis. On the other hand, *BSN-AS2* competes with *miR-193b*, *miR-195* and *miR-497*, thereby modulating *TGFBR3* mRNA, which was positively associated with OS. Interestingly enough, *TGFBR3* mRNA levels were found to be underexpressed in pheochromocytoma patients, therefore, we are still in need of explanation of divergent expression levels between *TGFBR3* mRNA and *BSN-AS2* lncRNA. The findings of this bioinformatics study also need to be validated experimentally.

A recently published study about the transcriptome analysis of lncRNAs in PPGL revealed lncRNA phenotypes that can distinguish PPGL subtypes [81]. In the *SDHx* subtype, a putative lncRNA *BC063866* was found to be able to distinguish between metastatic tumors and tumors that remain indolent. lncRNA *BC063866* was found to be related to some of the genes involved in metastatic signature of various tumors such as *CDH19*, *ERBB3*, *PLP1*, and *SOX10*. Interestingly, these genes are also involved in neural crest and glial development [82]. Furthermore, lncRNA *BC063866* was found to be an independent risk factor for poor outcome in *SDHx* mutants, although this marker should be replicated in large prospective cohorts, as well.

Additionally, in a more recent ceRNA bioinformatics study, the previously described *miR-195-5p* and *miR-34a-5p* were predicted to be involved in the following two lncRNA–miRNA–mRNA axes: *AP001486.2/hsa-miR-195-5p/RCAN3* and *AP006333.2/hsa-miR-34a-5p/PTPRJ* respectively, functioning as tumor suppressors [83]. Higher expression levels of *RCAN3* (regulator of calcineurin 3) and *PTPRJ* in PPGL compared with normal adjacent tissue were experimentally validated by immunohistochemistry analysis. Matching with normal adjacent tissue might bias the results, as it was outlined before. The ceRNA study also revealed *RCAN3* as a good prognostic marker. In contrast to the previous study [76], this bioinformatical approach revealed underexpressed PTPRJ to be related to unfavorable prognosis. The controversial results concerning the relevance of *PTPRJ* highlight the limitations of bioinformatical analyses and the need for focused translational studies to establish the marker potential of a given coding or non-coding RNA molecule. *PTPRJ* might be involved in malignancies at different levels acting both as a tumor suppressor, but also in the regulation of antitumoral T-cell activity [84,85]. In a similar manner, *RCAN3* is implicated in the calcineurin–nuclear factor of activated T cells (NFAT) pathway-mediated immune response and also acts as a tumor suppressor [86]. It is also noteworthy that *miR-483-5p*, *miR-195*, and *miR-34a* were shown to be differentially expressed in adrenocortical cancer, as well [79,87].

3.3. MicroRNA in PPGL

According to one of the first studies from our research group on the miRNA expression profiles in FFPE samples of PPGL of various genetic backgrounds, *miR-139-3p*, *miR-541* and *miR-765* in VHL showed significantly higher expression compared to sporadic benign pheochromocytomas [68]. Altered expression of *miR-139-3p* has been demonstrated in various types of cancer [88–90]. *miR-541* has been shown to be upregulated in VHL compared with sporadic recurring pheochromocytomas (Table 1). Another finding has been the overexpression of *miR-885-5p* in MEN2-related pheochromocytoma compared with VHL- NF1-, sporadic recurring, and sporadic benign pheochromocytomas. Upregulated expression of *miR-1225-3p* has been found in sporadic recurrent pheochromocytomas in comparison to benign pheochromocytomas that raised its potential as a marker of PPGL recurrence. By using a bioinformatics pathway analysis approach, we raised the relevance of Notch-signaling in pheochromocytoma recurrence, and there are in vitro data showing the anti-proliferative potential of Notch-modulation in pheochromocytoma [91].

The previously detailed ceRNA network study in pheochromocytoma revealed the up-regulation of *miR-137* and *miR-375* and down-regulation of *miR-193b*, *miR-195*, *miR-497*, and *miR-508* [76].

The aforementioned recent ceRNA study also shed light on *miR-148b-3p* and *miR-338-3p* in respect of favorable prognosis and overall survival in PPGL [83].

Studies aimed at understanding miR expression pattern changes between benign and metastatic PPGL are pivotal in order to be able to differentiate between these two entities. Whole-genome microarray profiling revealed eight miRNAs to be differentially expressed [74]. In this study, "malignancy" was established when there was clinical evidence of tumor from "extra-chromaffin" sites corresponding to the current WHO definition of metastatic PPGL, but also when there was extensive local invasion. Significantly altered expression of *miR-101*, *miR-183*, and *miR-483-5p* was revealed in metastatic pheochromocytoma tissues versus benign ones and validated by RT-qPCR. Among them, *miR-101* and *miR-183* significantly differed in *SDHB* mutant vs. wild type samples and interestingly, *miR-483-5p* had significantly lower expression in *SDHB* mutant malignant pheochromocytoma compared to all other malignant pheochromocytomas. Furthermore, *miR-101*, *miR-183*, and *miR-483-5p* were measurable from serum samples, as well. In practice, this might raise the possibility that a patient without *SDHB* mutation might be screened for miR expression profile changes to assess the risk of malignancy. In another study investigating snap-frozen samples, significantly higher expression of *miR-483-5p* in metastatic PPGL was found, as well, validated by RT-qPCR [72]. The definition of metastatic disease corresponded to the WHO definition in this study, i.e., only tumors with metastases at "extra-chromaffin" sites were considered metastatic. On the other hand, lower expression of the general tumor suppressor miRNAs *miR-15a* and *miR-16* were revealed in metastatic versus benign tumors. *miR-15* and *miR-16* were raised as potential therapeutic targets, as their restoration in expression promoted cell death, partly through the down-regulation of *CCND1* (Cyclin D1) in metastatic rat pheochromocytoma cells [72]. Up-regulation of *miR-483-5p* in metastatic tumors corresponded to the amplification of *IGF2* (insulin-like growth factor 2) mRNA due to their co-expression from the same locus [72]. *IGF2* protein and mRNA were shown to be significantly increased in metastatic PPGL, which is consistent with other studies investigating the relationship between *IGF2*, *miR-483-5p*, and adrenocortical carcinoma, where *miR-483-5p* is also overexpressed in comparison to benign adrenocortical adenomas [70,79]. Moreover, *miR-483-5p* is a marker of worse disease-free survival in metastatic pheochromocytoma [72].

As mentioned before, *miR-210* (a general hypoxamiR [92]) is a key molecule in pseudohypoxia-type PPGL functioning as a master regulator [77]. When PPGL was compared with normal adrenal medullary tissues, overexpressed *miR-210* was significantly associated with *SDHx* or *VHL* mutant genotypes known to exhibit the pseudohypoxia phenotype [78].

The aforementioned *miR-96* and *miR-183* were described to contribute to the differentiation block of cells of *SDHB* mutated tumors [93]. An integrative study of expression signatures of PPGL revealed that *miR-382* targeting *SOD2* (superoxide dismutase 2) and *C-MYC* was up-regulated in tumors of most genetic backgrounds (*VHL, SDHB, SDHD, RET*) except in MAX mutants [75]. Up-regulation of *miR-137* was also observed in most genetic backgrounds (*VHL, SDHB, SDHD, RET*) except in MAX. *miR-137* possibly down-regulates *RUNX2, KDM5B* (histone H3 Lys4 demethylase) and interferes with *IDH1–EGLN* pathway, thus regulating neuronal gene activity as it has been previously reported [94]. *miR-885-5p* (interestingly a tumor suppressor) and *miR-488* were specific to MEN2-related PPGLs. *miR-133b* was related to *VHL*-type PPGLs. Robust upregulation was identified with *miR-96* especially in *SDHB* mutants [75].

In neuronal pheochromocytoma 12 cells (PC-12) *miR-18a* is involved in hypoxic responses through down-regulation of lncRNA urothelial carcinoma associated 1 (UCA1), sex determining region Y-box 6 (SOX6), and hypoxia inducible factor 1 subunit α (HIF-1α) [95]. However, the regulatory functions of *miR-18a* on HIF-1α have only been described previously in lung cancer stem-like cells, choroidal endothelial cells, and in a breast cancer xenograft model [96–98]. Given the tissue-specific nature of miRNA expression and action, the interaction between *miR-18a* and HIF-1α in PPGL should be investigated in pheochromocytoma cells. Under hypoxic conditions, UCA1 is upregulated, making cells more prone to hypoxic injuries through the putative down-regulation of *miR-18a*. Down-regulation of UCA1 is associated with the attenuation of hypoxic injuries. Furthermore, UCA1 directly targets and down-regulates *miR-18a* and vice versa, and the up-regulation of *miR-18a* alleviates hypoxic injury through downregulation of UCA1. Similar to UCA1, SOX6 also acts as a provoking factor in hypoxic injuries and inhibition of SOX6 leads to an ease of hypoxic injury (Figure 3).

MiR profiling also holds therapy-modifying potential in precision medicine. A recent study revealed a new regulatory axis of *miR-21-3p*/TSC2/mTOR signaling pathway as a future target for treatment, as *miR-21-3p* showed significant association with sensitivity to rapamycin, thus, *miR-21-3p* could be a marker for mTOR inhibitor therapy (Figure 3) [73]. This study not only shed light on miR profiling as a tool in risk stratification in PPGL, but also gives us a predictive biomarker accessible via liquid biopsy to investigate in a larger cohort in the future.

It is quite intriguing that some microRNAs seem to be differentially expressed between both benign and metastatic PPGL and benign and malignant adrenocortical tumors. These include *miR-483-5p, miR-195,* and *miR-34a* [72,74,76,79,83,87]. As the adrenal cortex is of mesodermic origin, whereas the adrenal medulla is of ectodermic origin, these common changes in microRNA expression might even suggest some common adrenal-specific features in tumorigenesis. Confirmation in larger cohorts is warranted.

Based on these significant differences in expression profiles, miR, lncRNA, and circRNA profile analysis are still one of the chief candidates for an adjunct diagnostic marker for "hard-to-diagnose" tumors.

3.4. ncRNAs as Therapeutic Targets in PPGL

Currently, there are no clinical studies evaluating ncRNAs as therapeutic targets in PPGL. Since treatment options for metastatic PPGL are rather limited, novel molecular targets are intensively sought for. We can only hypothesize on the relevance of ncRNAs in the treatment of PPGL from specific observations. Some of the ncRNA detailed above might represent potential treatment targets or exploited as markers of therapy-modifying potential. For example, miR-21-3p was shown to be correlated with rapamycin sensitivity, thus, miR-21-3p could be a marker for mTOR inhibitor therapy in PPGL (Figure 3) [73]. Detailed preclinical molecular investigations will be necessary to define the ncRNA that could be exploited as treatment targets (e.g., restoration of underexpressed "tumor suppressor" ncRNA expression or targeting overexpressed oncogenic ncRNA by small interfering RNA), but there would be quite a long way ahead before the clinical application of any treatments targeting these pathways given the numerous difficulties in such treatment strategies (e.g., problems of administration, question of the vector, off-site effects, etc.) [99].

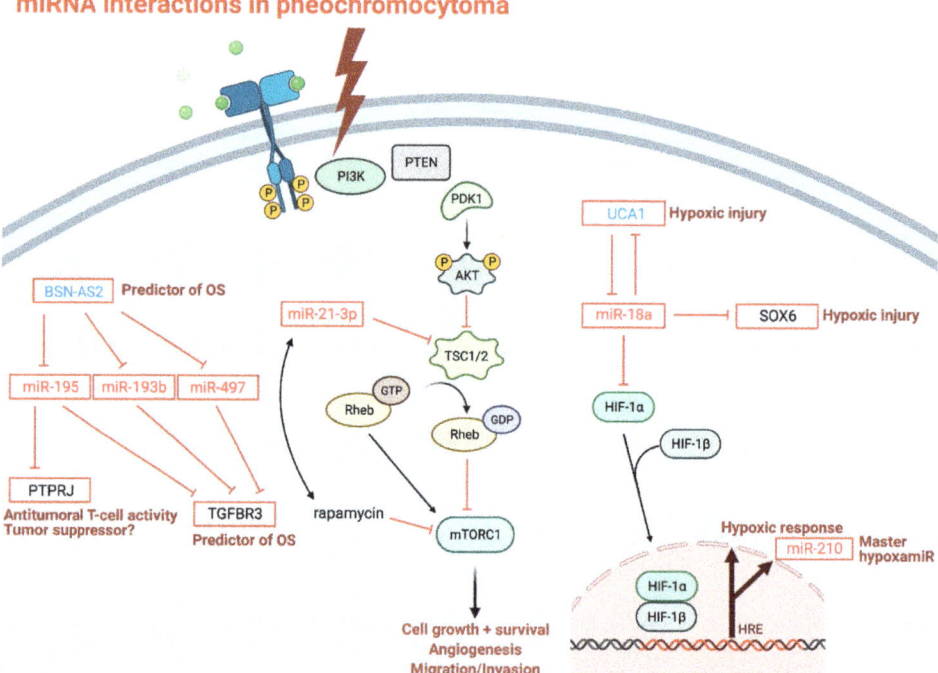

Figure 3. miRNA interactions in pheochromocytoma: Transmembrane tyrosine kinase receptor activation is the first step in the mTOR signaling pathway; thunderbolt represents activation of mTOR pathway in pheochromocytoma; P indicates phosphorylation sites; blunt-head lines indicate inhibition; faded arrows indicate downstream activation; solid arrows indicate direct activation; right-angle arrow indicates gene expression. Abbreviations: BSN-AS2: long non-coding RNA BSN-AS2; OS: overall survival; PTPRJ: receptor-type tyrosine-protein phosphatase eta; TGFBR3: transforming growth factor beta receptor 3; PI3K: phosphoinositide 3-kinase; PTEN: phosphatase and tensin homolog; PDK1: phosphoinositide-dependent kinase 1; AKT1: a serine/threonine protein kinase; TSC1/2: tuberous sclerosis complex subunit 1; Rheb: Ras homolog enriched in brain; GTP: guanosine triphosphate; GDP: guanosine diphosphate; mTROC1: mammalian target of rapamycin complex 1; rapamycin: mTOR inhibitor; UCA1: long non-coding RNA urothelial cancer associated 1; SOX6: SRY (sex determining region Y)-box 6; HIF-1 α/β: hypoxia inducible factor 1 subunit α/β; HRE: hypoxia response element; PC-12: pheochromocytoma 12 cell line, OS: overall survival. Note that miR-18 mediated down-regulation of HIF-1α has only been established in lung cancer stem-like cells, choroidal endothelial cells, and in breast cancer xenograft model and not yet in pheochromocytoma cells.

4. Conclusions

Pheochromocytoma was originally named after its microscopic and staining features and due to the complex nature of the disease, current diagnostics encompasses not only imaging and laboratory tests, but also the quest for new biomarkers on the horizon of an ever-evolving field of non-protein-coding ribonucleic acids. The emerging role of non-coding RNA in the setting of clinical evaluation and therapeutic approaches of clinically challenging tumors is an attractive candidate for precision medicine. By studying non-coding RNA, we might be able to double attack the therapeutic and the diagnostic ends of PPGL in our efforts towards making a reliable tool for the distinction and targeted therapy of metastatic and benign tumors.

Author Contributions: All authors have read and agreed to the published version of the manuscript.

Funding: Hungarian National Research, Development and Innovation Office (NKFIH) grant K134215 to Peter Igaz. The study was also financed by the Higher Education Institutional Excellence Program of the Ministry of Human Capacities in Hungary, within the framework of the molecular biology thematic program of the Semmelweis University.

Conflicts of Interest: The authors declare no conflict of interest.

References

1. Wong, C.C.; Qian, Y.; Yu, J. Interplay between epigenetics and metabolism in oncogenesis: Mechanisms and therapeutic approaches. *Oncogene* **2017**, *36*, 3359–3374. [CrossRef]
2. Beard, C.M.; Sheps, S.G.; Kurland, L.T.; Carney, J.A.; Lie, J.T. Occurrence of pheochromocytoma in Rochester, Minnesota, 1950 through 1979. *Mayo Clin. Proc.* **1983**, *58*, 802–804.
3. Ladroue, C.; Carcenac, R.; Leporrier, M.; Gad, S.; Le Hello, C.; Galateau-Salle, F.; Feunteun, J.; Pouysségur, J.; Richard, S.; Gardie, B. PHD2 Mutation and Congenital Erythrocytosis with Paraganglioma. *N. Engl. J. Med.* **2008**, *359*, 2685–2692. [CrossRef]
4. Pereira, B.D.; Luiz, H.V.; Ferreira, A.G.; Portugal, J. Genetics of Pheochromocytoma and Paraganglioma. In *Paraganglioma: A Multidisciplinary Approach*; Codon Publications: Brisbane, Australia, 2019; pp. 1–22.
5. Benn, D.E.; Robinson, B.G.; Clifton-Bligh, R.J. Clinical manifestations of paraganglioma syndromes types 1–5. *Endocr. Relat. Cancer* **2015**, *22*, T91–T103. [CrossRef] [PubMed]
6. Alrezk, R.; Suarez, A.; Tena, I.; Pacak, K. Update of Pheochromocytoma Syndromes: Genetics, Biochemical Evaluation, and Imaging. *Front. Endocrinol. (Lausanne)* **2018**, *9*, 515. [CrossRef] [PubMed]
7. Crona, J.; Taïeb, D.; Pacak, K. New perspectives on pheochromocytoma and paraganglioma: Toward a molecular classification. *Endocr. Rev.* **2017**, *38*, 489–515. [CrossRef] [PubMed]
8. Dahia, P.L.M. Pheochromocytoma and paraganglioma pathogenesis: Learning from genetic heterogeneity. *Nat. Rev. Cancer* **2014**, *14*, 108–119. [CrossRef]
9. Burnichon, N.; Vescovo, L.; Amar, L.; Libé, R.; de Reynies, A.; Venisse, A.; Jouanno, E.; Laurendeau, I.; Parfait, B.; Bertherat, J.; et al. Integrative genomic analysis reveals somatic mutations in pheochromocytoma and paraganglioma. *Hum. Mol. Genet.* **2011**, *20*, 3974–3985. [CrossRef]
10. Lenders, J.W.M.; Duh, Q.Y.; Eisenhofer, G.; Gimenez-Roqueplo, A.P.; Grebe, S.K.G.; Murad, M.H.; Naruse, M.; Pacak, K.; Young, W.F. Pheochromocytoma and paraganglioma: An endocrine society clinical practice guideline. *J. Clin. Endocrinol. Metab.* **2014**, *99*, 1915–1942. [CrossRef] [PubMed]
11. Ayala-Ramirez, M.; Feng, L.; Johnson, M.M.; Ejaz, S.; Habra, M.A.; Rich, T.; Busaidy, N.; Cote, G.J.; Perrier, N.; Phan, A.; et al. Clinical Risk Factors for Malignancy and Overall Survival in Patients with Pheochromocytomas and Sympathetic Paragangliomas: Primary Tumor Size and Primary Tumor Location as Prognostic Indicators. *J. Clin. Endocrinol. Metab.* **2011**, *96*, 717–725. [CrossRef] [PubMed]
12. Gimenez-Roqueplo, A.-P.; Favier, J.; Rustin, P.; Rieubland, C.; Crespin, M.; Nau, V.; Khau Van Kien, P.; Corvol, P.; Plouin, P.F.; Jeunemaitre, X.; et al. Mutations in the SDHB Gene Are Associated with Extra-adrenal and/or Malignant Phaeochromocytomas. *Cancer Res.* **2003**, *63*, 5615–5621.
13. Eisenhofer, G.; Bornstein, S.R.; Brouwers, F.M.; Cheung, N.K.V.; Dahia, P.L.; De Krijger, R.R.; Giordano, T.J.; Greene, L.A.; Goldstein, D.S.; Lehnert, H.; et al. Malignant pheochromocytoma: Current status and initiatives for future progress. *Endocr. Relat. Cancer* **2004**, *11*, 423–436. [CrossRef]
14. Fishbein, L.; Leshchiner, I.; Walter, V.; Danilova, L.; Robertson, A.G.; Johnson, A.R.; Lichtenberg, T.M.; Murray, B.A.; Ghayee, H.K.; Else, T.; et al. Comprehensive Molecular Characterization of Pheochromocytoma and Paraganglioma. *Cancer Cell* **2017**, *31*, 181–193. [CrossRef] [PubMed]
15. Huang, X.; Le, Q.T.; Giaccia, A.J. MiR-210—Micromanager of the hypoxia pathway. *Trends Mol. Med.* **2010**, *16*, 230–237. [CrossRef] [PubMed]
16. Lefebvre, M.; Foulkes, W.D. Pheochromocytoma and paraganglioma syndromes: Genetics and management update. *Curr. Oncol.* **2014**, *21*, e8. [CrossRef] [PubMed]
17. Stein, P.P.; Black, H.R. A simplified diagnostic approach to pheochromocytoma: A review of the literature and report of one institution's experience. *Medicine* **1991**, *70*, 46–66. [CrossRef]
18. Cotesta, D.; Petramala, L.; Serra, V.; Pergolini, M.; Crescenzi, E.; Zinnamosca, L.; De Toma, G.; Ciardi, A.; Carbone, I.; Massa, R.; et al. Clinical experience with pheochromocytoma in a single centre over 16 years. *High. Blood Press Cardiovasc. Prev.* **2009**, *16*, 183–193. [CrossRef] [PubMed]
19. Manger, W.M.; Gifford, R.W. Pheochromocytoma. *J. Clin. Hypertens* **2002**, *4*, 62–72. [CrossRef]
20. Newell, K.A.; Prinz, R.A.; Pickleman, J.; Braithwaite, S.; Brooks, M.; Karson, T.H.; Glisson, S. Pheochromocytoma Multisystem Crisis: A Surgical Emergency. *Arch. Surg.* **1988**, *123*, 956–959. [CrossRef] [PubMed]
21. Drenou, B.; Le Tulzo, Y.; Caulet-Maugendre, S.; Le Guerrier, A.; Leclerq, C.; Guilhem, I.; Lecoq, N.; Fauchet, R.; Thomas, R. Pheochromocytoma and secondary erythrocytosis: Role of tumour erythropoietin secretion. *Nouv. Rev. Fr. Hematol.* **1995**, *37*, 197–199.

22. Guller, U.; Turek, J.; Eubanks, S.; DeLong, E.R.; Oertli, D.; Feldman, J.M. Detecting pheochromocytoma: Defining the most sensitive test. *Ann. Surg.* **2006**, *243*, 102–107. [CrossRef]
23. Lenders, J.W.M.; Pacak, K.; Walther, M.M.; Marston Linehan, W.; Mannelli, M.; Friberg, P.; Keiser, H.R.; Goldstein, D.S.; Eisenhofer, G. Biochemical diagnosis of pheochromocytoma: Which test is best? *J. Am. Med. Assoc.* **2002**, *287*, 1427–1434. [CrossRef]
24. Sawka, A.M.; Jaeschke, R.; Singh, R.J.; Young, W.F. A comparison of biochemical tests for pheochromocytoma: Measurement of fractionated plasma metanephrines compared with the combination of 24-hour urinary metanephrines and catecholamines. *J. Clin. Endocrinol. Metab.* **2003**, *88*, 553–558. [CrossRef]
25. Grossrubatscher, E.; Dalino, P.; Vignati, F.; Gambacorta, M.; Pugliese, R.; Boniardi, M.; Rossetti, O.; Marocchi, A.; Bertuzzi, M.; Loli, P. The role of chromogranin A in the management of patients with phaeochromocytoma. *Clin. Endocrinol. (Oxf.)* **2006**, *65*, 287–293. [CrossRef] [PubMed]
26. Pacak, K.; Linehan, W.M.; Eisenhofer, G.; Walther, M.M.; Goldstein, D.S. Recent advances in genetics, diagnosis, localization, and treatment of pheochromocytoma. *Ann. Intern. Med.* **2001**, *134*, 315–329. [CrossRef] [PubMed]
27. Stenman, A.; Zedenius, J.; Juhlin, C.C. The value of histological algorithms to predict the malignancy potential of pheochromocytomas and abdominal paragangliomas—A meta-analysis and systematic review of the literature. *Cancers* **2019**, *11*, 225. [CrossRef] [PubMed]
28. Lam, A.K. Update on Adrenal Tumours in 2017 World Health Organization (WHO) of Endocrine Tumours. *Endocr. Pathol.* **2017**, *28*, 213–227. [CrossRef]
29. Hescot, S.; Lebouilleux, S.; Amar, L.; Vezzosi, D.; Borget, I.; Bournaud-Salinas, C.; de la Fouchardiere, C.; Libé, R.; Do Cao, C.; Niccoli, P.; et al. One-Year Progression-Free Survival of Therapy-Naive Patients With Malignant Pheochromocytoma and Paraganglioma. *J. Clin. Endocrinol. Metab.* **2013**, *98*, 4006–4012. [CrossRef] [PubMed]
30. Amar, L.; Servais, A.; Gimenez-Roqueplo, A.-P.; Zinzindohoue, F.; Chatellier, G.; Plouin, P.-F. Year of Diagnosis, Features at Presentation, and Risk of Recurrence in Patients with Pheochromocytoma or Secreting Paraganglioma. *J. Clin. Endocrinol. Metab.* **2005**, *90*, 2110–2116. [CrossRef]
31. Hamidi, O.; Young, W.F.; Iñiguez-Ariza, N.M.; Kittah, N.E.; Gruber, L.; Bancos, C.; Tamhane, S.; Bancos, I. Malignant pheochromocytoma and paraganglioma: 272 patients over 55 years. *J. Clin. Endocrinol. Metab.* **2017**, *102*, 3296–3305. [CrossRef]
32. Plouin, P.F.; Amar, L.; Dekkers, O.M.; Fassnach, M.; Gimenez-Roqueplo, A.P.; Lenders, J.W.M.; Lussey-Lepoutre, C.; Steichen, O. European Society of Endocrinology Clinical Practice Guideline for long-term follow-up of patients operated on for a phaeochromocytoma or a paraganglioma. *Eur. J. Endocrinol.* **2016**, *174*, G1–G10. [CrossRef]
33. Lloyd, R.V.; Osamura, R.Y.; Klöppel, G.; Rosai, J. *World Health Organization Classification of Tumours of Endocrine Organs*, 4th ed.; Lloyd, R.V., Osamura, R.Y., Klöppel, G., Rosai, J., Eds.; International Agency for Research on Cancer: Lyon, France, 2017; ISBN 978-92-832-4493-6.
34. Bisogni, V.; Petramala, L.; Oliviero, G.; Bonvicini, M.; Mezzadri, M.; Olmati, F.; Concistrè, A.; Saracino, V.; Celi, M.; Tonnarini, G.; et al. Analysis of short-term blood pressure variability in pheochromocytoma/paraganglioma patients. *Cancers* **2019**, *11*, 658. [CrossRef]
35. Prejbisz, A.; Lenders, J.W.M.; Eisenhofer, G.; Januszewicz, A. Mortality associated with phaeochromocytoma. *Horm. Metab. Res.* **2013**, *45*, 154–158. [CrossRef]
36. Huang, H.; Abraham, J.; Hung, E.; Averbuch, S.; Merino, M.; Steinberg, S.M.; Pacak, K.; Fojo, T. Treatment of malignant pheochromocytoma/paraganglioma with cyclophosphamide, vincristine, and dacarbazine: Recommendation from a 22-year follow-up of 18 patients. *Cancer* **2008**, *113*, 2020–2028. [CrossRef] [PubMed]
37. O'Kane, G.M.; Ezzat, S.; Joshua, A.M.; Bourdeau, I.; Leibowitz-Amit, R.; Olney, H.J.; Krzyzanowska, M.; Reuther, D.; Chin, S.; Wang, L.; et al. A phase 2 trial of sunitinib in patients with progressive paraganglioma or pheochromocytoma: The SNIPP trial. *Br. J. Cancer* **2019**, *120*, 1113–1119. [CrossRef]
38. Burotto Pichun, M.E.; Edgerly, M.; Velarde, M.; Bates, S.E.; Daerr, R.; Adams, K.; Pacak, K.; Fojo, T. Phase II clinical trial of axitinib in metastatic pheochromocytomas and paraganlgiomas (P/PG): Preliminary results. *J. Clin. Oncol.* **2015**, *33*, 457. [CrossRef]
39. Ferreira, C.V.; Siqueira, D.R.; Romitti, M.; Ceolin, L.; Brasil, B.A.; Meurer, L.; Capp, C.; Maia, A.L. Role of VEGF-A and its receptors in sporadic and MEN2-associated pheochromocytoma. *Int. J. Mol. Sci.* **2014**, *15*, 5323–5336. [CrossRef]
40. Nivolumab and Ipilimumab in Treating Patients With Rare Tumors—Full Text View—ClinicalTrials.gov. Available online: https://clinicaltrials.gov/ct2/show/NCT02834013 (accessed on 7 February 2021).
41. Frumovitz, M.; Westin, S.N.; Salvo, G.; Zarifa, A.; Xu, M.; Yap, T.A.; Rodon, A.J.; Karp, D.D.; Abonofal, A.; Jazaeri, A.A.; et al. Phase II study of pembrolizumab efficacy and safety in women with recurrent small cell neuroendocrine carcinoma of the lower genital tract. *Gynecol. Oncol.* **2020**, *158*, 570–575. [CrossRef] [PubMed]
42. Pang, Y.; Lu, Y.; Caisova, V.; Liu, Y.; Bullova, P.; Huynh, T.T.; Zhou, Y.; Yu, D.; Frysak, Z.; Hartmann, I.; et al. Targeting NAD$\flat$/PARP DNA repair pathway as a novel therapeutic approach to SDHB-mutated cluster I pheochromocytoma and paraganglioma. *Clin. Cancer Res.* **2018**, *24*, 3423–3432. [CrossRef]
43. Oh, D.-Y.; Kim, T.-W.; Park, Y.S.; Shin, S.J.; Shin, S.H.; Song, E.-K.; Lee, H.J.; Lee, K.; Bang, Y.-J. Phase 2 study of everolimus monotherapy in patients with nonfunctioning neuroendocrine tumors or pheochromocytomas/paragangliomas. *Cancer* **2012**, *118*, 6162–6170. [CrossRef] [PubMed]
44. Ilanchezhian, M.; Jha, A.; Pacak, K.; Del Rivero, J. Emerging Treatments for Advanced/Metastatic Pheochromocytoma and Paraganglioma. *Curr. Treat. Options Oncol.* **2020**, *21*, 1–18. [CrossRef]

45. Grillone, K.; Riillo, C.; Riillo, C.; Scionti, F.; Rocca, R.; Rocca, R.; Tradigo, G.; Guzzi, P.H.; Alcaro, S.; Alcaro, S.; et al. Non-coding RNAs in cancer: Platforms and strategies for investigating the genomic "dark matter". *J. Exp. Clin. Cancer Res.* **2020**, *39*, 117. [CrossRef]
46. Kaikkonen, M.U.; Lam, M.T.Y.; Glass, C.K. Non-coding RNAs as regulators of gene expression and epigenetics. *Cardiovasc. Res.* **2011**, *90*, 430–440. [CrossRef] [PubMed]
47. Ponting, C.P.; Oliver, P.L.; Reik, W. Evolution and Functions of Long Noncoding RNAs. *Cell* **2009**, *136*, 629–641. [CrossRef]
48. Kim, T.K.; Hemberg, M.; Gray, J.M. Enhancer RNAs: A class of long noncoding RNAs synthesized at enhancers. *Cold Spring Harb. Perspect. Biol.* **2015**, *7*, a018622. [CrossRef] [PubMed]
49. Jansson, M.D.; Lund, A.H. MicroRNA and cancer. *Mol. Oncol.* **2012**, *6*, 590–610. [CrossRef] [PubMed]
50. Chi, Y.; Wang, D.; Wang, J.; Yu, W.; Yang, J. Long Non-Coding RNA in the Pathogenesis of Cancers. *Cells* **2019**, *8*, 1015. [CrossRef]
51. Schmitt, A.M.; Chang, H.Y. Long Noncoding RNAs in Cancer Pathways. *Cancer Cell* **2016**, *29*, 452–463. [CrossRef]
52. Kung, J.T.Y.; Colognori, D.; Lee, J.T. Long noncoding RNAs: Past, present, and future. *Genetics* **2013**, *193*, 651–669. [CrossRef]
53. Hanahan, D.; Weinberg, R.A. Hallmarks of cancer: The next generation. *Cell* **2011**, *144*, 646–674. [CrossRef]
54. Memczak, S.; Jens, M.; Elefsinioti, A.; Torti, F.; Krueger, J.; Rybak, A.; Maier, L.; Mackowiak, S.D.; Gregersen, L.H.; Munschauer, M.; et al. Circular RNAs are a large class of animal RNAs with regulatory potency. *Nature* **2013**, *495*, 333–338. [CrossRef]
55. Li, W.; Zhong, C.; Jiao, J.; Li, P.; Cui, B.; Ji, C.; Ma, D. Characterization of hsa_circ_0004277 as a new biomarker for acute myeloid leukemia via circular RNA profile and bioinformatics analysis. *Int. J. Mol. Sci.* **2017**, *18*, 597. [CrossRef]
56. Zheng, Q.; Bao, C.; Guo, W.; Li, S.; Chen, J.; Chen, B.; Luo, Y.; Lyu, D.; Li, Y.; Shi, G.; et al. Circular RNA profiling reveals an abundant circHIPK3 that regulates cell growth by sponging multiple miRNAs. *Nat. Commun.* **2016**, *7*, 11215. [CrossRef]
57. Ashwal-Fluss, R.; Meyer, M.; Pamudurti, N.R.; Ivanov, A.; Bartok, O.; Hanan, M.; Evantal, N.; Memczak, S.; Rajewsky, N.; Kadener, S. CircRNA Biogenesis competes with Pre-mRNA splicing. *Mol. Cell* **2014**, *56*, 55–66. [CrossRef] [PubMed]
58. Salzman, J.; Chen, R.E.; Olsen, M.N.; Wang, P.L.; Brown, P.O. Cell-Type Specific Features of Circular RNA Expression. *PLoS Genet.* **2013**, *9*, e1003777. [CrossRef]
59. Enuka, Y.; Lauriola, M.; Feldman, M.E.; Sas-Chen, A.; Ulitsky, I.; Yarden, Y. Circular RNAs are long-lived and display only minimal early alterations in response to a growth factor. *Nucleic Acids Res.* **2016**, *44*, 1370–1383. [CrossRef] [PubMed]
60. Jeck, W.R.; Sharpless, N.E. Detecting and characterizing circular RNAs. *Nat. Biotechnol.* **2014**, *32*, 453–461. [CrossRef]
61. Li, Z.; Huang, C.; Bao, C.; Chen, L.; Lin, M.; Wang, X.; Zhong, G.; Yu, B.; Hu, W.; Dai, L.; et al. Exon-intron circular RNAs regulate transcription in the nucleus. *Nat. Struct. Mol. Biol.* **2015**, *22*, 256–264. [CrossRef]
62. Du, W.W.; Yang, W.; Liu, E.; Yang, Z.; Dhaliwal, P.; Yang, B.B. Foxo3 circular RNA retards cell cycle progression via forming ternary complexes with p21 and CDK2. *Nucleic Acids Res.* **2016**, *44*, 2846. [CrossRef]
63. Holdt, L.M.; Kohlmaier, A.; Teupser, D. Molecular roles and function of circular RNAs in eukaryotic cells. *Cell Mol. Life Sci.* **2018**, *75*, 1071–1098. [CrossRef] [PubMed]
64. Krol, J.; Loedige, I.; Filipowicz, W. The widespread regulation of microRNA biogenesis, function and decay. *Nat. Rev. Genet.* **2010**, *11*, 597–610. [CrossRef] [PubMed]
65. Guo, Z.; Maki, M.; Ding, R.; Yang, Y.; Zhang, B.; Xiong, L. Genome-wide survey of tissue-specific microRNA and transcription factor regulatory networks in 12 tissues. *Sci. Rep.* **2014**, *4*, 5150. [CrossRef] [PubMed]
66. Roberts, T.C. The MicroRNA biology of the Mammalian nucleus. *Mol. Ther. Nucleic Acids* **2014**, *3*, e188. [CrossRef]
67. Bartel, D.P. MicroRNAs: Genomics, biogenesis, mechanism, and function. *Cell* **2004**, *116*, 281–297. [CrossRef]
68. Tömböl, Z.; Éder, K.; Kovács, A.; Szabó, P.M.; Kulka, J.; Likó, I.; Zalatnai, A.; Rácz, G.; Tóth, M.; Patócs, A.; et al. MicroRNA expression profiling in benign (sporadic and hereditary) and recurring adrenal pheochromocytomas. *Mod. Pathol.* **2010**, *23*, 1583–1595. [CrossRef] [PubMed]
69. Igaz, I.; Igaz, P. Tumor surveillance by circulating microRNAs: A hypothesis. *Cell Mol. Life Sci.* **2014**, *71*, 4081–4087. [CrossRef]
70. Igaz, P.; Igaz, I.; Nagy, Z.; Nyírő, G.; Szabó, P.M.; Falus, A.; Patócs, A.; Rácz, K. MicroRNAs in adrenal tumors: Relevance for pathogenesis, diagnosis, and therapy. *Cell Mol. Life Sci.* **2015**, *72*, 417–428. [CrossRef]
71. Yu, A.; Li, M.; Xing, C.; Chen, D.; Wang, C.; Xiao, Q.; Zhang, L.; Pang, Y.; Wang, Y.; Zu, X.; et al. A Comprehensive Analysis Identified the Key Differentially Expressed Circular Ribonucleic Acids and Methylation-Related Function in Pheochromocytomas and Paragangliomas. *Front. Genet.* **2020**, *11*, 1. [CrossRef]
72. Meyer-Rochow, G.Y.; Jackson, N.E.; Conaglen, J.V.; Whittle, D.E.; Kunnimalaiyaan, M.; Chen, H.; Westin, G.; Sandgren, J.; Stålberg, P.; Khanafshar, E.; et al. MicroRNA profiling of benign and malignant pheochromocytomas identifies novel diagnostic and therapeutic targets. *Endocr. Relat. Cancer* **2010**, *17*, 835–846. [CrossRef]
73. Calsina, B.; Castro-Vega, L.J.; Torres-Pérez, R.; Inglada-Pérez, L.; Currás-Freixes, M.; Roldán-Romero, J.M.; Mancikova, V.; Letón, R.; Remacha, L.; Santos, M.; et al. Integrative multi-omics analysis identifies a prognostic miRNA signature and a targetable miR-21-3p/TSC2/mTOR axis in metastatic pheochromocytoma/paraganglioma. *Theranostics* **2019**, *9*, 4946–4958. [CrossRef]
74. Patterson, E.; Webb, R.; Weisbrod, A.; Bian, B.; He, M.; Zhang, L.; Holloway, A.K.; Krishna, R.; Nilubol, N.; Pacak, K.; et al. The microRNA expression changes associated with malignancy and SDHB mutation in pheochromocytoma. *Endocr. Relat. Cancer* **2012**, *19*, 157–166. [CrossRef]
75. De Cubas, A.A.; Leandro-García, L.J.; Schiavi, F.; Mancikova, V.; Comino-Méndez, I.; Inglada-Pérez, L.; Perez-Martinez, M.; Ibarz, N.; Ximénez-Embún, P.; López-Jiménez, E.; et al. Integrative analysis of miRNA and mRNA expression profiles in pheochromocytoma and paraganglioma identifies genotype-specific markers and potentially regulated pathways. *Endocr. Relat. Cancer* **2013**, *20*, 477–493. [CrossRef] [PubMed]

76. Liang, Y.-C.; Wu, Y.-P.; Chen, D.-N.; Chen, S.-H.; Li, X.-D.; Sun, X.-L.; Wei, Y.; Ning, X.; Xue, X.-Y. Building a Competing Endogenous RNA Network to Find Potential Long Non-Coding RNA Biomarkers for Pheochromocytoma. *Cell Physiol. Biochem.* **2018**, *51*, 2916–2924. [CrossRef] [PubMed]
77. Fasanaro, P.; Greco, S.; Lorenzi, M.; Pescatori, M.; Brioschi, M.; Kulshreshtha, R.; Banfi, C.; Stubbs, A.; Calin, G.A.; Ivan, M.; et al. An integrated approach for experimental target identification of hypoxia-induced miR-210. *J. Biol. Chem.* **2009**, *284*, 35134–35143. [CrossRef]
78. Tsang, V.H.M.; Dwight, T.; Benn, D.E.; Meyer-Rochow, G.Y.; Gill, A.J.; Sywak, M.; Sidhu, S.; Veivers, D.; Sue, C.M.; Robinson, B.G.; et al. Overexpression of miR-210 is associated with SDH-related pheochromocytomas, paragangliomas, and gastrointestinal stromal tumours. *Endocr. Relat. Cancer* **2014**, *21*, 415–426. [CrossRef]
79. Soon, P.S.H.; Tacon, L.J.; Gill, A.J.; Bambach, C.P.; Sywak, M.S.; Campbell, P.R.; Yeh, M.W.; Wong, S.G.; Clifton-Bligh, R.J.; Robinson, B.G.; et al. miR-195 and miR-483-5p identified as predictors of poor prognosis in adrenocortical cancer. *Clin. Cancer Res.* **2009**, *15*, 7684–7692. [CrossRef] [PubMed]
80. Aran, D.; Camarda, R.; Odegaard, J.; Paik, H.; Oskotsky, B.; Krings, G.; Goga, A.; Sirota, M.; Butte, A.J. Comprehensive analysis of normal adjacent to tumor transcriptomes. *Nat. Commun.* **2017**, *8*, 1–14. [CrossRef] [PubMed]
81. Job, S.; Georges, A.; Burnichon, N.; Buffet, A.; Amar, L.; Bertherat, J.; Bouatia-Naji, N.; De Reyniès, A.; Drui, D.; Lussey-Lepoutre, C.; et al. Transcriptome Analysis of lncRNAs in Pheochromocytomas and Paragangliomas. *J. Clin. Endocrinol. Metab.* **2020**, *105*, 898–907. [CrossRef]
82. Adameyko, I.; Lallemend, F.; Aquino, J.B.; Pereira, J.A.; Topilko, P.; Müller, T.; Fritz, N.; Beljajeva, A.; Mochii, M.; Liste, I.; et al. Schwann Cell Precursors from Nerve Innervation Are a Cellular Origin of Melanocytes in Skin. *Cell* **2009**, *139*, 366–379. [CrossRef]
83. Wang, Z.; Li, Y.; Zhong, Y.; Wang, Y.; Peng, M. Comprehensive analysis of aberrantly expressed competitive endogenous rna network and identification of prognostic biomarkers in pheochromocytoma and paraganglioma. *OncoTargets Ther.* **2020**, *13*, 11377–11395. [CrossRef] [PubMed]
84. Harrod, T.P.; Justement, L.B. Evaluating function of transmembrane protein tyrosine phosphatase CD148 in lymphocyte biology. *Immunol. Res.* **2002**, *26*, 153–166. [CrossRef]
85. Zhang, X.-F.; Tu, R.; Li, K.; Ye, P.; Cui, X. Tumor Suppressor PTPRJ Is a Target of miR-155 in Colorectal Cancer. *J. Cell Biochem.* **2017**, *118*, 3391–3400. [CrossRef] [PubMed]
86. Martínez-Høyer, S.; Solé-Sánchez, S.; Aguado, F.; Martínez-Martínez, S.; Serrano-Candelas, E.; Hernández, J.L.; Iglesias, M.; Redondo, J.M.; Casanovas, O.; Messeguer, R.; et al. A novel role for an RCAN3-derived peptide as a tumor suppressor in breast cancer. *Carcinogenesis* **2015**, *36*, 792–799. [CrossRef]
87. Patel, D.; Boufraqech, M.; Jain, M.; Zhang, L.; He, M.; Gesuwan, K.; Gulati, N.; Nilubol, N.; Fojo, T.; Kebebew, E. MiR-34a and miR-483-5p are candidate serum biomarkers for adrenocortical tumors. *Surgery* **2013**, *154*, 1224–1229. [CrossRef] [PubMed]
88. Corbetta, S.; Vaira, V.; Guarnieri, V.; Scillitani, A.; Eller-Vainicher, C.; Ferrero, S.; Vicentini, L.; Chiodini, I.; Bisceglia, M.; Beck-Peccoz, P.; et al. Differential expression of microRNAs in human parathyroid carcinomas compared with normal parathyroid tissue. *Endocr. Relat. Cancer* **2010**, *17*, 135–146. [CrossRef] [PubMed]
89. Liu, X.; Chen, Z.; Yu, J.; Xia, J.; Zhou, X. MicroRNA profiling and head and neck cancer. *Comp. Funct. Genom.* **2009**, *2009*, 837514. [CrossRef]
90. Guo, J.; Miao, Y.; Xiao, B.; Huan, R.; Jiang, Z.; Meng, D.; Wang, Y. Differential expression of microRNA species in human gastric cancer versus non-tumorous tissues. *J. Gastroenterol. Hepatol.* **2009**, *24*, 652–657. [CrossRef]
91. Adler, J.T.; Hottinger, D.G.; Kunnimalaiyaan, M.; Chen, H. Histone deacetylase inhibitors upregulate Notch-1 and inhibit growth in pheochromocytoma cells. *Surgery* **2008**, *144*, 956–962. [CrossRef]
92. Chan, S.Y.; Loscalzo, J. MicroRNA-210: A unique and pleiotropic hypoxamir. *Cell Cycle* **2010**, *9*, 1072–1083. [CrossRef]
93. Castro-Vega, L.J.; Letouzé, E.; Burnichon, N.; Buffet, A.; Disderot, P.H.; Khalifa, E.; Loriot, C.; Elarouci, N.; Morin, A.; Menara, M.; et al. Multi-omics analysis defines core genomic alterations in pheochromocytomas and paragangliomas. *Nat. Commun.* **2015**, *6*, 1–9. [CrossRef]
94. Tarantino, C.; Paolella, G.; Cozzuto, L.; Minopoli, G.; Pastore, L.; Parisi, S.; Russo, T. miRNA 34a, 100, and 137 modulate differentiation of mouse embryonic stem cells. *FASEB J.* **2010**, *24*, 3255–3263. [CrossRef] [PubMed]
95. Tian, J.; Xu, H.; Chen, G.; Wang, H.; Bi, Y.; Gao, H.; Luo, Y. Roles of lncRNA UCA1-miR-18a-SOX6 axis in preventing hypoxia injury following cerebral ischemia. *Int J. Clin. Exp. Pathol.* **2017**, *10*, 8187–8198.
96. Han, F.; Wu, Y.; Jiang, W. MicroRNA-18a decreases choroidal endothelial cell proliferation and migration by inhibiting HIF1a expression. *Med. Sci. Monit.* **2015**, *21*, 1642–1647. [PubMed]
97. Chen, X.; Wu, L.; Li, D.; Xu, Y.; Zhang, L.; Niu, K.; Kong, R.; Gu, J.; Xu, Z.; Chen, Z.; et al. Radiosensitizing effects of miR-18a-5p on lung cancer stem-like cells via downregulating both ATM and HIF-1α. *Cancer Med.* **2018**, *7*, 3834–3847. [CrossRef]
98. Krutilina, R.; Sun, W.; Sethuraman, A.; Brown, M.; Seagroves, T.N.; Pfeffer, L.M.; Ignatova, T.; Fan, M. MicroRNA-18a inhibits hypoxia-inducible factor 1α activity and lung metastasis in basal breast cancers. *Breast Cancer Res.* **2014**, *16*, R78. [CrossRef]
99. Verduci, L.; Strano, S.; Yarden, Y.; Blandino, G. The circRNA-microRNA code: Emerging implications for cancer diagnosis and treatment. *Mol. Oncol.* **2019**, *13*, 669–680. [CrossRef] [PubMed]

Article

A Multicenter Epidemiological Study on Second Malignancy in Non-Syndromic Pheochromocytoma/Paraganglioma Patients in Italy

Letizia Canu [1,2,†], Soraya Puglisi [3,†], Paola Berchialla [4], Giuseppina De Filpo [1], Francesca Brignardello [3,‡], Francesca Schiavi [5], Alfonso Massimiliano Ferrara [5], Stefania Zovato [5], Michaela Luconi [1,2,*], Anna Pia [3], Marialuisa Appetecchia [6], Emanuela Arvat [7], Claudio Letizia [8], Mauro Maccario [9], Mirko Parasiliti-Caprino [9], Barbara Altieri [10], Antongiulio Faggiano [11], Roberta Modica [12], Valentina Morelli [13], Maura Arosio [13], Uberta Verga [13], Micaela Pellegrino [14], Luigi Petramala [8], Antonio Concistrè [8], Paola Razzore [15], Tonino Ercolino [2,16], Elena Rapizzi [2,17], Mario Maggi [1,2], Antonio Stigliano [11], Jacopo Burrello [18,§] on behalf of AIRTUM Working Group Collaborators, Massimo Terzolo [3], Giuseppe Opocher [19], Massimo Mannelli [1,2] and Giuseppe Reimondo [3]

1. Department of Experimental and Clinical Biomedical Sciences "Mario Serio", University of Florence, 50139 Florence, Italy; letizia.canu@unifi.it (L.C.); giuseppina.defilpo@unifi.it (G.D.F.); mario.maggi@unifi.it (M.M.); massimo.mannelli@unifi.it (M.M.)
2. Centro di Ricerca e Innovazione sulle Patologie Surrenaliche, AOU Careggi, 50134 Florence, Italy; tonino.ercolino@unifi.it (T.E.); elena.rapizzi@unifi.it (E.R.)
3. Internal Medicine, Department of Clinical and Biological Sciences, San Luigi Gonzaga Hospital, University of Turin, Orbassano, 10043 Turin, Italy; soraya.puglisi@unito.it (S.P.); m.luconi@unifi.it (F.B.); a.pia@sanluigi.piemonte.it (A.P.); massimo.terzolo@unito.it (M.T.); giuseppe.reimondo@unito.it (G.R.)
4. Statistical Unit, Department of Clinical and Biological Sciences, University of Turin, Orbassano, 10143 Turin, Italy; paola.berchialla@unito.it
5. Familial Cancer Clinic, Veneto Institute of Oncology IOV – IRCCS, 35128 Padua, Italy; francesca.schiavi@iov.veneto.it (F.S.); massimiliano.ferrara@iov.veneto.it (A.M.F.); stefania.zovato@iov.veneto.it (S.Z.)
6. Oncological Endocrinology Unit, IRCCS-Regina Elena National Cancer Institute, 00128 Rome, Italy; marialuisa.appetecchia@ifo.gov.it
7. Oncological Endocrinology Unit, Department of Medical Sciences, University of Turin, 10126 Turin, Italy; emanuela.arvat@unito.it
8. Secondary Arterial Hypertension Unit, Department of Translational and Precision Medicine, Sapienza University of Rome, 00161 Rome, Italy; claudio.letizia@uniroma1.it (C.L.); luigi.petramala@uniroma1.it (L.P.); antonio.concistre@uniroma1.it (A.C.)
9. Endocrinology, Diabetology, and Metabolism Unit, Department of Medical Sciences, University of Turin, 10126 Turin, Italy; mauro.maccario@unito.it (M.M.); mirko.parasiliticaprino@gmail.com (M.P.-C.)
10. Division of Endocrinology and Diabetes, Department of Internal Medicine I, University Hospital, University of Würzburg, 97080 Würzburg, Germany; Altieri_B@ukw.de
11. Endocrinology, Department of Clinical and Molecular Medicine, Sant'Andrea Hospital, Sapienza University of Rome, 00189 Rome, Italy; antongiulio.faggiano@uniroma1.it (A.F.); antonio.stigliano@uniroma1.it (A.S.)
12. Division of Endocrinology, Department of Clinical Medicine and Surgery, ENETS Center of Excellence, University "Federico II" of Naples, 80138 Naples, Italy; robertamodica@libero.it
13. Endocrinology Unit, Fondazione IRCCS Ca' Granda Ospedale Maggiore Policlinico, Department of Clinical Sciences and Community Health, University of Milan, 20122 Milan, Italy; morellivale@yahoo.it (V.M.); maura.arosio@unimi.it (M.A.); uverga@gmail.com (U.V.)
14. Division of Endocrinology, Diabetology and Metabolism, Santa Croce and Carle Hospital, 12100 Cuneo, Italy; micaela13.pellegrino@gmail.com
15. Endocrinology, Diabetology and Metabolism Diseases Unit, AO Ordine Mauriziano, 10128 Turin, Italy; prazzore@mauriziano.it
16. Endocrinology Unit, AOU Careggi, 50134 Florence, Italy
17. Department of Experimental and Clinical Medicine, University of Florence, 50139 Florence, Italy
18. Division of Internal Medicine and Hypertension Unit, Department of Medical Sciences, University of Turin, 10126 Turin, Italy; jacopo.burrello@unito.it
19. Veneto Institute of Oncology, IRCCS, 35128 Padua, Italy; giuseppe.opocher@gmail.com
* Correspondence: michaela.luconi@unifi.it
† L.C. and S.P. equally contributed and should be considered as joint first authors.
‡ In memory.

§ Collaborators listed in the Appendix A.

Simple Summary: As no previous studies had assessed the risk of second malignant tumors in patients with pheochromocytomas/paragangliomas (PPGLs), we aimed to evaluate whether these patients could have an increased risk of additional malignancy, comparing them with patients in the general population who had a first malignancy and developed a second malignant tumor. We demonstrated that PPGL patients had higher incidence of additional malignant tumors and the risk of developing a second malignant tumor increased with age at diagnosis. As the main tumors were prostate, colorectal and lung/bronchial cancers in males, and breast cancer, differentiated thyroid cancer and melanoma in females, our findings could have an impact on the surveillance strategy.

Abstract: No studies have carried out an extensive analysis of the possible association between non-syndromic pheochromocytomas and paragangliomas (PPGLs) and other malignancies. To assess >the risk of additional malignancy in PPGL, we retrospectively evaluated 741 patients with PPGLs followed-up in twelve referral centers in Italy. Incidence of second malignant tumors was compared between this cohort and Italian patients with two subsequent malignancies. Among our patients, 95 (12.8%) developed a second malignant tumor, which were mainly prostate, colorectal and lung/bronchial cancers in males, breast cancer, differentiated thyroid cancer and melanoma in females. The standardized incidence ratio was 9.59 (95% CI 5.46–15.71) in males and 13.21 (95% CI 7.52–21.63) in females. At multivariable analysis, the risk of developing a second malignant tumor increased with age at diagnosis (HR 2.50, 95% CI 1.15–5.44, $p = 0.021$ for 50–59 vs. <50-year category; HR 3.46, 95% CI 1.67–7.15, $p < 0.001$ for >60- vs. <50-year). In patients with available genetic evaluation, a positive genetic test was inversely associated with the risk of developing a second tumor (HR 0.25, 95% CI 0.10–0.63, $p = 0.003$). In conclusion, PPGLs patients have higher incidence of additional malignant tumors compared to the general population who had a first malignancy, which could have an impact on the surveillance strategy.

Keywords: pheochromocytoma; paraganglioma; epidemiology; genetic analysis; mortality; surveillance

1. Introduction

Pheochromocytomas and paragangliomas (PPGLs) are rare tumors arising from the neural crest [1]. Pheochromocytomas (PCCs) and thorax/abdominal paragangliomas (PGLs) derive from sympathetic ganglia, whereas head and neck PGLs (HNPGLs) derive from parasympathetic ones [2].

Up to 70% of PPGLs are caused by germline or somatic genetic variants in one of the susceptibility genes [3]. Depending on the transcription profile, PPGLs are divided into two main clusters: cluster 1 includes genes involved in pseudohypoxia signaling (*SDHA, SDHB, SDHC, SDHD, SDHAF2, VHL, FH, EPAS1*), and cluster 2 includes genes related to the activation of kinase signaling (*NF1, RET, TMEM127, MAX, HRAS*) [3,4].

Until a few years ago, the association of PPGL with other solid tumors was reported only in neurofibromatosis type 1 (NF1), multiple endocrine neoplasia type 2 (MEN2) and von Hippel Lindau (VHL) syndrome. However, non-chromaffin tumors have recently been reported in patients with PPGL without any of these syndromic diseases. In fact, *SDHx* mutations have been associated with renal cell carcinomas (RCCs) [5], gastrointestinal stromal tumors (GISTs) [6,7] and pituitary adenomas (PAs) [6]. *SDHx* mutated RCCs represent less than 0.5% of all renal carcinomas [8], whereas 30% of GISTs are associated with *SDHA* mutations [9].

The presence of *SDHC* promoter hypermethylation has also been observed in patients affected by SDH-deficient GIST without somatic *SDHx* mutations [10]. *MAX* mutated patients are rarely affected by pituitary adenomas [11] and RCC has been reported in *TMEM127* [12] and *FH* [13] mutated patients. The prevalence of *SDHx* mutations in pituitary adenomas is very low (0.3–1.8%) [14] and the majority are functional macroadenomas [15].

The data on the association between non-chromaffin tumors and PPGLs with or without mutations in any of the PPGL susceptibility genes are heterogeneous. A great deal of interest has been placed on the association with *SDHx* mutations, and these tumors have been defined as *SDH*-deficient tumors [9]. Some studies have reported an association between PPGLs and other solid tumors in non-genotyped patients. On the other hand, other studies have reported the presence of GISTs, RCCs or pituitary adenomas in *SDH*-mutated patients, but without proving a causal relationship between the *SDHx* mutation and tumor occurrence.

We searched the current literature for studies (Supplemental Table S1 [16]) on patients affected by PPGL and/or other tumors, including patients who were carriers or not of mutations in any of the PPGL susceptibility genes. Any genetic alteration should be clear from the immunohistochemistry (IHC) and/or loss of heterogeneity (LOH) in tumor tissue. We found that IHC and LOH on tumor tissue revealed a mutation in 9.6% (784/8159) and 34% (143/420) of cases, respectively. IHC was more widely used, but LOH more frequently identified non-chromaffin tumors due to mutations in susceptibility genes.

The aims of this retrospective, multicentric study were to assess whether patients with PPGLs have an increased risk of additional malignant tumors compared with the general population, and to identify the predisposing factors.

2. Materials and Methods

2.1. Subjects

We evaluated the prevalence and incidence of an additional malignant tumor in 741 patients affected by PPGLs followed-up in 12 referral centers in Italy, listed in Appendix B. Patients with confirmed biochemical and/or histopathological diagnosis of PPGL were included, while those presenting with known hereditary syndromes, such as VHL, MEN2 and NF1, were excluded. The median duration of follow-up was 48 months (12–108).

Genetic analysis was considered as assessed if at least *SDHx*, *MAX* and *TMEM127* genes were analyzed. Data on patients diagnosed between 1990 and 2019 were collected retrospectively by local investigators in a computerized database. Most patients were diagnosed between 2009 and 2019 (46.8%). All patients gave their informed consent to the collection of data according to the local ethics committee indications (Registry and Repository of biological samples of the European Network for the Study of Adrenal Tumors (ENS@T).

We collected the following data: demographics, date of diagnosis, metanephrine (MN), normetanephrine (NMN) and methoxytyramine (MTX) levels, detection of malignant tumors before, after or within the same year of the PPGL diagnosis, family history of tumors, smoking (yes/no answers), drinking (female >1 alcholic unit (A.U.)/per day, male >2 A.U./per day) and toxic exposure (yes/no answers). Toxic exposure was classified as occupational exposure to toxic substances such as pesticides, polychlorinated biphenyls, asbestos, radon and lead-based paint.

The incidence of a second malignant tumor found in our series was compared to that of the general Italian population (data from Italian Network of Cancer Registries—AIRTUM registry 2019) [17]. Age was reported as a categorical variable in line with what is reported in the AIRTUM registry. The comparison was carried out considering the associated malignant tumors as a second event, taking into account that the 2017 World Health Organization (WHO) classification includes PPGLs among malignant tumors [18–20].

2.2. Statistical Analysis

Continuous variables were presented using the median and the interquartile range (IQR) as measure of variability; categorical variables were presented with frequencies and percentages. Differences between groups were analyzed with the Mann–Whitney test for continuous variables and the chi-squared test, or Fisher test when appropriate, for categorical variables. To evaluate the factors associated with the risk of second malignancy after the diagnosis of the chromaffin pathology, a univariable analysis was carried out to estimate the hazard ratio (HR) and the corresponding 95% confidence interval (95% CI) with the Cox proportional hazard model. In the Cox proportional hazard models, age was entered as a categorical variable. A final multivariable model was developed based on clinical discussion and statistical selection procedures. Model selection was performed using an automatic approach based on the Akaike Information Criteria (AIC) method [21]. Given the large number of covariates, a genetic algorithm was used to explore the candidate set of models. Model goodness of fit was computed with reference to the Brier score (the closer to 0, the better) and the Somers' Dxy Index, which assesses the predictive discrimination derived from the set of predictor variables included in the model. To compute the Somers' Dxy index, the predictive survival time was used. To account for the degree of optimism in model accuracy evaluations induced by the use of the same data source for training and testing purposes, all goodness of fit indexes were computed using a bootstrap procedure (1000 runs). The Schoenfeld residual-based method was used to verify the assumption of proportionality of the risks. The significance level was set at $p < 0.05$. Incidence of second malignant tumors in the study sample was compared with the incidence in Italian patients who had a first malignancy and developed a second malignant tumor. The standardized incidence ratio (SIR) was computed, which is the ratio of the observed number of second malignancies in the study sample to the number of the cases expected according to a set of reference incidence rates. The number of expected tumors was computed by multiplying the number of person-years in the cohort by the national cancer incidence rates, specified for sex and 5-year-age-group and calendar year. Incidence rates by sex and age and calendar year of second malignant tumor of the Italian population were obtained from the AIRTUM database [17]. An SIR greater than 1 means a higher incidence than expected in the reference population. Finally, exact Poisson 95% CIs were computed. Data were analyzed with R version 3.5.0.

3. Results

This study included 741 PPGL patients, of whom 415 (56.0%) were female, with a median age at diagnosis of 49 years (36–60).

Patients' characteristics are reported in Table 1.

Table 1. Patient characteristics.

Characteristics	n. of Evaluated Patients	N
Sex	741	
Female		415/741 (56.0%)
Male		326/741 (44.0%)
Age (years) at PPGL diagnosis, median	741	49 [IQR: 36–60]
Metastatic PPGL	612	54 (8.8%)
Functioning PPGL	572	379 (66.3%)
PPGL localization	741	
Abdominal PGL		172 (23.1%)
Mediastinal PGL		2 (0.3%)
HNPGL		3 (0.4%)
PCC		37 (5.0%)
Abdominal PGL + PCC		58 (7.8%)
Mediastinal PGL + HNPGL		56 (7.6%)
Abdominal PGL + HNPGL		5 (0.7%)
PCC + HNPGL		408 (55.1%)
Family history of tumor	727	264 (36.3%)
Risk factors		
Smoke	672	159 (23.7%)
Alcohol	678	32 (4.7%)
Exposure to toxic substances	625	29 (4.6%)
Genetic analysis	515	
Wild type		349 (67.8%)
SDHD		86 (16.7%)
SDHB		45 (8.7%)

Table 1. Cont.

Characteristics	n. of Evaluated Patients	N
MAX		12 (2.3%)
TMEM127		11 (2.1%)
SDHC		7 (1.4%)
SDHA		4 (0.8%)
SDHAF2		1 (0.2%)
Cluster 1	515	141 (26.6%)
Cluster 2	515	23 (4.5%)
Second malignant tumor	741	95 (12.8%)
Death		26 (3.5%)
Death for PCC/PGL		11 (1.5%)
Follow up months, median		48 [IQR: 12–108]

PPGL = pheochromocytoma and paraganglioma; IQR = interquartile range; PGL = paraganglioma; HNPGL = Head and neck paraganglioma; PCC = pheochromocytoma.

Genetic analysis was performed in 69.5% of patients and 32.2% were mutation carriers: 16.7% *SDHD*, 8.7% *SDHB*, 2.3% *MAX*, 2.1% *TMEM127*, 1.4% *SDHC*, 0.8% *SDHA* and 0.2% *SDHAF2*. A total of 26.6% of the patients belonged to cluster 1, and 4.5% to cluster 2. Patients' characteristics are reported in Table 2.

Table 2. Patient characteristics stratified by genetic mutation.

Characteristics	Patients with Mutation (n. 166)	Patients without Mutation (n. 349)	p Value
Sex			0.537
Female	92/166 (55.4%)	205/349 (58.7%)	
Male	74/166 (44.6%)	144/349 (41.3%)	
Age (years) at PPGL diagnosis, median	37 (IQR: 28–46.5)	52 (IQR: 41–61)	<0.001
Age (years) at second malignancy	57 (IQR: 47–65.5)	56.5 (IQR: 37.8–64)	0.527
Metastatic PPGL	21 (14.5%)	21 (6.8%)	0.014
Functioning PPGL	39 (30.5%)	202 (70.1%)	<0.001
HNPGL	92 (55.4%)	84 (24.1%)	<0.001
Family history of tumor	62 (38.5%)	174 (50.0%)	0.020
Risk factor: smoke	30 (20.5%)	90 (28.1%)	0.105
Risk factor: alcohol	4 (2.7%)	12 (3.7%)	0.781

Ninety-five (12.8%) patients developed a second malignant tumor: mainly breast cancer, differentiated thyroid cancer (DTC) and melanoma in females and prostate cancer, colorectal cancer and lung and bronchial cancer in males (Figure 1).

Twenty-nine (30.5%) of second malignant tumors were discovered after the diagnosis of PPGLs. Comparing our series with the general population [17], the standardized incidence ratio (SIR) of the whole series was 9.59 (95% CI 5.46–15.71) in males, and 13.21 (95% CI 7.52–21.63) in females. The same figure was also observed in the group of subjects who were genetically tested: 7.86 (95% CI 3.44–15.56) in males and 15.71 (95% CI 8.26–27.21) in females.

Only 18% of patients who developed a second malignancy carried a germ-line mutation, which was present in 34% of individuals without a second malignant tumor ($p = 0.01$). Comparing the 646 patients without second malignant tumors with the 95 patients who developed a second malignant tumor (Table 3), the latter patients were more frequently older ($p < 0.001$), had less frequently germline mutations ($p = 0.01$), with a minor frequency in genes involved in pseudohypoxia signaling (11.1% of patients with second malignant tumors belonging to cluster 1 vs. 29.8% of patients without second malignant tumors, $p = 0.006$). No significant difference was found considering the urinary metanephrine and normetanephrine levels comparing patients with and without second malignant tumors (p 0.873 and p 0.522, respectively).

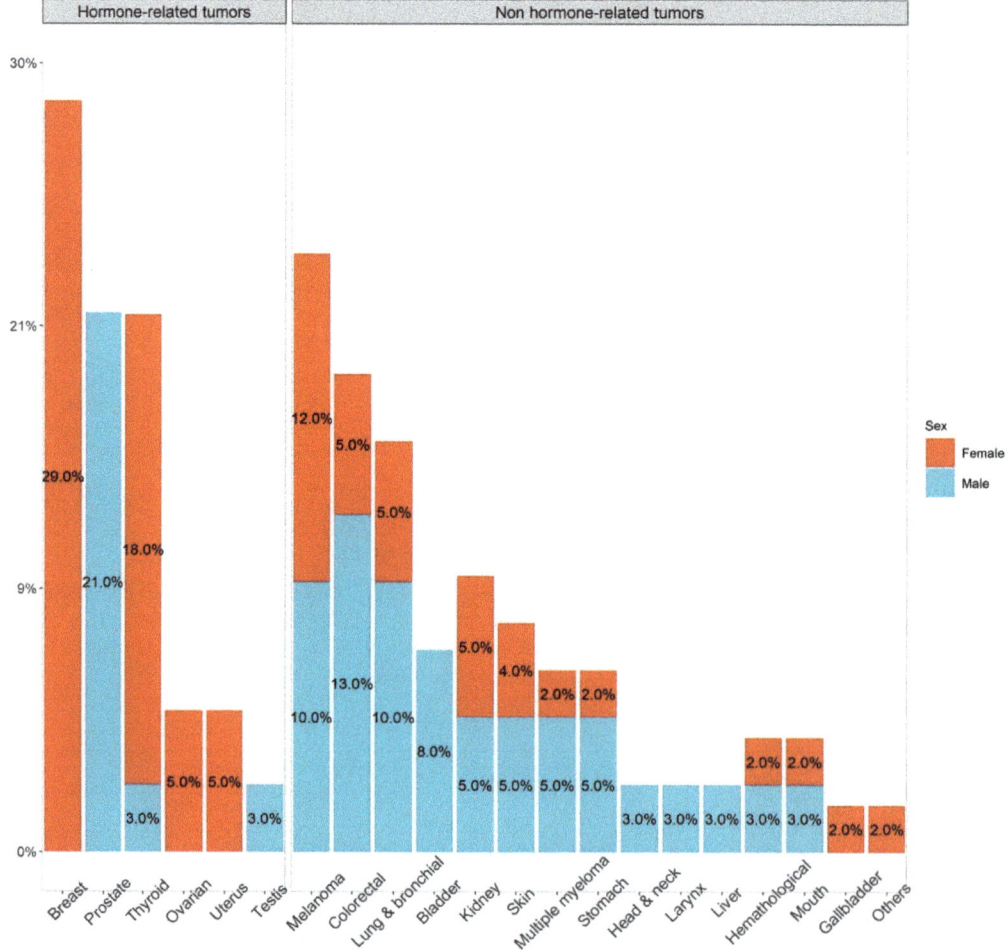

Figure 1. Frequency of second malignant tumor, according to gender (in red females, in blue males) divide into hormone-related and non-hormone-related tumors.

The risk factors associated with the development of second malignant tumors after the diagnosis of PPGLs were assessed by univariable analysis (Table 4). The analysis revealed an association with age (HR 2.27, 95% CI 1.13–4.53, $p = 0.021$ for the 50–59 age category vs. <50 age category; HR 2.22, 95% CI 1.05–4.69, $p = 0.036$ for the over 60 vs. <50 age category).

In the univariable analysis, germline mutations were associated with a lower risk of developing a second malignant tumor (HR 0.27, 95% CI 0.11–0.63, $p = 0.003$). The presence of mutations occurring in the susceptibility genes belonging to cluster 1 (HR 0.31, 95% CI 0.13–0.73, $p = 0.008$), but not to cluster 2, was also inversely associated with the risk of second tumors. Positive family history of cancer was associated with an increased risk of a second malignant tumor (HR 1.80, 95% CI 1.03–3.14, $p = 0.04$).

Table 3. Patient characteristics stratified by a second malignant tumor.

Characteristics	Patients with Second Malignant Tumors (n 95)	Patients without Second Malignant Tumors (n 646)	p Value
Sex			0.61
Female	56/95 (58.9%)	359/646 (55.6%)	
Male	39/95 (41.1%)	287/646 (44.4%)	
Age (years) at PPGL diagnosis, median	58 (IQR: 50–65.8)	47 (IQR: 35–58)	<0.001
Metastatic PPGL	5/76 (6.6%)	49/536 (9.1%)	0.60
Functioning forms	51/72 (70.8%)	328/500 (65.6%)	0.46
PPGL localization			0.43
Abdominal PGL	23/95 (24.3%)	149/646 (23.1%)	
Mediastinal PGL	0/95 (0.0%)	2/646 (0.3%)	
HNPGL	0/95 (0.0%)	3/646 (0.4%)	
PCC	2/95 (2.1%)	35/646 (5.4%)	
Abdominal PGL + PCC	4/95 (4.2%)	54/646 (8.4%)	
Mediastinal PGL + HNPGL	6/95 (6.3%)	50/646 (7.7%)	
Abdominal PGL + HNPGL	0/95 (0.0%)	5/646 (0.8%)	
PCC + HNPGL	60/95 (63.1%)	348/646 (53.9%)	
Positive family history of cancer	36/89 (40.4%)	228/638 (35.7%)	0.45
Risk factors			
Smoke	21/83 (25.3%)	138/589 (23.4%)	0.81
Alcohol	4/86 (4.7%)	28/592 (4.7%)	1.00
Exposure to toxic substances	3/77 (3.9%)	26/548 (4.7%)	0.97
Germ-line mutation	10/56 (17.9%)	156/459 (34.0%)	**0.01**
Genetic test			
Wild type	46/56 (82.1%)	303/459 (66.0%)	0.18
SDHA	0/56 (0.0%)	4/459 (0.9%)	1.00
SDHB	1/56 (1.7%)	44/459 (9.6%)	0.08
SDHC	0/56 (0.0%)	7/459 (1.5%)	0.73
SDHD	5/56 (8.3%)	81/459 (17.2%)	0.12
SDHAF2	0/56 (0.0%)	1/459 (0.2%)	1.00
MAX	2/56 (3.6%)	10/459 (2.2%)	0.86
TMEM127	2/56 (3.5%)	9/459 (2.0%)	0.79
Cluster 1	6/54 (11.1%)	137/459 (29.8%)	**0.006**
Cluster 2	4/54 (7.4%)	19/459 (4.1%)	0.45
Years between PPGL and second malignant tumor, median	6 (IQR: 2–14)		
Death	7/95 (7.4%)	19/646 (2.9%)	0.06
Death for PPGL	3/95 (3.2%)	8/646 (1.2%)	0.32
Follow up months, median	36 (IQR: 12–108)	48 (IQR: 15–108)	0.47

PPGL = pheochromocytoma and paraganglioma; IQR = interquartile range; PGL = paraganglioma; HNPGL = Head and neck paraganglioma; PCC = pheochromocytoma. Statistically significant p are indicated in bold.

In the multivariable analysis, the risk of developing a second malignant tumor increased with age at diagnosis (HR 2.50, 95% CI 11.5–5.44, $p = 0.021$ for 50–59 vs. <50; HR = 3.46, 95% CI 1.67–7.15, $p < 0.001$ for the over 60 vs. <50) (Table 5A). In the series of patients with an available genetic evaluation, the association between age and risk of second tumor weakened, whereas a positive genetic test was strongly protective against developing a second tumor (HR 0.25, 95% CI 0.10–0.63, $p = 0.003$) (Table 5B).

A median of 6 (2–14) years elapsed between the diagnosis of PPGLs and the appearance of a second malignant tumor with a progressive reduction in the risk of developing a second tumor of 7% per year (HR 0.94, 95% CI 0.90–0.97, $p < 0.001$).

Table 4. Univariable analysis for incident second malignant tumor.

	HR	95% CI		p Value
Males vs. females	0.79	0.45	1.39	0.42
Age category				
50–59 years vs. <50 years	2.27	1.13	4.53	**0.021**
>60 years vs. <50 years	2.22	1.05	4.69	**0.036**
Metastatic PPGLs (yes vs. no)	0.20	0.03	1.49	0.12
Functioning PPGLs (no vs. yes)	0.80	0.38	1.66	0.54
Parasympathetic vs. sympathetic lesions	0.89	0.50	1.60	0.71
Family history of cancer (yes vs. no)	1.80	1.03	3.14	**0.04**
Germ-line mutation vs. wild type	0.27	0.11	0.63	**0.003**
Cluster 1 (positive vs. negative)	0.31	0.13	0.73	**0.008**
Cluster 2 (positive vs. negative)	0.82	0.24	2.74	0.75
Risk factors (yes vs. no)				
Smoke	1.18	0.58	2.40	0.64
Alcohol	2.46	0.75	8.06	0.14
Exposure to toxic substances	0.57	0.01	4.11	0.67

PPGL = pheochromocytoma and paraganglioma. Statistically significant p are indicated in bold.

Table 5. Multivariable analysis for the risk of developing a malignant tumor excluding patients with a second tumor developed before or simultaneously with the chromaffin tumor (A) and limited to the patients with genetic evaluation (B).

	A (n. 741)			B (n. 515)		
	HR	95% CI	p Value	HR	95% CI	p Value
Age category						
50–59 years vs. <50 years	2.50	1.15 5.44	**0.021**	1.71	0.72 4.07	0.23
>60 years vs. <40 years	3.46	1.67 7.15	**<0.001**	1.46	0.54 3.94	0.46
Males vs. females	1.23	0.63 2.41	0.54	1.18	0.53 2.60	0.69
Smoker vs. non-smoker	2.10	0.82 5.39	0.12	1.64	0.57 4.72	0.36
Genetic test (positive vs. negative)				0.25	0.10 0.63	**0.003**

Statistically significant p are indicated in bold.

4. Discussion

In this study, we observed a higher risk of developing second malignant tumors in patients with PPGLs compared with the general population in Italy. The risk was greater in patients affected by sporadic PPGLs compared to genetically driven PPGLs. The presence of a known mutation in any of the susceptibility genes for PPGLs was actually a protective factor against developing a second malignant tumor.

The analysis revealed a higher incidence of second malignancies in our series, both in males and females, with an approximately 9 and 13 times higher risk, respectively, confirming previous preliminary findings in a small sample (110 PCC and 11 PGL) with sporadic and familial tumors [22]. The risk appears higher than expected since we compared the incidence of second malignant tumors in our population with that in the general population who had a first malignancy and developed a second malignant tumor. The comparison was conducted in view of the new WHO classification which includes all PPGLs among malignant tumors [18].

We focused on second malignant tumors both due to the greater clinical interest of these tumors compared to benign ones, together with the availability of incidence data on only malignant tumors in the general population [17]. The most frequently reported association in the literature concerns GIST, RCC and pituitary adenoma. The data reported in the literature are rather heterogenous, with studies conducted on patients suffering from non-chromaffin tumors with a negative history of PPGLs and lacking a genetic analysis for known susceptibility genes but with the tumor tissue analysis of *SDHx* mutations. Other authors have described the appearance of non-chromaffin tumors in patients with previously sporadic or familial PPGLs. Moreover, in some studies the association between PPGL and second tumors or between *SDHx* mutations and non-chromaffin tumors, was not supported by immunohistochemical analysis or tissue gene sequencing. In addition, the interpretation of the immunohistochemical analysis for SDHB and/or SDHA on PPGL tissues is not always univocal [23], as also happens in the tissues of other tumors. In our case series there was one GIST, one GH- secreting pituitary adenoma and five kidney lesions.

In the whole series, in females we found that the most frequent cancers associated with PPGLs were breast cancer, DTC and melanoma. In males, the most frequent tumors were prostate cancer, colorectal cancer and lung and bronchial cancer. In the general population, colorectal cancer is the second most frequent tumor (13%) after breast cancer (14%), followed by prostate, lung and bronchial cancer (all 11%) [17]. The high frequency of breast cancer is in line with findings observed in the general population, since it represents the most frequent neoplasia in the female population (30%), while DTC is the fourth (5%) [17]. The high incidence of DTC in our population may result from a selection bias of patients who were followed up in endocrinology care units, where thyroid evaluation is routinely performed. Melanoma, representing the third most frequent second neoplasia in our cohort, was in the youngest population (<50 years), the second most frequent in males (9%), immediately after testicular cancer (12%), whereas it was the third in females (7%), after breast cancer (40%) and DTC (16%) [17]. Interestingly, in our series almost 50% of patients with melanoma were older than 60. Melanoma has already been identified as one of the most frequent cancers associated with PPGLs in women in a study including 121 patients with PPGLs [22]. The association between PPGL and melanoma is interesting due to their common embryonic origin from the neural crest. The microphthalmia-associated transcription factor (MITF) is a transcription factor involved in the regulation of survival, proliferation and differentiation of the neural crest cells such as melanocytes [24]. Two studies [25,26] identified a germline variant of MITF, *p*.E318K, associated with an increased risk of melanoma and RCC. Castro-Vega et al. hypothesized that this variant might also contribute to the development of PPGL, which they found in 7 out of 555 patients with PPGL [27]. The breast cancer associated protein 1 (BAP1) gene is a tumor suppressor gene involved in cell cycle regulation, cell differentiation, cell death and DNA damage response [28]. Loss of BAP1 expression has been demonstrated in many other tumors including melanoma, mesothelioma and RCC. Maffeis et al. analyzed tissues of 56 PPGLs, demonstrating the loss of BAP1 expression also in PPGLs (2/22 PGL and 12/34 PCC) [29]. Only in a few cases has an association between DTC and sporadic/genetically inherited PPGL been described. To date, the relationship between DTC and PPGL remains to be clarified and is likely affected by a heterogeneous genetic background [30]. Currently only one case has been reported of prostate cancer SDHB negative at immunohistochemistry [31], while the association between prostate cancer and PPGLs has not been described. Interestingly, in our population one patient developed prostate cancer at 30 years old after a diagnosis of chromaffin disease.

Advanced age at diagnosis of PPGLs is a predisposing factor for the development of second malignant tumors, similarly to findings in the general population. However, a progressive 7% reduction per year in the risk of developing a second tumor has been observed with increasing time after a diagnosis of PPGL. We cannot exclude that the accurate diagnostic evaluation, starting from the initial diagnosis of chromaffin pathology, might facilitate the detection of unknown co-morbidities, including tumors in the early years of follow-up. Current data indicate a lifetime follow up in patients with PPGL familial forms and a 10-year follow up in patients with PPGL sporadic forms [32] which is also suitable for identifying incidentally detected second malignant tumors.

An intriguing result emerging from our analysis of the series is the role of the genetic profile. In the last decade, there has been growing interest in other tumors in patients with PPGLs. Most studies have evaluated the association between the second tumors and *SDHx* mutations. In line with the literature data, 30% of our patients were carriers of a germ-line mutation for PPGLs [5]. In view of the data on the association between *SDHx* and other tumors [33], we expected that second malignant tumors would be more frequent in patients with genetic forms of PPGLs, particularly belonging to cluster 1 with mutations of the *SDHx* genes. However, our analysis revealed that almost 82% of patients with second malignant tumors were affected by sporadic forms. This data could be explained by mutations in not yet identified PPGL susceptibility genes. Single nucleotide polymorphisms (SNPs) possibly play a protective role. SNPs are single nucleotide variations present in more than 1% of the population [34]. In Wilms' tumor, in squamous cell carcinoma of the head and neck [35], and in breast cancer [36], SNPs in genes appear to be involved in the base excision repair (BER) complex, which is the main DNA repair mechanism in damage induced by reactive oxygen species (ROS) [37]. The protective role of SNPs is thus highly selective for a specific type of tumor; in fact, SNPs that reduce the risk of developing a type of tumor, conversely may play a promoting action for other tumor histotypes [35]. Similarly, mutations in the susceptibility genes for PPGLs might predispose the development of chromaffin diseases, while reducing the risk of other malignant tumors.

Another unexpected finding is that patients affected by a second malignant tumor less frequently belonged to cluster 1, which in our series mainly included *SDHx* genes. *SDHx* mutated cells present an impaired mitochondrial electron transport chain with increased ROS production. Accordingly, SDHx mutated cells shift to aerobic glycolysis (Warburg effect) [38]. This also happens in non-tumor cells bearing *SDHx* mutations which were forced towards glycolysis to maintain low levels of ROS, resulting in a less oxidative mutational environment that could protect against the development of non-chromaffin malignancies. This might justify why patients from cluster 1 developed a second malignant tumor less frequently than in cluster 2.

Secondly, in our series, no patient affected only by non-secreting parasympathetic lesion (HNPGL) developed a second malignant tumor. This result is in line with previous studies showing the role of catecholamines in tumorigenesis [39,40]. Interestingly, this data could also explain why patients belonging to cluster 1 are less affected by second malignant tumors. In fact, patients with parasympathetic lesions belong to cluster 1 and are not present in cluster 2. Despite this, in our study no significant difference was found between urinary metanephrine and normetanephrine levels comparing patients with and without second malignant neoplasm, probably due to the limited number of events.

Despite the associations described in the literature, to date, there is no indication to check for the presence of second tumors in patients affected by PPGLs and/or carriers of mutations in one of the susceptibility genes. Of the three most frequently associated tumors reported in the literature, RCC is the only one that can be found during the routine follow-up of our patients. Highlighting the presence of kidney lesions with an abdomen ultrasound is straightforward, while to identify pituitary adenoma, a dedicated contrasted-MRI is necessary. However, these lesions are generally larger than one centimeter, and in most cases, secreting. These characteristics could lead to the discovery of the lesion despite the lack of dedicated investigations during the follow-up. In order to rule out the presence of a GIST, an abdominal CT scan with contrast medium would be necessary, which is not usually done in a routine follow up.

Our findings suggest some modifications could be made to improve the follow-up procedures in females: (a) for breast cancer, a surveillance program for women between 50 and 69 years-old, which includes a mammogram every two years; (b) for DTC and melanoma, a neck ultrasound and a dermatological examination would be sufficient. In males: (a) annual detection of prostate specific antigen (PSA) value might be suggested; (b) for colorectal cancer, fecal immunochemical testing every two years for men between 50 and 75 years old.

Our study has some limitations. Due to the retrospective nature of the study not all missing data could be recovered. Anamnestic data were not collected in a standardized manner and not all patients underwent genetic analysis. Furthermore, there are also methodological differences in the genetic tests performed: traditional Sanger sequencing vs. new next-generation sequencing methods. We did not make tissue analysis of associated tumors to assess whether the germline mutation was responsible for the appearance of a second non-chromaffin neoplasia. Finally, the duration of the median follow-up (48, 12–108, months) was limited.

5. Conclusions

We believe that our study represents the most extensive evaluation of the prevalence of second malignant tumors in patients with PPGLs. Our main finding was that there is a higher incidence of second malignancies in patients affected by PPGLs compared to the general population.

Appropriate changes in the follow-up of patients with sporadic chromaffin tumors should thus be fostered, in order to identify a second tumor early. Finally, our results suggest the need for further efforts to identify new PPGL susceptibility genes.

Supplementary Materials: The following are available online at https://www.mdpi.com/article/10.3390/cancers13225831/s1, Available in FigShare (10.6084/m9.figshare.14737494). Table S1: Association between non-chromaffin tumors and PCC/PGL and/or mutations in one of the PCC/PGL susceptibly genes doi.10.6084/m9.figshare.14737494.

Author Contributions: Conceptualization, L.C., S.P. and G.R.; methodology, P.B.; software, not applicable; validation, P.B.; formal analysis, P.B.; investigation, L.C., S.P., G.D.F., F.B., F.S., A.M.F., S.Z., M.L., A.P., M.A., E.A., C.L., M.M. (Mauro Maccario), M.P.-C., B.A., A.F., R.M., V.M., M.A., U.V., M.P., L.P., A.C., P.R., T.E., E.R., M.M. (Mario Maggi), A.S., J.B., M.T., G.O. and M.M. (Massimo Mannelli); resources, G.R., M.L., M.M. (Massimo Mannelli) and M.T.; data curation, L.C., S.P., G.D.F., F.B., F.S., A.M.F., S.Z., M.L., A.P., M.A., E.A., C.L., M.M. (Mauro Maccario), M.P.-C., B.A., A.F., R.M., V.M., M.A., U.V., M.P., L.P., A.C., P.R., T.E., E.R., M.M. (Mario Maggi), A.S., J.B., M.T., G.O. and M.M. (Massimo Mannelli); writing—original draft preparation, L.C., S.P., P.B., M.L. and G.R.; writing—review and editing, L.C., S.P., G.D.F., F.B., F.S., A.M.F., S.Z., M.L., A.P., M.A., E.A., C.L., M.M. (Mauro Maccario), M.P.-C., B.A., A.F., R.M., V.M., M.A., U.V., M.P., L.P., A.C., P.R., T.E., E.R., M.M. (Mario Maggi), A.S., J.B., M.T., G.O. and M.M. (Massimo Mannelli) and G.R.; visualization, L.C., S.P., P.B., M.L. and G.R.; supervision, M.L. and G.R.; project administration, M.L. and G.R.; funding acquisition, G.R., M.L., M.M. (Massimo Mannelli) and M.T. AIRTUM Working Group Collaborators provided data of the general Italian population. All authors have read and agreed to the published version of the manuscript.

Funding: This research was funded by AIRC—IG-2020-ID.24820; MIUR—Departments of Excellence 2018–2022; Ricerca Locale Università di Torino 2020—RILO 2020; AIRC IG2019-23069.

Institutional Review Board Statement: The study was conducted according to the guidelines of the Declaration of Helsinki. Ethical review and approval were waived for this study, due to the retrospective nature of the study and use of anonymized data.

Informed Consent Statement: Patient consent was waived due to the retrospective nature of the study and use of anonymized data.

Data Availability Statement: The data presented in this study are available in this article.

Conflicts of Interest: All the authors declare no conflict of interest.

Appendix A

AIRTUM Working Group—Collaborators.

Bisceglia, I.; Candela, G.; Carozzi, G.; Cavallo, R.; Celesia, M.V.; Cirilli, C.; Citarella, A.; Contiero, P.; Cuccaro, F.; Dal Maso, L.; Fusco, M.; Galasso, R.; Giuliani, O.; Mangone, L.; Marani, E.; Maule, M.; Mazzoleni, G.; Melcarne, A.; Michiara, M.; Musolino, A.; Paderni, F.; Palma, F.; Piffer, S.; Pompili, M.; Quarta, F.; Ravaioli, A.; Rizzello, R.; Rugge, M.; Sacerdote, C.;

Sciacchitano, C.G.; Serraino, D.; Sferrazza, A.; Sutera Sardo, A.; Tagliabue, G.; Tumino, R.; Valenti Clemente, S.; Vincenzi, R.; Vitale, M.F.; Vitarelli, S.; Vittadello, F.

NAME	SURNAME	TUMOR REGISTRY
Guido	Mazzoleni	South Tyrol Tumour Registry, Italy
Fabio	Vittadello	South Tyrol Tumour Registry, Italy

NAME	SURNAME	TUMOR REGISTRY
Rosario	Tumino	Cancer Registry, Provincial Health Authority (ASP) Ragusa, Italy
Ausilia	Sferrazza	Cancer Registry, Provincial Health Authority (ASP) Ragusa, Italy
Marco	Pompili	Cancer Registry Marche, Italy
Susanna	Vitarelli	Cancer Registry Marche, Italy
Francesco	Cuccaro	Cancer Registry of Puglia, Italy
Giuseppa	Candela	Cancer Registry Trapani-Agrigento ASP Trapani, Italy
Roberto	Rizzello	Trento Province Cancer Registry, Trento, Italy
Silvano	Piffer	Trento Province Cancer Registry, Trento, Italy
Maria	Michiara	Cancer Registry of Parma, Parma, Italy
Antonino	Musolino	Cancer Registry of Parma, Parma, Italy
Milena	Maule	Unit of Cancer Epidemiology, Turin, Italy
Carlotta	Sacerdote	Unit of Cancer Epidemiology, Turin, Italy
Alessandra	Ravaioli	Cancer Registry Romagna, Italy
Orietta	Giuliani	Cancer Registry Romagna, Italy
Maria Vittoria	Celesia	Cancer Registry Liguria, Italy
Enza	Marani	Cancer Registry Liguria, Italy
Diego	Serraino	Oncology referral Center Aviano, Italy
Luigino	Dal Maso	Oncology referral Center Aviano, Italy
Fernando	Palma	Cancer Registry Foggia, Section Cancer Registry Puglia, Italy
Mario	Fusco	Napoli 3 South Cancer Registry, Italy
Maria Francesca	Vitale	Napoli 3 South Cancer Registry, Italy
Giuliano	Carozzi	Modena Cancer Registry, Italy
Claudia	Cirilii	Modena Cancer Registry, Italy
Giovanna	Tagliabue	Lombardy Cancer Registry, Italy
Paolo	Contiero	Lombardy Cancer Registry, Italy
Santa	Valenti Clemente	Reggio Calabria Tumour Registry, Italy
Romina	Vincenzi	Reggio Calabria Tumour Registry, Italy
Rocco	Galasso	Regional Cancer Registry Basilicata, Italy
Fabrizio	Quarta	Lecce Tumour Registry, Italy
Anna	Melcarne	Lecce Tumour Registry, Italy
Rossella	Cavallo	Salerno Tumour Registry, Italy
Lucia	Mangone	Reggio-Emilia Tumour Registry, Italy
Isabella	Bisceglia	Reggio-Emilia Tumour Registry, Italy
Carlo Giacomo	Sciacchitano	CT-ME-EN Tumour Registry, Italy
Fiorella	Paderni	CT-ME-EN Tumour Registry, Italy
Annarita	Citarella	Benevento Tumour Registry, Italy
Antonella	Sutera Sardo	Catanzaro Tumour Registry, Italy
Massimo	Rugge	Veneto Tumour Registry, Italy

Appendix B

List of 12 referral centers in Italy involved in the study.
1. Istituto Oncologico Veneto IRCCS, Padova;
2. Dipartimento di Scienze Biomediche Sperimentali e Cliniche, AOU Careggi, Firenze;
3. Centro Specialistico Ipertensioni Secondarie, Dipartimento di Medicina Interna e Specialità Mediche, Università di Roma "Sapienza", Policlinico Umberto I, Roma;
4. Endocrinologia, Diabetologia e Metabolismo, Dipartimento di Scienze Mediche, Università di Torino, Città della Salute e della Scienza, Torino e Endocrinologia Oncologica, Dipartimento di Scienze Mediche, Università di Torino, Città della Salute e della Scienza, Torino;
5. Medicina Interna ed Endocrinologia, Dipartimento di Scienze Cliniche e Biologiche, Università di Torino, AOU San Luigi, Orbassano Torino;
6. Unità di Endocrinologia e Malattie Metaboliche Fondazione IRCCS Cà Granda Ospedale Maggiore Policlinico, Milano;
7. Dipartimento di medicina Clinica e Chirurgia, Divisione di Endocrinologia Università Federico II Napoli;
8. Endocrinologia AO S. Croce e Carle, Cuneo;
9. Unità di Endocrinologia Istituto Nazionale Tumori Regina Elena, Roma;
10. Medicina Interna e Ipertensione, Dipartimento di Scienze Mediche, Università di Torino, Città della Salute e della Scienza, Torino;
11. Endocrinologia, Dipartimento di Medicina Clinica e Molecolare, Università Roma "Sapienza", Ospedale Sant'Andrea, Roma;
12. Endocrinologia, AO Ordine Mauriziano, Torino

References

1. Lenders, J.W.; Eisenhofer, G.; Mannelli, M.; Pacak, K. Phaeochromocytoma. *Lancet* **2005**, *366*, 665–675. [CrossRef]
2. Andrews, K.A.; Ascher, D.B.; Pires, D.E.V.; Barnes, D.R.; Vialard, L.; Casey, R.T.; Bradshaw, N.; Adlard, J.; Aylwin, S.; Brennan, P.; et al. Tumour risks and genotype–phenotype correlations associated with germline variants in succinate dehydrogenase subunit genes SDHB, SDHC and SDHD. *J. Med. Genet.* **2018**, *55*, 384–394. [CrossRef]
3. Dahia, P.L.M. Pheochromocytoma and paraganglioma pathogenesis: Learning from genetic heterogeneity. *Nat. Rev. Cancer* **2014**, *14*, 108–119. [CrossRef]
4. Currás-Freixes, M.; Piñeiro-Yañez, E.; Montero-Conde, C.; Apellániz-Ruiz, M.; Calsina, B.; Mancikova, V.; Remacha, L.; Richter, S.; Ercolino, T.; Rogowski-Lehmann, N.; et al. PheoSeq: A Targeted Next-Generation Sequencing Assay for Pheochromocytoma and Paraganglioma Diagnostics. *J. Mol. Diagn.* **2017**, *19*, 575–588. [CrossRef] [PubMed]
5. Renella, R.; Carnevale, J.; Schneider, K.A.; Hornick, J.L.; Rana, H.Q.; Janeway, K.A. Exploring the association of succinate dehydrogenase complex mutations with lymphoid malignancies. *Fam. Cancer* **2014**, *13*, 507–511. [CrossRef]
6. Vanharanta, S.; Buchta, M.; McWhinney, S.R.; Virta, S.K.; Pęczkowska, M.; Morrison, C.D.; Lehtonen, R.J.; Januszewicz, A.; Järvinen, H.; Juhola, M.; et al. Early-Onset Renal Cell Carcinoma as a Novel Extraparaganglial Component of SDHB-Associated Heritable Paraganglioma. *Am. J. Hum. Genet.* **2004**, *74*, 153–159. [CrossRef] [PubMed]
7. Miettinen, M.; Lasota, J. Succinate dehydrogenase deficient gastrointestinal stromal tumors (GISTs)—A review. *Int. J. Biochem. Cell Biol.* **2014**, *53*, 514–519. [CrossRef]
8. Ugarte-Camara, M.; Fernandez-Prado, R.; Lorda, I.; Rossello, G.; Gonzalez-Enguita, C.; Cannata-Ortiz, P.; Ortiz, A. Positive/retained SDHB immunostaining in renal cell carcinomas associated to germline SDHB-deficiency: Case report. *Diagn. Pathol.* **2019**, *14*, 42. [CrossRef]
9. Gill, A.J. Succinate dehydrogenase (SDH)-deficient neoplasia. *Histopathology* **2018**, *72*, 106–116. [CrossRef] [PubMed]
10. Killian, J.K.; Miettinen, M.; Walker, R.L.; Wang, Y.; Zhu, Y.J.; Waterfall, J.J.; Noyes, N.; Retnakumar, P.; Yang, Z.; Smith, W.I.; et al. Recurrent epimutation of SDHC in gastrointestinal stromal tumors. *Sci. Transl. Med.* **2014**, *6*, 268ra177. [CrossRef]
11. Roszko, K.L.; Blouch, E.; Blake, M.; Powers, J.; Tischler, A.; Hodin, R.; Sadow, P.; Lawson, E.A. Case Report of a Prolactinoma in a Patient With a Novel MAX Mutation and Bilateral Pheochromocytomas. *J. Endocr. Soc.* **2017**, *1*, 1401–1407. [CrossRef]
12. Hernandez, K.G.; Ezzat, S.; Morel, C.F.; Swallow, C.; Otremba, M.; Dickson, B.; Asa, S.; Mete, O. Familial pheochromocytoma and renal cell carcinoma syndrome: TMEM127 as a novel candidate gene for the association. *Virchows Arch.* **2015**, *466*, 727–732. [CrossRef]
13. Muller, M.; Ferlicot, S.; Guillaud-Bataille, M.; Le Teuff, G.; Genestie, C.; Deveaux, S.; Slama, A.; Poulalhon, N.; Escudier, B.; Albiges, L.; et al. Reassessing the clinical spectrum associated with hereditary leiomyomatosis and renal cell carcinoma syndrome in French FH mutation carriers. *Clin. Genet.* **2017**, *92*, 606–615. [CrossRef] [PubMed]

14. Xekouki, P.; Brennand, A.; Whitelaw, B.; Pacak, K.; Stratakis, C.A. The 3PAs: An Update on the Association of Pheochromocytomas, Paragangliomas, and Pituitary Tumors. *Horm. Metab. Res.* **2019**, *51*, 419–436. [CrossRef]
15. O'Toole, S.M.; Dénes, J.; Robledo, M.; A Stratakis, C.; Korbonits, M. 15 YEARS OF PARAGANGLIOMA: The association of pituitary adenomas and phaeochromocytomas or paragangliomas. *Endocr. -Related Cancer* **2015**, *22*, T105–T122. [CrossRef]
16. Canu, L.; Puglisi, S.; Berchialla, P.; De Filpo, G.; Brignardello, F.; Schiavi, F.; Ferrara, A.M.; Zovato, S.; Luconi, M.; Pia, A.; et al. Depositated in Figshare 5 June 2021. [CrossRef]
17. AIOM-AIRTUM. I Numeri del Cancro in Italia. Available online: https://www.aiom.it/wp-content/uploads/2019/09/2019_Numeri_Cancro-operatori-web.pdf (accessed on 1 February 2021).
18. Lam, A.K.-Y. Update on Adrenal Tumours in 2017 World Health Organization (WHO) of Endocrine Tumours. *Endocr. Pathol.* **2017**, *28*, 213–227. [CrossRef]
19. Tischler, A.; de Krijger, R. Phaeocromocytoma. In *WHO Classification of Tumours of Endocrine Organs*, 4th ed.; International Agency for Research on Cancer (IARC): Lyon, France, 2017; pp. 183–189.
20. Kimura, N.; Cappella, C. Extraadrenal paraganglioma. In *WHO Classification of Tumours of Endocrine Organs*, 4th ed.; International Agency for Research on Cancer (IARC): Lyon, France, 2017; pp. 190–195.
21. Burnham, K.P.; Anderson, D.R. *Model Selection and Multimodel Inference*, 2nd ed.; Springer: New York, NY, USA, 2002.
22. Khorram-Manesh, A.; Jansson, S.; Wangberg, B.; Nilsson, O.; Tisell, L.-E.; Ahlman, H. Mortality Associated with Pheochromocytoma: Increased Risk for Additional Tumors. *Ann. N. Y. Acad. Sci.* **2006**, *1073*, 444–448. [CrossRef] [PubMed]
23. Papathomas, T.G.; Oudijk, L.; Persu, A.; Gill, A.J.; Van Nederveen, F.; Tischler, A.; Tissier, F.; Volante, M.; Matias-Guiu, X.; Smid, M.; et al. SDHB/SDHA immunohistochemistry in pheochromocytomas and paragangliomas: A multicenter interobserver variation analysis using virtual microscopy: A Multinational Study of the European Network for the Study of Adrenal Tumors (ENS@T). *Mod. Pathol.* **2015**, *28*, 807–821. [CrossRef] [PubMed]
24. Bertolotto, C.; Abbe, P.; Hemesath, T.J.; Bille, K.; Fisher, D.E.; Ortonne, J.-P.; Ballotti, R. Microphthalmia Gene Product as a Signal Transducer in cAMP-Induced Differentiation of Melanocytes. *J. Cell Biol.* **1998**, *142*, 827–835. [CrossRef]
25. Bertolotto, C.; Lesueur, F.; Giuliano, S.; Strub, T.; De Lichy, M.; Bille, K.; Dessen, P.; D'Hayer, B.; Mohamdi, H.; Remenieras, A.; et al. A SUMOylation-defective MITF germline mutation predisposes to melanoma and renal carcinoma. *Nature* **2011**, *480*, 94–98. [CrossRef] [PubMed]
26. Yokoyama, S.; Woods, S.L.; Boyle, G.M.; Aoude, L.G.; MacGregor, S.; Zismann, V.; Gartside, M.; Cust, A.E.; Haq, R.; Harland, M.; et al. A novel recurrent mutation in MITF predisposes to familial and sporadic melanoma. *Nature* **2011**, *480*, 99–103. [CrossRef]
27. Castro-Vega, L.J.; Kiando, S.R.; Burnichon, N.; Buffet, A.; Amar, L.; Simian, C.; Berdelou, A.; Galan, P.; Schlumberger, M.; Bouatia-Naji, N.; et al. The MITF, p.E318K Variant, as a Risk Factor for Pheochromocytoma and Paraganglioma. *J. Clin. Endocrinol. Metab.* **2016**, *101*, 4764–4768. [CrossRef] [PubMed]
28. Carbone, M.; Yang, H.; Pass, H.; Krausz, T.; Testa, J.R.; Gaudino, G. BAP1 and cancer. *Nat. Rev. Cancer* **2013**, *13*, 153–159. [CrossRef]
29. Maffeis, V.; Cappellesso, R.; Nicolè, L.; Guzzardo, V.; Menin, C.; Elefanti, L.; Schiavi, F.; Guido, M.; Fassina, A. Loss of BAP1 in Pheochromocytomas and Paragangliomas Seems Unrelated to Genetic Mutations. *Endocr. Pathol.* **2019**, *30*, 276–284. [CrossRef]
30. Bugalho, M.J.; Silva, A.L.; Domingues, R. Coexistence of paraganglioma/pheochromocytoma and papillary thyroid carcinoma: A four-case series analysis. *Fam. Cancer* **2015**, *14*, 603–607. [CrossRef]
31. Miettinen, M.; Sarlomo-Rikala, M.; Cue, P.M.; Czapiewski, P.; Langfort, R.; Waloszczyk, P.; Wazny, K.; Biernat, W.; Lasota, J.; Wang, Z. Mapping of Succinate Dehydrogenase Losses in 2258 Epithelial Neoplasms. *Appl. Immunohistochem. Mol. Morphol.* **2014**, *22*, 31–36. [CrossRef]
32. Plouin, P.F.; Amar, L.; Dekkers, O.M.; Fassnacht, M.; Gimenez-Roqueplo, A.P.; Lenders, J.W.M.; Lussey-Lepoutre, C.; Steichen, O. European Society of Endocrinology Clinical Practice Guideline for long-term follow-up of patients operated on for a phaeochromocytoma or a paraganglioma. *Eur. J. Endocrinol.* **2016**, *174*, G1–G10. [CrossRef]
33. Mannelli, M.; Canu, L.; Ercolino, T.; Rapizzi, E.; Martinelli, S.; Parenti, G.; De Filpo, G.; Nesi, G. DIAGNOSIS of ENDOCRINE DISEASE: SDHx mutations: Beyond pheochromocytomas and paragangliomas. *Eur. J. Endocrinol.* **2018**, *178*, R11–R17. [CrossRef] [PubMed]
34. Matsuda, K. PCR-Based Detection Methods for Single-Nucleotide Polymorphism or Mutation. *Adv. Clin. Chem.* **2017**, *80*, 45–72. [CrossRef]
35. Mitra, A.; Singh, S.V.; Garg, V.K.; Sharma, M.; Chaturvedi, R.; Rath, S.K. Protective association exhibited by the single nucleotide polymorphism (SNP) rs1052133 in the gene human 8-oxoguanine DNA glycosylase (hOGG1) with the risk of squamous cell carcinomas of the head & neck (SCCHN) among north Indians. *Indian J. Med. Res.* **2011**, *133*, 605–612.
36. Hoffman, J.; Fejerman, L.; Hu, D.; Huntsman, S.; Li, M.; John, E.M.; Torres-Mejía, G.; Kushi, L.H.; Ding, Y.C.; Weitzel, J.; et al. Identification of novel common breast cancer risk variants at the 6q25 locus among Latinas. *Breast Cancer Res.* **2019**, *21*, 3. [CrossRef]
37. Zhu, J.; Jia, W.; Wu, C.; Fu, W.; Xia, H.; Liu, G.; He, J. Base Excision Repair Gene Polymorphisms and Wilms Tumor Susceptibility. *EBioMedicine* **2018**, *33*, 88–93. [CrossRef] [PubMed]
38. Neumann, H.P.H.; De Herder, W. Energy and metabolic alterations in predisposition to pheochromocytomas and paragangliomas: The so-called Warburg (and more) effect, 15 years on. *Endocr.-Relat. Cancer* **2015**, *22*, E5–E7. [CrossRef] [PubMed]

39. Mravec, B.; Dubravicky, J.; Tibensky, M.; Horvathova, L. Effect of the nervous system on cancer: Analysis of clinical studies. *Bratisl. Lek. List.* **2019**, *120*, 119–123. [CrossRef]
40. Mravec, B.; Horvathova, L.; Hunakova, L. Neurobiology of Cancer: The Role of β-Adrenergic Receptor Signaling in Various Tumor Environments. *Int. J. Mol. Sci.* **2020**, *21*, 7958. [CrossRef] [PubMed]

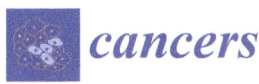

Article

Targeting the Redox Balance Pathway Using Ascorbic Acid in *sdhb* Zebrafish Mutant Larvae

Margo Dona [1,*], Maaike Lamers [1], Svenja Rohde [1], Marnix Gorissen [2] and Henri J. L. M. Timmers [1]

[1] Department of Internal Medicine, Radboud University Medical Center, 6525 GA Nijmegen, The Netherlands; mhg.lamers@gmail.com (M.L.); srohde.99@gmail.com (S.R.); henri.timmers@radboudumc.nl (H.J.L.M.T.)
[2] Department of Animal Ecology and Physiology, Radboud Institute for Biological and Environmental Sciences, Radboud University, 6525 AJ Nijmegen, The Netherlands; M.Gorissen@science.ru.nl
* Correspondence: margo.dona@radboudumc.nl

Simple Summary: Thus far, no curative therapies are available for malignant *SDHB*-associated phaeochromocytomas and paragangliomas (PPGLs). Therapy development is severely hampered by the limited availability of suitable animal models. In this study, we investigated the potential of the *sdhb*^{rmc200} zebrafish model to study *SDHB*-associated PPGLs using a drug screening approach. One of the key features of cancer initiation and progression is redox imbalance. First, we identified increased reactive oxygen species levels in homozygous *sdhb*^{rmc200} larvae at baseline. Next, we tested the effect of anti- and pro-oxidant ascorbic acid (Vitamin C) on these larvae. We validated the *sdhb*^{rmc200} zebrafish model as a powerful drug screening tool to provide valuable insights into pathomechanisms, which may lead to novel therapeutic targets and therapy development in the future.

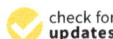

Citation: Dona, M.; Lamers, M.; Rohde, S.; Gorissen, M.; Timmers, H.J.L.M. Targeting the Redox Balance Pathway Using Ascorbic Acid in *sdhb* Zebrafish Mutant Larvae. *Cancers* **2021**, *13*, 5124. https://doi.org/10.3390/cancers13205124

Academic Editor: Peter Igaz

Received: 17 September 2021
Accepted: 11 October 2021
Published: 13 October 2021

Publisher's Note: MDPI stays neutral with regard to jurisdictional claims in published maps and institutional affiliations.

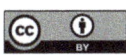

Copyright: © 2021 by the authors. Licensee MDPI, Basel, Switzerland. This article is an open access article distributed under the terms and conditions of the Creative Commons Attribution (CC BY) license (https://creativecommons.org/licenses/by/4.0/).

Abstract: Patients with mutations in the β-subunit of the succinate dehydrogenase (*SDHB*) have the highest risk to develop incurable malignant phaeochromocytomas and paragangliomas (PPGLs). Therapy development is hindered by limited possibilities to test new therapeutic strategies in vivo. One possible molecular mechanism of *SDHB*-associated tumorigenesis originates in an overproduction of reactive oxygen species (ROS) due to mitochondrial dysfunction. Ascorbic acid (Vitamin C) has already been shown to act as anti-cancer agent in several clinical trials for various types of cancer. In this study, the potential of the *sdhb*^{rmc200} zebrafish model to study *SDHB*-associated PPGLs using a drug screening approach was investigated. First, we identified increased basal ROS levels in homozygous *sdhb* larvae compared to heterozygous and wild-type siblings. Using a semi high-throughput drug screening, the effectiveness of different dosages of anti- and pro-oxidant Vitamin C were assessed to evaluate differences in survival, ROS levels, and locomotor activity. Low-dosage levels of Vitamin C induced a decrease of ROS levels but no significant effects on lifespan. In contrast, high-dosage levels of Vitamin C shortened the lifespan of the homozygous *sdhb*^{rmc200} larvae while not affecting the lifespan of heterozygous and wild-type siblings. These results validated the *sdhb*^{rmc200} zebrafish model as a powerful drug screening tool that may be used to identify novel therapeutic targets for *SDHB*-associated PPGLs.

Keywords: phaeochromocytoma; paraganglioma; cancer; mitochondrial complex II; zebrafish; therapy; drug discovery; redox balance pathway; Vitamin C

1. Introduction

The mitochondrial enzymatic succinate dehydrogenase (SDH) complex, also called mitochondrial complex II, has an essential role in ATP production. The dysfunction of the SDH complex is linked to several diseases, varying from severe neuromuscular disorders [1] to different types of cancer including phaeochromocytomas and paragangliomas (PPGLs), gastrointestinal stromal tumour, renal cell carcinoma (RCC), pituitary adenoma, and pancreatic neuroendocrine tumours [2,3].

PPGLs are rare neuroendocrine tumours originating from chromaffin cells in the adrenal medulla or from extra-adrenal paraganglia, respectively [4]. The incidence of PPGLs is up to eight per million persons per year [5]. Although the majority of the tumours are benign, genetic predisposition can be a risk factor for metastasis development, resulting in poor prognosis [6–9]. The most prevalent *succinate dehydrogenase subunit B* (*SDHB*) germline mutations are especially known to play a crucial role in the pathogenesis of aggressive PPGLs, with a metastatic rate of 50–97% [9–11]. In general, the curative surgical removal of the tumour is no longer valid when metastases develop. Although not curative, chemotherapy, radionuclide therapy, and anti-angiogenic drugs might lead to the stabilisation of the disease for months to years, improved quality of life, and prolonged survival. To develop more effective and targeted treatment detailed insight into the pathomechanisms is essential [12].

Several hypotheses of the predisposition for the malignancy of *SDHB*-mutated PPGLs have been proposed [13,14]. Upon the dysregulation of the SDH complex, the oncometabolite succinate accumulates, which leads to the reprogramming of cellular metabolic pathways including hypermethylation, the activation of the HIF pathway, and decreased DNA repair [14]. In addition, the substantial loss of complex II activity impairs electron transfer to oxygen and thus leads to the increased formation of reactive oxygen species (ROS) and redox imbalance [9,15–19]. Increased ROS levels can cause defects in cell signalling, DNA damage, and lipid peroxidation [20]. The ability of ROS to cause genomic instability is a well-established cause of carcinogenesis. In this study, we investigated the potential of the *sdhb^{rmc200}* zebrafish model to study *SDHB*-associated PPGLs using a drug screen approach.

High-dosage levels of ascorbic acid (Vitamin C) have already been shown to act as anti-cancer agent for several types of cancer [21]. Vitamin C can act as an antioxidant, reducing ROS levels, but it can also function as pro-oxidant to kill cancer cells in vitro and slow tumour growth in vivo. Pharmacologic levels of Vitamin C have been shown to aggravate the ROS-mediated toxicity in *SDHB^{KD}* mouse phaeochromocytoma (MPC) cells, thus leading to genetic instability and apoptotic cell death [19]. Moreover, these *SDHB^{KD}* MPC cells were injected into athymic nude mice, establishing metastatic PPGL tumours in vivo; the supplementation of high-dosage levels of Vitamin C strongly delayed metastatic lesions and thereby improved disease outcome [19].

Recently, we generated and characterised a systemic *sdhb^{rmc200}* knockout zebrafish model that mimics the metabolic properties of *SDHB*-associated PPGLs [22]. Homozygous *sdhb^{rmc200}* mutant larvae display a decreased lifespan due to decreased mitochondrial complex II activity and significant succinate accumulation, and they mimic important genomic and metabolic effects observed in *SDHB*-associated PPGL tumours [22]. In addition, a decreased mobility attributed to energy deficiency is observed. These phenotypic read-outs in 6-day-old zebrafish larvae can be used to evaluate the effects of candidate drugs and could facilitate the (semi) high-throughput in vivo testing of potential therapeutic agents for *SDHB*-associated PPGLs.

In this study, we investigated redox homeostasis in larvae of the *sdhb^{rmc200}* zebrafish model, and we evaluated the effect of both low-dosage and high-dosage levels of Vitamin C by using an in vivo zebrafish drug screen.

2. Results

2.1. sdhb^{rmc200} Zebrafish Larvae as Drug Screening Model for SDHB-Associated PPGLs

2.1.1. Homozygous *sdhb^{rmc200}* Zebrafish Larvae Exhibit Increased Reactive Oxygen Species (ROS) Levels

To investigate whether *sdhb^{rmc200}* larval zebrafish mutants possess an unbalanced cellular redox state, whole-mount ROS-detection was used to determine ROS levels at baseline. At day 6 post fertilization (dpf), increased levels of ROS were observed in homozygous *sdhb* compared to their heterozygous *sdhb* and wild-type siblings (Figure 1).

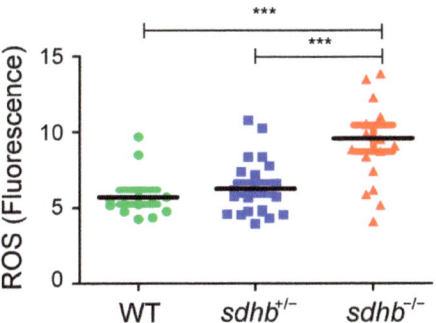

Figure 1. Reactive oxygen species (ROS) measurements showed a significant increase in homozygous *sdhb* larvae (n = 17) compared to their heterozygous (n = 22) and wild-type siblings (n = 12) at 6 dpf. One-way ANOVA with Tukey's post hoc test, *** $p < 0.001$.

2.1.2. Successful Design of Drug Screening Protocol

To test the effect of Vitamin C on zebrafish larvae, an optimal drug screening protocol was established (Figure 2). First, the offspring of the incross of heterozygous adult *sdhb* mutants were collected. At day 2 post fertilization (dpf), hatched larvae were assembled in 48-well plates with either an E3 control egg medium or E3 medium supplemented with Vitamin C (20, 500, or 1000 mg·L^{-1}). Different read-outs to assess the effect of the vitamin were developed. Lethality scores were performed to assess the effect of Vitamin C on overall survival. In addition, at day 6, ROS levels were measured to check the effect of supplementation of the anti- and pro-oxidant Vitamin C. As quick read-out for general health and toxicity, locomotor activity was evaluated using DanioVision at day 6.

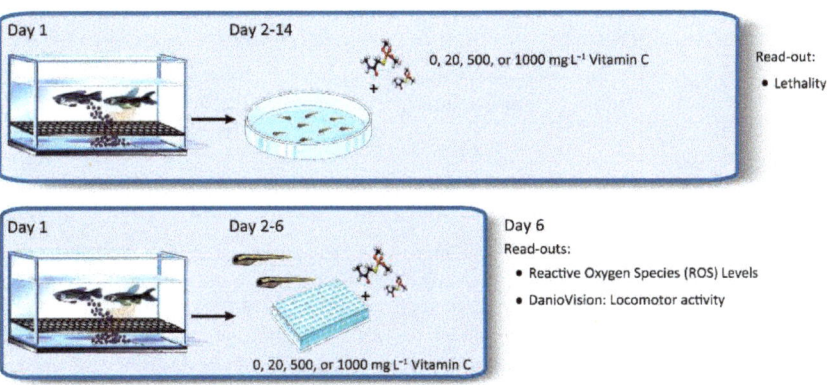

Figure 2. Schematic overview of zebrafish drug screening set-up.

2.2. Effects of Vitamin C as Anti- and Pro-Oxidant on Sdhb Zebrafish Larvae

2.2.1. High-Dosage Levels of Vitamin C Decreases Lifespan of Homozygous *sdhb*^{rmc200} Larvae

Heterozygous adult *sdhb* mutants were used to generate a mixed offspring following Mendelian inheritance. The larvae were checked at least twice a day to determine lethality. At baseline, homozygous *sdhb* larvae showed an enhanced mortality compared to heterozygous and wild-type siblings (Figure 3A,C,E). Low dosages of Vitamin C (20 mg·L^{-1}) did not have an significant effect on the survival of homozygous *sdhb*, heterozygous *sdhb*, or wild-type larvae measured until two weeks of age. High dosage levels of Vitamin C

(500 and 1000 mg·L^{-1}) significantly decreased the survival rate of the homozygous *sdhb* mutants (Figure 3F; $p < 0.01$) while not having a significant effect on heterozygous and wild-type siblings (Figure 3B–D).

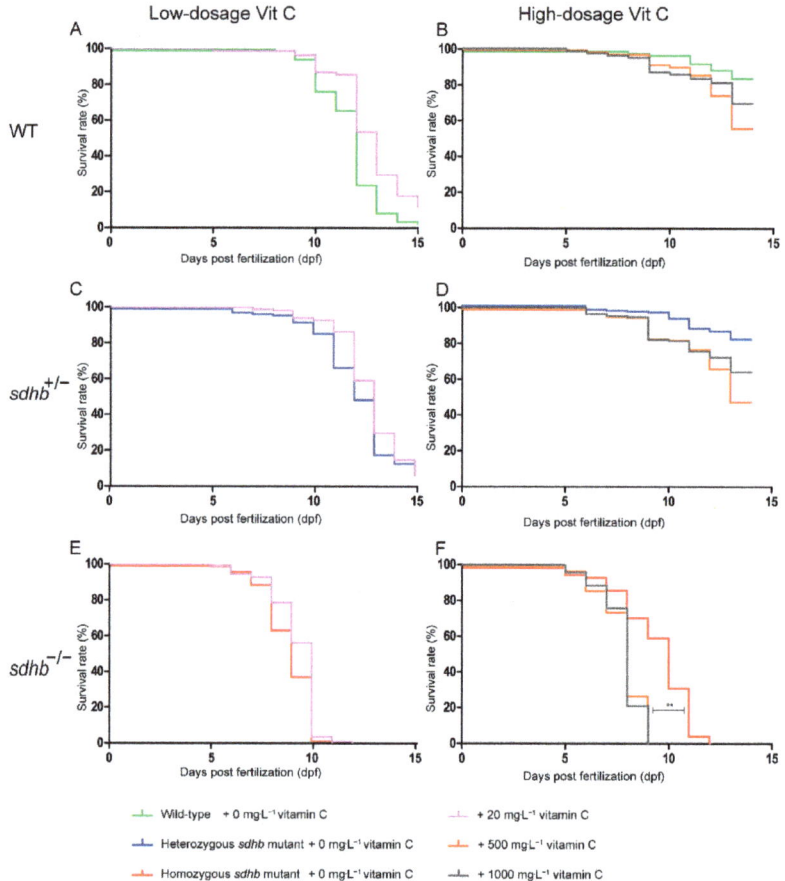

Figure 3. Survival in WT siblings (**A,B**), heterozygous *sdhb* mutants (**C,D**), and homozygous *sdhb* mutants (**E,F**) presented for control (0 mg·L^{-1} green, blue, and red lines, respectively); low dosage ((**A,C,E**) 20 mg·L^{-1}, purple line) and high dosage ((**B,D,F**) 500 mg·L^{-1}, orange line; 1000 mg·L^{-1}, grey line) Vitamin-C-treated larvae. (**A,C,E**) Survival rate (%) was not significantly prolonged after the low-dosage treatment of Vitamin C *sdhb* larvae compared to control (E3 medium supplemented; 0 mg·L^{-1}) larvae (control: $n = 95$ homozygous *sdhb* larvae, $n = 126$ heterozygous *sdhb* larvae, and $n = 85$ WT larvae; 20 mg·L^{-1} Vitamin C: $n = 112$ homozygous *sdhb* larvae, $n = 190$ heterozygous *sdhb* larvae, and $n = 91$ WT larvae from two replicates). (**B,D,F**) Survival rate (%) was significantly reduced in homozygous *sdhb* mutants after treatment with high dosages of Vitamin C (500 and 1000 mg·L^{-1}) compared to control (E3 medium supplemented) larvae (control: $n = 72$ homozygous *sdhb* larvae, $n = 198$ heterozygous *sdhb* larvae, and $n = 87$ WT larvae; 500 mg·L^{-1} Vitamin C: $n = 84$ homozygous *sdhb* larvae, $n = 195$ heterozygous *sdhb* larvae, and $n = 70$ WT larvae; 1000 mg·L^{-1} Vitamin C: $n = 90$ homozygous *sdhb* larvae, $n = 172$ heterozygous *sdhb* larvae, and $n = 86$ WT larvae from two replicates). No significant differences were observed between *sdhb* heterozygous and WT siblings at either low or high dosage Vitamin C treatment. Log-rank (Mantel–Cox) test, ** $p < 0.01$.

2.2.2. Effects of Vitamin C Treatment on ROS Levels

The effect of low-dosage and high-dosage levels of Vitamin C was measured compared to an untreated control group. In Figure 4, the ROS levels after the supplementation of either the E3 medium control medium (0 mg·L^{-1}) or low-dosage levels of Vitamin C (20 mg·L^{-1}) and high-dosage Vitamin C levels of Vitamin C (500 and 1000 mg·L^{-1}) are shown. Low-dosage Vitamin C levels significantly decreased ROS levels in the heterozygous and homozygous *sdhb* mutant group compared to the untreated control group, while no significant differences were identified in the wild-type group without low-dosage levels of Vitamin C. High-dosage levels of Vitamin C possessed a more heterozygous effect in heterozygous and homozygous *sdhb* larvae. No significant differences were identified high-dosage levels of Vitamin C supplementation.

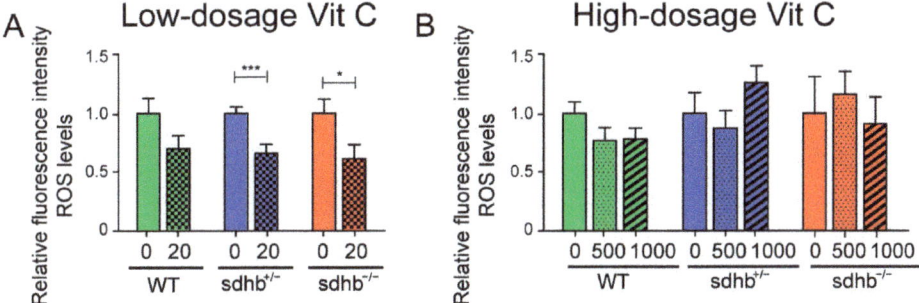

Figure 4. Reactive oxygen species (ROS) measurements after a low- and high-dosage Vitamin C treatment. Relative average fluorescence levels are shown normalised to control levels without Vitamin C supplementation. (**A**) Larvae were supplemented with 20 mg·L^{-1} Vitamin C homozygous *sdhb* ($n = 22$), heterozygous sibling ($n = 33$), and wild-type sibling ($n = 21$) compared to the control group (indicated with 0 mg·L^{-1}) consisting of homozygous *sdhb* larvae ($n = 24$), heterozygous sibling ($n = 38$), and wild-type sibling ($n = 18$) from two different replicates measured at 6 dpf. Low-dosage levels of Vitamin C significantly decreased ROS levels in heterozygous and homozygous *sdhb* larvae compared to the untreated control group. (**B**) Larvae were supplemented with 500 mg·L^{-1} Vitamin C homozygous *sdhb* ($n = 12$), heterozygous sibling ($n = 24$), and wild-type sibling ($n = 18$); 1000 mg·L^{-1} Vitamin C homozygous *sdhb* ($n = 8$), heterozygous sibling ($n = 22$), and wild-type sibling ($n = 22$) compared to the control group (indicated with 0 mg·L^{-1}) consisting of homozygous *sdhb* larvae ($n = 10$), heterozygous sibling ($n = 14$), and wild-type sibling ($n = 16$) from three different replicates measured at 6 dpf. High-dosage levels of Vitamin C did not alter ROS levels in all three genotypes compared to the untreated control group. Two-tailed unpaired Student's *t*-test, * $p < 0.05$ and *** $p < 0.001$.

2.2.3. Behavioural Assessment as Quick Read-Out of Toxicity of the Larvae

We previously identified that homozygous *sdhb* mutant larvae possess a lower basal activity and reduced endurance compared to heterozygous and wild-type siblings [22]. We designed a short protocol (<5 min) with randomized tapping stimuli to induce a robust startle response. In Figure 5A, the maximum distance moved is plotted against time in seconds, all peaks reflect a startle response induced by the tapping stimulus. At baseline, homozygous *sdhb* mutant larvae possessed a decreased startle response compared to heterozygous and wild-type siblings. Low-dosage levels of Vitamin C induced a significantly decreased startle response in heterozygous *sdhb* and wild-type larvae but did not alter the startle response of homozygous *sdhb* larvae (Figure 5B). Furthermore, both high-dosage levels of Vitamin C decreased the startle response of heterozygous *sdhb* larvae, but only 1000 mg·L^{-1} had a significant decreased in startle response in homozygous *sdhb* larvae and none of the high-dosage levels significantly affected the startle response of the wild-type larvae (Figure 5C).

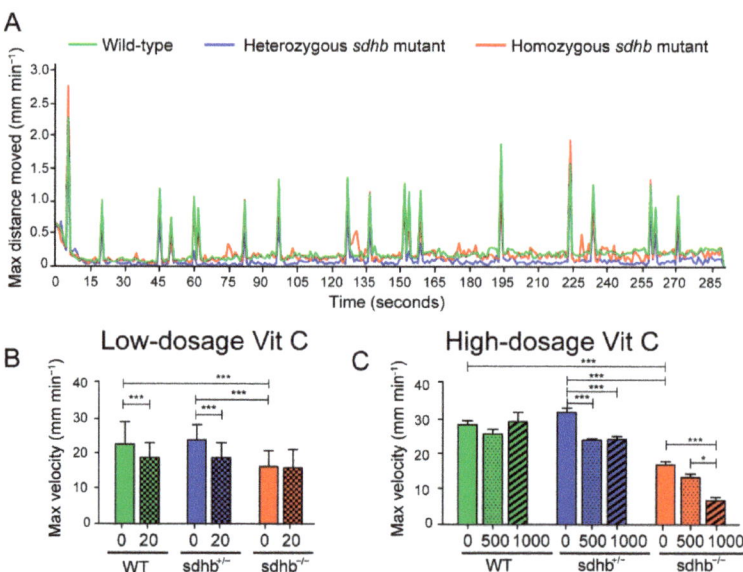

Figure 5. Startle response measurements at basal level and after low- and high-dosage levels of Vitamin C. (**A**) Optimized short protocol (<5 min in total) to quickly assess startle responses as a toxicity indicator induced by tapping stimuli with random intervals varying between 2 and 35 s. The max distance moved (mm min^{-1}) is plotted against time per seconds. Between the wild-type (green line) and heterozygous mutants (blue line), no differences were observed, while homozygous *sdhb* mutants (red line) showed a decrease in moved distance. (**B**) Quantification of the average of the maximum velocity of three startle responses with or without the supplementation of low-dosage levels of Vitamin C (20 mg·L^{-1}). Low-dosage levels of Vitamin C decreased the startle response of wild-type and heterozygous *sdhb* larvae while not affecting homozygous *sdhb* larvae. Larvae were supplemented with 20 mg·L^{-1} Vitamin C homozygous *sdhb* (n = 106), heterozygous sibling (n = 244), and wild-type sibling (n = 137) compared to the control group (indicated with 0 mg·L^{-1}) consisting of homozygous *sdhb* larvae (n = 91), heterozygous sibling (n = 227), and wild-type sibling (n = 100) from five different replicates measured at 6 dpf. (**C**) Quantification of the average of the maximum velocity of three startle responses with or without supplementation of high-dosage levels of Vitamin C (500 and 1000 mg·L^{-1}). Both 500 and 1000 mg·L^{-1} concentrations of Vitamin C induced a decreased startle response in heterozygous *sdhb* larvae, while only the 1000 mg·L^{-1} concentration of Vitamin C induced a decreased startle response in homozygous *sdhb* larvae and none of the high-dosage levels of Vitamin C significantly altered the startle response of the wild-type larvae. Larvae were supplemented with 500 mg·L^{-1} Vitamin C homozygous *sdhb* (n = 73), heterozygous sibling (n = 139), and wild-type sibling (n = 55), 1000 mg·L^{-1} Vitamin C homozygous *sdhb* (n = 20), heterozygous sibling (n = 37), and wild-type sibling (n = 19) compared to the control group (indicated with 0 mg·L^{-1}) consisting of homozygous *sdhb* larvae (n = 32), heterozygous sibling (n = 48), and wild-type sibling (n = 40) from at least two different replicates measured at 6 dpf. One-way ANOVA with Tukey's post hoc test, * $p < 0.05$ and *** $p < 0.001$.

3. Discussion

The development of novel therapeutic targets for metastatic *SDHB*-associated PPGLs is hampered by the limited availability of suitable in vivo models. In this study, we investigated the effects of Vitamin C in the *sdhb*^{rmc200} zebrafish model and thereby tested the suitability for drug screening experiments in this validated PPGL cancer model [22]. First, we revealed an imbalance in cellular redox homeostasis in homozygous *sdhb* zebrafish larvae by increased levels of ROS at baseline. Next, we successfully tested the effect of different dosages of Vitamin C treatment: aqueous solutions of Vitamin C were added to the swim water of the larvae, and we showed that although low-dosage levels (20 mg·L^{-1}) of Vitamin C did not increase the lifespan of homozygous *sdhb* larvae, ROS was decreased. High-dosage levels of Vitamin C (500 and 1000 mg·L^{-1}) significantly shortened the lifespan of homozygous *sdhb* larvae while not altering the lifespan of their heterozygous *sdhb* and wild-type siblings regardless of unchanged levels of ROS.

As previously reported, homozygous *sdhb* larvae have a shortened lifespan (maximal two weeks of age) compared to heterozygous *sdhb* and wild-type siblings [22]. Additionally, these homozygous *sdhb* larvae display key metabolic characteristics of *SDHB*-associated PPGLs such as impaired mitochondrial complex II function and vastly increased succinate levels [22]. The heterozygous *sdhb* larvae revealed no differences in mitochondrial function and metabolite levels compared to wild-types siblings.

Here, we identified increased ROS levels in homozygous *sdhb* larvae compared to heterozygous and wild-type siblings. Redox imbalance by increased levels of ROS is known to play a critical role in carcinogenesis [23–25], as has also been suggested for PPGLs [14,26,27]. Although no alternative relevant systemic *Sdhb* knockout animal model is available, different cell lines and graft models have been created. Our findings are in line with increased ROS levels in the mitochondria of *SDHB*-deficient mouse phaeochromocytoma cells [19], confirmed by two *SDHB*-silenced cell lines and one *SDHC*-mutated transgenic mouse cell line [17,28,29]. On the other hand, two other studies reported no increased ROS levels in cell lines silenced for *SDHB* [30,31], despite hypoxia-inducible factor (HIF) stabilisation. The usage of different cell lines and the variations of different assays for measuring ROS could be reasons for this discrepancy.

Zebrafish models possesses unique advantages for investigating the effect of drugs to unravel pathomechanisms and test the therapeutic efficacy of re-purposing drugs from related types of cancer such as neuroblastoma and RCC [32]. Zebrafish can produce a large number of offspring, rapidly develop, and still have a high grade of similarity with humans; approximately 70% of human genes have at least one obvious zebrafish orthologue [33]. The use of larval zebrafish as a model organism in semi high-throughput drug screens is rapidly expanding [34–36]. This drug screen approach enables one to test a high number of potential targets, evaluate toxicity, and evaluate compound efficiency to select the most promising drugs to be validated in pre-clinical tumour models. The read-outs we optimized for our drug screen are lethality measurements, which are the most important and direct values used to check effects on lifespan, a protocol to assess locomotion activity as read-out for toxicity and possible other negative side-effects, and ROS levels.

Vitamin C is a natural compound with a high safety profile that was previously positively tested in pre-clinical studies for non-PPGL types of cancer [37]. The efficiency of Vitamin C has also been assessed in clinical trials, such as renal cell carcinoma in a phase-II clinical trial [21]. Often, Vitamin C is used supplementary to other types of treatment such as chemotherapy and radiation therapy. The exact mechanism of its action remains unclear since multiple critical pathways are targeted including redox imbalance, epigenetic reprogramming, and oxygen-sensing regulation, thereby preventing ROS-mediated toxicity [21]. Pharmacological levels of Vitamin C aggravated the oxidative burden of *SDHB*-deficient PPGLs, leading to genetic instability and apoptotic cell death [19]. Furthermore, in a preclinical animal model with PPGL allografts, high-dosage levels of Vitamin C suppressed metastatic lesions and prolonged overall subject survival [19].

We investigated the effects of low- and high-dosage levels of Vitamin C as pro- and antioxidants in the *sdhb* zebrafish larvae. Low-dosage levels of Vitamin C induced a decrease of ROS levels in homozygous mutants but no significant effects on lifespan. In contrast, high-dosage levels of Vitamin C further shortened the lifespan of the homozygous *sdhb* larvae while not affecting heterozygous and wild-type siblings. This is in line with previous findings obtained in the allografted mice model treated, with high-dosage levels of Vitamin C inducing ROS-medicated toxicity in tumour cells [19]. We detected no increase in basal ROS levels in the homozygous *sdhb* larvae supplemented with high-dosage levels of Vitamin C at 6 dpf. This discrepancy could be explained by the timing of the ROS measurement. We performed ROS measurements by using the fluorescent dye CM-H2DCFDA analysed by microscopy at 6 dpf. Fluorescence-activated cell sorting (FACs) analysis could optimise the quantification of the total ROS value in an entire larvae, and the measurements also could be performed at later time points to identify possible differences. Since in all other studies, HIF stabilisation was detected regardless of whether increased or normal ROS levels were detected, in follow up studies, other ROS indicators and HIF stabilisation could be measured as well.

Despite the fact that homozygous *sdhb* zebrafish larvae mimic the metabolic human tumour environment, the major limitation of using this zebrafish model is the absence of tumours at the age of 14 days. The translational value to predict the effect in human PPGLs therefore remains challenging and requires further investigation. For this, the allograft mice model and rat xenograft model are currently the best used alternatives [19,38]. Currently, the homozygous *sdhb* zebrafish larvae possess resemblance to patients with bi-allelic *SDHB* mutations with a Leigh-syndrome-like phenotype, resulting in severe progressive neurodegeneration and myopathy with the onset in infancy and poor prognosis [1,39]. The supplementation of low-dosage levels of Vitamin C was also shown to be effective in pre-clinical studies for neuropathy [40], and other anti-oxidants showed a beneficial effect for patients with mitochondrial disorders [41]. More research is required to investigate the therapeutic potential of low-dosage levels of Vitamin C for Leigh-syndrome-like patients.

To follow up the PPGL research, we will investigate whether adult heterozygous *sdhb* fish develop tumours in comparison to human *SDHB* mutations, which are at risk of developing PPGLs. If successful, this zebrafish tumour model can be complementarily used to test the potential of the most promising compounds identified in the larval drug seen for the effectiveness on tumour growth and to further unravel the mode of action behind its pathomechanism. Additionally, the onset of tumorigenesis and the prevention of tumour formation could be investigated in more detail.

In this study, we identified increased ROS levels in our homozygous *sdhb* larvae at baseline. Further, we validated the zebrafish larvae drug screen as tool to screen for therapeutic compounds and possible combination of compounds to target pathways involved in the tumorigenesis of *SDHB*-associated PPGLs. The most powerful advantage of this zebrafish model is its ability to screen many targets for possible new therapeutics in a cheap and cost-effective manner. This enables us to narrow down possible therapeutics to test for effectiveness in a more advanced tumour model. Patient-derived xenografts (PDXs) or cancer "Avatars" could attribute to personalized medicine in the future. In addition to mouse and rat PDXs [38,42], zebrafish Avatars are emerging as a cheaper and faster alternative [43,44] to hopefully accelerate personalised drug discovery for currently incurable metastatic *SDHB*-associated PPGLs.

4. Materials and Methods

4.1. Zebrafish Maintenance and Husbandry

Experimental procedures were conducted in accordance with institutional guidelines and National and European laws. Ethical approval of the experiments was granted by Radboud University's Institutional Animal Care and Use Committee (IACUC, application numbers RU-DEC 2015-0098 and RU-DEC 2020-0030). Wild-type adult Oregon AB* zebrafish (*Danio Rerio*) and heterozygous adult $sdhb^{rmc200}$ mutants were used [22]. Eggs were obtained from natural spawning. Larvae were maintained and raised by standard methods [45].

4.2. Genotyping

Larvae were briefly anesthetised in 2-phenoxyethanol (0.1%, *v/v*). Genomic DNA isolation and PCR amplification and analysis were performed as previously described [22].

4.3. ROS Measurements

ROS levels were assessed in 6 dpf zebrafish larvae using the 2′,7′-dichlorodihydrofluorescein diacetate (CM-H2DCFDA) dye (Fisher Scientific). When oxidized, this non-fluorescent dye is converted into a fluorescent compound, 2′,7′-dichlorofluorescein (DCF) [33]. The ROS levels were measured according to protocol [33]. In brief, each larva was individually placed in a well of a 96-well plate with 100 µL of an E3 embryo medium at 6 dpf. A working solution of H2DCFDA (500 µg/mL in dimethyl sulfoxide (DMSO, 14.1 M)/E3 medium (5 mM NaCl, 0.17 mM KCl, 0.33 mM CaCl2, and 0.33 mM MgSO4)) was prepared, and 100 µL were added to each well. Then, the solutions were mixed for 20 s at 150 rpm and incubated for 3.5 h at 28 °C in the dark. After incubation, the plates were analysed with the use of a fluorescence microscope (EVOS M5000 Imaging System) for the low-dosage levels of Vitamin C and a fluorescence microscope (Leica MZFL-III) for the high-dosage levels of Vitamin C. The level of fluorescence was calculated with the use of ImageJ [34].

4.4. Vitamin C Treatments

Fertilised eggs originating from a heterozygous $sdhb^{rmc200}$ incross were reared in petri dishes filled with E3 medium supplemented with 0.1% methylene blue (Sigma-Aldrich) and incubated at 28 °C with a day/night rhythm. At 2 dpf, the hatched larvae were put in a 48-wells plate containing 200 µL of medium with or without Vitamin C (A4544, Sigma-Aldrich) until 6 dpf. At day 5, the medium was replaced with E3 medium without or with appropriate concentrations of Vitamin C. All working solutions (20, 500, or 1000 mg·L^{-1}) were freshly prepared in E3 medium, and the pH was adjusted using 0.5 M NaOH between 6.8 and 8.5 [46].

4.5. Lethality Score Analysis

Heterozygous $sdhb^{rmc200}$ adult fish were crossed to collect eggs. The larvae were divided into two groups. An E3 medium was added for the control group, and a Vitamin C dosage (20, 500, or 1000 mg·L^{-1}) was added from 2 dpf onwards. Larvae were either raised in petri dishes (max 60 larvae per dish) for low-dosage levels of Vitamin C experiments or transferred to 1 L tanks for high-dosage levels of Vitamin C experiments. Minimally, twice a day, the larvae were checked to collect death larvae. Death larvae were collect in 75 µL of lysis buffer (40 mM NaOH and 0.2 mM EDTA) and then genotyped. Every day, the medium was refreshed, and in the afternoon, the larvae were fed with Gemma micro 75 ZF for the low-dosage level Vitamin C experiments and with rotifers for the high-dosage level Vitamin C experiments.

4.6. Behavioural Assessment: Locomotion Assay

Using DanioVision (Noldus Information Technologies, Wageningen, The Netherlands), the locomotion of 6 dpf larvae was tracked. Each larva was individually placed in a well of a 48-well plate with 200 µL of an E3 embryo medium. The study was conducted at a constant 28 °C and 3000 lux. The short protocol (<5 min in total) to induce startle responses consisted of tapping stimuli with random intervals varying between 2 and 35 s. Afterward, the complete larval body was used for genotyping. Larvae were pooled based on genotype and data grouped per phenotype were exported to Microsoft Excel (version 1906). The max velocity was used as read-outs for startle response to detect possible differences between the three different genotypes and Vitamin C treatment.

4.7. Statistical Analysis

GraphPad Prism software (Version 5.03 for Windows, GraphPad Software, La Jolla, CA, USA) was used to generate scatter plots, calculate mean values, and perform statistical analyses. The Log-rank (Mantel–Cox) test was used for the survival curve analysis. The one-way ANOVA with Tukey's post hoc test was used for the ROS basal levels and startle response quantification. A two-tailed unpaired Student's t-test was used for ROS levels without or with Vitamin C treatment.

5. Conclusions

In this study, we showed that the *sdhb* zebrafish model possesses an unbalanced redox homeostasis, as indicated by elevated ROS levels at baseline. Further, we evaluated the utility of *sdhb* zebrafish larvae to test drugs for their therapeutic potential for *SDHB*-associated PPGLs. We demonstrated that high-dosage levels of Vitamin C shortened the lifespan of homozygous *sdhb* larvae. This zebrafish model could potentially be used for preclinical drug screening and the identification of new therapeutic targets.

Author Contributions: Conceptualization, M.D. and M.G.; formal analysis, M.D., M.L. and S.R.; funding acquisition, M.D. and H.J.L.M.T.; investigation, M.D., M.L. and S.R.; writing—original draft, M.D.; writing—review and editing, M.G. and H.J.L.M.T. All authors have read and agreed to the published version of the manuscript.

Funding: This research was funded by the Paradifference Foundation.

Institutional Review Board Statement: Experimental procedures were conducted in accordance with institutional guidelines and National and European laws. Ethical approval of the experiments was granted by Radboud University's Institutional Animal Care and Use Committee (IACUC, application numbers RU-DEC 2015-0098 and RU-DEC 2020-0030).

Informed Consent Statement: Not applicable.

Data Availability Statement: The data presented in this study are available on request from the corresponding author.

Acknowledgments: The authors would like to thank Antoon Horst, Jeroen Boerrigter, and Jan Zethof for excellent zebrafish husbandry and experiment guidance.

Conflicts of Interest: The authors declare no conflict of interest. The funders had no role in the design of the study; in the collection, analyses, or interpretation of data; in the writing of the manuscript, or in the decision to publish the results.

References

1. Alston, C.L.; Davison, J.E.; Meloni, F.; van der Westhuizen, F.H.; He, L.; Hornig-Do, H.T.; Peet, A.C.; Gissen, P.; Goffrini, P.; Ferrero, I.; et al. Recessive germline SDHA and SDHB mutations causing leukodystrophy and isolated mitochondrial complex II deficiency. *J. Med. Genet.* **2012**, *49*, 569–577. [CrossRef] [PubMed]
2. Saxena, N.; Maio, N.; Crooks, D.R.; Ricketts, C.J.; Yang, Y.; Wei, M.H.; Fan, T.W.; Lane, A.N.; Sourbier, C.; Singh, A.; et al. SDHB-Deficient Cancers: The Role of Mutations That Impair Iron Sulfur Cluster Delivery. *J. Natl. Cancer Inst.* **2016**, *108*. [CrossRef]
3. Gill, A.J. Succinate dehydrogenase (SDH)-deficient neoplasia. *Histopathology* **2018**, *72*, 106–116. [CrossRef] [PubMed]
4. Jochmanova, I.; Pacak, K. Pheochromocytoma: The First Metabolic Endocrine Cancer. *Clin. Cancer Res.* **2016**, *22*, 5001–5011. [CrossRef] [PubMed]
5. Fishbein, L.; Leshchiner, I.; Walter, V.; Danilova, L.; Robertson, A.G.; Johnson, A.R.; Lichtenberg, T.M.; Murray, B.A.; Ghayee, H.K.; Else, T.; et al. Comprehensive Molecular Characterization of Pheochromocytoma and Paraganglioma. *Cancer Cell* **2017**, *31*, 181–193. [CrossRef]
6. Fishbein, L.; Nathanson, K.L. Pheochromocytoma and paraganglioma: Understanding the complexities of the genetic background. *Cancer Genet.* **2012**, *205*, 1–11. [CrossRef] [PubMed]
7. Zelinka, T.; Musil, Z.; Dušková, J.; Burton, D.; Merino, M.J.; Milosevic, D.; Widimský, J., Jr.; Pacak, K. Metastatic pheochromocytoma: Does the size and age matter? *Eur. J. Clin. Investig.* **2011**, *41*, 1121–1128. [CrossRef]
8. Else, T.; Greenberg, S.; Fishbein, L. Hereditary Paraganglioma-Pheochromocytoma Syndromes. In *GeneReviews((R))*; University of Washington: Seattle, WA, USA, 1993.
9. Fliedner, S.M.J.; Lehnert, H.; Pacak, K. Metastatic paraganglioma. *Semin. Oncol.* **2010**, *37*, 627–637. [CrossRef]
10. Brouwers, F.M.; Eisenhofer, G.; Tao, J.J.; Kant, J.A.; Adams, K.T.; Linehan, W.M.; Pacak, K. High frequency of SDHB germline mutations in patients with malignant catecholamine-producing paragangliomas: Implications for genetic testing. *J. Clin. Endocrinol. Metab.* **2006**, *91*, 4505–4509. [CrossRef]
11. van Hulsteijn, L.T.; Dekkers, O.M.; Hes, F.J.; Smit, J.W.; Corssmit, E.P. Risk of malignant paraganglioma in SDHB-mutation and SDHD-mutation carriers: A systematic review and meta-analysis. *J. Med. Genet.* **2012**, *49*, 768–776. [CrossRef]
12. Martucci, V.L.; Pacak, K. Pheochromocytoma and paraganglioma: Diagnosis, genetics, management, and treatment. *Curr. Probl. Cancer* **2014**, *38*, 7–41. [CrossRef]
13. Dona, M.; Neijman, K.; Timmers, H. MITOCHONDRIA: Succinate dehydrogenase subunit B-associated phaeochromocytoma and paraganglioma. *Int. J. Biochem. Cell Biol.* **2021**, *134*, 105949. [CrossRef] [PubMed]

14. Cascon, A.; Remacha, L.; Calsina, B.; Robledo, M. Pheochromocytomas and Paragangliomas: Bypassing Cellular Respiration. *Cancers* **2019**, *11*, 683. [CrossRef] [PubMed]
15. Sun, F.; Huo, X.; Zhai, Y.; Wang, A.; Xu, J.; Su, D.; Bartlam, M.; Rao, Z. Crystal structure of mitochondrial respiratory membrane protein complex II. *Cell* **2005**, *121*, 1043–1057. [CrossRef] [PubMed]
16. Huang, J.; Lemire, B.D. Mutations in the C. elegans succinate dehydrogenase iron-sulfur subunit promote superoxide generation and premature aging. *J. Mol. Biol.* **2009**, *387*, 559–569. [CrossRef]
17. Ishii, T.; Yasuda, K.; Akatsuka, A.; Hino, O.; Hartman, P.S.; Ishii, N. A mutation in the SDHC gene of complex II increases oxidative stress, resulting in apoptosis and tumorigenesis. *Cancer Res.* **2005**, *65*, 203–209.
18. Smith, E.H.; Janknecht, R.; Maher 3rd, L.J. Succinate inhibition of alpha-ketoglutarate-dependent enzymes in a yeast model of paraganglioma. *Hum. Mol. Genet.* **2007**, *16*, 3136–3148. [CrossRef]
19. Liu, Y.; Pang, Y.; Zhu, B.; Uher, O.; Caisova, V.; Huynh, T.T.; Taieb, D.; Vanova, K.H.; Ghayee, H.K.; Neuzil, J.; et al. Therapeutic Targeting of SDHB-Mutated Pheochromocytoma/Paraganglioma with Pharmacologic Ascorbic Acid. *Clin. Cancer Res.* **2020**, *26*, 3868–3880.
20. Purohit, V.; Simeone, D.M.; Lyssiotis, C.A. Metabolic Regulation of Redox Balance in Cancer. *Cancers* **2019**, *11*, 955. [CrossRef]
21. Ngo, B.; Van Riper, J.M.; Cantley, L.C.; Yun, J. Targeting cancer vulnerabilities with high-dose vitamin C. *Nat. Rev. Cancer* **2019**, *19*, 271–282. [CrossRef] [PubMed]
22. Dona, M.; Waaijers, S.; Richter, S.; Eisenhofer, G.; Korving, J.; Kamel, S.M.; Bakkers, J.; Rapizzi, E.; Rodenburg, R.J.; Zethof, J.; et al. Loss of sdhb in zebrafish larvae recapitulates human paraganglioma characteristics. *Endocr. Relat. Cancer* **2020**, *28*, 65–77. [CrossRef]
23. Storz, P. Reactive oxygen species in tumor progression. *Front. Biosci.* **2005**, *10*, 1881–1896. [CrossRef]
24. Weinberg, F.; Hamanaka, R.; Wheaton, W.W.; Weinberg, S.; Joseph, J.; Lopez, M.; Kalyanaraman, B.; Mutlu, G.M.; Budinger, G.R.; Chandel, N.S. Mitochondrial metabolism and ROS generation are essential for Kras-mediated tumorigenicity. *Proc. Natl. Acad. Sci. USA* **2010**, *107*, 8788–8793. [CrossRef] [PubMed]
25. Weinberg, F.; Ramnath, N.; Nagrath, D. Reactive Oxygen Species in the Tumor Microenvironment: An Overview. *Cancers* **2019**, *11*, 1191. [CrossRef]
26. Kluckova, K.; Tennant, D.A. Metabolic implications of hypoxia and pseudohypoxia in pheochromocytoma and paraganglioma. *Cell Tissue Res.* **2018**, *372*, 367–378. [CrossRef] [PubMed]
27. Gottlieb, E.; Tomlinson, I.P. Mitochondrial tumour suppressors: A genetic and biochemical update. *Nat. Rev. Cancer* **2005**, *5*, 857–866. [CrossRef]
28. Saito, Y.; Ishii, K.A.; Aita, Y.; Ikeda, T.; Kawakami, Y.; Shimano, H.; Hara, H.; Takekoshi, K. Loss of SDHB Elevates Catecholamine Synthesis and Secretion Depending on ROS Production and HIF Stabilization. *Neurochem. Res.* **2016**, *41*, 696–706. [CrossRef] [PubMed]
29. Guzy, R.D.; Hoyos, B.; Robin, E.; Chen, H.; Liu, L.; Mansfield, K.D.; Simon, M.C.; Hammerling, U.; Schumacker, P.T. Mitochondrial complex III is required for hypoxia-induced ROS production and cellular oxygen sensing. *Cell Metab.* **2005**, *1*, 401–408. [CrossRef]
30. Selak, M.A.; Armour, S.M.; MacKenzie, E.D.; Boulahbel, H.; Watson, D.G.; Mansfield, K.D.; Pan, Y.; Simon, M.C.; Thompson, C.B.; Gottlieb, E. Succinate links TCA cycle dysfunction to oncogenesis by inhibiting HIF-alpha prolyl hydroxylase. *Cancer Cell* **2005**, *7*, 77–85. [CrossRef]
31. Cervera, A.M.; Apostolova, N.; Crespo, F.L.; Mata, M.; McCreath, K.J. Cells silenced for SDHB expression display characteristic features of the tumor phenotype. *Cancer Res.* **2008**, *68*, 4058–4067. [CrossRef]
32. Argentiero, A.; Solimando, A.G.; Krebs, M.; Leone, P.; Susca, N.; Brunetti, O.; Racanelli, V.; Vacca, A.; Silvestris, N. Anti-angiogenesis and Immunotherapy: Novel Paradigms to Envision Tailored Approaches in Renal Cell-Carcinoma. *J. Clin. Med.* **2020**, *9*, 1594. [CrossRef] [PubMed]
33. Howe, K.; Clark, M.D.; Torroja, C.F.; Torrance, J.; Berthelot, C.; Muffato, M.; Collins, J.E.; Humphray, S.; McLaren, K.; Matthews, L.; et al. The zebrafish reference genome sequence and its relationship to the human genome. *Nature* **2013**, *496*, 498–503. [CrossRef] [PubMed]
34. Rennekamp, A.J.; Peterson, R.T. 15 years of zebrafish chemical screening. *Curr. Opin. Chem. Biol.* **2015**, *24*, 58–70. [CrossRef] [PubMed]
35. MacRae, C.A.; Peterson, R.T. Zebrafish as tools for drug discovery. *Nat. Rev. Drug. Discov.* **2015**, *14*, 721–731. [CrossRef]
36. Cully, M. Zebrafish earn their drug discovery stripes. *Nat. Rev. Drug. Discov.* **2019**, *18*, 811–813. [CrossRef]
37. Luchtel, R.A.; Bhagat, T.; Pradhan, K.; Jacobs, W.R., Jr.; Levine, M.; Verma, A.; Shenoy, N. High-dose ascorbic acid synergizes with anti-PD1 in a lymphoma mouse model. *Proc. Natl. Acad. Sci. USA* **2020**, *117*, 1666–1677. [CrossRef]
38. Powers, J.F.; Cochran, B.; Baleja, J.D.; Sikes, H.D.; Pattison, A.D.; Zhang, X.; Lomakin, I.; Shepard-Barry, A.; Pacak, K.; Moon, S.J.; et al. A xenograft and cell line model of SDH-deficient pheochromocytoma derived from Sdhb+/− rats. *Endocr. Relat. Cancer* **2020**, *27*, 337–354. [CrossRef]
39. Gronborg, S.; Darin, N.; Miranda, M.J.; Damgaard, B.; Cayuela, J.A.; Oldfors, A.; Kollberg, G.; Hansen, T.V.O.; Ravn, K.; Wibrand, F.; et al. Leukoencephalopathy due to Complex II Deficiency and Bi-Allelic SDHB Mutations: Further Cases and Implications for Genetic Counselling. *JIMD Rep.* **2017**, *33*, 69–77.

40. Passage, E.; Norreel, J.C.; Noack-Fraissignes, P.; Sanguedolce, V.; Pizant, J.; Thirion, X.; Robaglia-Schlupp, A.; Pellissier, J.F.; Fontes, M. Ascorbic acid treatment corrects the phenotype of a mouse model of Charcot-Marie-Tooth disease. *Nat. Med.* **2004**, *10*, 396–401. [CrossRef]
41. Janssen, M.C.H.; Koene, S.; de Laat, P.; Hemelaar, P.; Pickkers, P.; Spaans, E.; Beukema, R.; Beyrath, J.; Groothuis, J.; Verhaak, C.; et al. The KHENERGY Study: Safety and Efficacy of KH176 in Mitochondrial m.3243A>G Spectrum Disorders. *Clin Pharmacol. Ther.* **2019**, *105*, 101–111. [CrossRef]
42. Verginelli, F.; Perconti, S.; Vespa, S.; Schiavi, F.; Prasad, S.C.; Lanuti, P.; Cama, A.; Tramontana, L.; Esposito, D.L.; Guarnieri, S.; et al. Paragangliomas arise through an autonomous vasculo-angio-neurogenic program inhibited by imatinib. *Acta Neuropathol.* **2018**, *135*, 779–798. [CrossRef] [PubMed]
43. Costa, B.; Estrada, M.F.; Mendes, R.V.; Fior, R. Zebrafish Avatars towards Personalized Medicine-A Comparative Review between Avatar Models. *Cells* **2020**, *9*, 293. [CrossRef] [PubMed]
44. Fazio, M.; Ablain, J.; Chuan, Y.; Langenau, D.M.; Zon, L.I. Zebrafish patient avatars in cancer biology and precision cancer therapy. *Nat. Rev. Cancer* **2020**, *20*, 263–273. [CrossRef] [PubMed]
45. Kimmel, C.B.; Ballard, W.W.; Kimmel, S.R.; Ullmann, B.; Schilling, T.F. Stages of embryonic development of the zebrafish. *Dev. Dyn.* **1995**, *203*, 253–310. [CrossRef]
46. Goodwin, N.; Westall, L.; Karp, N.A.; Hazlehurst, D.; Kovacs, C.; Keeble, R.; Thompson, P.; Collins, R.; Bussell, J. Evaluating and Optimizing Fish Health and Welfare During Experimental Procedures. *Zebrafish* **2016**, *13*, S127–S131. [CrossRef] [PubMed]

MDPI
St. Alban-Anlage 66
4052 Basel
Switzerland
Tel. +41 61 683 77 34
Fax +41 61 302 89 18
www.mdpi.com

Cancers Editorial Office
E-mail: cancers@mdpi.com
www.mdpi.com/journal/cancers

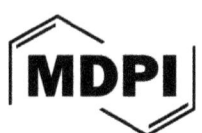

www.ingramcontent.com/pod-product-compliance
Lightning Source LLC
LaVergne TN
LVHW070505100526
838202LV00014B/1792